Advanced Practice Nursing in

Psychiatric and

Mental Health Care

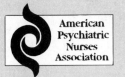

American Psychiatric Nurses Association

$\mathcal{A}$DVANCED PRACTICE NURSING *in*

PSYCHIATRIC *and*

MENTAL HEALTH CARE

Edited by

Carole A. Shea, PhD, RN, CS, FAAN
Associate Dean for Academic Affairs
Bouvé College of Health Sciences
Northeastern University
Boston, Massachusetts

Luc R. Pelletier, MSN, RN, CS, CPHQ
Healthcare Consultant
Editor, *Journal for Healthcare Quality*
Washington, DC

Elizabeth C. Poster, PhD, RN
Dean and Professor
School of Nursing
University of Texas at Arlington
Arlington, Texas

Gail W. Stuart, PhD, RN, CS, FAAN
Professor of Nursing and Psychiatry
Center for Health Care Research
Medical University of South Carolina
Charleston, South Carolina

Marilyn P. Verhey, PhD, RN, CS
Professor, School of Nursing
San Francisco State University
San Francisco, California

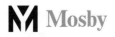 Mosby

St. Louis Baltimore Boston Carlsbad Chicago Minneapolis New York Philadelphia Portland
London Milan Sydney Tokyo Toronto

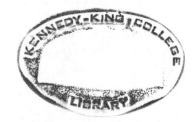

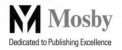

Editor-in-Chief: Sally Schrefer
Executive Editor: Barbara Nelson Cullen
Senior Developmental Editor: Sandra Clark Brown
Project Manager: Dana Peick
Senior Production Editor: Jeffrey Patterson
Designer: Amy Buxton
Manufacturing Manager: David Graybill

RC
440
.A3365
1999

Mosby, Inc.
A Harcourt Health Sciences Company
11830 Westline Industrial Drive
St. Louis, Missouri 63146

Printed in the United States of America
Composition by PRD Group
Printing/binding by Maple-Vail

Library of Congress Cataloging in Publication Data

ISBN 0-323-00352-4

99   00   01   02 / 9 8 7 6 5 4 3 2 1

About the Editors

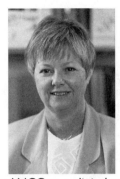

Dr. Carole Shea is a tenured professor of nursing in the Northeastern University Bouvé College of Health Sciences and an adjunct associate professor of socio-medical sciences and community medicine in the Boston University School of Medicine. She received her BSN from William Paterson College in New Jersey, her MS in advanced psychiatric nursing from Rutgers University, and her PhD in medical sociology from Rutgers University in New Jersey. She had a fellowship from the Arthritis Foundation to support her doctoral study of how urban residents cope with rheumatoid arthritis. Her post-doctoral studies include certificates from Boston University's Alcohol Studies Program and the Wellesley College Management Institute for Women in Higher Education. She is certified by the ANCC as a clinical specialist in adult psychiatric and mental health nursing.

Currently, Dr. Shea is the associate dean for academic affairs in the Bouvé College of Health Sciences at Northeastern University in Boston, with responsibility for nursing, pharmacy, and allied health programs. As a nurse educator and academic administrator, she has more than 20 years of experience in teaching, program development, and academic administration. As a faculty member and board director of the Center for Community Health Education, Research and Service (CCHERS), her collaborative efforts with university faculty, community health center providers, and urban residents resulted in an interdisciplinary, community-based, primary care curriculum for health professions students, which has received national attention. She has presented her work on curriculum and mental health issues nationally and internationally. Her writings and consultations reflect her practice in education, management, and psychiatric nursing. As a member of the ANA Task Force, she authored sections of the *Statement of Psychiatric-Mental Health Clinical Nursing Practice and Standards of Psychiatric-Mental Health Clinical Nursing Practice.* On the state level she has worked with the Massachusetts Alliance for the Mentally Ill and the Department of Mental Health's Central Office of Research Review Committee. Dr. Shea is a past-president of the APNA, a current member of the editorial board of the *Journal of the American Psychiatric Nurses Association,* and has served as chair of APNA's Annual Conference Committee. She is a Fellow of the American Academy of Nursing and a recipient of the APNA Excellence in Education Award and the Leadership Award of the Sigma Theta Tau International, Gamma Epsilon Chapter.

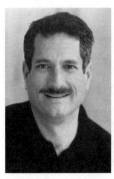

Luc R. Pelletier is a healthcare consultant in Washington, DC. He is also editor of the *Journal for Healthcare Quality.* He has 20 years of experience in the behavioral health care field, having held staff, management, executive, and consultative positions in various care delivery settings, including public and private health care facilities, academic medical centers, psychiatric homecare, and managed behavioral healthcare. He holds a BSN from Fairfield University and an MSN from Yale University. Mr. Pelletier's consultative expertise encompasses the areas of psychiatric-mental health nursing, clinical informatics, quality management, policy development, and regulatory compliance. He was an assistant clinical professor at UCLA from 1982 to 1990, where he provided guest lectures and thesis advisement. An avid writer, Mr. Pelletier has published over 70 critical scholarly works, including psychiatric nursing texts, directories of psychiatric-mental health nurses in California, chapters in nursing texts, articles in refereed professional journals, research abstracts, book reviews, and invited works. His research has been in the areas of client needs in an AIDS service organization, nurses in private practice, falls in psychiatric hospitals, medication errors, and symptom profiling (outcomes management). He is a reviewer/editorial board member of several professional journals. Mr. Pelletier belongs to and has held various offices in several professional associations and societies.

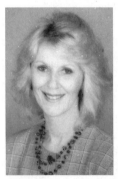

Formerly, **Dr. Elizabeth Poster** was the director of nursing research and education at UCLA's Neuropsychiatric Hospital and assistant clinical professor at the UCLA School of Nursing. She received her BS and MS in child psychiatric nursing from Boston University and her doctorate in educational psychology from Boston College.

Dr. Poster has practiced nursing for 30 years as a clinician, researcher, faculty member, administrator, and journal editor.

Her areas of research include patient assault, children's drawings, children's concept of mental illness, nursing quality management, and the evaluation of psychiatric patient outcomes. She has published extensively in these areas and has authored over 50 articles and a variety of books, chapters, media reviews, and monographs. She has also presented her research and clinical work nationally and internationally at over 100 conferences.

Dr. Poster has been active in leadership positions in a number of national organizations: the Society for Education and Research in Psychiatric Nursing, the Association of Psychiatric Health Care Systems, and the American Psychiatric Nurses Association. In 1997, she was appointed, by Governor Bush, to be a member of the Texas Board of Nurse Examiners for a 6-year term.

Dr. Poster is also actively involved in editorial service for numerous psychiatric and nursing journals and was the founding co-editor of the *Journal of Pediatric Nursing*. Currently, she is the editor of the *Journal of Child and Adolescent Psychiatric Nursing*.

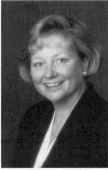

Dr. Gail Stuart is a tenured professor in the College of Nursing and a professor in the College of Medicine in the Department of Psychiatry and Behavioral Sciences at the Medical University of South Carolina. She received her BSN from Georgetown University, her MS in adult psychiatric nursing from the University of Maryland, and her PhD in behavioral sciences from Johns Hopkins University, School of Hygiene and Public Health. She is an ANCC certified specialist in psychiatric and mental health nursing, a Fellow in the American Academy of Nursing, a member of the American College of Mental Health Administrators, and a past president of the American Psychiatric Nurses Association.

Her current position at the Medical University of South Carolina is as Associate Director of the Center for Health Care Research where Dr. Stuart works as a member of an interdisciplinary research team focusing on issues of access, resource utilization, outcomes, and health care delivery systems. She most recently was administrator and chief executive officer of the Institute of Psychiatry at the Medical University where she was responsible for all clinical, fiscal, and human operations across the continuum of psychiatric care. Dr. Stuart has taught in undergraduate, graduate, and doctoral programs in nursing and maintains a clinical practice in the Department of Psychiatry. She serves on numerous academic, pharmaceutical, and governmental boards and represents nursing on a variety of National Institute of Mental Health policy and research panels. She is a strong advocate for the specialty and is in great demand to speak and consult throughout the United States and Canada. Dr. Stuart is a prolific writer and has numerous publications of articles, textbooks, and media productions. She has received many awards, including the American Nurses' Association Distinguished Contribution to Psychiatric Nursing—Current Impact on Innovations in Health Care Delivery Systems and the Health Policy Award. Dr. Stuart's clinical and research interests involve the study of depression, anxiety disorders, and mental health delivery systems.

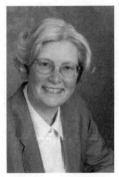

Dr. Marilyn P. Verhey is a professor in the School of Nursing, coordinator of assessment in the College of Health and Human Services, and faculty coordinator for assessment in the Public Research Institiute at San Francisco State University. She received her BSN, an MS in psychiatric and community mental health nursing, and a PhD in curriculum, instruction, and administration from Boston College. Dr. Verhey also holds an MS in library science from the University of Illinois. She is certified as a clinical specialist in psychiatric and mental health nursing by the ANCC.

As co-investigator and co-project director of the innovative nurse-managed, school-based Mission High School Health Center in San Francisco, she developed and implemented mental health services, an extensive interdisciplinary clinical training program, the quality management program, and the computerized information management system, and she served as the program evaluator. She also has a strong interest in information literacy for lifelong learning in nursing and developed the *InformationRN* learning package for searching the literature in nursing and health care. She has worked as a librarian, both in public libraries and at the Biomedical Library at the University of California, Los Angeles.

Dr. Verhey has consulted, written, and presented extensively in the areas of patient education, staff development, quality management, and program planning and evaluation. She is an active member of the American Psychiatric Nurses Association, having served as national treasurer and as a member of the Education Committee and the Public Action and Advocacy Task Force. Currently, she is chair of the Archives Task Force and media editor of the *Journal of the American Psychiatric Nurses Association.* In 1998 she was awarded the APNA Innovation Award.

CONTRIBUTORS

Deborah Antai-Otong, MS, RN, CS
Consultant
Private Practice
Dallas, Texas
antai-otong.deborah_Y@dallas.va.gov
21 *Continued Professional Development*

Linda M. E. Auton, RN, JD
President, AdvoGuard, Inc.
Attorney and Counsellor at Law
Private Practice
Rockland, Massachusetts
auton19@idt.net
8 *Legal and Regulatory Issues in Advanced Practice Nursing*

Karen S. Babich, PhD, RN, FAAN
Health Scientist Administrator
National Institute of Mental Health
Rockville, Maryland
K_BABICH@nih.gov
22 *Knowledge Dissemination and Utilization*

Katharine P. Bailey, RN, MS, CS
Assistant Professor, School of Nursing
Yale University
New Haven, Connecticut;
Private Practice
New Haven, Connecticut
Katharine.Bailey@yale.edu
13 *Framework for Prescriptive Practice*

Anne Bateman, EdD, RN, CS
Assistant Professor, School of Nursing
Bouvé College of Health Sciences
Northeastern University
Boston, Massachusetts
abateman@lynx.neu.edu
16 *Acute Care and Crisis Management*

Christy L. Beaudin, PhD, LCSW, CPHQ
Vice President, Research and Development
Magellan Behavioral Health
Columbia, Maryland
cbeaudin@compuserve.com
2 *Mental Health Services Delivery and Managed Care*

Wailua Brandman, MSN, APRN, CS, NP
Clinical Instructor
Manoa School of Nursing
University of Hawaii
Honolulu, Hawaii;
President, Hawaii Chapter of American
Psychiatric Nurses Association;
Media Committee Chair, HNA Council on
Advanced Nursing Practice
WAILUA@prodigy.net
11 *Complementary Therapies and Practices*

Carolyn Chambers Clark, EdD, ARNP, FAAN, HNC
Mental Health and Complementary Specialist
Bay Area Psychological Services
St. Petersburg, Florida;
Faculty, Graduate School
Schiller International University
Dunedin, Florida
cccwellness@earthlink.net
11 *Complementary Therapies and Practices*

Victoria S. Conn, RN, MN, MA
Alliance for the Mentally Ill Training Institute
Harrisburg, Pennsylvania
17 *Working with Families*

Phyllis M. Connolly, PhD, RN, CS
Professor, School of Nursing
San Jose State University
San Jose, California
ConnollyDr@aol.com
18 *Consumer Advocacy*

Judith Gregorie D'Afflitti, MSN, CS
Mental Health Department
Harvard Vanguard Medical Associates
Wellesley, Massachusetts
Judith_DAfflitti@harvardpilgrim.org
6 *Collaboration and Partnership in Managed Care*

Anne Fishel, PhD, RN, CS
Professor, School of Nursing
University of North Carolina,
Chapel Hill
Chapel Hill, North Carolina
afishel.uncson@mhs.unc.edu
9 *Psychosocial and Behavioral Health Care*

Donna A. Gaffney, RN, DNSc, FAAN
Director, Center for Women and
Children at Risk
School of Nursing
Columbia University
New York, New York
DAG1@columbia.edu
4 *Marketing Mental Health Services*

Judith Haber, PhD, APRN, CS, FAAN
Visiting Professor and Director
Master's Program and Post-Master's
Advanced Certificate Programs
Division of Nursing, New York University
New York, New York;
Private Practice
Stamford, Connecticut
drjudih@aol.com
7 *Health Policy, Politics, and Advanced Practice
Nursing*

Suzanne Sayle Jimerson, MS, RN, CS
Mental Health Department
Harvard Vanguard Medical Associates
Wellesley, Massachusetts
Suzanne_Jimmerson@harvardpilgrim.org
6 *Collaboration and Partnership in Managed Care*

Barbara Krainovich-Miller, EdD, RN, CS
Psychotherapist, Private Practice
Garden City, New York;
Visiting Professor, Division of Nursing,
Graduate Program
New York University
New York, New York
rubmil@aol.com
15 *Behavioral Health Home Care*

Michele T. Laraia, PhD, RN, CS
Assistant Professor, Department of Psychiatry
College of Medicine
Colleges of Nursing and Graduate Studies
Medical University of South Carolina
Charleston, South Carolina
laraiamt@musc.edu
23 *Scientific Advancement through Clinical Trials*

Diane T. Marsh, PhD
Professor of Psychology
University of Pittsburgh at Greensburg
Greensburg, Pennsylvania
dtm3@pop.pitt.edu
17 *Working with Families*

Sandra J. McElhaney, MA
Director of Prevention
National Mental Health Association
Alexandria, Virginia
smcelhaney@nmha.org
14 *Prevention in Mental Health and Substance
Abuse Services*

Geoffry McEnany, PhD, RN, CS
Medical Science Manager in Neuroscience
Bristol-Myers Squibb Company
Boston, Massachusetts
10 *Psychobiologic Influences: Chronobiology*

Patricia A. Murphy, PhD, CS, RN, FAAN
Clinical Ethics and Consultation
University Hospital
University of Medicine and Dentistry of
New Jersey
Newark, New Jersey;
Member, ANA Board of Directors
Member, American Nurses Credentialing
Center Board of Directors
crisisclub@aol.com
19 *Ethical Perspectives and Issues in Advanced
Practice Nursing*

Luc R. Pelletier, MSN, RN, CS, CPHQ
Healthcare Consultant
Editor, *Journal for Healthcare Quality*
Washington, DC
lucpell@ix.netcom.com
2 *Mental Health Services Delivery and Managed
Care*
25 *Envisioning the Future in Mental Health Care*

Elizabeth C. Poster, PhD, RN
Dean and Professor
School of Nursing
University of Texas at Arlington
Arlington, Texas
poster@uta.edu
25 *Envisioning the Future in Mental Health Care*

David M. Price, PhD
Ethics Consultant
UMDNJ—New Jersey Medical School
Newark, New Jersey
19 *Ethical Perspectives and Issues in Advanced Practice Nursing*

Mary Gannon Rosedale, MS, RN
Director, Psychiatric Behavioral
Home Care Services
Priority Home Care
New York, New York
15 *Behavioral Health Home Care*

Carole A. Shea, PhD, RN, CS, FAAN
Associate Dean for Academic Affairs
Bouvé College of Health Sciences
Northeastern University
Boston, Massachusetts
cshea@lynx.neu.edu
1 *Careers in Advanced Practice Psychiatric Nursing*
20 *Graduate Education for Advanced Practice*
25 *Envisioning the Future in Mental Health Care*

George B. Smith, ARNP, C, MSN, Cm
Doctoral Student, College of Nursing
University of South Florida
Tampa, Florida;
Secretary
American Psychiatric Nurses Association
GBSmith@earthlink.net
12 *Practice Guidelines and Outcome Evaluation*

Sharon Mindlin Steinberg, MS, RN, CS
Department of Ambulatory Care
and Prevention
Harvard Medical School and Harvard Pilgrim
Health Care
Boston, Massachusetts
Sharon_Steinberg@harvardpilgrim.org
6 *Collaboration and Partnership in Managed Care*

Maureen Beirne Streff, MS, RN, CS
Assistant Professor, Department of Nursing
Regis College
Boston, Massachusetts;
Private Practice
Boston, Massachusetts
streff@ma.utranet.com
7 *Health Policy, Politics, and Advanced Practice Nursing*

Gail W. Stuart, PhD, RN, CS, FAAN
Professor of Nursing and Psychiatry
Center for Health Care Research
Medical University of South Carolina
Charleston, South Carolina
stuartGW@musc.edu
24 *Mental Health Services Research*
25 *Envisioning the Future in Mental Health Care*

Nancy M. Valentine, RN, PhD, MPH
Special Assistant to the Secretary and Advisor
to the Undersecretary
Department of Veterans Affairs
Washington, DC
Valena@mail.va.gov
14 *Prevention in Mental Health and Substance Abuse Services*

Marilyn P. Verhey, PhD, RN, CS
Professor, School of Nursing
San Francisco State University
San Francisco, California
mverhey@sfsu.edu
3 *Technology, Information, and Data Management*
25 *Envisioning the Future in Mental Health Care*

Maria R. Warda, PhD, RN
Assistant Dean for Academic Services and
Diversity Enhancement
School of Nursing
University of California at San Francisco
San Francisco, California
5 *Cultural Diversity in Health Care Delivery*

FOREWORD

The American Psychiatric Nurses Association (APNA) is a professional organization for all psychiatric nurses, at all levels of practice, and in all sub-specialties. The APNA's mission is to provide leadership to advance psychiatric-mental health nursing practice; improve mental health care for individuals, families, groups, and communities; and shape health policy for the delivery of mental health services. Its vision is that all people will have accessible, effective, and efficient psychiatric-mental health care in delivery systems that fully utilize the skills and expertise of psychiatric nurses.

The APNA is proud to sponsor *Advanced Practice Nursing in Psychiatric and Mental Health Care* as part of its efforts to achieve the APNA's mission and vision. The book is intended for nurses who are currently practicing in advanced roles, those who are studying to become advanced practice registered nurses, those who have a special interest in the broad field of psychiatric nursing and mental health care, and anyone who is passionate about wanting to work together to make a difference in the lives of those who suffer from mental illness.

American Psychiatric Nurses Association

PREFACE

In concert with its mission statement, the American Psychiatric Nurses Association (APNA) advocates that advanced practice registered nurses (APRNs) in psychiatric-mental health nursing take a lead role in improving mental health care and transforming the specialty of psychiatric nursing for the next century. This book is one step toward accomplishing this mission.

Advanced Practice Nursing in Psychiatric and Mental Health Care is a state-of-the-art-and-science analysis of the transforming mental health care environment, issues in advanced clinical practice, and developments in professional scholarship within psychiatric nursing. It is a resource book for all nurses in advanced practice, faculty, graduate students, and psychiatric nurses who aspire to the advanced practice role in psychiatric nursing. The book is intended to:

- Prepare nurses for advanced practice roles as leaders, clinicians, managers, educators, consultants, policy makers, and researchers
- Present the scientific knowledge and contextual base of emerging psychiatric and mental health care for APRNs seeking to deliver holistic nursing care at an advanced level
- Examine the clinical trends and issues that have a critical impact on the specialty practice of psychiatric nursing
- Provide information about resources and connections to enhance professional development

Reverberations from health care reform are still sweeping the country on the threshold of the new millennium. There are major changes in health care delivery; revolutionary developments in the sciences related to nursing, medicine, and health care; and strong recommendations from both public and private sources that call for the transformation of professional practice and education in all health care disciplines. Nurses in advanced practice need to be in the forefront of the reform movement to ensure access, quality, and effective health care at affordable cost for all patients, their families, and communities. To take their rightful place, APRNs have to embrace the new science, navigate the complexities of the work environment, and anticipate the trends and issues that influence advanced practice.

Five trends continue to have a significant impact on health care and advanced nursing practice:

1. The movement toward cost-contained managed care and capitation systems to deliver health care services
2. The emphasis on primary care as the focal point of treatment
3. The expectation that treatment outcomes will be specified and measurable
4. A greater concern for consumer/patient satisfaction in an era of consumerism
5. Cross-training of health care providers to prepare them for new roles, different responsibilities, and interdisciplinary collaboration

In addition to the trends in general health care, there are developments within mental health care and psychiatric nursing to consider. Some examples are breakthroughs in the sciences related to mental health and psychiatric illness; new communication technologies and information systems; improved treatment options; new provider roles; empowerment of patients and families; different service settings; new models for outcome-oriented practice; the evolution of quality management principles and practices toward performance excellence; changes in mental health policy; and professional/consumer pressures for parity in funding. Nurses must be able to carefully analyze advanced practice in psychiatric nursing and mental health care in light of these developments and their implications for management, clinical practice, education and research. In this book, the editors and contributing authors discuss these important subjects in depth and suggest ways to make a difference in advanced practice nursing.

Professional nursing organizations (e.g.,

APNA, American Nurses Association, American Association of Colleges of Nursing, and the National League for Nursing), private foundations (e.g., the W. K. Kellogg Foundation, the Robert Wood Johnson Foundation, and the Pew Health Professions Commission), and governmental bodies (e.g., U.S. Congress, National Institute of Mental Health, and state legislatures) are also vital forces for change. These institutions study the ways in which health professionals are educated, deployed, reimbursed, and evaluated. Although the reports, demonstration projects, regulations, standards, and guidelines from these organizations do not always specify recommendations for psychiatric nursing and mental health care, they do point the direction in which health care providers will be expected to practice. Consensus has emerged from these various think tanks that mental health care must converge with health care in general to provide quality comprehensive health services yet contain costs and to prepare providers who are knowledgeable about managed care systems and skilled in providing culturally-sensitive, community-based primary care. The contributing authors, who are experts from across the country, present the knowledge, skills, and competencies necessary to make these high expectations into a practical reality for APRNs in psychiatric and mental health care.

Traditionally, psychiatric and mental health care has been outside the mainstream of health care delivery. Today, mental health care is no longer impervious to the same pressures being exerted on general health care to restructure and redesign its services. However, to include mental health care under the same reform umbrella is a struggle. There are still profound differences between mental illness and physical illness in terms of the philosophy of science, treatment modalities, service delivery, reimbursement, public acceptance, and many other factors. Therefore, the current ideas driving the transformation of health care need to be translated and adapted to make them meaningful to APRNs engaged in the delivery of mental health care. The authors use models, examples, and case studies to illustrate how APRNs in various settings with diverse populations can provide effective mental health services. Diversity is reflected in terms of the patient's age, gender, ethnicity, and diagnosis, as well as the clinical practice settings and interdisciplinary approaches to care depicted in the examples. Therefore, this book is relevant to all nurses who are seeking to understand the momentous changes in health care and to update their knowledge and skills in areas related to the phenomena of psychiatric nursing and mental health care.

The book is organized in three units: The Health Care Environment, Advanced Clinical Practice, and Professional Scholarship. Chapter one presents the overarching theme of career evolution. This is the process of being and becoming as nurses develop and grow toward their own ideal of the consummate nurse. It represents the continuous professional journey on which nurses embark to find their niche, improve their fit, break the mold, pioneer in new territory, or simply endure the tremors that emanate from rapidly changing systems. It is a journey taken by those who identify themselves first and foremost as psychiatric nurses but also by those nurses who have other allegiances and roles, yet frequently cross paths with those needing psychiatric and mental health care. The chapters in this book reflect the theme of an evolving career by presenting different perspectives and new roles for psychiatric nurses to meet the opportunities and challenges of the next century.

In Unit One, *The Health Care Environment*, the chapters set the stage for practice by describing the organizational context for mental health care (i.e., the structures and processes that influence how nurses provide care and deliver mental health services). The general concepts and principles of managed care and the specific features of managed behavioral healthcare are discussed in detail to lay the foundation for contemporary practice. The use of information systems, technology, and marketing techniques shows APRNs how to improve their practice and service delivery. A chapter on cultural diversity addresses this important issue from a management perspective. The chapters on collaborative partnerships, politics and policy, and legal issues present examples from a health care organization, a professional association, and private practice that demonstrate the knowledge base and interpersonal skills necessary for successful practice in the complex health care system.

In Unit Two, *Advanced Clinical Practice*, the chapters address the broad scope of advanced practice in terms of its science, defining competencies, delivery models, and special roles. This book is unique in its presentation of evidence-based research for scientific nursing practice. There are groundbreaking chapters that synthesize the research on psychosocial therapies, chronobiology, complementary and alternative health care practices, and mental health promotion. The authors enrich the theoretical discussion with examples drawn from their own practice. Chapters on practice guidelines and prescriptive practice provide a framework for competent practice by APRNs. These chapters are followed by descriptions of models of mental health care delivery in behavioral home care, crisis and acute care, rehabilitation, and in working with families and consumers. Special emphasis is given to the advocacy role and to the ethical dimensions of practice in the concluding chapters of Unit Two.

Unit Three, *Professional Scholarship*, presents the educational and research aspects of advanced practice nursing. The chapter on graduate education examines the effect of history and current trends on the role development of the clinical nurse specialist, including the controversy about the nurse practitioner role for psychiatric nurses in advanced practice. Doctoral education is discussed as a means for continuing professional development as well as advancing the science of the psychiatric nursing specialty. Continuing education is also presented as a professional commit-

ment to life-long learning. Chapters on research knowledge, clinical trials, and mental health services research inform the reader of the latest developments and suggest areas for future research to build the science of psychiatric nursing.

In the final chapter, as editors we have woven the strands of organization, science, practice, education, and research into a tapestry that forecasts the future of psychiatric and mental health care. From our collective perspective, we envision a future that, while fraught with challenges, is still brimming with potential for the specialty of psychiatric nursing. Our hope is that by "pushing the edge of the envelope," we will stimulate APRNs to think creatively about new ways to meet the challenge of today's complex problems, continue to improve mental health care, and engender a progressive future for the specialty of psychiatric nursing.

Acknowledgments

We, the editors, welcome the opportunity to acknowledge our gratitude to the American Psychiatric Nurses Association for its enthusiastic support of this project. We also wish to express our appreciation for the collaborative spirit with which the Mosby editors—Barbara Cullen, Sandra Brown, and Jeffrey Patterson—participated in developing this publication. We offer well-deserved recognition to Valerie Clough and Stephen Doherty for their special assistance in preparing the manuscript. To our families, friends, mentors, and colleagues, we extend our heartfelt thanks for their inspiration and sustaining support as we continue to evolve in our careers and fulfill our professional commitment to psychiatric nursing.

Carole A. Shea
Luc R. Pelletier
Elizabeth C. Poster
Gail W. Stuart
Marilyn P. Verhey
July 1999

To psychiatric nurses everywhere, to our colleagues and mentors, to the future generation of nurses, and most of all to patients, consumers, and families who deserve the very best psychiatric and mental health care.

The editors of this book join the American Psychiatric Nurses Association and the chorus of countless voices throughout the world in paying tribute to the legacy of Dr. Hildegard E. Peplau, the founder of psychiatric nursing.

Hildegard E. Peplau, 89, one of the world's leading nurses, known to many as the "Nurse of the Century," died March 17, 1999, at her home in Sherman Oaks, California. Dr. Peplau is the only nurse to serve the American Nurses Association as Executive Director and later as President. She was also elected to serve two terms on the Board of the International Council of Nurses (ICN). In 1997 she received the world of nursing's highest honor, the Christiane Reimann Prize, at the ICN Quadrennial Congress. This award is given once every 4 years for outstanding national and international contributions to nursing and health care. In 1996, the American Academy of Nursing honored Peplau as a "Living Legend," and in 1998 the American Nurses Association inducted her into the ANA Hall of Fame.

Dr. Peplau is universally regarded as the "mother of psychiatric nursing." Her theoretical and clinical work led to the development of the distinct specialty field of psychiatric nursing. Dr. Peplau's seminal book, Interpersonal Relations in Nursing (1952), was completed in 1948. Publication was delayed for 4 years, however, because at that time it was considered too revolutionary for a nurse to publish a book without a physician co-author. Peplau's book has been widely credited with the transformation of nursing from a group of skilled workers to a full-fledged profession. Since the publication of Peplau's work, interpersonal process has been universally integrated into nursing education and nursing practices throughout the United States and abroad. It has been argued that Dr. Peplau's life and work produced the greatest changes in nursing practice since Florence Nightingale.

Dr. Peplau was awarded honorary doctoral degrees from universities including: Alfred, Duke, Indiana, Ohio State, Rutgers, and the University of Ulster in Ireland. Dr. Peplau was named one of "50 Great Americans" in Who's Who in 1995 by Marquis. She was an elected fellow of the American Academy of Nurses and of Sigma Theta Tau, the national nursing honorary society.

Hilda Peplau was born September 1, 1909, in Reading, Pennsylvania, the second daughter of immigrants Gustav and Ottylie Peplau. She was one of six children, having two sisters and three brothers. As a child, she witnessed the devastating flu epidemic of 1918. This personal experience greatly influenced her understanding of the impact of illness and death on families.

Peplau began her career in nursing in 1931 as a graduate of the Pottstown, Pennsylvania School of Nursing. She then worked as a staff nurse in Pennsylvania and New York City. A summer position as nurse for the New York University summer camp led to a recommendation for Peplau to become the school nurse at Bennington College in Vermont. There she earned a bachelor's degree in interpersonal psychology in 1943. At Bennington and through field experiences at Chestnut Lodge, a private psychiatric facility, she studied psychological issues with Erich Fromm, Frieda Fromm-Reichmann and Harry Stack Sullivan. Peplau's lifelong work was largely focused on extending Sullivan's interpersonal theory for use in nursing practice.

From 1943–1945 she served in the Army Nurse Corps and was assigned to the 312th Field Station Hospital in England where the American School of Military Psychiatry was located. Here she met and worked with all the leading figures in British and American psychiatry. After the war, Peplau was at the table with many of these same men as they worked to reshape the mental health system in the United States through the passage of the National Mental Health Act of 1946.

Peplau held master's and doctoral degrees from Teachers College, Columbia University. She was also certified in psychoanalysis by the William Alanson White Institute of New York City. In the early 1950s, Peplau developed and taught the first classes for graduate psychiatric nursing students at Teachers College. Dr. Peplau was a member of the faculty of the College of Nursing at Rutgers University from 1954–1974. At Rutgers, Peplau created the first graduate level program for the preparation of clinical specialists in psychiatric nursing. She was a prolific writer and was equally well known for her presentations, speeches, and clinical training workshops. Peplau vigorously advocated that nurses should become further educated so they could provide truly therapeutic care to patients rather than the custodial care that was prevalent in the mental hospitals of that era. During the 1950s and 1960s, she conducted summer workshops for nurses throughout the United States, mostly in state psychiatric hospitals. In these seminars, she taught interpersonal concepts and interviewing techniques, as well as individual, family, and group therapy. Peplau was an advisor to the World Health Organization and was a visiting professor at universities in Africa, Latin America, Belgium, and throughout the United States. A strong advocate for graduate education and research in nursing, she served as a consultant to the U.S. Surgeon General, the U.S. Air Force, and the National Institutes of Mental Health. She participated in many government policy making groups. After her retirement from Rutgers, she served as a visiting professor at the University of Leuven in Belgium in 1975 and 1976. There she helped establish the first graduate nursing program in Europe.

Peplau once said that the test of a good idea was whether or not it had staying power. Her original book from 1952 has been translated into nine languages and in 1989 was reissued in Great Britain by Macmillan of London. In 1989, Springer published a volume of selected works of Peplau from previously unpublished papers. The archives of her work and life are housed at the Schlesinger Library at Harvard University. Peplau's ideas have, indeed, stood the test of time.

CONTENTS

■ UNIT III

PROFESSIONAL SCHOLARSHIP

Careers in Advanced Practice Psychiatric Nursing

CAROLE A. SHEA

■ INTRODUCTION

Health care in the new millennium is characterized by opportunity, challenge, and uncertainty. These characteristics make this an exciting time to be an advanced practice nurse. *Crisis theory* states that opportunities for growth and change are greater at major turning points in life (Aguilera, 1994). *Social learning theory* supports the idea that challenges in life strengthen our sense of mastery and competence (Bandura, 1986). *Chaos theory* suggests that uncertainty, unpredictability, surprise, instability, and lack of control are the natural characteristics of complex, open systems such as human beings and health care organizations (Vicenzi, White, & Begun, 1997; Wilson, 1998).

Seen from these perspectives, advanced psychiatric nursing is the specialty practice for these uncertain times. Some of its key concepts are stress, anxiety, crisis, trust, accountability, competency, coping, adaptation, and change. Its science focuses on human behavior at all system levels: the cognitive, emotional, and behavioral processes of individuals; interpersonal relationships; group and family dynamics; organizational behavior; and community attitudes and actions. Its practice offers a combination of mind, body, and spirit interventions to deal with distress and improve the overall mental health and general well-being of individuals, families, and communities. Box 1-1 lists psychiatric-mental health nursing's phenomena of concern.

In studying human behavior, advanced practice registered nurses (APRNs) in psychiatric-mental health nursing seek to answer fundamental questions: "Why do people do what they do?" and its corollary, "How can we help people to adapt positively or change their behavior?" APRNs acknowledge that there are multiple answers to these questions because human behavior is so complex. People do what they do because of who they are and where they are, past and present influences, future hopes and aspirations, the times in which they live, and unseen and unpredictable forces that have a continuously changing effect in both minor and major ways (Butterfield, 1996; Prager & Scallet, 1992).

Understanding the human condition and providing effective mental health care requires specialized knowledge, competencies, and skills (Dee, van Servellen, & Brecht, 1998; Stuart, 1997). Given the daily pressures, constant uncertainty, and escalating rate of change in modern society, there is an increasing need for advanced practice nurses who have in-depth knowledge of mental health and illness and the skills to affect behavioral change. These qualities are the bedrock of the advanced practice of psychiatric-mental health nursing.

box 1-1

PSYCHIATRIC-MENTAL HEALTH NURSING'S PHENOMENA OF CONCERN

Actual or potential mental health problems of clients pertaining to:

- Maintenance of optimal health and well-being and the prevention of psychobiologic illness
- Self-care limitations or impaired functioning related to mental and emotional distress
- Deficits in the functioning of significant biological, emotional, and cognitive systems
- Emotional stress or crisis components of illness, pain, and disability
- Self-concept changes, developmental issues, and life process changes
- Problems related to emotions such as anxiety, anger, sadness, loneliness, and grief
- Physical symptoms that occur with altered psychologic functioning
- Alterations in thinking, perceiving, symbolizing, communicating, and decision making
- Difficulties in relating to others
- Behaviors and mental states that indicate that the client is a danger to self or others or has a severe disability
- Interpersonal, systemic, sociocultural, spiritual, or environmental circumstances or events that affect the mental and emotional well-being of the individual, family, and community
- Symptom management of side effects or toxicities associated with psychopharmacologic intervention and other aspects of the treatment regimen

Reprinted with permission from ANA,1994.

PSYCHIATRIC-MENTAL
■ HEALTH NURSING PRACTICE
Historical Background

Psychiatric nursing is a specialty area within the discipline of nursing. The specialty developed along an alternative path (Church, 1985) at about the same time as Nightingale's work to establish nursing as a profession. In its early years, psychiatric nursing was based on postgraduate, on-the-job training to provide custodial care and to manage the institutional environment. However, even then psychiatric nurses were beginning to appreciate the reciprocal effect of mind and body and the value of psychotherapy. In the first published psychiatric nursing text, Bailey (1920) advised, "Listen patiently to all the patient will tell, for to unburden the mind affords great relief, and be sympathetic with the patient but not with the symptoms." Providing nurturing care, attending to daily activities, observing symptom patterns, and carrying out medical orders for somatic therapies comprised the role of the psychiatric nurse in the first half of the twentieth century.

According to Fox (1992), psychiatric nursing did not enter the modern era of nursing until after World War II with the passage of the Mental Health Act in 1946. Federal support for mental health education and services, enlightened mental health policy, public optimism about new treatments, and most importantly, the discovery of psychiatric nursing theory and practice by Peplau gave fresh impetus to psychiatric nursing as an advanced practice specialty. The first master's program in a *clinical* nursing specialty was established by Peplau at Rutgers University in 1952. This program focused on teaching the role of the psychotherapist and fostering the autonomy and leadership of the clinical nurse specialist. In the ensuing decades, other graduate programs in psychiatric nursing followed this innovative model. Many of nursing's greatest clinicians, theorists, administrators, educators, and leaders emerged from these programs in the 1960s and 1970s.

In the 1980s, the specialty both waxed and waned, responding to the trends that influenced the delivery and financing of psychiatric-mental health care. Many nurses with a psychiatric nursing background pursued their careers in leadership roles as expert clinicians in independent

practice, executives of health care organizations, academic deans, researchers, consultants, and presidents of professional organizations. This provided high-profile visibility for psychiatric nursing, especially when the leaders acknowledged their specialty roots. However, the overall growth in numbers of psychiatric nurses at the advanced practice level did not meet the expectations of those in the specialty (Pothier et al., 1990) or the public need. Some of the factors cited for the decline in the number of nurses entering the field of psychiatric nursing in the late 1980s were 1) the integrated undergraduate nursing curriculum, which provided little specialty content and few clinical experiences with psychiatric patients; 2) dwindling federal support for education and services; 3) refocused attention on the needs of the deinstitutionalized seriously mentally ill; 4) nursing shortages; and 5) competition from high-tech, high-status nursing specialties such as critical care nursing (Fox, 1992). The "Decade of the Brain" in the 1990s, however, brought a resurgence of interest in the specialty of psychiatric nursing that continues today. The factors for this trend are described in more detail later in this chapter.

Scope of Practice

Given its relatively short history, psychiatric-mental health nursing has made remarkable progress in defining and expanding its scope of practice to meet the needs of society and the profession. In its most recent iteration, *A Statement on Psychiatric-Mental Health Clinical Nursing Practice and Standards of Psychiatric-Mental Health Clinical Nursing Practice* (ANA, 1994), the scope of practice is described according to levels of practice, role of the nurse, and the work setting.

There are two levels of practice—basic and advanced. These levels are distinguished by educational preparation, professional experience, type of practice, role functions, and certification.

Basic level of practice. At the *basic level,* psychiatric-mental health nurses are registered nurses

(RNs) with a baccalaureate degree who demonstrate skills beyond the beginning RN or novice to the specialty. These nurses are nationally certified by the American Nurses Credentialing Center (ANCC) within the specialty (i.e., designated as RN, C). RN, Cs engage in the full range of professional nursing interventions with individuals, groups, families, and communities who seek psychiatric and mental health services. Their activities include health promotion and maintenance, intake screening and evaluation, case management, milieu therapy, assistance with self-care activities, psychobiologic interventions, health teaching, crisis intervention, counseling, home visits, community action, and advocacy (ANA, 1994). The practice of RN, Cs may be based in psychiatric facilities, community-based agencies, managed care organizations, and entrepreneurial ventures.

Advanced level of practice. At the *advanced level*, those who specialize in psychiatric-mental health nursing must have educational preparation leading to a minimum of a master's degree. This preparation includes indepth knowledge of theory and practice, supervised clinical practice, and competence in advanced clinical skills in the specialty area. At this level, the traditional designation for psychiatric nurses is *clinical specialist.* Currently, national certification by the ANCC as a certified specialist (CS) is required for advanced clinical practice in psychiatric-mental health nursing. In the future, national certification as a nurse practitioner (NP) in psychiatric-mental health nursing will be available also. (See Chapter 20 for a discussion of the CS and NP roles.) Certification is necessary to become eligible for prescriptive authority, admission privileges, and third-party reimbursement, depending on individual state nursing regulations.

Titling of the psychiatric-mental health nurse at the advanced level continues to vary regionally. Efforts to designate all advanced practice nurses (e.g., clinical specialists, nurse practitioners, nurse midwives, and nurse anesthetists) as APRNs have not achieved consensus among the nursing specialties to date. However, 50 nursing groups signed the proposal endorsing the APRN designation, and many states and Congress prefer to use this term in their legislation (Cronenwett, 1995). In this book the term *APRN* will be used when referring to the CS or NP who is practicing psychiatric-mental health nursing at the advanced level.

APRNs can perform all of the clinical role functions and interventions of the basic level RN, C nurse. However, when doing so, APRNs apply their expertise in cases of greater severity and with more complex systems or in situations requiring leadership and interdisciplinary collaboration. In advanced clinical practice, APRNs diagnose and treat mental disorders using a wide range of psychotherapeutic and psychobiologic interventions, including prescribing medication where nursing regulations permit. Most notably, APRNs take on the role of primary therapist, engaging in psychotherapy with individuals, groups, couples, and families. Additional roles include providing supervision and educational consultation for other mental health therapists and being a consultation-liaison nurse in working with those who have psychiatric and psychosocial problems as well as physical illness and disability.

APRNs may also subspecialize (i.e., define their practice according to a specific patient population, mental disorder, role, or function). Subspecialization requires graduate study, additional training and experience, and judgment on the APRN's part about standards and appropriate practice. At this time additional certification is not necessary (ANA, 1994). For example, APRNs may subspecialize in the group therapy modality; in the consultation-liaison role; in the forensic system; or in working with children, elders, the chronically mentally ill, or addicted mothers with AIDS.

APRNs may function in the role of educator, administrator, consultant, or researcher in conjunction with the clinician role or as their primary role. When one of these indirect (i.e., nonclinical) roles is the primary role, the APRN may find that further education, including a doctorate in nursing or another field, and related professional experience is required. Certification for advanced practice in the indirect roles is not required.

APRNs work in all settings—institutional, community-based, and private practices (Merwin et al., 1997). They are qualified to establish independent practices by virtue of their professional expertise and legally-sanctioned autonomy. However, in this turbulent era of health care, most APRNs choose to maintain an affiliation with a health care organization or are employed by a mental health care agency. Having an organizational tie allows APRNs to take advantage of a greater access to patients, established reimbursement mechanisms, administrative support, centralized risk management, colleagueship with other APRNs, and opportunities for interdisciplinary collaboration in patient care and research.

These descriptions of the scope of psychiatric-mental health practice at the basic and advanced levels are reflected in *Nursing's Social Policy Statement* (ANA, 1995). Although both levels encompass specialty practice, the advanced level is characterized by specialization, expansion, and advancement (Cronenwett, 1995). In psychiatric-mental health nursing, *specialization* refers to a concentration or focus on psychiatric illness and mental health, as part of the whole field of health care and nursing. *Expansion* is the acquisition of new practice knowledge and skills that enable the APRN to practice autonomously and in areas that traditionally border on medical practice (e.g., psychotherapy, differential diagnosis, and prescription of medication). *Advancement* is the integration of theory, research, and practice that occurs through graduate education in nursing and achievement of a master's or doctoral degree in psychiatric-mental health nursing. By conceptualizing advanced practice in a way that does not specify roles such as nurse practitioner or clinical specialist, the development of new roles will be possible as health care evolves. For example, the crafting of innovative roles for the APRN is a subject of discussion in many chapters in this book.

Psychiatric Nurses in Advanced Practice

Who are the psychiatric-mental health nurses in advanced nursing practice? The most recent national study, conducted by the Society for Education and Research in Psychiatric-Mental Health Nursing (SERPN, 1997), presented a profile of certified APRNs in practice (Merwin et al., 1997). APRNs are highly educated, with 51% holding a master's degree in psychiatric nursing and the other 49% holding master's degrees in another area of nursing or a related field; 13% also hold doctoral degrees. They are very experienced, with an average of 17.1 years in psychiatric nursing and an average of 11.1 years as APRNs. Most APRNs work full-time and identify their primary place of employment as hospitals (32%), ambulatory clinics or outpatient settings (22%), solo or group independent practice (22%), and academia (15%). About 24% are self-employed. Overall, 44% report that they practice in solo or group independent practice in a secondary setting with fee-for-service as the predominant mode of payment. About 38% work in the public sector, 33% in private for-profit organizations, and 29% in private nonprofit organizations. About 74% are salaried, and 94% have a day work schedule. Most work in direct care as clinical specialists in the primary therapist role with adult patients. Individual psychotherapy and psychiatric assessment are the predominant activities. The five most commonly treated conditions as reported by the survey respondents are affective disorders (95%), anxiety disorders (88%), personality disorders (78%), adjustment disorders (77%), and dually-diagnosed mental health and substance abuse problems (71%). Although the total range of conditions is broad, only 55% reported that they had treated persons with schizophrenia and other major psychoses within the previous 2 months. This suggests a need for the specialty to rethink priorities so that those with the most serious mental illnesses will have access to the expert care of the APRN.

Three of the SERPN survey's findings are particularly troubling. First, 77% of those surveyed in 1994 were between the ages of 40 and 59, with an average age of 47. The researchers relate the aging of the APRN workforce to the following factors: the decrease in the number of graduate students entering the specialty of psychiatric-mental health nursing, the decline in funding for graduate education, the extended length of time to complete part-time master's programs, and the certification requirements for extensive post-master's supervised practice (Merwin et al., 1997). These same factors apply to all nursing specialties, except primary care nurse practitioners, which has seen a dramatic increase in the last five years (AACN, 1998).

Second, as in all areas of nursing, there is little diversity among APRNs—most are Caucasian women. There are few men (about 5%) and very few APRNs of ethnic or racial backgrounds other than Caucasian (i.e., 2% African-American, 1% Asian, 1% Hispanic, and 1% other, according to the SERPN survey). Although 7% to 10% of APRNs speak a second language, the lack of ethnic or racial diversity may compromise the ability of those in the specialty to provide culturally competent care to the increasingly diverse population in the United States. Federally funded initiatives to address the disparity have yet to produce a significant shift toward increased diversity (Market forces, 1997).

The third area for concern is the geographic maldistribution of the APRN workforce. Although there are certified APRNs in all states, the number of APRNs is not proportional to the state's geographic size or population density. For example, a small east-coast state such as Massachusetts had 799 APRNs, whereas a large western state such as Texas had 176 APRNs (SERPN, 1997). In part, this is a reflection of the historical location of specialized psychiatric treatment facilities, medical training centers, and graduate education programs. For example, the first psychiatric nursing training program was located at McLean Hospital in Massachusetts. Currently there are five psychiatric-mental health nursing master's programs that prepare APRNs in Massachusetts; three are in Boston. Another distribution factor is that nurses tend to practice in the same community in which they live, work, and attend school. Their mobility is restricted by such factors as family interests, job seniority, and the convenience of local employment. However, as practice patterns change in the new health care era, there may be more opportunities for APRNs to practice in community-based primary care settings that are more widely dispersed according to the population needs. The expansion of mental health care into these settings may help redistribute the APRN workforce, thereby increasing access to mental health services by vulnerable populations (Cotroneo et al., 1997).

In summary, the practice attributes evident in the APRN's profile is encouraging in terms of the educational preparation and experiential quality of the clinicians. There are strong indications for future employment opportunities. However, certain findings suggest that the delivery of quality mental health services may be jeopardized in the future unless there is an increase in recruitment to the field, especially among men and ethnically diverse groups, and a more widespread deployment of APRNs across the country.

Characteristics of Psychiatric Nursing

The study of human behavior, with all its ambiguity and intricate complexity, both attracts and repels individuals to the field of psychiatric and mental health care (Pothier et al., 1990; Skovholt & Rønnestad, 1992). In the past, nurses who chose a career in this field had to step out of the mainstream of nursing and medical care. Today, psychiatric nursing is rapidly moving back into the mainstream (Shea, 1993). At the basic level of practice, the nurse who pursues a career in psychiatric nursing may prefer to concentrate on psychosocial interventions versus physiologically based care. At the advanced level, the APRN often seeks greater autonomy in practice (Schutzenhofer & Musser, 1994).

APRNs need to embrace a world view distinguished by meaningful inner and outer dimensions, expansive time frames, and a pervading sense of the importance of relationships. Aspiring APRNs must welcome the cognitive stimulation provided by studying genetics, neurophysiology, neuroendocrinology, immunology, epidemiology, psychology, sociology, and anthropology. These are the sciences that describe the intricate relationships of biopsychosocial systems. In practice, APRNs are intrigued by the search for patterns and meaning in seemingly unpredictable and often risky behavior. On an emotional level, APRNs' feelings may resonate with the pain and vulnerability of special persons who lead unstable lives in a world that prizes normality, control, and balance. Above all, APRNs value the therapeutic interpersonal relationship as a principal means for promoting, maintaining, and restoring health and preventing disease (Williams et al., 1998).

In contrast, nurses attracted to other specialties of nursing may share these same characteristics to a lesser degree or hardly at all. Possibly influenced by popular conceptions of the "bedside nurse" and media portrayals of dramatic roles for nurses such as the highly-rated *ER* television show (Rice & Smith, 1997), they choose careers in fields exemplified by critical care and emergency nursing. The nature of their practice reflects a more linear, physiologically based, high-tech, fast-paced, episodic approach to care and the nurse-patient relationship. They draw upon the focus, time-orientation, work environment, and tools of their practice from the mainstream of nursing and medical care and long-established nursing traditions regarding professional roles, responsibilities, and service (Rice & Smith, 1997). For example, Schutzenhofer and Musser (1994) found that spe-

cialty and employment setting were related to a difference in autonomy, with critical care nurses demonstrating a lower level of autonomy when compared with psychiatric nurses.

In the continuously transforming health care environment, the different work worlds of advanced practice nursing are converging as new paradigms take shape. Despite traditions, professional practice preferences, and personal character differences, all specialties of nursing are designing patterns for advanced practice that incorporate a more holistic, community-based, collaborative, interdisciplinary approach to care (McCloskey & Maas, 1998). The designs must be appropriate for delivery systems that reward evidenced-based or best practices, cost-effective outcomes, and patient satisfaction. Moreover, to achieve the goals for significant improvement in the nation's health, interventions need to be targeted toward helping people make difficult changes in lifestyle and behavioral health practices, as well as manage their complex health problems. As a result, there are new alternatives for nursing careers in psychiatric and behavioral health care as direct care providers (Cotroneo et al., 1997; Shea et al., 1997) and a variety of indirect roles. There are also new opportunities for advanced practice nurses in other fields to collaborate with APRNs in psychiatric nursing to provide specialized mental health care through creative practice arrangements.

CAREER PATHS IN ■ PSYCHIATRIC NURSING

A career in nursing is the lifelong pursuit of work that is of service and benefit to others, fosters self-actualization in personal and professional ways, and nurtures the development of future generations of nurses (McBride, 1996). The attributes of a "career" clearly differentiate it from a "job." A career is meaningful, satisfying, advancing work that is rewarding to society, the individual nurse, and the profession. A job is characterized by regular activity or tasks done for pay. In its fullest sense, a career is the means for achieving the goals of Erikson's (1968) generativity stage of life, using all of a person's wisdom and talents in service to others.

Nurses may embark on a career in psychiatric nursing from different routes, depending on their educational background and work experience. The multiple entry routes and various career paths to advanced practice roles are depicted in Fig. 1-1.

Entry Routes

Without professional consensus about the degree required for entry into practice, potential nurses may seek education in diploma, associate, bachelor, master's, or doctoral programs. Most psychiatric nurses have a bachelor or associate degree. However, because of its long history of custodial care, the field of psychiatric nursing also includes a significant number of licensed practical nurses (LPN) and nursing assistants (NA) who may consider themselves to be "psychiatric nurses." Many LPNs and NAs obtain an associate or bachelor degree to enhance their career options in psychiatric nursing.

Work experience also shapes career choice and development. There are three main pathways to becoming a psychiatric nurse. The traditional path is taken by the nurse who first seeks a time-limited experience in medical-surgical nursing. The nontraditional path is the direct pursuit of experience in psychiatric nursing. The third path is taken by the nurse who has more extensive experience in general nursing or another specialty before turning to psychiatric nursing.

Medical-surgical beginnings. Graduates of professional nursing programs who wish to become psychiatric nurses upon graduation face stiff opposition. For years those in education and service have decreed that new graduate RNs must have "one year of med-surg experience" in an acute care setting before moving to their chosen nursing specialty (Fox, 1992). This mandate is based on the conventional wisdom of the profession that the work experience of an RN should be based in

a traditional general hospital, on a unit where the practice is broad-based, illness-oriented, and technologically focused. There is an assumption that socialization to the role of the RN should take place within a bureaucratic structure where close supervision and perhaps precepting by an experienced medical-surgical nurse can inculcate the knowledge, policies, and values of the institution. A major emphasis of this first year is on-the-job training to become facile in performing technical skills, using high-tech equipment, and practicing nursing according to the policies and standards of the institution.

There are several problems with this scenario. Today most hospital units function in a similar way to intensive care units because of the acuity of the patients' conditions and the shortened lengths of stay. With the downsizing of hospitals and medical centers, patients are admitted more ill and must be treated and discharged more quickly. These hospitalized patients require and deserve highly skilled nursing care from nurses who have honed their expertise over many years. Therefore how can new graduates learn to practice in this environment? The nurses with expertise may have difficulty precepting novice RNs because of their own increased patient load and time pressures. With the changes in the staffing mix caused by economic pressures, the more experienced nurses are often charged with administrative responsibilities that take them away from the bedside. Furthermore, Benner (1984) suggests that expert nurses may not be the appropriate ones to orient novice nurses because their intuitive level of practice is too far removed from the basic principles and processes that guide entry-level practice.

The new graduate typically has a long, slow learning curve that requires intensive orientation and practice over time in an atmosphere that accepts mistakes as an inevitable part of the learning process. Often this is not feasible in the pressured environment of the modern hospital. Also, downsizing has led to fewer openings for nursing positions in the general hospital,

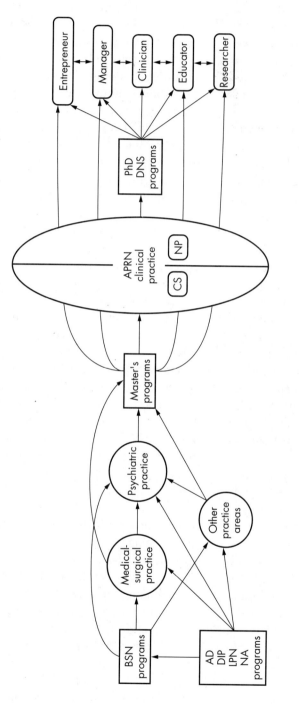

Figure 1-1 Career paths to psychiatric nursing.

although the number of positions fluctuates depending on periodic "nursing shortages." For these reasons, it is much more difficult for a newly graduated RN with limited experience to obtain such a position. Instead, many new graduates find their first nursing position in a skilled nursing facility, nursing home, or sub-acute unit, often very different from their desired specialty area (Fetter & Grindel, 1997).

Starting in psychiatric nursing. New graduates who would like to become psychiatric nurses may lose their way when they have to begin their career working with other patient populations (McBride, 1996). There are, however, nurses who ignore the "one year med-surg" advice and proceed to build their career in psychiatric nursing directly upon graduation. Those seeking to become a psychiatric nurse usually take a position in a psychiatric facility or social agency that serves a psychiatric population. The main focus of their work is the use of interpersonal skills with less emphasis on the traditional technical skills. They are actively engaged in making comprehensive assessments, doing counseling and teaching, and managing the therapeutic environment. However, their nursing practice must also include care of common health problems and both acute and chronic physical illnesses experienced by psychiatric patients in hospital and ambulatory settings.

Benner (1984) would applaud this approach to career development because she believes in early specialization as an efficient and necessary way to acquire a sufficient experiential base for advanced clinical practice. In order to become experts, nurses must have the opportunity to practice with many cases of a similar nature over time so that they learn to distinguish nuances and respond to subtle cues in the patient's response to health, illness, and treatment. Therefore specializing at an early stage in a nursing career allows for both a shorter learning curve and a greater depth of knowledge in the specialty practice.

When RNs take their first nursing position in a psychiatric setting, they become socialized to an "alternative" culture, one that has evolved through the delivery of mental health care outside the traditional medical system. Many times this culture has evolved within a locked unit away from the general medical population or in a separate building with its own rules and norms. Socialization to the specialty role tends to occur within the subculture of the specialty rather than the general institutional culture because the specialized practice takes precedence in forming the professional identity. In this way RNs become steeped in the theories, practices, beliefs, values, and mores of the specialty at an early stage in their career.

New graduates may be hired directly upon graduation for entry-level positions in psychiatric facilities. However, with the move to providing comprehensive care to psychiatric patients in primary care settings, they must possess the knowledge and skills to promote general health, prevent disease, and carry out interventions for general medical problems as well. Most basic nursing programs now prepare their graduates to perform these functions at a competent level (Stuart, 1997).

Coming from other areas. A third pathway to becoming a psychiatric nurse is that taken by experienced nurses who are seeking to expand their practice into the psychosocial realm. These nurses may come from another area of specialty practice or general medical-surgical nursing. They bring a wealth of nursing knowledge and skills but have to adjust to the different world of psychiatric nursing practice. In that sense they are somewhat like the new graduate. For these experienced RNs, the learning curve may be steep but short as they gain knowledge and experience in the specialty. Re-socialization to the norms and values of psychiatric nursing, however, may take longer because of the previously ingrained socialization to general nursing and medical care.

The diversity in education and experience of psychiatric nurses contributes to the strength of the specialty. Fig. 1-1 shows the career paths psychiatric nurses pursue to become an APRN and the areas of service and various roles that evolve from the synergy of education and practice.

Moving Toward Advanced Practice

After some years in practice with psychiatric patients, many nurses are motivated to move toward advanced practice. The impetus may come from several sources. Based on their research, Skovholt and Rønnestad (1992) identified the following motives:

1. Challenging clinical experiences with patients and families, which stimulate a need for greater knowledge and skills
2. Increased satisfaction with the counselor or therapist role
3. Encouragement from peers, other professional colleagues, or a mentor
4. Opportunities for career advancement, which require the master's degree credential
5. Personal experience in dealing with mental illness with a family member or friend
6. Less conscious motives, such as wanting to resolve personal issues by learning how to do therapy with others

In the instance of motives 5 and 6, the desire to become a therapist to resolve personal problems and help others may be viewed as part of the nurse's attempt to improve the fit between self-concept and occupation. However, Skovholt and Rønnestad (1992) suggest that personal suffering and family crisis are not sufficient to sustain an individual in a counseling career over a lifetime. Therefore there is an expectation that APRN therapists will examine their career motives and resolve personal problems that might affect their practice as part of their own continuing professional development.

Regardless of the entry route and motives for a career move, nurses who wish to practice at an advanced level today must pursue a master's degree in psychiatric nursing as indicated in Fig. 1-1. The master's degree program offers not only the necessary knowledge and skills for advanced practice but also makes graduates of the program eligible for ANCC certification in the specialty. As of 1998, a master's degree in psychiatric nursing is required for certification at the advanced level.

However, in the past, the ANCC regulations allowed applicants to hold graduate degrees in a related field such as psychology, counseling, and social work. For example, as reported in the SERPN survey (Merwin et al., 1997), about 21% of certified specialists have master's degrees and 57% have doctoral degrees in a health-related field other than nursing. CSs without a *nursing* master's degree, who took the examination and maintained their certification before 1998, retain their eligibility for recertification in the future. This cadre of CSs has been grandfathered by the ANCC and will not be lost to the specialty.

The ANCC took the measure of changing the education requirement to a master's degree in nursing to strengthen the bond between advanced specialty practice and nursing as a discipline. Nursing policy-makers recognized that the profession has matured to the point that nurses need to be educated and socialized within their own discipline for advanced practice. Standardizing the educational qualifications for CSs and nurse practitioners also benefits the public (e.g., by allowing regulatory consistency among states, thereby enhancing the geographic mobility of APRNs [ANA, 1995]). Political advocates have used the standardization of educational preparation to good advantage in lobbying with legislators on behalf of advanced practice nursing and the public's health care interests.

Chapter 20 describes the programs in graduate education that prepare nurses for advanced practice in psychiatric nursing and discusses the controversies about role preparation as a CS or NP. In this next section, role models in psychiatric nursing are presented briefly to show the wide range of professional contributions that APRNs make to the profession and society.

Role Models

The major roles for advanced practice nurses are clinician, manager, educator, researcher, consultant, advocate, and entrepreneur. One of the best ways to envision a role model is to study the careers of nurses with high visibility within the profession. No discussion of role models can fail to mention the preeminent psychiatric nurse, Hildegard Peplau EdD, RN. Peplau has been called the "Mother of Psychiatric Nursing." Clinician, theorist, educator, author, professional leader, supervisor, mentor—the list of prominent roles that she played throughout her long career is awe-inspiring. She is recognized for her "firsts" and for her leadership by all nurses within and outside the specialty. A representative sample of her achievements includes the following:

1. Creator of the first theoretical framework for psychiatric nursing and author of *Interpersonal Relations in Nursing* (Peplau, 1952)
2. Developer of the first master's program for advanced clinical preparation of psychiatric nurses
3. Professor emeritus of Rutgers University and recipient of 11 honorary degrees
4. Star of films and training videos on psychotherapy
5. The only nurse who served as both president and executive director of the American Nurses Association
6. Namesake of the ANA's Peplau Award for the most significant contributions to psychosocial and psychiatric aspects of nursing care delivery
7. Fellow of the American Academy of Nursing
8. 1998 inductee into the ANA Nursing Hall of Fame
9. Recipient of the Christiane Reimann Prize, an eminent international award
10. One of the 50 greatest Americans, as designated by President Bill Clinton

At the heart of these accolades of success is her role as clinician and critical thinker. Peplau practiced psychotherapy with patients who had the most serious mental illnesses in the era before modern psychopharmacology. She was an astute therapist. She not only provided effective therapy, but she passed on her pearls of wisdom to future generations as well. Peplau taught what she learned from her patients and colleagues during World War II and at the Chestnut Lodge with Frieda Fromm-Reichman and Harry Stack Sullivan in countless workshops conducted at state mental hospitals and clinics across the country. She expounded upon her insights in her interpersonal theory, graduate teaching, and professional publications. Peplau's lectures and writings have influenced the advanced practice of thousands of nurses and other mental health providers. While her historical memories of the early days in psychiatric nursing are a national treasure, her work continues to have special relevance today as she continues to engage in the continuing dialogue about the profession.

Psychiatric nursing is replete with excellent leaders who have made their mark in one or several roles at the advanced level of practice. To select only a few for special mention here would do a great injustice to the myriad of leaders who have a national reputation. However, there is a *set* of psychiatric nurses who serve as a representative sample of the specialty, making contributions to the profession as expert clinicians, educators, researchers, executives, consultants, entrepreneurs, and pathfinders. This set is composed of the first nine presidents of the American Psychiatric Nurses Association (APNA) (Box 1-2). Highlights of their professional careers and their achievements as APNA presidents demonstrate how they have used their special talents and interests not only to shape the organization, but to have a lasting influence on improving mental health care as well.

Fernando Duran, the founding president of the APNA, was a pathfinder and innovative administrator. His career embodies the American dream. A native of the Basque region in Spain, he was educated in Spain and England as a psychiatric nurse before coming to the United States to escape postwar oppression in Spain. Once here, he plunged into the fledgling community mental health movement, pioneering the development of the geographic unit system for mental health centers, a system that is still used across the United States and in many other countries for the delivery of community-based mental health care. Over the course of his career, in which he spanned the

1-2

ROLE MODELS: PEPLAU AND THE PRESIDENTS OF THE AMERICAN PSYCHIATRIC NURSES ASSOCIATION (APNA)

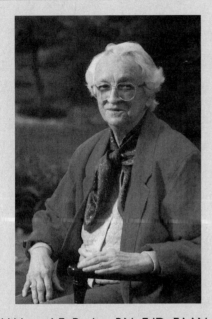

Hildegrad E. Peplau, RN, EdD, FAAN
Clinician and Educator
Mother of Modern Psychiatric Nursing

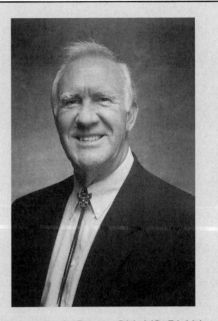

Fernando A. Duran, RN, MS, FAAN
Administrator and Pathfinder
First APNA president, 1986–1990

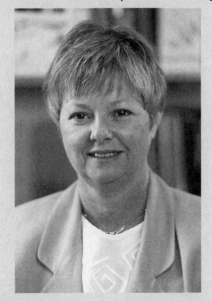

Carole A. Shea, RN, PhD, CS, FAAN
Academic Administrator and Consultant
Second APNA president, 1990–1992

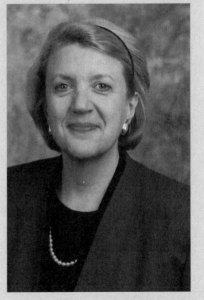

Ann Marie Brooks, RN, DNSc, MBA, FAAN
Nurse Executive and Consultant
Third APNA president, 1992–1993

continued

box 1-2

ROLE MODELS: PEPLAU AND THE PRESIDENTS OF THE AMERICAN PSYCHIATRIC NURSES ASSOCIATION (APNA)—cont'd

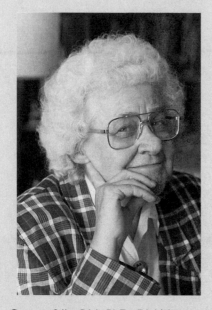

Grayce Sills, RN, PhD, FAAN
Educator and Consultant
Fourth APNA president, 1993–1994

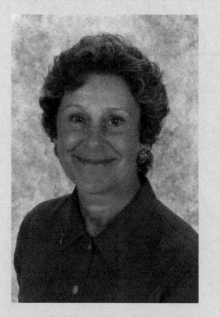

Karen S. Babich, RN, PhD, FAAN
Researcher and Policy Maker
Fifth APNA president, 1994–1995

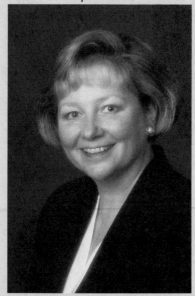

Gail W. Stuart, RN, PhD, CS, FAAN
Clinician and Researcher
Sixth APNA president, 1995–1996

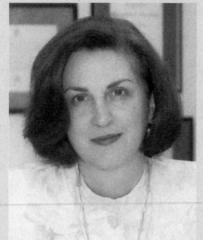

Nancy A. Valentine, RN, PhD, FAAN
Nurse Executive and Policy Maker
Seventh APNA president, 1996–1997

continued

box 1-2

ROLE MODELS: PEPLAU AND THE PRESIDENTS OF THE AMERICAN PSYCHIATRIC NURSES ASSOCIATION (APNA)—cont'd

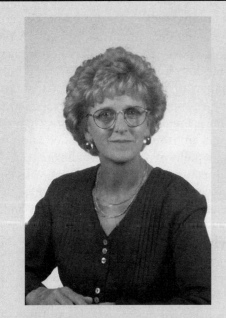

Phyllis M. Connolly, RN, PhD, CS
Educator and Advocate
Eighth APNA president, 1997–1998

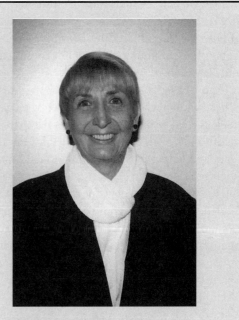

Jane Ryan, RN, MN, CNAA
Clinician and Consultant
Ninth APNA president, 1998–1999

country from New Mexico to Vermont, Duran served in administrative roles such as director of nursing, assistant commissioner of mental health, and superintendent of a large community mental health center. His professional accomplishments include being elected as president of the Iowa State Nurses Association, becoming a charter member of the American Academy of Nursing, and serving as a consultant to the National Institute of Mental Health and the World Health Organization. As a founding member of APNA, Duran was chosen by his fellow founders to be the first president of the Association, a position he held for 4 years because of his national stature and leadership qualities.

Carole Shea, the second APNA president, was the first president to be elected by the membership. With a background in nursing education and academic administration, she took as her theme,

"building an identity" (Shea, 1990; 1991). During her years on the APNA's Board of Directors, the membership of the APNA rose dramatically. She also worked to enhance the presence of the APNA at policy-making tables such as the interdisciplinary and consumer-oriented National Mental Health Leadership Forum, sponsored by the National Institute of Mental Health, which held national hearings in the early 1990s on the plight of mental illness; the National Federation of Specialty Nursing Organizations, composed of professional organizations representing the different nursing specialties, which seeks to speak in a collective voice on specialty nursing practice issues; and the National Organization Liaison Forum, the select group of nursing organizations that enjoy a formal affiliation with the ANA. She strengthened the dialogue with the Coalition of Psychiatric Nursing Organizations to work toward a more unified psychiatric nursing voice on behalf of mental health issues. She took a lead role in writing the statement and standards of clinical practice in psychiatric-mental health nursing (ANA, 1994). She is a Fellow of the American Academy of Nursing and a founding board member of the Center for Community Health Education, Service, and Research in Boston.

Ann Marie Brooks, the third APNA president, is best known as a nurse executive with a strong track record in some of the premier psychiatric institutions, such as the Shepard-Pratt Institute in Maryland and the Strong Memorial Hospital in Rochester, New York. She is a distinguished consultant who has traveled the world, spending extended time in Russia and Saudi Arabia, sharing her expertise on nursing service management, quality improvement practices, and transformational leadership skills. During her tenure on the Board of Directors, she brought strong management practices to the young organization, such as instituting a strategic plan as well as a business plan. She was also instrumental in moving the APNA headquarters to Washington, DC. A believer in team efforts, Brooks brought the key stakeholders together at an invitational conference sponsored by the APNA to devise effective strategies for dealing with mental health issues during the early days of the health care reform movement (Brooks, Polis, & Sills, 1993). Because of her efforts on the national level, Dr. Brooks was invited by President Bill Clinton to a memorable ceremony honoring nurses at the White House. She has also served as president of the American Organization of Nurse Executives and is a member of the accrediting body for private psychiatric hospitals and a Fellow of the American Academy of Nursing.

Grayce Sills, the fourth APNA president, has had a distinguished career as an educator, dean, consultant, editor, mentor, and policy maker. She has received many awards for teaching and service. She was a founding member of the APNA and served on its first Board of Directors. She was a prime mover in the development of chapters in APNA, with her home state of Ohio becoming the first APNA chapter. Her leadership is evident in the number of other boards on which she has served, within academia and in the community at large. One of her most significant accomplishments occurred when she chaired the Governor's Study Committee on Mental Health Services. Drawing on her extensive experience in practice, teaching, and policy-making, she worked with the Committee to reorganize the way that mental health care is provided in Ohio. This required an exquisite sense of systems and politics in order to balance sound professional practice and ethical care with political necessity and finance. A Fellow of the American Academy of Nursing, Sills enjoys sharing her professional wisdom and perspectives on life as a mentor to graduate students and colleagues. She also sends her message in editorial columns (Sills, 1998) and as editor of the *Journal of the American Psychiatric Nurses Association,* which she helped found while serving on the APNA Board. She is a model for productivity in retirement as she continues to provide consultation to schools of nursing and chairs the Board of Directors of a large university hospital.

Karen Babich, a founding member of the APNA, became its fifth president. She brought to the Board experience and insights gleaned from a distinguished career that successfully blended roles in education, practice, and research in leading institutions in New York, Chicago, Colorado, and Maryland. As a research administrator and senior policy officer for the National Institute of Mental Health, Babich was instrumental in promoting knowledge exchange and programs of research on victims of violence. During her presidential tenure, she gave priority to developing the APNA's organizational infrastructure, establishing the APNA as the nation's recognized authority on scientific, clinical, and policy issues pertaining to psychiatric nursing. (See the APNA Position Statements and Congress materials in the Appendix of this book.) By establishing innovative partnerships with diverse corporate entities, Babich was particularly successful in obtaining funds to support the development of educational materials for clinicians and consumers, thereby increasing public access to the APNA's professional services. Her energetic leadership resulted in the creation of committees to respond to the political challenges and opportunities that affect nursing practice and quality patient care. She is a Fellow of the American Academy of Nursing.

Gail Stuart's term in office as the sixth APNA president marked the tenth anniversary of the APNA as an organization. A psychiatric nurse for all seasons, Stuart brought her talents as an expert clinician, administrator, collaborator, researcher, educator, and author to the Board as the APNA began its second decade. Her keen business sense, skill in transforming plans into action, and drive for accountability put the APNA on a sound financial basis. The Congress on Advanced Practice in Psychiatric Nursing convened to bring together nurses from each state to develop a strategic plan addressing political, legislative, educational, and practice issues. Her vision for the APNA and the value she placed on communication resulted in the creation of the APNA website (www.apna.org) and the expansion of the *APNA Newsletter;* she continues as editor of both media. A Fellow of the American Academy of Nursing, she also provides great external visibility for psychiatric nursing as she travels around the country to present papers and workshops. Her scholarly expertise is sought by numerous national research and organizational boards, interdisciplinary work groups, and clinical guideline development panels. She has clearly left her mark on the APNA and the psychiatric nursing specialty through these activities, perhaps most lastingly in her textbook *Principles and Practice of Psychiatric Nursing* (Stuart & Laraia, 1998), which has been translated into several languages and is used throughout the world.

Nancy Valentine, the seventh APNA president, has an extensive background in nursing administration and health care policy. Her APNA presidency coincided with her major policy position in the Department of Veterans Affairs, so that she was able to capitalize on her knowledge of the macro trends in health care and apply them to the needs of the APNA. Her action plan focused on a commitment to increasing APNA member satisfaction, gaining a voice in expanded policy and legislative arenas, and building a communications network among the members. During her term, the APNA sponsored a government relations position and successfully lobbied for passage of the Medicare bill, which provides reimbursement for services by CSs and NPs. With its greater visibility, APNA membership grew by 15%, seven new chapters were formed, a national network of volunteers was identified to form a legislative task force with state affiliates, the website posted a calendar of events, and a nationwide Survival Skills Program for the staff nurse was offered. Valentine worked to establish important new alliances with the American Academy of Nursing, the Friends of the National Institute of Nursing Research, and Sigma Theta Tau International. Through these connections and others, the APNA became one of the originators of the Mental Health Patients' Bill of Rights. Valentine is a Fellow of the Academy of Nursing and Treasurer of the American College of Mental Health Administrators.

Phyllis Connolly, the eighth APNA president, came to office with a distinguished academic career as an educator and administrator. She is dedicated to serving the needs of families and consumers living with serious mental illness in the community. Using her organization and advocacy skills, she supported the development of the APNA Public Relations Task Force, which led to a Marketing for Mission Board Retreat. The detailed marketing plan that evolved provides the framework for achieving the mission and goals of the APNA well into the twenty first century. She also initiated the Functional Networking Groups in response to members' needs for better communication and more interaction. She was instrumental in establishing closer ties between the APNA and the National Alliance for the Mentally Ill so that APNA members could more easily join in the work of both organizations. Connolly is fearless when it comes to technology. Her presentations reflect the latest multimedia and set a wonderful example of modern communication techniques at professional conferences. Her grants to fund the use of computer technology in caring for psychiatric patients in the community reap benefits for nursing students and consumers alike. Mindful that clinical innovations need to be disseminated, she has published and presented her work, nationally and internationally, on the Transdisciplinary Collaboration Project, an outgrowth of a Psychiatric Nurse Managed Center at her university.

Jane Ryan, the ninth APNA president, is highly regarded for her achievements as a nurse executive, clinician, and researcher at a major west coast academic medical center. Her energy and dynamic presentation made her successful in securing influential positions that tied together service and education. Through her work as a consultant for the U.S. Department of Justice, she has improved the nursing care of patients in public sector mental hospitals. She has also worked tirelessly as a volunteer on behalf of children's mental health. Her election as president, without a doctoral degree, demonstrates that the APNA is an inclusive organization that represents all nurses. She took as her theme "dialogue and diversity" to signify that she values these concepts. She traveled to all the APNA chapters to converse with members as a source of empowerment and as a means to give members a strong voice in shaping the future of the APNA. She also emphasized diversity among the membership in such areas as education and work experience, practice roles and settings, gender, and ethnicity by encouraging the concept of councils within the structure of the APNA. Ryan also strengthened the strategic alliance between the APNA and the National Mental Health Association at both the national and local levels.

These outstanding role models are successful in their complex roles because they are skilled communicators, risk takers, creative innovators, and able to think "outside the box." Countless others could have been chosen to demonstrate cherished role models in psychiatric nursing. For further examples, see the descriptions of the influence and contributions of renown psychiatric nurses that authors have included in their chapters in this book. Influential role models are also to be found in local

communities where APRNs live and work as nursing colleagues, employers, friends, and family. They too shape the professional growth of advanced practice and help support APRNs through transitional stages in their careers.

MODELS OF CAREER
■ DEVELOPMENT

Models of career development are useful in describing the normative stages through which nurses must pass to forge a new professional identity. Like other developmental models, career models focus on making systematic changes in a progressive direction over time. There is a presumption that the growth process is adaptive and qualitative as well as quantitative in nature (Skovholt & Rønnestad, 1992). Three models of career development are presented. Benner's (1984) model describes the evolution in clinical practice expertise and has relevance for all nurses. Skovholt and Rønnestad's (1992) model has particular relevance for APRN psychotherapists. The Professional Career Model, a general organizational model for professionals, has application for APRNs in any role and stresses planning for a career over a lifetime (Dalton, Thompson, & Price, 1977). The Professional Career Model has been applied to nursing by several authors (Davidhizar & Stewart, 1996; McBride, 1993, 1996).

Novice to Expert Model

One of the most influential models of career development in nursing is that of Benner and colleagues. Benner's Novice to Expert Model (1984) is an application in nursing of the Dreyfus Model of Skill Acquisition. As in the Dreyfus model, there are five levels of proficiency: novice, advanced beginner, competent, proficient, and expert. As nurses progress through levels of proficiency, Benner proposes that their skill performance changes in three essential ways:

1. Nurses move from relying on abstract principles to using their past experience with signifi-

cant cases (i.e., paradigms) to inform their practice.

2. Their perceptions change from seeing the clinical situation in terms of parts to viewing the situation as a complex whole.
3. They shift from being a detached observer to being an involved performer.

Benner's seminal contribution to nursing is her insistence on the fundamental importance of the nurse's perceptions and the relation of experience in a particular clinical practice to expertise in that specialty. She defines *experience* as the "refinement of preconceived notions and theory through encounters with many actual practical situations that add nuances or shades of differences to theory" (Benner, 1984). Experience, then, is the outcome when the nurse's preconceived notions and expectations are challenged, refined, or disconfirmed by the actual practice situation.

Using qualitative research methods, Benner elicited narratives about their practice experiences from nurses at different levels of proficiency. She found that most nurses could give exemplars (i.e., narrative examples of cases that held particular significance for them). These exemplars conveyed more than one intent, meaning, function, or outcome and could easily be compared with or translated to other clinical situations whose objective characteristics might be quite different (Benner, 1984). Very experienced nurses described paradigm cases in which a past concrete experience changed their perceptions and subsequently transformed their practice. At the highest levels, the nurse's performance was characterized by knowledge embedded in intuitive perceptions that were dependent on the context of the situation. Because of the intuitive, contextually driven nature of their practice, expert nurses had difficulty articulating exactly how and why they made certain clinical judgments. However, there was general consensus among their colleagues and peers that they "knew expert practice when they saw it."

Benner developed her Novice to Expert Model from the narrative exemplars and paradigms of the nurses in her study. The model delineates five stages through which a novice nurse who has theoretical knowledge (the "know-what") may be transformed into an expert nurse who has extensive practical knowledge (the "know-how"). Table 1-1 describes the distinguishing features of each stage. The transformation from novice to expert takes place through sustained clinical experience over time within a defined area of nursing practice.

The appeal of the Novice to Expert Model is its premise that nurses acquire skill and develop expertise through a largely intuitive process that becomes ever more acute and refined throughout their years of practice. It refutes the argument that the rules and principles learned at earlier stages of a career become the unconscious, inevitable building blocks of later, more experienced practice. Instead, the model suggests that because perceptions change with experience and mastery, performance actually improves when rule-based behavior is replaced by the nurse's perceptions of the salient aspects of complex practice situations. The contextual perceptions of the expert rather than the abstract rules of the textbook or protocol become the driving force for clinical judgments and professional behavior (Benner, 1984).

Benner's model is generic for all nurses. Nurses in the field of psychiatric nursing could place themselves in any stage of Benner's model, depending on their level of theoretical know-what and practical know-how. To do so would give them an indication of the context, characteristics, intentions, expectations, and outcomes for practice at a particular level of proficiency. It is important to remember that the level of proficiency is not determined simply by the number of years of experience in the field but rather by a combination of experience with a designated patient population and skill performance in various roles and functions. Also, it would be a serious misconception to equate the intuitive perceptions of expert nurses with the sense of intuition people speak of in everyday life.

The general aspects of skill performance and Benner's model of professional development are applicable to psychiatric nursing. Novice nurses

table 1-1

BENNER'S NOVICE TO EXPERT NURSING MODEL

STAGE	YEARS OF EXPERIENCE	PERCEPTION OF CONTEXT	NURSING PRACTICE
Novice	Classroom and laboratory experience No prior clinical experience New to the field	Unable to perceive aspects and attributes of clinical situation Focuses on context-free rules and measurable phenomena	Relies on rules to govern practice Performs procedures and tasks Is inflexible with limited range of responses
Advanced beginner	New graduate to 1 year of clinical practice	Recognizes recurring aspects of situations and overall global characteristics Makes context-based judgments	Performs according to experience-based principles and guidelines Is unable to differentiate importance among aspects and attributes
Competent	2 to 3 years of clinical experience	Sees actions in terms of goals and plans: present and future Makes conscious, deliberate analysis of important aspects and attributes	Performs with increased mastery, organization, and efficiency Carries out plans for the present and future Able to cope with contingencies
Proficient	3 to 5 years of clinical practice	Perceives situations as contextual wholes Has holistic understanding of normal and abnormal	Fixes on the problem without complex analysis Learns from experience how to modify plans in response to the situation and patient events
Expert	More than 5 years of clinical practice	Embeds knowledge in own perceptions Has intuitive grasp of contextual situation Maintains a sense of the possibilities	Acts on intuitive knowledge Focuses on the most pertinent phenomenon or problem Performs on the basis of context and meaning

Adapted from Benner, 1984.

often rely on communication principles and formulaic techniques to engage in a therapeutic interview. Their use and application of principles and techniques prevent the exchange from becoming a social conversation, but the communication is often stilted and not effective in forging a therapeutic alliance. For instance, the novice nurse may repeat the patient's statements in an attempt to reflect a mutual understanding. The expert nurse may also use reflection with that same patient but effect a positive outcome. By weaving together concepts and past experience with the application of theory, the evidence from research and best practices, and present understandings of the contextual situation, the expert nurse creates an eclectic framework for dialogue that fits the individual patient's need for meaningful relatedness and relevant insights. A key to success is the full and active participation of the expert nurse within the therapeutic relationship.

Benner's model is not specific in terms of differentiating the stages of basic and advanced practice nursing, however. A psychiatric nurse might be accorded expert status as a RN, C with a bachelor degree and many years of experience in working with the seriously mentally ill in a day treatment program. This same individual might be termed an advanced beginner or competent APRN after graduating from a master's program with limited supervised experience as a psychotherapist. In contrast, the Counseling Model of Skovholt and Rønnestad (1992) can be applied to understand the stages of career development for the APRN.

Counseling Model

Skovholt and Rønnestad's (1992) research-based model of professional development is specific to the counseling disciplines (psychiatry, psychology, social work, and nursing). In complex detail, the Counseling Model shows the evolution of the therapist's professional cognition, affect, and behavior over the course of a career. The central assumption of the model is that the intertwining of personal and professional functioning has an effect on the professional development and competence of the counselor/therapist. In their qualitative study, Skovholt and Rønnestad used focused interviews with 100 counselor/therapists divided into five groups by education and experience to collect data about the development process. Through inductive analysis they created an eight-stage model of professional development:

1. Conventional
2. Transition to professional training
3. Imitation of experts
4. Conditional autonomy
5. Exploration
6. Integration
7. Individuation
8. Integrity

Table 1-2 gives an illustration abstracted from the model to show the progressive changes that occur as an individual moves through three of the stages, from a trainee to an experienced therapist (e.g., stage 2, stage 5, and stage 7). There are also eight categories that define aspects of each stage of career development:

1. Definition of the stage
2. Central task
3. Predominant effect
4. Sources of influence
5. Role and working style
6. Conceptual ideas used
7. Learning process
8. Measures of effectiveness and satisfaction

The Skovholt and Rønnestad Counseling Model is similar to Benner's model in three ways. First, it concentrates on the lived experience of the clinician in practice as the primary means of professional development and competence. Second, the stages of each model are comparable, although the Counseling Model has distinguished more stages over the course of a whole professional career. Third, both suggest that a constriction of thought, affect, and behavior takes place during training and the early stages of develop-

table 1-2

COUNSELING MODEL OF PROFESSIONAL DEVELOPMENT

CATEGORIES	TRANSITION TO PROFESSIONAL TRAINING	EXPLORATION	INDIVIDUATION
Definition/time period	First year of graduate school	New graduate, 2 to 3 years	10 to 30 years
Central task	Assimilate information from many sources and apply it in practice	Explore beyond the known	Deeper authenticity
Predominant affect	Enthusiasm and insecurity	Confidence and anxiety	Satisfaction and distress
Predominant sources of influence	Sense of being overwhelmed because of many interacting new and old data bases	New databases (i.e., new work setting, sees self as professional, multiple other sources)	Experience-based generalizations and accumulated wisdom are becoming primary; earlier sources of influence are internalized, sees self as professional elder
Role and working style	Uncertain and shifting while struggling to fit practice with theory	Modifying externally imposed professional style	Increasingly is oneself within competent professional boundaries
Conceptual ideas	Urgency in learning conceptual ideas and techniques	Personal rejection of some earlier mastered conceptual ideas	Individualized and personalized
Learning process	Cognitive processing and introspection	Reflection	Personally chosen methods
Measures of effectiveness	Visible client improvement and supervisor reaction	Increasingly realistic and internalized criteria	Realistic and internal

Adapted from Skovholt & Rønnestad, 1992.

ment that, while necessary, must be released during subsequent stages in order for the nurse or therapist to soar to the heights of expertise and professional fulfillment.

The models differ significantly in their emphasis on the need to explicate the personal realm of phenomena that affect practice and competence.

Benner seems content to accept that the deeply intuitive perceptions of expert nurses cannot be articulated and examined. Skovholt and Rønnestad (1992) maintain that the therapist's difficult life experiences, normative experiences, and professional experiences, although at times partially unconscious, painful, or elusive, must be illuminated and fully integrated into professional practice to benefit patients and to remain authentic to the self. Engaging in continuous self-reflection, participating in the supervisory process with more experienced colleagues, and moving to clarify boundaries within and across the personal self and the professional self are some of the ways that therapists come to terms with the necessity of examining the effect of personal and professional integration on practice. According to Skovholt and Rønnestad (1992), the main factors that affect therapists' ability to remain open and receptive to new growth, as opposed to stagnation, are as follows:

1. Intensity of motives to choose and stay in the profession
2. Dangers of countertransference activated by career motives
3. Excessive self-healing focus
4. Attitude toward appreciation of complexity and challenge
5. Ability to tolerate and modulate negative affect
6. Degree to which "personal anchoring" and internal integration occur
7. Awareness of a developmental, long-term, overarching goal

The stages in the Counseling Model are meant to serve as guides to providing appropriate learning experiences throughout a counseling career. They can also serve as benchmarks for tracking progressive professional development. However, education and work experience are not the only determinants of progress. Individual characteristics and environmental influences also affect the rate and stage of progress in a career.

Professional Career Model

The Professional Career Model is another stage model that was developed to describe how professionals in organizations can plan their careers and adapt to changing roles in their work over time (Dalton, Thompson, & Price, 1977). The four stages are 1) apprenticeship, 2) colleagueship, 3) mentorship, and 4) sponsorship. The salient fea-

tures of each stage are presented in Table 1-3. Davidhizar and Stewart (1996) have used this model as a framework to understand the tasks and issues involved in midlife career changes in nursing. They point out that not all nurses will progress through all stages regardless of the length of their career. There is an element of choice. Some nurses choose to move to the next stage and succeed because they have the necessary professional preparation and personal skill set. Others overreach their ability and do not succeed because of their lack of preparation, unrealistic expectations about their knowledge base and skills, or premature timing. Some voluntarily choose to stay at a particular stage, to make a lateral move, to take time out for family and personal reasons, or even to leave the world of work. Moving to the next stage requires a certain degree of professional maturity, but progress may be dependent on educational preparation, work experience, and opportunities of time and place.

With a clear understanding of the four stages, APRNs can use the model to plan for career advancement. Davidhizar and Stewart (1996) suggest several steps for nurses who are examining their careers and trying to make decisions about the future. First, individuals must recognize what stage of career development they are in currently, paying attention to their achievements and sources of satisfaction and dissatisfaction. Next, they must assess their abilities particularly in terms of knowledge, skills, credentials, experience, and personal strengths. Then they are ready to set goals that are strategic in nature, match the requirements of the next career stage, and draw upon their personal determination. At this point, in order to advance, they might have to move to a higher-level position, another institution, different work setting, or other geographic location. They must make an effort to take care of their own physical and emotional health so that they have the physical energy and mental stamina to pursue their goals and adapt to the new setting. Particularly when a major move is involved, they must learn to manage the increased stress, perhaps

table **1-3**

PROFESSIONAL CAREER MODEL

SALIENT FEATURES	STAGES OF PROFESSIONAL DEVELOPMENT			
	APPRENTICESHIP	COLLEAGUESHIP	MENTORSHIP	SPONSORSHIP
Focus	Learn knowledge, skills, and values of the profession	Hone high-level skills and achieve competence in specialty	Take care of others and help them grow by sharing knowledge	Use knowledge and influence beyond immediate setting
Key roles	Student Novice nurse Team member	Expert practitioner Colleague Team leader Subordinate in organization	Mentor Protector Principal investigator Superior in organization	Consultant Theorist Change agent Entrepreneur
Level of autonomy	Dependent	Dependent to independent	Independent to inter-dependent	Independent
Examples of activities	Routine tasks and functions Standard nursing care	Expert nursing care Special projects Publications	Teaching Research Staff/faculty development	Policy making Theory development System change
Level of leadership	Follower	Coordinator	Manager	Executive

Adapted from Davidhizar & Stewart, 1996.

by trying to create some balance in life and enjoying diversionary activities. At all steps along the way, they must maintain a sense of optimism by focusing on the positive and putting the negative into perspective. Finally, they must have a vision about the future, which includes a long-term plan with specific goals and achievements. Having a vision is invigorating and sustaining when events in the present threaten to sidetrack or overwhelm the best-laid career plans.

Role Transition

Professional growth in APRNs requires a combination of certain personal characteristics, learning resources, a cohort of peers and colleagues, role models, a practice arena, and the strength to sustain themselves during the transition of a career stage or the development of a new role.

A role is the set of expected and actual behaviors associated with a position in a social structure (Hardy & Hardy, 1988). A role requires a partner who plays the same role (nurse and nurse) or a complementary one (nurse and patient); it is not a solo part or solitary action. As part of a role-set, enacting a role requires relationship and negotiation skills for satisfactory performance. Therefore creating new roles or even maintaining essential roles in an organizational system often leads to the conditions of role stress (resulting from external environmental factors) and role strain (the internal, subjective state of distress). Nowhere is this more evident than in a rapidly changing social structure such as the health care delivery system. Still, nurses seem eager to pursue new and different roles at the advanced level of practice.

In the process of learning a new role, few people stop to consider that making the transition from old to new may have profound effects on their life. Barba and Selder (1995) describe this experience as a life transition that is characterized by a shift or disruption in the person's reality. As a result, the carefully crafted sense of "who I am" and "how the world is" becomes uncertain and loses meaning. The task then is to "build a bridge from the disrupted reality to one of the possible realities that can be created" (Barba & Selder, 1995).

The first step on the transition bridge to a new role is to relinquish the old reality (in this case, former roles and professional identities). This usually activates a grief process because of the perceived and actual losses. It may entail achieving closure with people and institutions, integrating life events into an historical context, and letting go of a lifestyle. The second step is to confront personal vulnerability and take a personal inventory (i.e., the nurse in transition needs to come to grips with weaknesses and deficiencies and acknowledge strengths and coping mechanisms in order to regain integrity of the self). The third step is to actively engage in the transition process by seeking information that supports the new role, testing new conceptions and ideas, practicing new behaviors with role partners, taking risks in new situations, and assimilating the beliefs and values associated with the new role. Over time, the combination of a structured learning process with opportunities for practice in the role and the professional socialization process facilitate the nurse's transition to the APRN role.

On a more practical level, people who are going through a transition often find that the established pattern of relationships and routines of daily life are very difficult to maintain yet cannot be relinquished. For example, the stresses and strains of role transition are very obvious when nurses are in graduate school, taking courses and carrying a difficult case load within an intensive clinical practicum, perhaps continuing to work part-time and managing a young family. They are also evident in the lives of APRNs who are maintaining a full career—engaged in clinical practice, research, and professional activities. McBride (1993) cautions that stress will occur invariably, but nurses must manage the pressures by taking care of themselves. She recommends health promotion such as good nutrition, exercise, rest, and relaxation. As a psychiatric nurse, she also pays attention to the value of maintaining a positive attitude, using humor, seeking support from others, and recognizing that time, energy, and resources are limited so that perfection in pursuit of a career is *not* an option.

In today's dynamic health care environment, role options for the APRN are virtually limitless. It is important to embrace the concept of "value added" and understand the nature of social exchange (i.e., have the ability to acquire and provide necessary resources in a reciprocal manner with a variety of role partners). In a cost-conscious world, trying to negotiate new roles in relatively uncharted waters requires the ability to deliver an excellent product or service, with meticulous market research to substantiate the nurse's worth as an APRN. As Lego (1997) suggests, there are many reasons why this is the right time to be a psychiatric nurse. With advanced practice competencies, personal conviction, strength of character, and a sense of humor, APRNs have the "right stuff" for the future health care delivery system.

IMPLICATIONS FOR
■ THE FUTURE

There are three "macro" and five "micro" influences that will continue to have a major effect on psychiatric nursing and mental health care in the future. The *macro influences* are the economics and financing of health care, information technology, and the new millennium. The *micro influences,* those particular to psychiatric-mental health nursing, are managed behavioral healthcare, the psychobiologic paradigm shift, accountability in practice, education trends, and mental health research. The macro and micro influences are discussed in relation to implications for future advanced practice, education, and research.

Macro Influence: Economics and Financing of Health Care

The economics and financing of health care was front-page news throughout the 1990s. Despite the failure of the health care reform movement, the effort to contain health care costs (to "manage"

care) took on a life of its own (Gabel, 1997; Millenson, 1997). As the "mainstream method of financing health care" (Millenson, 1997), managed care now dominates every aspect of health care services. Managed care financing affects who gets care; who provides care, what care may be provided, how care is paid for, what and how data are collected, how clinical effectiveness is determined, how quality is measured, how satisfied patients are with the care they receive, and so on. The essence of managed care financing is the link between the cost of services and the clinical effectiveness or outcomes of treatment. This sweeping transformation has led to a radical difference in the practice of nursing and medicine (Barrell, Merwin, & Poster, 1997; Millenson, 1997). There has been a power shift from the provider (supplier of services) to the payer (buyer of services). Today's clinicians must learn to function using evidence-based practices, clinical pathways and guidelines, treatment protocols, standard formularies, and other methods designed to standardize practice at a quality level while remaining cost-effective. Practicing according to the clinician's own judgment and spending health care dollars without regard for treatment results are no longer tolerated in managed care systems. In addition, the federal government has identified cases of fraudulent billing and other illegal practices, which have tainted the perception of health providers' ability to uphold the fiduciary trust that underpins the public's confidence in health professionals and the health care system (Gray, 1997).

These changes have engendered great controversy among providers, consumers, payers, policy makers, legislators, professional organizations, and other stakeholders. In an effort to correct for the excesses of the 1980s, the pendulum may have swung too far in the direction of managed care. It will be the work of the stakeholders in the next few years to evaluate the global effects of managed care financing. Whether this will be a case for fine-tuning or a major overhaul of the system will depend on the copious data presently being gathered and analyzed by those in the health care market, health policy forums, governmental agencies, and academic institutions. It will also be important for the public and the health professions to engage in the debate about how health care services should be structured and financed.

Micro Influence: Managed Behavioral Healthcare

American society has always viewed mental illness as distinct from physical illness. From the earliest precolonial times, American society has subscribed to a strong belief in the Cartesian mind/body dichotomy. People regarded mental illness and physical illness as separate entities in terms of areas for scientific study, causal attribution, disease process, symptom manifestation, treatments, practices, care facilities, providers, health policies, and their effects on society itself. As a result, the psychiatric specialty disciplines, psychiatric care systems, mental health policies and regulations, and even the mentally ill patient population, to some extent, remained outside the mainstream of modern medicine and medical care (Grob, 1973; McCrone, 1996).

The effects of this dualism persist to a great degree today. The stigma of mental illness is so pervasive that it is an uphill battle to obtain parity for mental health care. The advent of managed care systems has helped address the long-standing disparity between mental health care and physical health care. Managed care organizations (MCOs) emphasize ambulatory primary health care, access, cost-effective outcomes, and quality measures (Chisholm et al., 1997). In MCOs, persons with mental illness have access to a broader range of health services through their "primary care provider" who may make referrals within the same MCO for specialized psychiatric care or to an outside contractor as needed. MCO services are different from community mental health centers or state mental hospitals, which do not treat most physical illness or problems.

The rise of "for-profit" and "not-for-profit" managed behavioral healthcare organizations (MBHOs) may spell the demise of government-sponsored care for the seriously mentally ill. A legacy from the days of institutionalization, state-funded and state-controlled mental health care is being replaced by a system of privatization, in which states contract with MCOs and MBHOs to provide direct services for mental health and substance abuse disorders. These changes in mental health services delivery are very controversial among the mental health disciplines, however. Problems of access, utilization, effectiveness, quality, and benefits still exist. Service providers, administrators, researchers, and consumer groups must address these problems or the mentally ill will continue to fall through the cracks.

Another trend affecting the parity of mental health services and benefits involves the changes in the legislation and regulation of professional practice. Federal and state laws have expanded the types of service provider and mandated reimbursement mechanisms for disciplines other than medicine. For example, APRNs are now authorized to prescribe drugs and are reimbursed as primary providers in most states. This regulatory change gives the consumer greater access to service and choice of provider. It also enhances the professional opportunities for APRNs to participate in meeting the need for mental health promotion and disease prevention, as well as diagnosing and treating serious mental illness in a variety of settings and practice configurations.

The pervasive effects of managed care and managed behavioral healthcare on psychiatric nursing are recurring themes throughout this book. The authors of many chapters discuss the effects of managed care on practice and the profession and give examples of how APRNs deal with the system changes. The chapters in Unit One focus in particular on these issues in terms of organization management, information systems, marketing, diversity in the workforce, partnerships, health policy, and legal issues.

Macro Influence: Information Technology

The second macro influence is information technology in its broadest sense. Without information technology, managed care could not have developed so quickly or spread into so many arenas. Technology has provided all kinds of new information, often described as the "knowledge explosion." Technology also has allowed the use of traditional types and sources of information in new ways. For example, Millenson (1997) forecasts that "infomedicine will inexorably become the mainstream method of making medical decisions." By this he means that physicians and patients will communicate through computer/satellite link-ups, and physicians will access a clinical algorithm database to decide about the diagnosis and treatment of the patient. Although this is occurring in several locations, it is not yet the main method of diagnosis and treatment.

In addition to creating a new language, (e.g., infomedicine, telehealth, informatics, facsimile, Internet, e-mail), information technology has had a profound effect on how people communicate and in what time frame. Instant access and immediate response is now the expected norm for social and business interaction. Unwarranted access and unrealistic expectations about response time are a frequent source of social stress, examples of the unintended consequences of modern information technology.

The widespread acceptance of computers and electronic forms of communication is revolutionizing both professional and personal life. Many more people now have access to information about health care from a wide variety of sources. With knowledge comes power. As a result, better-informed consumers are prepared to take a greater role in making decisions about their health care. This shifts the power balance between provider and patient, changing the nature of the relationship. Under mandates to be more accountable, both individual providers and MCOs must strive for continuous improvement. Internal quality management and improvement systems, institutional report cards, and patient satisfaction surveys are sources of documentation about clinical and management performance, which serve the public's interest and may be used as marketing tools. Managed care systems

also have access to much more information about their enrolled members. The issues about patient confidentiality and right to privacy have sparked a national debate that may result in legislation restricting who has access to what information about whom.

These are just a few instances of the effects of information technology on health care in general. Since communication and health care information is their "stock in trade," APRNs will need to be in the forefront of using and studying the effects of information technology (Sandelowski, 1997). This field has wide applicability in terms of therapy, clinical outcomes, patient teaching, and research. Specific information about its use and effects in psychiatric nursing is provided in Chapter 3 and in several other chapters. Each chapter provides a resource section that is intended to guide the reader to websites, organizations, and printed material of particular interest.

Micro Influence: Biopsychosocial Paradigm Shift

A micro influence that has had a transforming effect on the discipline of psychiatric nursing is the shift in the basic paradigm from a psychodynamic perspective to the comprehensive biopsychosocial model (McEnany, 1991). Signaling the integrated philosophy, there is renewed interest in biologic, psychopharmacologic, spiritual, and complementary therapies, which are often used in combination with psychosocial interventions.

Advances made in neuroscience, especially in the later years of the twentieth century, have overturned the exclusive reliance on practices such as long-term, insight-oriented psychotherapy and set aside psychoanalytic concepts in the treatment of most serious mental disorders (McCrone, 1996). Not all scientific breakthroughs have been translated into clinical applications, but many have resulted in more effective forms of intervention. Notable examples are the latest generations of antidepressant and antipsychotic medications, which manage the symptoms very effectively without causing the debilitating side effects. Some of the genetic discoveries hold future promise for the management and prevention of serious mental disorders.

The scientific revolution in psychiatry caught the mental health disciplines unaware. Unlike their European counterparts, most American practitioners had focused almost exclusively on the behavioral and social sciences in studying mental illness (Betemps & Ragiel, 1994). In their education and training programs, they learned about psychoanalysis and psychotherapy. Therefore they lacked the training and tools for "bench science" on the brain. However, the discovery of neurotransmitters and the creation of sophisticated imaging technology has fostered a renewed interest in studying the reciprocal effects of brain and body, and mind and body. As a consequence, more funding has been allocated to the sciences for research on genetics, neuropsychoimmunology, psychobiology, psychopharmacology, and alternative therapies related to mental illness and health. Scientists from several disciplines, including nursing, have joined the search for a better understanding of the functioning of the brain, the integrated systems of the body, and holistic practices (McEnany, 1991).

Some chapters in Unit Two present these new scientific developments and their relevance for advanced practice nursing in psychiatric and mental health care. Other chapters discuss the application of various theories and findings within an integrative biopsychosocial framework.

Micro Influence: Accountability in Practice

Accountability in practice is another important factor influencing changes in psychiatric nursing. Accountability can take many forms, but it is most evident in the shift from process to outcomes by APRNs who have especially treasured the "process" and "processing" aspects of their practice. For instance, Barrell and colleagues (1997) provide a comprehensive list of the outcomes APRNs strive to facilitate with their patients. Dee and colleagues (1998) use Johnson's Behavior Systems Model and validated measures to examine the nursing care problems, functional levels, and impairment at discharge of seriously mentally ill, hospitalized patients.

APRNs are in the forefront of improving access to mental health care by delivering quality services when and where they are needed, such as in crisis mobile units and home care. Their use of practice guidelines, "best practices," critical pathways, professional standards of clinical care, and quality indicators are examples of how APRNs take account of their responsibilities in practice. APRNs are also accountable when they take the lead to promote mental health and prevent mental illness by developing and evaluating programs that are sensitive to the community's needs and responsive to epidemiologic trends. It is no longer sufficient to meet the needs of their own patients and families; APRNs must anticipate the needs of and develop health promotion and prevention strategies for whole populations. By adhering to the highest ethical standards and upholding the law, APRNs provide role models for other health professionals and maintain the nursing profession's reputation with the public. Advocating for patients and consumers in a politically savvy way and sharing responsibility with patients and families are also ways that APRNs keep account of the public's trust (Gray, 1997).

Accountability for "doing the right thing and doing the right thing *right*" is the challenge for those in clinical practice (Millenson, 1997). In Unit Two, the chapters provide ample evidence that APRNs are meeting that challenge.

Micro Influence: Education Trends

Is practice driving changes in education, or is education influencing how APRNs practice? The answer is both. Just as the health care industry is transforming itself to be more effective, consumer-oriented, and accountable, nursing education programs and academia itself are adapting to new ways to deliver innovative, student-centered programs and product-oriented outcomes (Shea, 1994). Nursing education programs have always responded to the needs of the public and the profession, although not always in a timely way. In today's fast-paced environment, the development and revision of curricula is proceeding with unheard of speed. Master's programs are proliferating, and specialty offerings, including psychiatric nursing, are on the rise (AACN, 1998; Market forces, 1997). Some of the trends that will influence those programs include managed care, information technology, the scientific discoveries that demand more research, prescriptive practice, and the biopsychosocial paradigm. There is passionate discourse at conferences and in print about resolving the perceived contradictions between the role of the psychiatric CS and the psychiatric NP (SERPN, 1997; Stuart, 1997; Williams et al., 1998). Nurse educators have taken creative approaches in designing curriculum that prepare APRNs for the CS, NP, or a blended role. Aspiring APRNs wishing to expand their scope of practice are enrolling in expanded master's degree programs, certificate programs, and continuing education offerings. To prepare for the indirect roles of management, teaching, and research, APRNs are entering doctoral programs in increasing numbers. These trends are discussed in Chapters 20 and 21.

APRNs are also involved in providing education for patients and families in new and different ways. The chapters in Units Two and Three give examples of some of the ways that APRNs deliver cost-effective, quality health care services and develop educational programs for mental health patients, families, and consumers to help them understand and manage their mental health needs.

Micro Influence: Research

All of the macro and micro influences come to bear on research, which is the scholarly investigation of phenomena from the cellular to the societal level. In psychiatric nursing the phenomena of interest have behavioral manifestations or organizational system features, such as depressive reactions, management of negative symptoms, crisis intervention techniques, brief therapies, psychopharmacologic strategies, mental health services, patient outcomes, effective communication, and so on.

Research is the profession's greatest need and its greatest hope. APRNs are perfectly positioned to identify the pivotal research questions that can improve care and advance the profession (Buerhaus, 1998). They have the knowledge and skills to collaborate on multidisciplinary studies seeking to answer fundamental but complex system research problems (e.g., how best to engage a psychiatric patient and family or significant other in an effective treatment plan). Psychiatric nurses have made great strides in developing their ability to use a variety of research methods, including everything from phenomenologic studies to clinical trials. They are becoming more experienced in seeking funding for studies that try to discover new knowledge, as well as studies that apply knowledge in clinical situations to define best practices.

However, there is a long way to go before advanced practice in psychiatric nursing lives up to its full promise. For example, literature reviews used to develop clinical practice guidelines in the field rarely include nursing research (i.e., compare the references cited in the Agency for Health Care and Policy Research Guideline documents). This is due primarily to the fact that psychiatric nursing research designs often fail to include the elements of randomized, controlled clinical trials that are viewed as the "gold standard" in health sciences. Thus one of the mandates for APRNs for the immediate future is to subject the process and outcomes of their clinical work with patients to more rigorous study designs.

The chapters in Unit Three suggest how APRNs can use research findings to improve their practice and engage in the change process in an informed, effective way. The chapters describing the intricacies of clinical trials and mental health services research provide insight into how these methods can be implemented to benefit psychiatric nursing and advanced practice.

Macro Influence: The New Millennium

Almost every chapter in this book begins with a reference to the new millennium or next century. The authors take notice of this dramatic turning point because they are living in the spirit of the times and can envision a different future in the new age. The last chapter in this book gives some predictions about the future for advanced practice and suggestions about how APRNs can thrive in the new millennium.

While the environment is rife with change, there is optimism, hope, economic prosperity, and promising scientific discoveries. Prospects for the future are challenging but filled with opportunities (Aiken & Fagin, 1992). There is almost a mythic quality about people's investment in witnessing the birth of a new millennium. Their investment in hope for the future speaks to the human desire to know more and live a better life. Within such a climate of positive thinking, people may be more willing to take risks and tolerate ambiguity, to embrace change and discovery, and to strive for a new world peace.

Of course there are those doom sayers who forecast an apocalypse at the turn of the century. Their vision may be colored by the environmental cataclysms, brutal civil wars, terrorism, unimagined family violence, government scandals, and rapid pace of change in modern everyday life that have characterized the 1990s. Resisting change or capitulating to the darker side of human nature may be reasonable given their perspective, but their negative thinking does not help repair environmental damage, right social injustices, or advance civilization.

Psychiatric nursing is a microcosm of these two perspectives. After 100 years of development, the specialty is poised to move in new directions of growth and expansion. The outcome is still uncer-

tain, but there is clear cause for optimism. There are those who are excited by the possibilities and those who loath the impending changes. Both groups need to mourn the loss of the good that was inherent in the old ways. Both groups can contribute to the new nursing art and science by retaining their bedrock values, adapting relevant theories and concepts to fit within new structures and processes, building systems and alliances, developing innovative roles, working collaboratively within the discipline and across disciplines, and participating energetically in professional organizations. This will create tensions and disagreements, but the diversity will ultimately strengthen and enrich the advanced practice of psychiatric nursing in mental health care.

RESOURCES AND CONNECTIONS

PROFESSIONAL NURSING ORGANIZATIONS

American Academy of Nursing
600 Maryland Avenue, S.W., Suite 100 West
Washington, DC 20024-2571
202-651-7238 (phone) 202-554-2641 (fax)
www.nursingworld.org/aan

American Association of Colleges of Nursing
One Dupont Circle, N.W., Suite 530
Washington, DC 20036-1120
202-463-6930 (phone) 202-785-8320 (fax)
www.aacn.nche.edu

American Association of Neuroscience Nurses
218 N. Jefferson Street, Suite 204
Chicago, IL 60606
312-993-0043 (phone) 312-993-0362 (fax)
www.aann.org

American Nurses Association
600 Maryland Avenue, S.W., Suite 100 West
Washington, DC 20024-2571
202-651-7000 (phone) 202-651-7006 (fax)
www.nursingworld.org

American Nurses Credentialing Center
600 Maryland Avenue, S.W., Suite 100 West
Washington, DC 20024-2571
202-651-7277 (phone) 202-651-7004 (fax)
www.nursingworld.org/ancc

American Psychiatric Nurses Association
1200 19th Street, N.W., Suite 300
Washington, DC 20036-2422
202-857-1133 (phone) 202-223-4579 (fax)
www.apna.org

Association for Child and Adolescent Psychiatric
 Nursing
1211 Locust Street
Philadelphia, PA 19107
800-826-2950 (toll-free) 215-545-8107 (fax)
www.acapn.org

International Society of Psychiatric Consultation Liaison Nurses
7794 Grow Drive
Pensacola, FL 32514
7850-474-4147 (phone) 850-484-8762 (fax)
www.ispcln@aol.com

National League for Nursing
61 Broadway
New York, NY 10006
800-669-9656 (toll-free) 212-812-0393 (fax)
www.nln.org

National Nursing Society on Addictions
4101 Lake Boone Trail, Suite 201
Raleigh, NC 27607
919-787-5181 (phone) 919-787-4916 (fax)
www.nnsa.org

Sigma Theta Tau International
550 West North Street
Indianapolis, IN 46202
888-634-7575 (toll-free) 317-634-8188 (fax)
www.stti@stti.iupui.edu

Society for Education and Research in Psychiatric-
 Mental Health Nursing
7794 Grow Drive
Pensacola, FL 32514
850-474-9024 (phone) 850-484-8762 (fax)
www.serpn2aol.com

PSYCHIATRIC NURSING JOURNALS

Archives of Psychiatric Nursing
 www.wbsaunders.com
Issues in Mental Health Nursing
 www.tandf.co.uk/JNLS/mhn.htm
Journal of the American Psychiatric Nurses Association www.mosby.com/psychnurs

Journal of Child and Adolescent Psychiatric Nursing
 www.nursecom.com
Journal of Psychosocial Nursing
 www.slackinc.com/jpn.htm
Perspectives in Psychiatric Care www.nurse.com

CAREER-RELATED NEWSLETTERS, GUIDES, AND MISCELLANEOUS RESOURCES

American Nurse www.nursingworld.org
APNA News www.apna.org
Bureau of Labor Statistics: *Occupational Handbook*:
 stats.bls.gov/oco/ocos083.htm
Nursing Spectrum: Regional career and employment
 information: www.nursingspectrum.com
Reflections: Career moves:
 www.stti@stti.iupui.edu/publications
The 1998 Health Network & Alliance Sourcebook:
 Resource guide:
 www.faulknergray.com/healthcare
The Riley Guide: General career advice:
 www.dbm.com/jobguide
State Boards of Registration in Nursing: Licensure and
 nurse practice acts in Massachusetts:
 www.state.ma.us/reg
US Census Bureau: Impact of demographic data:
 www.census.gov

References

Aguilera, D.C. (1994). *Crisis intervention: theory and methodology* (ed. 7). St. Louis: Mosby.

Aiken, L.H., & Fagin, C.M. (Eds.). (1992). *Charting nursing's future: agenda for the 1990s*. Philadelphia: J.B. Lippincott.

American Association of Colleges of Nursing. (1998, February). With demand for RNs climbing and shortening supply, forecasters say what's ahead isn't typical "nursing shortage." *Issue Bulletin*. Washington, DC: Author.

American Nurses Association. (1994). *A statement on psychiatric-mental health clinical nursing practice and standards of psychiatric-mental health clinical nursing practice*. Washington, DC: American Nurses Publishing.

American Nurses Association. (1995). *Nursing's social policy statement*. Washington, DC: American Nurses Publishing.

Bailey, H. (1920). *Nursing mental disorders*. New York: McMillan.

Bandura, A. (1986). *Social foundations of thought and action: a social cognitive theory*. Englewood Cliffs, NJ: Prentice-Hall.

Barba, E., & Selder, F. (1995). Life transitions theory. *Nursing Leadership Forum, 1*, 4–11.

Barrell, L.M., Merwin, E.I., & Poster, E.C. (1997). Patient outcomes used by advanced practice psychiatric nurses to evaluate effectiveness of practice. *Archives of Psychiatric Nursing, 11*, 184–197.

Benner, P. (1984). *From novice to expert: excellence and power in clinical nursing practice.* Menlo Park, CA: Addison-Wesley.

Betemps, E.J., & Ragiel, C. (1994). Psychiatric epidemiology: facts and myths on mental health and illness. *Journal of Psychosocial Nursing, 32*(5), 23–28.

Brooks, A.M., Polis, N.S., & Sills, G.M. (Eds.). (1993). Mental health care reform [Special issue]. *Journal of Psychosocial Nursing, 31*(8).

Buerhaus, P.I. (1998). Medicare payment for advanced practice nurses: what are the research questions? *Nursing Outlook, 46*, 151–153.

Butterfield, P.G. (1996). Thinking upstream: nurturing a conceptual understanding of the societal context of health behavior. In Kenney, J.W. (Ed.). *Philosophical and theoretical perspectives for advanced nursing practice.* Boston: Jones and Bartlett.

Chisholm, M., et al. (1997). Quality indicators for primary mental health within managed care: a public health focus. *Archives of Psychiatric Nursing, 11*, 167–181.

Church, O.M. (1985). Emergence of training programs of asylum nursing at the turn of the century. *Advances in Nursing Science, 7*(1), 35–46.

Cotroneo, M., et al. (1997). Opportunities for psychiatric-mental health nurses in a reforming health care system. *Journal of Psychosocial Nursing, 35*(10), 21–27.

Cronenwett, L.R. (1995). Molding the future of advanced practice nursing. *Nursing Outlook, 43*, 112–118.

Dalton, G., Thompson, P., & Price, R. (1977). The four stages of professional careers: a new look at performance by professionals. *Organizational Dynamics, 6*(1), 19–42.

Davidhizar, R., & Stewart, J. (1996). Maintaining a satisfying nursing career in midlife. *Nursing Leadership Forum, 2*, 108–112.

Dee, V., van Servellen, G., & Brecht, M.L. (1998). Managed behavioral healthcare patients and their nursing care problems, level of functioning, and impairment on discharge. *Journal of the American Psychiatric Nurses Association, 4*, 57–66.

Erikson, E.H. (1968). *Identity, youth, and crisis.* New York: Norton.

Fetter, M.S., & Grindel, C.G. (1997). Recent changes and current issues in medical-surgical nursing practice. In McCloskey, J.C., & Grace, H.K. (Eds.). *Current issues in nursing* (ed. 5). St. Louis: Mosby.

Fox, J.C. (1992). Psychiatric nursing: directions for the future. In Aiken, L.H., & Fagin, C.M. (Eds.). *Charting nursing's future: agenda for the 1990s.* Philadelphia: J.B. Lippincott.

Gabel, J. (1997). Ten ways HMOs have changed during the 1990s. *Health Affairs, 16*(3), 134–145.

Gray, B.H. (1997). Trust and trustworthy care in the managed care era. *Health Affairs, 16*(1), 34–49.

Grob, G.N. (1973). *Mental institutions in America: social policy to 1875.* New York: The Free Press.

Hardy, M.E. & Hardy, W.L. (1988). Role stress and role strain. In Hardy, M.E., & Conway, M.E. (Eds.). *Role theory: perspectives for health professionals* (ed. 2). Norwalk, CT: Appleton & Lange.

Lego, S. (1997). Top ten reasons why psychiatric nurses are a great resource. *Journal of the American Psychiatric Nurses Association, 3*, 191–195.

Market forces: are they working for the nation's vulnerable? (1997, Summer). *HRSA Health Workforce Newslink, 3*(2), 1–2.

McBride, A.B. (1993). Sustaining a career. *Journal of Psychosocial Nursing, 31*(10), 3.

McBride, A.B. (1996). Psychiatric-mental health nursing in the twenty-first century. In McBride, A.B., & Austin, J.K. (Eds.). *Psychiatric-mental health nursing.* Philadelphia: W.B. Saunders.

McCloskey, J.C., & Maas, M. (1998). Interdisciplinary team: the nursing perspective is essential. *Nursing Outlook, 46*, 157–163.

McCrone, S.H. (1996). The impact of the evolution of biological psychiatry on psychiatric nursing. *Journal of Psychosocial Nursing, 34*(1), 38–46.

McEnany, G.W. (1991). Psychobiology and psychiatric nursing: a philosophical matrix. *Archives of Psychiatric Nursing, 5*, 255–261.

Merwin, E.I., et al. (1997). Advanced practice psychiatric nursing: a national profile. *Archives of Psychiatric Nursing, 11*, 182–183.

Millenson, M.L. (1997). *Demanding medical excellence.* Chicago: University of Chicago Press.

Peplau, H. (1952). *Interpersonal relations in nursing.* New York: GP Putnam's Sons.

Pothier, P., et al. (1990). Dilemmas and directions for psychiatric nursing in the 1990s. *Archives of Psychiatric Nursing, 4*, 284–291.

Prager, D.J., & Scallet, L.J. (1992). Promoting and sustaining the health of the mind. *Health Affairs, 11*(3), 118–124.

Rice, M., & Smith, D.S. (1997). Recent changes and current issues in emergency nursing. In McCloskey, J.C., & Grace, H.K. (Eds.). *Current issues in nursing* (ed. 5). St. Louis: Mosby.

Sandelowski, M. (1997). (Ir)reconcilable differences? the debate concerning nursing and technology. *Image: Journal of Nursing Scholarship, 29*, 169–174.

Schutzenhofer, K.K., & Musser, D.B. (1994). Nurse characteristics and professional autonomy. *Image: Journal of Nursing Scholarship, 26*, 201–205.

Shea, C.A. (1990). President's address. *Journal of Psychosocial Nursing, 28*(2), 35.

Shea, C.A. (1991). APNA: building a strong identity. *Journal of Psychosocial Nursing, 30*(2), 7–9.

Shea, C.A. (1993). APNA convention address: moving into the mainstream. *Journal of Psychosocial Nursing, 31*(3), 5–7.

Shea, C.A. (1994). The three "R's" in nursing education. *Journal of Psychosocial Nursing, 32*(5), 7–8.

Shea, N. M., et al. (1997). The effects of an ambulatory collaborative practice model on process and outcome of care for bipolar disorder. *Journal of the American Psychiatric Nurses Association, 3*, 49–57.

Sills, G.M. (1998). Keeping the faith [Editorial]. *Journal of the American Psychiatric Nurses Association, 4*, 39–40.

Skovholt, T.M., & Rønnestad, M.K. (1992). *The evolving professional self: stages and themes in therapist and counselor development.* Chichester, England: John Wiley & Sons.

Society for Education and Research in Psychiatric-Mental Health Nursing. (1997). *Primary mental health and advanced practice nursing.* Pensacola, FL: SERPN.

Stuart, G.W. (1997). Recent changes and current issues in psychiatric nursing. In McCloskey, J.C., & Grace, H.K. (Eds.). *Current issues in nursing* (ed. 5). St. Louis: Mosby.

Stuart, G.W., & Laraia, M. (1998). *Principles and practices in psychiatric nursing* (ed. 6). St. Louis: Mosby.

Vicenzi, A.E., White, K.R., & Begun, J.W. (1997). Chaos in nursing: making it work for you. *American Journal of Nursing, 97*(10), 26–31.

Williams, C.A., et al. (1998). Toward an integration of competencies for advanced practice mental health nursing. *Journal of the American Psychiatric Nurses Association, 4*, 48–56.

Wilson, E.O. (1998). Back from chaos. *Atlantic Monthly, 281*(3), 41–62.

THE HEALTH CARE ENVIRONMENT

chapter 2

Mental Health Services Delivery and Managed Care

LUC R. PELLETIER and CHRISTY L. BEAUDIN

■ INTRODUCTION

Behavioral health services (mental health, substance abuse, and employee assistance) are being provided in various settings and systems throughout the country. Managed behavioral healthcare is a strategy for modifying reimbursement structures and delivery systems with an expanded focus on quality care, clinical outcomes evaluation, and consumer input. To work in this environment, advanced practice registered nurses (APRNs) in psychiatric and mental health care need to under-

stand the mechanics of managed care in behavioral health because employers and health plans will continue to seek ways to contain or reduce the costs of care. The programs, services, and delivery systems in which APRNs practice are influenced by managed care and will increase as the efforts in the private sector are translated to Medicaid behavioral health programs. In fact, the number of covered lives in Medicaid managed care programs has increased almost 500% from 1991 to 1996 (HCFA, 1996).

The process of managing care within the constraints of the health care benefit involves advocating for access and flexibility in service consumption. This chapter presents the different aspects of mental health services delivery and managed care and will introduce the reader to managed behavioral healthcare organizations (MBHOs), their development, and future implications for APRNs and the delivery of mental health and substance abuse services.

MANAGED BEHAVIORAL ■ HEALTHCARE DELIVERY

Managed care concerns in the behavioral health care industry are based in the provision of accessible and appropriate care while containing costs. Utilization of inpatient acute care is discouraged, and the use of least-restrictive treatment and maintenance of community support is encouraged. In behavioral health, managed care ensures that benefits are managed through pre-certification, concurrent review, and benefit design controls (calendar year, lifetime maximums, copayments, deductibles, and preexisting conditions). Specifically, managed care is defined as "a system of managing and financing health care delivery to ensure that services provided to managed care plan members are necessary, efficiently provided, and appropriately priced. Through a variety of techniques, such as preadmission certification, concurrent review, financial incentives, or penalties, managed care attempts to control access to provider sites where services are received, contain costs, manage utilization of services and resources, and ensure favorable patient outcomes" (Hart, 1995).

Factors Influencing the Development of Managed Care

Since the 1980s, there have been several paradigm shifts with the managed care evolution. These shifts include the following (Goodwin & Hill, 1997):

Treatment of illness and sickness	⇒	Prevention of illness, promotion of wellness
Fee-for-service	⇒	Capitation; case rates
Fragmented care	⇒	Integrated delivery systems/continuum/ focused factory
Responsibility	⇒	Accountability
Crisis management	⇒	Complex care management
Inpatient care	⇒	Ambulatory and alternative delivery systems
Solo practice	⇒	Group practice/integrated systems/ focused factory
Recidivism as statistic	⇒	Administrative and clinical outcomes
Symptom management	⇒	Disease management
Revenue maximization	⇒	Cost minimization and value maximization
Management of cases/individuals	⇒	Management of populations
Management of costs	⇒	Management of quality, outcomes, and offsets

What becomes important to the success of managed care is access, availability, quality of care, and quality of service. Addressing member preference and the cultural competency of providers cannot be overlooked. There are critics who argue that managed care is not the practice of ensuring that patients get necessary and appropriate care but a withholding of treatment to reduce expenditures (Mechanic, 1997). Others argue that quality, not managed care itself, is the concern. While there are forces at work promoting cost containment, the consumer is a reluctant recipient of the consequences (Brook, 1997).

A recent emphasis of managed care is the development or enhancement of population- and community-based delivery systems, a trend that is expected to continue into the twenty-first century. Managed behavioral healthcare will continue to be a strategy for modifying reimbursement structures and delivery systems, but it will also promulgate an expanded focus on quality care, clinical outcomes evaluation, and consumer input. The role of the MBHO and the implications of managed care are of particular importance to APRNs.

Underlying Assumptions

Assumptions about managed care incorporate aspects of care delivery that operate beyond the constructs of practice within fee-for-service reimbursement. Both the redefinition of what constitutes health as well as what is considered appropriate inform these assumptions, including the following (ANA, 1993):

1. Managed care is based on a health, rather than an illness, paradigm.
2. Managed care increases patient access to appropriate mental health services.
3. Managed care ensures cost effectiveness through the development of clear boundaries with regard to targeting, planning, and delivering needed mental health services.
4. Managed care ensures quality control through a utilization review process.
5. Managed care offers availability of a choice of providers based on the type of care required.

Roles in Managed Care

The role of any managed care organization (MCO) is to manage health care benefits wisely, reduce unnecessary or duplicative care, and budget a specified amount of dollars allocated to health care. There are many stakeholders who have had input and advocated for these and other objectives to be met in a managed care environment. The primary stakeholders are listed in Table 2-1.

According to the Foundation for Accountability (FACCT), the role of practitioners, providers, and health plans is to "understand what consumers want; monitor and improve performance in the areas that matter most to the public; mobilize consumers to become partners in their care; and compete on quality as well as price." The role of the purchaser is to "hold the health system accountable for quality and value; give employees and beneficiaries real health care choices; provide information and support for quality-based deci-

table 2-1

PRIMARY STAKEHOLDERS IN MANAGED CARE

CONSUMERS	DELIVERY AND SUPPORT SYSTEMS
• Patients	• Practitioners
• Families	• Support systems (e.g., family members, caregivers)
• Communities	• Institutes for mental disease (IMDs)
	• State, county, private, and Veterans Administration hospitals
PAYERS AND POLICYMAKERS	• Child and public welfare programs
• Health plans (e.g., indemnity, HMOs)	• Criminal justice systems
• Employer groups and unions	• Providers
• Accreditation commissions and committees	• Community mental health centers
• Advocacy groups	• Board and care and residential care facilities
• Politicians	• Skilled nursing facilities (SNFs)
• Taxpayers	

sion making; and create health-focused partnerships with beneficiaries, providers and the community." The consumer's role is to "understand the importance of quality in health care; make decisions based on clear, reliable quality information; provide direction to the health care system about what's important; and balance personal and societal goals in the decisions they make" (FACCT, 1998).

Behavioral Health Statistics

Participation in managed behavioral healthcare programs has increased since the mid-1980s. In 1997, it was reported that approximately 168.5 million Americans (75%) with some type of health plan were enrolled in a managed care program. Of these persons, 149 million were managed by specialty managed behavioral healthcare programs, and 19.5 million were managed within health maintenance organizations (HMOs)(*Psychiatric Services*, 1997). By 1998, the number of MBHO enrollees increased by 9% to 162.2 million, representing 72% of an estimated 225 million Americans with health insurance (*Open Minds*, 1998b). Some cities have HMO enrollment of more than 50%, and in newer markets the number of HMOs is doubling every 1 to 2 years (Carter Center, 1997). To work in this environment, APRNs need to understand the mechanics of managed care in behavioral health because employers and health plans will continue to seek ways to rein in or reduce the costs of care. MCOs that serve persons with behavioral problems cannot ignore the interests of the consumers that relate to accessible care, affordable care, and quality of care. The efficiencies and savings that have been realized in a managed care model are being used to develop parity legislation and resultant reimbursement models that will enable many Americans to receive the care that they vitally need.

The costs associated with the effective treatment of behavioral disorders are difficult to ascertain because individuals seek help from primary care providers as well as behavioral health providers. Because most cost savings associated with managed care strategies have already been extracted, managed behavioral healthcare entities will be increasingly emphasizing cost savings in relationship to quality (Manderscheid & Henderson, 1997). There are enormous economic and societal costs associated with untreated and ineffective treatment of mental disorders. However, managed care is a strategy designed to provide necessary services and effective treatment at an affordable cost to payers and consumers. The Substance Abuse and Mental Health Services Administration (SAMHSA) suggests that within the context of managed health care, quality standards can be maintained while treatment costs can be controlled. Effective treatment of mental health and substance abuse disorders can also contribute to cost savings in other medical areas (SAMHSA, 1995).

MANAGED BEHAVIORAL HEALTHCARE ■ ORGANIZATIONS

MBHOs grew out of the need for employers to curtail the upward spiraling costs of specialty health care for their employees and their dependents. Employers and health plans entrusted MBHOs to develop and implement strategies to cut the costs of mental health and substance abuse care. This has been accomplished by applying the same managed care principles associated with medical benefits to behavioral health services. Since most employers and health plans had little experience with redefining benefit plan designs for behavioral health using managed care principles, they looked to MBHOs for guidance. Ultimately, these organizations have assisted with managing benefits, managing the financial risk of providing such benefits, managing care, and reducing overall costs. An MBHO can be characterized by the following elements:

- Behavioral health care benefits for a defined population to include child and adolescent mental health services, adult mental health services, substance abuse and chemical dependency services, workplace services (employee assistance programs, short-term and long-term disability, legal advice), and preventive health services

- Delivery systems that include inpatient, residential, partial hospital, outpatient settings, and home care for commercial and public sector populations
- Centralized operations (utilization management and claims), contracted provider networks (practitioners and provider organizations), formalized quality management programs, and management information systems to support operations (JCAHO, 1997; NCQA, 1998)

Mental health services have historically been provided from a covered service menu, which has not always been able to meet continuum of care needs. The challenge is to build upon those services that meet the needs of the individual and create provisions to fill service gaps. An additional challenge is creating plans for community-based care that will address the unique mental health needs of the individual. From a continuity perspective, care should be managed from assessment and evaluation to termination of services as the symptoms are resolved and the benefit from treatment has been achieved. Whenever possible, individuals should always be included in planning their treatment and rehabilitation. Treatment flexibility should be such that a person achieves a higher and more stable functional status and receives the community support necessary to maintain the least restrictive living situation while promoting the independence of the consumer.

Birth and Growth of MBHOs

There has been a proliferation of MBHOs that provide oversight of behavioral health benefits in both the public and private sectors. The impetus for the growth of these organizations was federal policy changes in health care, the introduction of managed care mechanisms in employer-based

health insurance, and a more general public acceptance that managed care would contribute to lower costs for the consumer. Concurrently, purchasers wanted "value-added" management of benefits, which in health care means quality over price with no perceived or actual barriers to the care experienced by consumers.

MBHOs are relatively new in the managed care industry when compared with their MCO counterparts. The first company, Managed Health Network, Inc., was formed in 1987. Since then the number of MBHOs grew as employers, health plans, and government programs expressed increasing interest in contracting for the management of behavioral health benefits. In 1997, there were over 30 MBHOs in operation in the United States managing more than 136 million covered lives (*Open Minds*, 1998a). In 1998, the number of covered lives rose to 162.2 million (*Open Minds*, 1998b). During that time, several major mergers and acquisitions took place. For example, the acquisition by Magellan Health Services, Inc. of Merit Behavioral Care Corporation, Green Spring Health Services, Inc., and Human Affairs International resulted in a market share of 36% of the overall behavioral managed care business. A second major consolidation in 1998 was the purchase of Value Behavioral Health, Inc. by First Hospital Corporation/Options. This new entity, named ValueOptions, Inc., represents 27,111,000 lives. These two new entities now represent 85,810,000 persons, or 53% of the total market of behavioral managed care (*Open Minds*, 1998b).

MBHO Services

Many management products and services are offered by MBHOs to employers, health plans, unions, and both state and federal agencies. These include mental health and substance abuse (MHSA) services; employee assistance programs (EAP), which are now a range of programs referred to in the industry as workplace services (WPS); integrated models (MHSA services and WPS as a continuum); risk-based products; public sector products; and utilization review services. These products are briefly described as follows.

Mental health and substance abuse care.

Mental health and substance abuse services are provided by credentialed practitioners and contracted facilities. Financing is either fee-for-service or risk-based (i.e., per employee per month premiums). Various providers within a panel or network are allowed to provide services as long as they meet medical or clinical necessity criteria. These criteria, based upon scientific sources, are used by MBHO staff and practitioners to monitor the progress of care and the transition of patients from higher to lower levels of care. The purpose of this type of care management is to allow the individual to continue to participate in daily activities with the least amount of disruption while structuring a safe, healing environment through MHSA services. Critical components of any MHSA managed care program include the following:

- 24 hour access
- Assessment, triage, and referral
- Care management: the process of managing discreet episodes of care that encompasses treatment planning, discharge planning, and planning for treatment termination; it occurs within the context of the illness-wellness continuum for the individual or in coordination with other caregivers, family, and other support systems; different from traditional "utilization review/management," which focuses on an episode of care and management of the health care benefit
- Customer service: a core MBHO department consisting of customer service representatives who answer technical or administrative questions of practitioners, providers, enrollees, and recipients of care
- Management of complaints, grievances, and appeals
- Claims processing and adjudication: the process of receiving, confirming, and researching missing data, and paying claims; accurate claims adjudication allows the MBHO to analyze utilization data and determine trends by book-of-business, geographical regions, provider types, plan types, and population characteristics

- Network management: the process of selecting, credentialing, and recredentialing a panel of practitioners and contracting with facilities; also ensuring that there are an adequate number and types of practitioners and providers available for a specific geographic region or population
- Quality and outcome management

Employee Assistance Programs and Workplace Services.

EAP and WPS are specialty services for problems such as consultation, counseling and referrals, dependent care, critical incident debriefing, regulatory interventions, and training to assist employers and employees with workplace or life-management issues. The focus of these programs is often wellness, prevention, health risk appraisal, and the promotion of health and well-being in the workplace. The typical benefit includes a certain number of free visits for the employee and dependents (e.g., a range from three to eight visits per episode or case).

The WPS program is often the "front door" to MHSA services. Employees seek these services before accessing their MHSA benefit. Assistance is obtained from designated WPS staff who address the presenting problems of the employee and/or their dependents and make referrals to the appropriate service. Issues could include, but may not be limited, to the following:

- Personal performance and relationships (both professional and personal)
- Identification of a disease process, such as depression and drug and alcohol use
- Health and wellness (e.g., weight management, smoking cessation, exercise and fitness, self-management of health conditions, and complementary care)
- Long- and short-term disability management
- Child and elder care
- Financial guidance and legal consultation
- Training and educational needs in the workplace (e.g., balancing work and personal life,

time management and organizational skills, managing during stressful times, and enhancing communication skills)

Problem resolution-oriented services provided by WPS staff for these issues include 24-hour crisis lines, short-term counseling, links to existing internal and external resources, supervisory training (e.g., management and supervisory consultations, cultural diversity, and change management), and the prevention of violence in the workplace. Consultation may be provided to the employee or dependent, manager or supervisor, and groups of employees or managers. The services are provided by the MBHO to the employer by charging either per employee per month or a service fee per unit.

Some MBHOs contract to outside vendors for components of their workplace services programs. National vendors provide telephonic and Internet access to a wide variety of workplace or life management services for real-time counseling and support. For example, employees or dependents requiring health and wellness assistance may have access to companies that offer an array of personalized counseling, education, and referral services. These are delivered by health and wellness professionals and through educational self-help information. The goal is to assist the individual with attaining a healthier lifestyle. This can contribute to the reduction of an employer's health care costs, improve the health of a given workplace community, and increase employee productivity and morale.

The National Depression Screening Project (NDSP) is another example of an EAP program that can complement mental health and substance abuse services. This program is part of the National Mental Illness Screening Project and is sponsored in part by Eli Lilly. The program encompasses an interactive computerized system that allows employees and their family members access to a free, anonymous, self-administered telephone screening test for depression. The program provides the caller with immediate feedback and provides specific referral information for EAP services.

Integrated models. The term *integrated model* is used to describe a comprehensive continuum of services provided to an employer that includes both MHSA services and WPS within the same delivery arrangement. An integrated model provides access to a comprehensive behavioral health care delivery system composed of EAP clinicians, behavioral health clinicians, and contracted programs and facilities. This option is attractive to many employers who prefer a seamless approach to rendering EAP and behavioral health services to its employee population. Instead of dealing with a MBHO and an EAP vendor, they only need to develop systems using a single MCO. Fig. 2-1 provides an illustration of this managed care model.

One objective of an integrated model is to optimize treatment outcomes by facilitating referrals to the most appropriate resource at the point of access. This minimizes the number of levels of care or provider transitions that an individual might experience. The role of care management is to identify the treatment needs of the caller and make a referral to the appropriate resource. If the presenting problems can be addressed by the EAP clinician through short-term counseling, then the behavioral health referral may be bypassed. Persons presenting with a higher intensity of service need or severity of illness may be referred directly into the behavioral health delivery system for more long-term treatment.

Public sector products. Public sector products that are designed to effectively and efficiently manage the behavioral health benefits for Medicaid recipients and Medicare beneficiaries are growing. Government-sponsored programs are attempting to achieve what has been successful with commercial (or private sector) markets in cost-containment. Since 1995, over 36 states and the District of Columbia have entered into some type of managed care arrangement for their eligible members (Rosenbaum, Silver, & Wehr, 1997).

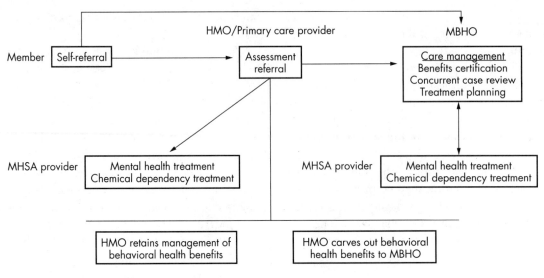

Figure 2-1   Integrated product.

MBHOs have changed their strategies, core systems, and competencies to accommodate the special needs of Medicaid and Medicare populations.

The MBHO provider network developed for carve-out programs capitalizes on the exceptional work done by community mental health centers over the years. The systems have proven themselves effective at managing the needs of the chronically mentally ill adults and severely emotionally disturbed children and adolescents. There are partnerships with the MBHOs to provide culturally sensitive and linguistically appropriate services. Care management can be delegated to clinical partners who are local, community-based, traditional providers, with the services being monitored by the MBHO. National accreditation standards provide guidelines for the delegated functions and activities.

States may modify the way they deliver care through a Health Care Financing Administration (HCFA) waiver process. Section 1115 of the Social Security Act allows states to petition the Secretary of the U.S. Department of Health and Human Services (USDHHS) through the HCFA in the form

of HCFA waivers for exclusion from various Medicaid requirements. HCFA waivers are one strategy used by individual states to reform health care delivery for those eligible for Medicaid. As of the Spring of 1998, over 17 states had such waivers implemented (Smiddy, 1998). Two waivers were approved but are pending implementation: program waivers and research and demonstration waivers. The rationale behind the waiver is to request permission to redesign programs, which will result in no additional cost to the government. Section 1115 allows the Secretary of the USDHHS to grant permission for states to conduct "pilot, or demonstration projects, which, in the judgment of the Secretary, are likely to assist in promoting the objectives of the Medicaid statute" (CMHS, 1995). Waivers that can be used for Section 1115 requirements are summarized in Table 2-2. The status of health care reform demonstrations is exhibited in Fig. 2-2.

The Center for Mental Health Statistics (1995) conducted a study of five state programs and found that all five states chose a managed care model for service delivery. Among the most significant

table 2-2

SECTION 1115 WAIVERS

REQUIREMENT	WAIVER
Comparability	Permit certain benefits to be provided to a particular group and not another.
Statewide uniformity	Permit variations in the program in different areas of the state.
Eligibility	Permit a state to revise Medicaid eligibility standards and criteria.
Provider choice/freedom of choice	Permit the state to restrict recipients' freedom of provider choice and require that they enroll in cost-saving managed care plans.
MCOs	Permit states to deliver Medicaid-funded services through delivery systems not currently recognized by Medicaid as a result of existing state and federal requirements
Reimbursement	Permit "reasonable alterations" in Medicaid payment requirements

From CMHS, 1995.

findings from the study was that seriously mentally ill adults and children with serious emotional disturbance received more flexible and richer services within the demonstration projects compared with the general Medicaid population.

Utilization review. Utilization review is the process of applying medical necessity criteria to the clinical situation to determine both the approval and payment of services rendered to a consumer. Utilization review includes precertification authorization, concurrent review, and retrospective review. This MBHO function is provided to health plans and employers that contract for administrative services only, which means that triage, care management, and discharge planning are not routinely provided as part of the contract. This has become increasingly less common as payers seek MBHOs to manage their care as well as their benefits.

Alternative services. Alternative services address wellness and health promotion, outreach and linkage, home-based care, ambulatory care, emergency care, and acute care. Levels of care

are arranged in a manner that not only ensures community maintenance but also facilitates the community-based management of personal and family crises and emergencies. The MBHO effectively encourages the integration of services by the following:

- Continually assessing and understanding the behavioral health needs of individuals
- Establishing appropriate clinical and operations policies and procedures for mental health organizations
- Coordinating the clinical components of care through effective primary and behavioral health care linkages
- Reducing barriers to accessibility to and availability of a credentialed provider network
- Integrating organizational financing through appropriate cost-management strategies
- Using an integrated information system that combines clinical, financial, and utilization data

There are types of alternative services that are not covered but, by their provision, may prevent a hospitalization or unnecessary removal from

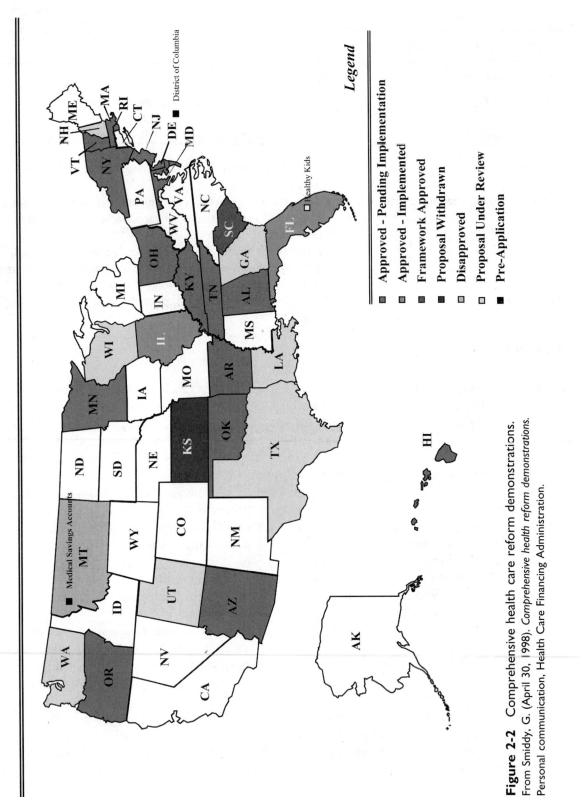

Figure 2-2 Comprehensive health care reform demonstrations.
From Smiddy, G. (April 30, 1998). *Comprehensive health reform demonstrations.*
Personal communication, Health Care Financing Administration.

home-based care. A continuum of care delivery model of traditional and alternative service is proposed that will, on some level, provide for supported living services, 24-hour crisis services, observation beds, development of community living skills, social rehabilitation services, personal networking, supportive counseling, and crisis residential services. Through a multidisciplinary approach to targeted and intensive care management, treatment will be clinically appropriate and will build a better service network for rural and urban areas. It is important to differentiate the met and unmet needs of persons with biologically based mental illness from those with situational disorders.

Networking to Promote a Continuum of Care

In managed care, networking traditional and alternative behavioral health services encourages the effective and efficient use of community-based care while minimizing the need for more restrictive care, such as acute hospitalization. Services need to be arranged and delivered so that they are consistent, compatible, continuous, and accountable to the consumer. Managing crises and promoting individual stability in a noninstitutionalized environment are achieved through the careful consideration of cognitive, emotional, and social conditions. Consumers, their support system, and behavioral health care providers desire the least restrictive treatment settings.

In the MBHO, care is managed through the linkage and development of relationships with existing facilities, programs, and providers in rural and urban areas. Provider arrangements enable the MBHO to ensure availability and accessibility to the different levels of care. Integrating traditional and alternative service is important to the overall goal of providing a continuum-of-care approach to behavioral health. Levels of care are arranged to facilitate the community-based management of personal and family crises and emergencies as well as maintenance of daily life. In addition to the traditional services, many behavioral health services are available that promote continuity of care. These are listed in Table 2-3.

The use of alternative approaches advances the achievement of desired outcomes, which include reduced symptomatology and relapse, increased duration of independent living, enhanced satisfaction with life, decreased psychosocial distress, and improved instrumental function (e.g., employment, social relations, and activities of daily living [ADLs]). Additionally, by providing an array of services and supports, opportunities for progress and success will be maximized over time (Budson, 1994; Carling, 1990; Fenton et al., 1998; Manderscheid & Sonneschein, 1997; Munetz & Geller, 1993; Stein & Test, 1980; Test, 1992). Finally, integration promotes a continuum of care where services are available and accessible, of acceptable quality to the purchaser and the consumer, and provided at the lowest cost in the least restrictive environment.

Challenges to MBHOs

Funding arrangements. The number of financial arrangements has burgeoned over the years. The manner in which an employer, health plan, or government agency pays the MBHO for its services varies. Common arrangements are indemnity plans, HMOs, preferred provider organizations (PPOs), and point-of-service plans (POS), as well as direct contracting arrangements between employers and providers. One mechanism for funding is capitation, with a prepaid, per-member, per-month payment that covers contracted services. The practitioner agrees to provide service for this fixed amount for a predetermined amount of time, regardless of service utilization. Capitation rates can be adjusted for age, sex, and diagnosis, based on previous claims data and future projected utilization.

Specialty services, such as behavioral health, are sometimes a part of the medical package and managed by the medical MCO. When services are managed and delivered internally by the MCO,

table 2-3

BEHAVIORAL HEALTH SERVICES THAT PROMOTE CONTINUITY OF CARE

CARE DOMAIN	SERVICE TYPES
Wellness and health promotion	Medication management; information clearinghouse; regionalized educational programs; peer support groups/self-help; family support groups; independent living skills; vocational rehabilitation counseling; targeted care management; intensive care management; individual and group psychotherapy; toll-free crisis phone line; social rehabilitation
Outreach and linkage	Screening; information and referral; rural and urban telemedicine; community buddy program; emergency mobile response system; transportation; 24-hour crisis intervention; case management with social service programs, targeted case management, or intensive case management; family-centered service programs
Home-based care	Psychiatric nursing; rehabilitation specialist (occupational and physical therapy); respite care; medication management
Ambulatory care	Outpatient psychotherapy (group and individual); partial hospitalization; day treatment; detoxification (medical and acupuncture); primary care provider interface and linkages
Acute care	Emergency room evaluation; 23-hour bed hold; crisis residential housing; mobile emergency response team; detoxification
Extended care	Board and care; intermediate care facility; skilled nursing facility; apartments; group homes

they are referred to as *carve-in* services. Staff employed by the company is specially trained in behavioral health, or the behavioral health vendor's staff is co-located with the medical plan. The advantage in this arrangement is that staff can use a single information system in which medical as well as mental health records can be accessed and reviewed. The review of the health of the individual or family is easily accessible to the care manager, who makes decisions about medical necessity. Conceptually, the interface between the behavioral health practitioner and the primary care provider is enhanced. Medical offset research, which is the ability of the organization to measure the savings in medical spending resulting from mental health service utilization, is easier to perform in a carve-in model. All the data reside in single or complementary management information systems.

When services are outsourced to a specialty vendor, such as an MBHO, the services are said to be a *carve-out*. These plans provide MHSA services only, and basic medical services are provided under an entirely separate plan and benefits management structure. The MBHO offers a network of credentialed practitioners and contracted facilities; assessment, triage, and referral services; case review and care management; and claims processing and payment. Fig. 2-3 provides an illustration of HMO carve-out arrangements with an MBHO.

Further, the American Managed Behavioral Healthcare Association (AMBHA) defines a *carve-out* as "a management approach where a defined

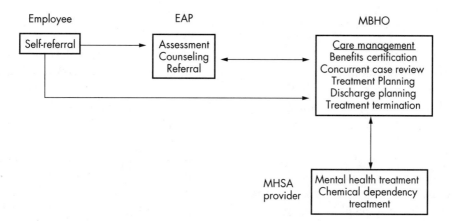

Figure 2-3 HMO carve-outs for managed behavioral healthcare.

category of health benefits are placed under the supervision of experts who understand that category of services and are better prepared to manage the associated costs" (AMBHA, 1997). Advantages of a carve-out program are the number of specialty resources available to the consumer and the reliance on the expertise of the MBHO in managing behavioral health benefits.

The use of different information systems and the need for interface between the behavioral health practitioner and primary care provider are potential weaknesses in this arrangement. It may be more difficult to perform health services research, especially related to medical cost offset, when the clinical and financial information systems data are housed separately by the HMO and the MBHO. The sharing and aggregation of health data for analysis and reporting become more cumbersome in this arrangement, particularly given the laws protecting the confidentiality of behavioral health treatment. It is critical in this model for there to be a shared understanding about the accountability for reimbursing for services where specific circumstances ("mixed services") might apply. For example, with a patient presenting with anorexia, the MBHO and MCO would need to have a clear agreement about who would pay for life-sustaining care, such as nourishment and medical observation, as well as who would pay for psychiatric care.

Health plans and employers have alternated positions in their preferred approach to the management of specialty services. Although carve-outs were popular in the 1980s, the MCOs tended to prefer carve-in services in the late 1990s for commercial sector products. For the public sector business, carve-outs have become more prevalent than carve-in programs. A driving force of choosing a carve-in or carve-out program is financial. Carve-outs have saved companies significant mental health care dollars and can be very appealing to some, but other companies may find the administrative costs of carve-outs to be higher than those of carve-in arrangements.

Vulnerable populations. Subpopulations may present any behavioral health practitioner or MBHO with unique challenges as a result of intrinsic or extrinsic characteristics. Many times treatment planning is more complex because consumer needs may not be self-defined or there is a brokering of services required that extend beyond the boundaries of traditional behavioral health (e.g., social services, educational institutions, health care, and housing). Vulnerable subpopulations include children and adolescents, persons with severe and persistent mental illness, persons with comorbid conditions (including disabilities), older adults, racial and ethnic minorities, the terminally ill, and veterans. These populations are "especially vulnerable to health care quality problems, differential experiences in the health system, or increased burden of poor health" (USDHHS, 1997). Several population characteristics and factors contribute to vulnerability. These include economic status; geographic location (rural or urban); health, functional, and developmental status; communication barriers; and age, sex, race, and ethnicity.

Vulnerability affects demand and use. Successful care management of children, adolescents, and older adults, as well as persons with mental illness, depends on an accessible continuum of care. Difficulties with accessing care, having a usual source of care, and affordability are common problems cited by Americans. Sometimes practitioners are not available when needed (e.g., child psychiatrists or APRNs with a speciality focus). In addition, persons who do have a usual source of care are more likely to receive preventive services and treatment for both acute and chronic conditions.

MBHO Performance Standards

Standards are built into the behavioral healthcare program design and developed according to the specifications of the customer (patient or employer), standards established by accrediting organizations, or standards promoted by professional associations. Current efforts underway in the measurement of performance in managed behavioral healthcare include the following:

- AMBHA PERMS 2.0
- Joint Commission on the Accreditation of Healthcare Organizations (JCAHO) National Health Library of Indicators (NHLI)
- National Committee on Quality Assurance (NCQA) Accreditation Standards: preventive clinical activities; nonpreventive clinical activities; health management systems; service activities
- American College of Mental Health Administration (ACMHA) Key Indicators
- NCQA Health Plan Employer Data Information Set (HEDIS) 3.0
- FACCT Performance Measures

- Mental Health Statistics Improvement Program (MHSIP)
- Institute for Behavioral Healthcare (IBH) Performance Indicators in Behavioral Healthcare
- American Public Health Association (APHA) Healthy Communities 2000 Model Standards
- Digital HMO Performance Standards (Third Edition).

Standards are based on the program requirements, administrative performance requirements, quality measures, and additional customized performance standards. Requirements include a plan for monitoring, tracking, and reporting on each performance measure: how data are tracked (source); who in the organization is responsible (accountability); how often tracking reports will be generated (reporting frequency); and the development and implementation of a corrective action plan when performance is substandard. However, there are also standards that the MBHO promotes as part of its daily operations, independent of external influence. These standards are exhibited in Table 2-4.

Performance standards related to MBHO core processes. Table 2-5 identifies performance standards and benchmarks related to various internal MBHO functions. Although there may be a core set of standards that the MBHO develops and monitors, there are standards that are account or health plan specific. These standards are tracked monthly, and MBHOs place a portion of their administrative fee at risk (from 1% to 25%), depending on the critical nature of the measure and relative importance to the payer. The reconciliation of fees and performance penalties is conducted quarterly and reported on an annual basis. Current trends include penalties for not meeting NCQA accreditation requirements.

ROLE OF CONSUMERS AND FAMILIES IN MANAGED ■ BEHAVIORAL HEALTHCARE

The role of consumers and the input of families are more visible as behavioral health care organizations develop and refine their programs. The

table 2-4

MBHO PERFORMANCE DOMAINS

DOMAIN	DEFINITION
Accessibility and availability	Timely and geographically appropriate provision of services and treatment as defined by the needs of the consumer.
Care management	Telephone assessment, triage, and referral; provision of referrals that meet consumer needs, ensuring appropriate clinical certification, and providing information to consumers and providers to optimize efficiency and quality of service and care.
Workflow management	Interface with all care providers in the fee-for-service and HMO settings, including, but not limited to, coordination of treatment planning, discharge planning, establishing clear access and lines of authority for care coordination, and follow-up between the manager and providers.
Internal and external resources	Internal and external resources must be adequate to support the behavioral health program (e.g., information technology, staff resources dedicated to quality management, and an adequate provider network).
Satisfaction	Systematic evaluation and measurement of consumer satisfaction with access, availability, appropriateness of care, coordination of care, cultural and linguistic competence of provider network, and outcome of services.
Outcomes of treatment	Clinician-assessed and self-assessed improvement in general health and well-being. Utilization is also examined as an administrative outcome of treatment.

issues of consumers, families, and advocates are described in detail in Chapters 17 and 18, but the importance of consumer input related to care delivered in behavioral managed care settings is discussed here. As business continues to be developed in the public sector, consumers and families play a critical role in ensuring that the services proposed are appropriate and accessible.

The NCQA requires consumer representation on MBHO quality improvement committees. MBHOs are also required to seek consumer input related to the development of the quality management program and quality initiatives. The most omnipresent advocacy group is the National Alliance for the Mentally Ill (NAMI), a grassroots organization that has been gaining momentum and influence in national policy and managed care issues. NAMI (1998) has developed and published

principles for managed care. The context within which these principles were developed is the ongoing restructuring and shifting of the delivery system architecture to enhance the public health care system. NAMI and other consumer-focused groups were also influential in the ongoing struggle for mental health benefits to be at par with other medical benefits. These principles are exhibited in Box 2-1. A discussion of parity legislation follows.

Parity

The Mental Health Parity Act (MHPA) of 1996, named "H.R. 3666, Title VII—Parity in the Application of Certain Limits to Mental Health Benefits" was signed by President Bill Clinton on September 26, 1996. This legislation, introduced by Senators

text continues on p. 56

table **2-5**

EXAMPLES OF MBHO PERFORMANCE STANDARDS

INDICATOR/DEFINITION	PERFORMANCE STANDARD
CARE MANAGEMENT	
Access standards: the plan's ability to be compliant with access to network practitioners and facilities (in locations with minimum population concentrations)	*Industry standards:* Drive time: 30 minutes from outpatient practitioners 45 minutes from facilities Appointment availability: Emergencies: immediate (within 30 minutes) Urgent: within 48 hours Nonurgent/routine: within 10 working days
Care management audits: audits of a representative sample of case records to measure adherence and consistency of clinical decision-making	*NCQA/MBHO standards:* completed at least annually
TELEPHONE ACCESS	
Average speed of answer: the amount of time it takes for a call to be answered on average (in seconds)	*NCQA/MBHO standards:* 100% of callers must reach a non-recorded voice within 30 seconds
Abandonment rate: the percentage of calls, on average, that do not reach an automated attendant or a person	*NCQA/MBHO standards:* abandonment rate of less than 5%
CLAIMS ADMINISTRATION	
Overall accuracy: percentage of claims processed correctly in every aspect (correct amount paid to correct person with correct coding [practitioner or provider, diagnosis, procedures, assignment of payment to type of service])	*Industry standards:* overall accuracy will be 90%
Payment accuracy: reflects the number of correct payments, irrespective of the total dollar impact, measured on a payment basis	*Industry standards:* payment accuracy will be at least 95% to 99%
Financial accuracy: the total claim dollars paid correctly, divided by the total claim dollars actually processed, measured on a dollar basis	*Industry standards:* financial accuracy will be at least 99% to 99.5%

Turnaround time: the number of calendar days from the date a claim is received by the MBHO to the date a response is issued (a claim benefit payment, a statement to claimant providing reasons for no benefit payment, or a request for additional information or documentation)

Industry standards: 85% to 90% within 10 to 14 calendar days 90% to 95% within 15 to 30 calendar days

Preprocessed claim turnaround time (for MBHOs that do not pay claims): a preprocessed claim submitted by the practitioner or facility is reviewed by the MBHO that is responsible for determining the amount of covered expense using authorized treatment guidelines and negotiated rates; the preprocessed claim is then sent to the claims administrator for payment

Industry standards: 85% of preprocessed claims are forwarded to the claims administrator within 3 business days; 100% within 5 business days

INQUIRIES, COMPLAINTS, AND GRIEVANCES

Inquiries: oral or written communication from a consumer or practitioner requesting information or an action (check eligibility, clarification of benefits, explanation of a process, checking on claim payment status)

Industry standards: 98% of all telephone inquiries resolved or followed up by a letter within 2 business days; 100% within 60 days

Complaints: an oral or written communication expressing dissatisfaction by a member or his or her representative or a practitioner or facility

Grievances: a formal request, written or oral, from a practitioner, consumer, or the consumer's representative, for the MBHO to change an administrative decision rendered after a response to a complaint (such as a benefit or claim payment denial, an administrative noncertification, or other administrative action)

continued

table 2-5

EXAMPLES OF MBHO PERFORMANCE STANDARDS—cont'd

DENIALS AND APPEALS

Denials: the clinical information presented by the practitioner or facility does not meet preestablished medical necessity criteria; only physicians and licensed clinical psychologists can make denials

Appeals: requests by the practitioner or facility for the MBHO to reconsider the decision made regarding denial of care

American Accreditation Healthcare Commission (AAHC), formerly the Utilization Review Accreditation Commission (URAC), Health Utilization Management standards (1997):

An attending provider can request and receive reconsideration by a clinical peer reviewer within 1 business day of the denial

An attending provider can request and receive an expedited appeal if the reconsideration results in the denial being upheld

95% of expedited appeals will be resolved within 1 business day

The initial written notification of the denial will describe the reconsideration and appeal procedure

The MBHO will maintain complete documentation of each case involving a denial disputed by a provider, patient, or plan member for audit purposes

Aggregate denial and appeal data will be reported to the payer at preestablished frequencies

CONSUMER SATISFACTION

The MBHO must have a process in place to measure patient satisfaction, including availability of consumer-specific information, description of sample, sample size, sample methodology, timing of satisfaction measurement, and response rate; AMBHA domains for patient satisfaction measurement include the following:

Access: satisfaction with time interval to first appointment

Intake: satisfaction with intake clinician

Clinical care: satisfaction with therapist

Outcome: consumer-based assessment of outcome

Global satisfaction: overall satisfaction with MBHO

American Managed Behavioral Healthcare Association (AMBHA); Industry standards:

Response rate: >25%

Satisfaction level: >80% to 90% overall satisfaction

Box 2-1

NATIONAL ALLIANCE FOR THE MENTALLY ILL'S PRINCIPLES FOR MANAGED CARE

1. State government must continue to be accountable for the delivery of treatment and services for persons with severe and persistent brain disorders (mental illnesses).
2. State government cannot relinquish this responsibility, even when contracting out the services.
3. The priority population for treatment and services shall be persons with severe and persistent brain disorders. In adults, these include schizophrenia, bipolar disorder, major depression, obsessive-compulsive disorder, panic disorder, and borderline personality disorder. In children, these disorders include autism, pervasive developmental disorders, Tourette's syndrome, and attention-deficit hyper-activity disorder (ADHD).
4. There must be continued eligibility for persons who are employed but cannot obtain health coverage through their employers.
5. State government must develop and maintain a comprehensive community support system of treatment and services for those disabled by a severe brain disorder. Services must, at a minimum, be those required in a state mental health plan by Public Law 99–660.
6. There must be meaningful participation of consumers and families at every stage of the redesign, implementation, evaluation, and monitoring of the managed care system.
7. All planning and delivery of services must be culturally sensitive to ethnically diverse populations and the communities in which they are located.
8. States that contract with for-profit MCOs or other entities for the management and/or delivery solely of Medicaid-funded services for the severely and persistently mentally ill must exercise great caution lest they inadvertently divide the mental health system and cause dumping of chronic heavy users of costly services back onto a public system that is likely underfunded.
9. Public resources saved by reduced utilization of state hospitals must be committed to those who used these facilities or who would have met the threshold for admission. Funds generated through other system efficiencies should also be reallocated to expand services to the priority population.
10. Provider personnel, both administrators and treatment staff, must have an understanding of serious and persistent brain disorders; have training to work with the priority population (including training in the family and consumer perspective), and must accept accountability for the quality of services.
11. All provider staff must be rigorously and appropriately credentialed by the state mental health authority.
12. For individuals who meet the priority definition and either have a Global Assessment Functioning (GAF) scale score of 50 or below or who are at risk of declining to this level, a comprehensive array of community support services must be available. This must include new-generation medications, inpatient treatment, intensive case management, psychosocial rehabilitation, and consumer-run services. Outpatient services must be mobile.
13. MCOs must be accountable for linkages to housing with supportive services and to employment services.
14. There must be consumer and family involvement in individual treatment planning, including choice of provider, treatment delivery, and appropriate access to peer support groups.
15. Appeal and grievance procedures must be in place that are user friendly and time sensitive to the life-threatening nature of psychotic episodes.
16. The state must report quarterly to the public on the number of recipients who fail to present for services, are in jail or prison, have been placed in a state hospital, or have died.

continued

box 2-1

NATIONAL ALLIANCE FOR THE MENTALLY ILL'S PRINCIPLES FOR MANAGED CARE—cont'd

17. Outcome measurement for persons with severe and persistent brain disorders must be included in the contracts with MCOs and be required by the states or counties in the public sector. Outcomes should include clinically relevant, person-centered, and scientifically sound measures of clinical status, general health status, functioning, quality of life (such as housing status, employment status, education, treatment status, substance abuse, involvement with the criminal justice system, and involvement with meaningful activities), and measures reflecting consumers' and family members' satisfaction or dissatisfaction.

From NAMI, 1998.

Pete Domenici (R-NM) and Paul Wellstone (D-MN), gained wide bipartisan support because it tackled the issue of brain disorders. The MHPA is limited in scope because it only requires that coverage dollar limits for mental health be at parity with medical benefits. Highlights of the bill include the following (Public Law 104–204, 1996):

- It does not require employers who currently do not offer coverage to offer mental health benefits.
- The MHPA applies to both self-insured Employee Retirement Income Security Act of 1974 (ERISA) plans, insured health plans, coverage of federal employees under the Federal Employee Health Benefits Act (FEHBA), and collective bargaining plans. The MHPA does not apply to individual health insurance policies, Medicare, Medicare Select, Medicare Cost, or Medicare Risk contracts. Finally, it does not apply to Medicaid or privatized versions of Medicaid.
- Small employers (50 employees or less) are exempt from its provisions, and the law exempts benefit plans if the cost increase as a result of parity exceeds 1% of total medical costs.
- If a lifetime limit is not imposed for medical benefits, a lifetime limit can not be imposed for mental health benefits. Wording is similar for annual limits. If lifetime and annual limits are imposed, they shall be the same for medical and mental health coverage.

- The bill covers the period from January 1, 1998 through September 30, 2001.
- The provisions shall not apply if the cost of providing the mental health benefit at parity with the medical benefit results in a cost increase of over 1% of total costs. Exemptions are allowed on a prospective forecasting basis. The proposal must be certified, however, by a member of the American Academy of Actuaries using generally accepted actuarial practices.
- The provisions of the MHPA are related to mental health services, excluding coverage for substance abuse or chemical dependency.
- The principal beneficiaries of the legislation will be those severely and persistently mentally ill who typically exceed annual and lifetime maximum benefits.

As of May 1998, 16 states had enacted laws related to parity of mental health benefits. State laws differ from each other in conditions served, specificity of parity, minimum benefits, approved providers, managed care usage, exemptions, and populations covered (Sing et al., 1998).

The MPHA received support from consumers, provider organizations, and professional associations. These groups hoped that employers would take the opportunity to review their total benefits coverage plan to ensure adequate resources for mental health issues. Amendments to the MHPA have already surfaced and will target the exemptions clause (of greater than 1% premium increase). Currently the law stipulates that a prospective accounting is allowed; amendments to the law would stipulate that only retrospective accounting would be allowed for an exemption. Consumer groups favor the retrospective accounting because it would be based on actual expenditures and not projected expenses. A national coalition was developed expressly to work through MHPA issues. The Coalition for Fairness in Mental Illness Coverage is composed of the following organizations: AMBHA, American Medical Association (AMA), American Psychiatric Association (APA), American Psychological Association (APA), Federation of American Health Systems (FAHS), NAMI, National Association of Psychiatric Health Systems (NAPHS), and the National Mental Health Association (NMHA).

The National Advisory Mental Health Council (NAMHC) has chartered a work group that is developing "a new comparative empirical database that can inform economic assumptions and models for estimating national effects of parity and managed care on the costs of mental health services" (NAMHC, 1998). Findings so far suggest that experience with parity implementation and the application of managed care techniques have lowered costs and premiums. Thus the findings refute the idea that parity would result in higher overall costs for medical coverage. Previous econometrics relied on fee-for-service estimates, which have since been replaced by managed care. State systems that have implemented parity legislation propose that a national plan would force the adoption of managed behavioral healthcare techniques by plans that do not currently embrace these concepts. The focus on parity will impel MBHOs and others to focus on access to services and the quality and outcomes of services rendered.

Research on the effect of parity on overall costs has shown that utilization actually is lower in the parity model. A study performed by United Behavioral Health (an MBHO), the University of California—Los Angeles (UCLA), and RAND (a research and development company) was conducted using data from 1988 to 1996. Before the carve-out model, costs had increased 30% (Goldman, McCulloch, & Sturm, 1998). The overall decrease in costs had much to do with the application of managed care principles and techniques and the resultant decrease in outpatient visits, the reduced use of restrictive inpatient services (but when used, shorter hospital stays), and reduced costs per units of service overall. Costs decreased by 40% after implementing a managed care model and continued decreasing over the years of the study. Previous fears about the potential increase of costs with implementing parity, based on old statistics from a fee-for-service era, were not confirmed.

A later report published by SAMHSA addressed the issue of costs and effects of parity mandates (Sing et al., 1998). The study summarized the laws of current state parity programs, conducted case study analysis of five states, analyzed actuarial estimates of the cost of parity, and provided updated estimates of premium increases as a result of full or partial parity implementation. Key findings of the study included the following:

- Most state parity laws are limited in scope and application.
- State parity laws have had a small effect on premiums.
- Employers have not attempted to avoid parity laws by becoming self-insured, and they do not tend to pass on the costs of parity to employees.
- Costs have not shifted from the public to the private sector.
- Previous actuarial predictions of premium increases resulting from MHSA parity ranged from 3.2% to 11.4%, primarily because of differences in their assumptions.
- Based on an updated actuarial model, full parity for mental health and substance abuse services is estimated to increase premiums by 3.6% on average.
- Premium increases vary by type of plan.

- Projected premium increases do not reflect potential market responses.
- Premium increases are greater for plans that are limited to children.

In a 1997 letter written to the Subcommittee on Consumer Rights, Protections, and Responsibilities of the Advisory Commission on Consumer Protection and Quality in the Health Care Industry, Jay Cutler, J.D., Director of the APA's Division of Government Relations, suggested that full parity coverage for mental illness would result in only modest increases in health plan deductibles and premiums. Cutler noted that the nonpartisan Congressional Budget Office estimated that full parity coverage would increase premiums by only 4%. In addition, a study by the actuarial firm Milliman and Robertson estimated the cost of full parity as an additional 3.9% per member per month. Finally, the National Institutes of Health concluded that the nondiscriminatory coverage of mental disorders is affordable. With parity, increased expenditures are certain to result in medical-cost offsets in areas such as employee productivity. The National Advisory Mental Health Council estimated in 1993 that parity coverage would save businesses as much as $2.2 billion a year (*Psychiatric News*, 1997). Other consumer-driven initiatives developed in the late 1990s are described next.

Consumer Bills of Rights

Quality first: better health care for all Americans. A consumer advisory commission was appointed by President Bill Clinton in March of 1997 with the express goal to "advise the President on changes occurring in the health care system and recommend measures as may be necessary to promote and assure health care quality and value, and protect consumers and workers in the health care system" (USDHHS, 1997). The Advisory Commission on Consumer Protection and Quality in the Health Care Industry, cochaired by the U.S. Secretary of the Department of Labor and the U.S. Secretary of the USDHHS, produced an Interim Report to the President on November 20, 1997, entitled "A Consumer Bill of Rights and Responsibilities." Eight areas of consumer rights and responsibilities were identified:

1. Information disclosure
2. Choice of providers and plans
3. Access to emergency services
4. Participation in treatment decisions
5. Respect and nondiscrimination
6. Confidentiality of health information
7. Complaints and appeals
8. Consumer responsibilities

The work of the commission and implementation of its recommendations will continue into the twenty first century.

Mental health Bill of Rights. In February of 1997, a mental health Bill of Rights (Box 2-2) was disseminated by leaders of nine professional organizations representing over 600,000 health and mental health professionals (APA, 1997). The Bill of Rights was the result of the first large scale national effort to reach a consensus on a set of principles declaring an American's right to safe, quality mental health care. The Bill of Rights was commended by the National Mental Health Consortium.

Previously, in January of 1997, AMBHA drafted a similar Bill of Rights for Consumers Accessing Behavioral Health Services" (AMBHA, 1998). AMBHA's Bill of Rights addressed the following:

- Parity
- Choice
- Confidentiality
- Determination of treatment
- Right to know
- Benefit usage
- Compliance with state statutes
- Disclosure
- Discrimination
- Appeals
- Accountability
- Continuity of care
- Timelines for authorization for reimbursement of care

2-2

PRINCIPLES FOR THE PROVISION OF MENTAL HEALTH AND SUBSTANCE ABUSE SERVICES: A BILL OF RIGHTS

Our commitment is to provide quality mental health and substance abuse services to all individuals without regard to race, color, religion, national origin, gender, age, sexual orientation, or disabilities.

RIGHT TO KNOW

Benefits. Individuals have the right to be provided information from the purchasing entity (such as employer, union, or public purchaser) and the insurance or third party payer describing the nature and extent of their mental health and substance abuse treatment benefits. This information should include details on procedures to obtain access to services, on utilization management procedures, and on appeal rights. The information should be presented clearly in writing with language that the individual can understand.

Professional expertise. Individuals have the right to receive full information from the potential treating professional about that professional's knowledge, skills, preparation, experience, and credentials. Individuals have the right to be informed about the options available for treatment interventions and the effectiveness of the recommended treatment.

Contractual limitations. Individuals have the right to be informed by the treating professional of any arrangements, restrictions, and/or covenants established between the third party payer and the treating professional that could interfere with or influence treatment recommendations. Individuals have the right to be informed of the nature of information that may be disclosed for the purposes of paying benefits.

Appeals and grievances. Individuals have the right to receive information about the methods they can use to submit complaints or grievances regarding provision of care by the treating professional to that profession's regulatory board and to the professional association. Individuals have the right to be provided information about the procedures they can use to appeal benefit utilization decisions to the third party payer systems, to the employer or purchasing entity, and to external regulatory entities.

Confidentiality. Individuals have the right to be guaranteed the protection of the confidentiality of their relationship with their mental health and substance abuse professional, except when laws or ethics dictate otherwise. Any disclosure to another party will be time limited and made with the full written, informed consent of the individuals. Individuals shall not be required to disclose confidential, privileged, or other information other than diagnosis, prognosis, type of treatment, time and length of treatment, and cost. Entities receiving information for the purposes of benefits determination, public agencies receiving information for health care planning, or any other organization with legitimate right to information will maintain clinical information in confidence with the same rigor and be subject to the same penalties for violation as is the direct provider of care. Information technology will be used for transmission, storage, or data management *only* with methodologies that remove individual identifying information and ensure the protection of the individual's privacy. Information should not be transferred, sold, or otherwise utilized.

Choice. Individuals have the right to choose any duly licensed or certified professional for mental health and substance abuse services. Individuals have the right to receive full information regarding the education and training of professionals, treatment options (including risks and benefits), and cost implications to make an informed choice regarding the selection of care deemed appropriate by the individual and the professional.

continued

box 2-2

PRINCIPLES FOR THE PROVISION OF MENTAL HEALTH AND SUBSTANCE ABUSE SERVICES: A BILL OF RIGHTS—cont'd

Determination of treatment. Recommendations regarding mental health and substance abuse treatment shall be made only by a duly licensed or certified professional in conjunction with the individual and his or her family as appropriate. Treatment decisions should not be made by third party payers. The individual has the right to make final decisions regarding treatment.

Parity. Individuals have the right to receive benefits for mental health and substance abuse treatment on the same basis as they do for any other illnesses, with the same provisions, co-payments, lifetime benefits, and catastrophic coverage in both insurance and self-funded or self-insured health plans.

Nondiscrimination. Individuals who use mental health and substance abuse benefits shall not be penalized when seeking other health insurance or disability, life, or any other insurance benefit.

Benefit usage. The individual is entitled to the entire scope or the benefits within the benefit plan that will address his or her clinical needs.

Benefit design. Whenever both federal and state law and/or regulations are applicable, the professional and all payers shall use whichever affords the individual the greatest level of protection and access.

Treatment review. To ensure that treatment review processes are fair and valid, individuals have the right to be guaranteed that any review of their mental health and substance abuse treatment shall involve a professional having the training, credentials, and licensure required to provide the treatment in the jurisdiction in which it will be provided. The reviewer should have no financial interest in the decision and is subject to the section on confidentiality.

Accountability. Treating professionals may be held accountable and liable to individuals for any injury caused by gross incompetence or negligence on the part of the professional. The treating professional has the obligation to advocate for and document necessity of care and to advise the individual of options if payment authorization is denied. Payers and other third parties may be held accountable and liable to individuals for any injury caused by gross incompetence or negligence or by their clinically unjustified decisions.

Participating groups:
American Association for Marriage and Family Therapy
American Counseling Association
American Family Therapy Academy
American Nurses Association
American Psychiatric Association
American Psychiatric Nurses Association
American Psychological Association
Clinical Social Work Federation
National Association of Social Workers

- Enrollee right to appeal denials
- Nonformulary alternatives
- Consumer access to ombudsman programs
- Mandatory choice of health plans
- Public disclosure of medical loss-ratio
- Liability of health plan management agents

- Mandatory point-of-service
- Provider privileges

The groups differed on some issues, primarily as a result of their disagreements related to managed care. Table 2-6 highlights the divergent points of each Bill of Rights.

table 2-6

BILL OF RIGHTS COMPARISONS

AMBHA BILL OF RIGHTS FOR CONSUMERS ACCESSING BEHAVIORAL HEALTH SERVICES (TRADE ORGANIZATION)	PRINCIPLES FOR THE PROVISION OF MENTAL HEALTH AND SUBSTANCE ABUSE TREATMENT SERVICES—A BILL OF RIGHTS (PROFESSIONAL ASSOCIATIONS)
CHOICE	
Consumers shall have access to services and a choice of providers within a full continuum of network-based services, including recovery and peer support programs.	Individuals have the right to choose any duly licensed or certified professional for mental health and substance abuse services.
CONFIDENTIALITY	
The exchange of information between treating professionals and managed-care organizations for third-party clinical review for clinical effectiveness, authorization of payment, and care coordination for the purpose of improving the quality and efficiency of health care delivery shall be held in the strictest confidence.	Individuals shall not be required to disclose confidential, privileged, or other information other than diagnosis, prognosis, type of treatment, time and length of treatment, and cost.
DETERMINATION OF TREATMENT	
Decisions regarding behavioral health treatment shall be made by the duly certified and/or licensed behavioral health professionals in conjunction with the patient or his or her family as appropriate. Organizations providing care review or care authorization function as clinical consultants to the professional-patient relationship, and they authorize payment according to established criteria available to providers and consumers	Recommendations regarding mental health and substance abuse treatment shall be made only by a duly licensed professional in conjunction with the individual and his or her family as appropriate. Treatment decisions should not be made by third-party payers. The individual has the right to make final decisions regarding treatment.

Adapted from Kertesz, 1997.

INSIDE THE MBHO: ANATOMY OF A CASE

MBHOs are usually organized under two major organizational structures—clinical operations and service operations. Functions that might fall under clinical operations include clinical affairs, utilization management, and care management. Functions encompassed by service operations include customer service and claims (processing and adjudication). Other functions that support clinical and service operations include quality management and improvement, provider relations and network management (including credentialing, recredentialing, and quality of care monitoring), management information services, sales and marketing, and human resources. To describe core components of these functions, workflows are presented that show the process of care from the initial call to claims payment. This case assumes that the beneficiary is managed under a carve-out arrangement previously described (Fig. 2-4).

Assessment, Triage, and Referral

Initially, if a patient wishes to access services, he or she calls the toll-free number. Employees at the MBHO staff the toll-free help line available 24 hours a day, 7 days a week, 365 days a year. Either an automated interactive voice response (IVR), or auto-attendant (AA), or a "live" person answers the phone inquiry. The decision to have either an AA or a live person is made by the purchaser. Some employers want their employees to speak to a live person first; others do not find this as important and choose the AA option. The AA guides the consumer through a list of options. The first option is to be connected with a clinician if the call is an emergency. In the case of an emergency, the person is connected with a clinician who has a master's degree (e.g., LCSW, APRN). The clinician is part of an assessment, triage, and referral unit of clinical operations. The clinician asks relevant questions of the caller to ascertain

the presenting problem and the urgency of the situation.

In a customer-focused MBHO, the caller is encouraged to define the urgency of the situation. If the caller states that his or her situation is emergent, meaning that significant harm could come to the patient if he or she is not seen within 30 minutes, the company follows its usual emergent care protocols. The clinician follows internal policies related to the determination of medical or clinical necessity that includes the application of intensity of service and severity of illness criteria. In the case of an emergency, the clinician will assist the consumer to reach an emergency room, often with the assistance of 911, the police, or a psychiatric emergency response team.

Once the consumer is safe and has been evaluated, the care management staff follows the case to ensure a smooth transition from a high-intensity setting to a less restrictive level of care or treatment. The clinician follows up with the evaluating practitioner or facility to ensure arrangements for an appropriate disposition. If the case is urgent (patient should be seen within 48 hours) or routine (patient should be seen within 5 business days), the clinician reviews the unique needs of the caller and matches these needs to a practitioner close to the patient's home or workplace. The clinician follows up with the patient to ensure that the consumer has been connected successfully with the practitioner.

An initial certification of approved visits or days is made by the clinician. For benefits to be certified, medical necessity criteria are applied to the clinical information supplied by the practitioner or facility to decide if the information meets the criteria. The review process relates to the individualized treatment plan proposed by the treating practitioner. It does not always mean that the claims will be paid for the services rendered. Noncertification is the process whereby a psychiatrist or clinical psychologist is unable to render a certification based

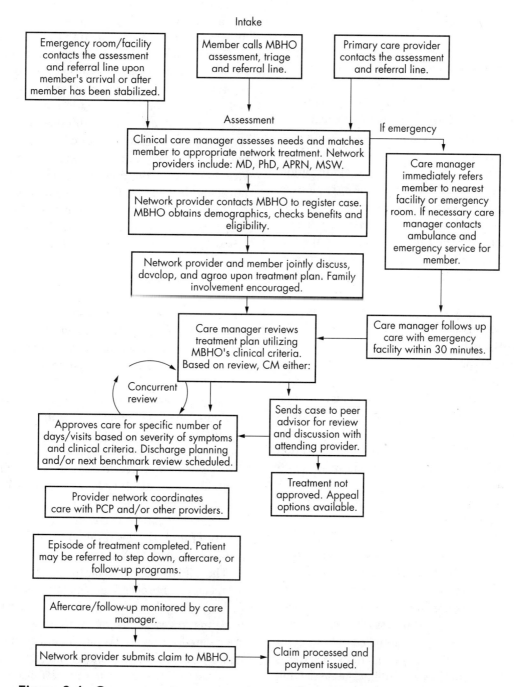

Figure 2-4 Care management process-integrated model.

upon medical necessity. The requested care is not approved, and a letter with this information is sent to the practitioner who originally requested certification for services. This does not refer to all benefits being denied; it refers to the particular level of care and treatment approach proposed by the practitioner on behalf of his or her patient.

Care Management

Once the referral has been made, the MBHO awaits further clinical information on details of treatment progress. The practitioner calls or sends paperwork to register the case, and further concurrent review is performed at preestablished time intervals with the care manager. MBHOs are currently upgrading their information systems to keep up with the wave of new communication technologies. The 1980s were a time of exploiting telephone communication such as facsimile machines instead of mail correspondence, whereas the 1990s have been a time to maximize the use of interactive voice response systems and Internet technologies to help manage complex clinical information and care management functions.

Denials and appeals.   There are situations where a care manager is unable to make a certification decision based on the information provided by the practitioner or facility. The care manager will forward these cases to a peer advisor (PA), who is either a board-certified psychiatrist or a clinical psychologist, for review. The PA reviews the case and consults with the attending practitioner or treatment facility. More information is gathered about the case through an in-depth inquiry about the clinical situation, and the PA provides technical and clinical assistance to the practitioner in formulating a treatment plan.

If the PA determines that the clinical situation does not meet medical necessity criteria, care is not certified at the level of treatment requested and the PA proposes alternatives. Denials occur for the plan of treatment or level of care proposed by the practitioner, not necessarily for the care itself. It is the treating practitioner's right to agree or disagree with the recommendations. A letter is sent to the practitioner describing the denial and reasons for the denial. The practitioner is alerted at the time of the denial that he or she has the right to appeal the decision. Explicit instructions on how to appeal are given. The appeals information is received by the MBHO, and the information is then reviewed by the appeals committee accountable for rendering a decision. The results of this review are communicated to the practitioner.

Customer service and claims. Customer service representatives answer calls related to general information, benefits, eligibility, and claims issues (see Fig. 2-5 for an illustration of processes). These representatives have a thorough orientation regarding the company, its functions, and the systems used to carry out daily tasks. Customer service lines are monitored for quality assurance purposes; in general, the call is monitored with hardware that allows a supervisor or auditor to listen in on the call as it occurs. Employees are oriented to the telephone monitoring procedures and receive feedback on aggregate scores of the department's compliance with preestablished criteria. If a customer service representative cannot resolve an issue, an inquiry can be entered into an inquiry system and routed to the appropriate department for resolution (e.g., claims, provider relations, care management, eligibility, and clinical affairs).

An important function in customer service is verifying benefits eligibility. This involves checking the information system to determine if the caller was covered by the employer during the time that services were rendered. Employers provide eligibility tapes to MBHOs on a regular basis to update information on covered employees and dependents. If a patient is covered, and medical necessity criteria review resulted in a certification decision, then the claim is usually paid.

The MBHO claims department is responsible for receipt and processing of claims. Issues identified by either the member or practitioner related to claims are researched by the claims staff. Claims are entered into a claims-paying information system. Data are brought forward from other information system modules, such as certification data from the care management system. Claims audits are performed on a percentage of the total number of claims processed for a specified time (e.g., 10% for the previous month). Inquiries related to claims processing issues are referred to customer service representatives for resolution.

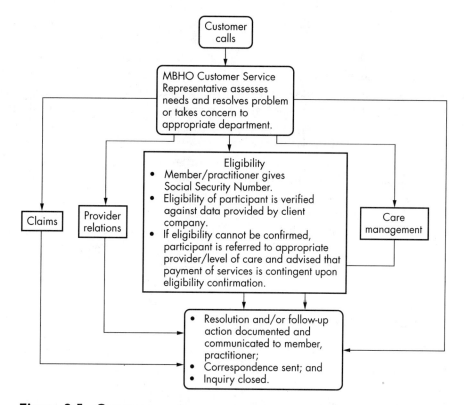

Figure 2-5 Customer service management.

Provider credentialing. The provider relations department is responsible for network management, which includes the credentialing and recredentialing of practitioners and providers, provider training, site reviews, treatment record reviews, and disenrollments. A practitioner is a behavioral health provider (duly credentialed by the MBHO and licensed by the state in which he or she practices) to render mental health and/or substance abuse services. A provider is an organization, facility, or agency (duly credentialed by the MBHO and licensed by the state in which services are rendered) that provides mental health and substance abuse services (NCQA, 1998).

The MBHO ensures that practitioners and providers are of sufficient number and type to treat the issues related to a particular geographic area or member population. Provider relations staff perform primary source verification (PSV) on various components of the application submitted by practitioners. PSV is the credentialing function whereby an MBHO verifies a license, degree, certification, training, and professional experience with the original credentialing body or organization (e.g., getting confirmation from the school of nursing that an advanced degree was conferred for an APRN). Provider relations staff also review inquiries that have been attributed to a particular practitioner in the recredentialing process. Various categories of information are evaluated, including consumer complaints or compliments, consumer satisfaction, utilization information, grievance and appeals rates, and other quality indicators. Credentialing standards for APRNs include, but may not be limited to, the following:

1. Possession of a master's degree or higher in psychiatric nursing from an accredited college or university
2. Possession of a current and valid license as a registered nurse and state clinical specialist

or advanced practice nurse certification (as applicable)

3. Certification as a Certified Specialist (CS) by the American Nurses Credentialing Center

4. Minimum of 5 years full-time post-master's experience in the direct provision of mental health or substance abuse care, 2 years of which were under the supervision of an APRN or MD/DO

5. Possession of professional liability insurance coverage of at least $1 million/$1 million

6. Work requirement of a minimum of 20 hours per week in the direct provision of behavioral health care

ROLE OF NURSES IN MANAGED BEHAVIORAL ■ HEALTHCARE

Psychiatric-mental health nurses at both the basic and advanced practice levels are uniquely qualified to serve in both indirect and direct care roles within managed care systems. Nurses at the basic level of preparation interact with managed care companies indirectly, but their documentation of care is critical. Utilization review nurses at facilities use nurses' notes to describe progress or lack of progress with the patient's care. Nurses at the advanced level speak to managed care companies directly in providing clinical information. Nurses alone among the various mental health disciplines combine biopsychosocial knowledge, psychopharmacologic competency, physical and psychiatric assessment skills with an intrinsic perspective of patient advocacy, and 24-hour accountability. Psychiatric nurses are experts at evaluating complex psychiatric, substance abuse, and physical health needs and problems of patients over the life span. Their systems knowledge and expertise also allow them to manage and monitor complex service delivery issues. Nurses assess and treat psychosocial consequences of physical illness (APNA, 1997). Further, the American Nurses Association (ANA) "endorses the utilization of psychiatric-mental health nurses as highly qualified professional participants in both indirect and direct care roles within psychiatric-mental health managed care systems. As the managed care industry evolves, we believe that it will be important for the professional to monitor the operationalization of the managed care concept to assure that its original objectives are fulfilled" (ANA, 1998).

Although there is great variability of nursing activity based on service setting and geographic location, the advanced practice nurse and basic practice nurse can assume a number of roles in managed care systems. As adapted from Stuart (1998), roles can include the following:

- *Psychiatric-mental health clinician.* Nurses with various levels of preparation serve as direct care providers in contracted facilities and practices. These include staff nurses; managers and administrators; practitioners in psychiatric home health and community mental health settings; primary care providers; and independent providers of psychotherapy to individuals, groups, and families across the life span. Advanced practice nurses have prescriptive authority in 48 states, and all registered nurses administer, provide teaching, and monitor pharmacologic agents and their effects.

- *Clinical care manager.* Nurses in this role assess the intensity of symptoms and severity of illness. Depending on the presenting problems and needs (emergent, urgent, or routine), treatment plans are developed and referrals are coordinated to facilitate access to the appropriate level of treatment. The care manager manages continuum of care resources over the episode of care and is skilled in managing psychiatric rehabilitation as well as relapse prevention.

- *Assessment, evaluation, triage, and referral nurse.* In this role, the nurse evaluates patients in direct encounters or by telephone to triage the patient to the most appropriate level of care, including referrals to credentialed providers, contracted facilities, and community resources.

- *Utilization review nurse.* Many managed care companies employ psychiatric nurses to function as utilization reviewers. They review different aspects of the individual's treatment plan and make decisions about treatment certification. In this role, the nurse focuses on the current episode of care, serves as "gatekeeper" to behavioral health services, and manages the mental health benefit.
- *Patient educator.* Some settings hire nurses who are responsible for patient and family education. This role encompasses an increasing emphasis on patient compliance, self-management of symptoms, and disease management programs. In public sector programs, this role can include prevention, education, and outreach.
- *Risk manager.* Nurses who work as risk managers are charged with the task of decreasing the probability of adverse outcomes related to patient care. They engage in identifying risk factors, individual and system-wide problems, corrective actions, and the implementation of strategies to reduce risk and prevent loss to the MBHO and its customers.
- *Chief quality officer.* These nurses assume primary responsibility for formulating and implementing comprehensive quality management and improvement programs for managed care companies. They train MBHO staff, synthesize data related to performance improvement and outcomes management, and facilitate other health services research activities.
- *Marketing and development specialist.* Some psychiatric nurses work in the managed care growth areas of sales (proposal writing), marketing, and program development. In these roles, they interface with consumers, employers, providers, and regulators, and they make recommendations for furthering the mission and goals of the MCO.
- *Corporate managers and executives.* Psychiatric nurses are also present in middle management and senior management positions where they participate in the development of corporate policy and strategic planning. Nurses hold positions in various departments including Provider Relations, Quality Management, Care Management and Clinical Operations, Service Operations, and Clinical Affairs.

CURRENT RESEARCH IN MANAGED BEHAVIORAL ■ HEALTHCARE

There is a great need for nursing research in the area of psychiatric and substance abuse care in a managed care setting. Population-based studies will continue to be needed for planning and program development, as will research to support evidence-based care. For example, the National Institute of Mental Health has funded several health service research sites to study managed care. UCLA and RAND published findings related to outcomes for adult outpatients treated for depression in 1993. They concluded from an observational study of 617 depressed outpatients that outcomes did not differ for patients under fee-for-service or prepaid plans such as indemnity plans and HMOs (Rogers et al, 1993).

The American Association of Health Plans (AAHP) maintains an inventory of studies that have been completed or are in progress. Through consumer-driven fact sheets, they describe health service research results related to care delivered in managed care delivery settings. The following examples are of such research related to behavioral health, which have been taken from the AAHP website (AAHP, 1998):

- Development of a specialized human immunodeficiency virus (HIV) resource team at Harvard Vanguard Associates in Boston to identify and care for patients with HIV or acquired immunodeficiency syndrome (AIDS) through home interventions, education, and prevention programs for caregivers.
- Development of episode of care (EOC) disease management programs at Lovelace Health System for chronic illnesses including depression.

Disease-specific teams are made up of specialists, nurse care managers, education specialists, pharmacists, and quality measurement specialists to provide multidisciplinary care.

- Evidence from the Group Health Cooperative (GHC) of Puget Sound that self-management training and support services resulted in the improvement and attainment of positive clinical outcomes in patients with chronic illness (GHC, 1998). Other research currently in progress at GHC includes the following:
  - A randomized trial examining whether a systemic care monitoring and feedback system will affect the outcomes and treatment costs of primary care patients treated with antidepressant medication. This population-based quality improvement program will include a registry of patients treated for depression, routine monitoring of patient outcomes, and support of the primary care practice by a dedicated "population manager." The computerized registry will include real-time information on medication use and follow up visits (Simon, G; Von Korff, M).
  - An observational study exploring the management of patients treated for bipolar disorder and the relationship to expert recommendations regarding medication dosing, laboratory monitoring, and frequency of follow-up visits (Simon, G).
  - A randomized trial examining whether a coordinated program of depression treatment will improve quality of life and reduce overall health care costs among HMO members who are frequent users of outpatient medical services and are depressed. This collaborative project will enroll members from GHC, Harvard Vanguard Associates in Boston, and DeanCare HMO in Wisconsin (Simon, G).
- Development by the Kaiser Permanente Medical Center at Santa Teresa of reconditioning, behavioral, and relaxation therapies in the management of chronic pain through their "Skills Not Pills" program. Data show that medical utilization fell by 57% among the program's graduates based upon 1-year follow-up and that utilization of pain-related visits declined by 84%.
- Development by Health Partners in Minnesota of flexible benefit packages to allow for increased coordination of services, access to an expanded care management process, and linkages to community support agencies for chronically ill children.

Future research will include the collaboration of academic medical centers, universities, and private enterprise in the forming of research consortia to support health service research on behavioral managed health care. APRNs are extremely well positioned to participate in such research activity. Future research by APRNs and other health care professionals should address the following areas:

- Effects of the intensity of care management on reduced recidivism and readmissions to the same level or higher levels of care
- Identification of vulnerable subpopulations within a geographic area and testing of prevention strategies for depression or other high-volume or high-risk disorders
- Effects of interventions in the home on family preservation
- Case finding and prevention programs designed to address HIV- or AIDS-associated depression and cognitive deficits
- Benefits of the utilization of APRNs in prepaid and fee-for-service arrangements and impact on functional and clinical outcomes

More ideas about potential opportunities for behavioral health research can be found in Chapter 24.

IMPLICATIONS FOR ■ THE FUTURE

As managed care continues to be a driving force in the financing of behavioral healthcare, nurses must educate new professionals about its theories, practices, and principles. For example, the American Nurses Foundation and ANA developed a "Managed Care Curriculum for Baccalaureate Nursing Programs" in 1995. The curriculum is designed to teach the baccalaureate nurse to assume a leadership role in existing or emerging managed care delivery systems (Hart, 1995). Meeting the revolving expectations of a reformed health care system requires professional expertise, particularly specialized knowledge, and skills. According to Yurick and Kobert (1997), graduate programs in nursing will need to focus on effectively preparing practitioners for the care management of complex medical and psychiatric problems of consumers. To accomplish this, training is needed that extends beyond direct, clinical practice and addresses role definition, reimbursement, prescriptive authority, credentialing and admitting privileges, practice environment, and professional networking. Chapters 20 and 21 discuss these issues in greater detail.

Graduate and continuing education needs to be flexible in a way that continued self-directed learning continues throughout the APRN career. Changes in the way behavioral health care is financed and organized, as well as the influence of external accrediting and advocacy organizations, provides many opportunities for advanced training and education. These include the following:

- Health care financing and financial management principles
- Managed care principles and delivery systems
- Role of primary care linkages, coordination of care, and continuity of care in managed behavioral healthcare
- Utilization management principles such as development of clinical criteria for APRN management of behavioral health disorders
- National standards of practice related to behavioral health management, such as credentialing, treatment record documentation, accessibility and availability, and effective clinical care
- Design and methods for evaluation research; outcomes evaluation methodologies for patient-

centered care and population-based primary care (Grimes & Garcia, 1997)
- Behavioral psychopharmacotherapy that takes into consideration pharmacodynamics, pharmacokinetics, and pharmacotherapeutics (Schwertz et al, 1997)
- Public policy that will promote the role of advanced practice nursing in health care reform efforts, ultimately improving patient well-being (Beyers et al, 1997)
- Database management to enable informed contributions to the design, development, and evaluation of information systems
- Clinical practica that reflect the current state of managed care and effects on practice
- Ongoing exploration of the various opportunities in advanced practice nursing enabling the mapping of a career pathway (Price, 1998)

Economic, societal, and political forces will continue to affect the American health care delivery system. Specifically, the processes associated with managed behavioral healthcare will not be exempt from change. There will be continued focus on the provision of quality care to individuals and populations. Prevention, health promotion, and disease management will be components of care, and MBHOs will seek to provide these at a reasonable cost. Therefore it is in the interest of APRNs in psychiatric and mental health care to understand the emerging approaches to managing behavioral healthcare so they can contribute not only to the structuring of delivery models, but also provide guidance in the development of care management systems.

RESOURCES AND CONNECTIONS

PROFESSIONAL AND TRADE ORGANIZATIONS

American Association of Health Plans www.aahp.org
American Association of Managed Care Nurses www.aamcn.org
American Health Information Management Association www.ahima.org
American Managed Behavioral Healthcare Association www.ambha.org

American Nurses Association
  www.nursingworld.org
American Psychiatric Nurses Association
  www.apna.org
Institute for Behavioral Healthcare
  www.ibh.com
National Association of Psychiatric Health Systems
  www.naphs.org

ACCREDITATION
Joint Commission on Accreditation of Healthcare Organizations www.jcaho.org
National Committee for Quality Assurance
  www.ncqa.org
Psychotherapy Finances and Managed Care Strategies
  www.psyfin.com
Substance Abuse and Mental Health Services Administration www.samhsa.gov

RESEARCH
Agency for Health Care Policy and Research
  www.ahcpr.gov
Association for Health Services Research
  www.ahsr.org
Foundation for Accountability www.facct.org
Kaiser Family Foundation www.kff.org
National Center for Health Statistics
  www.cdc.gov/nchswww/nchshome.html
Robert Wood Johnson Foundation
  www.rwjf.org

WORKPLACE SERVICES
Employee Assistance Professionals Association
  eap-association.com
Employers Resource Association hrexperts.com
Dependent Care Connection www.dcclifecare.com

References

American Accreditation Healthcare Commission. (1997). *National utilization management standards.* Washington, DC: Author.

American Association of Health Plans. (1998). *Fact sheets.* www.aahp.org.

American Managed Behavioral Healthcare Association. (1997). *AMBHA media kit: questions and answers.* www.ambha.org.

American Managed Behavioral Healthcare Association. (1998). Press release: *AMBHA proposes expanded consumer rights, suggests clinically appropriate access to clinical records.*

American Nurses Association. (1998). ANA board adopts nursing's principles for managed care environment. *The American Nurse, 30*(1), 19.

American Nurses Association. (1993). *Position statement: psychiatric mental health nursing and managed care.* www.nursingworld.org/readroom/position/practice/prpsymen.htm.

American Psychiatric Nurses Association. (1997). [Brochure] *Advanced practice registered nurses in psychiatric and mental health care.* Washington, DC: Author.

Beyers, M., et al. (1997). Policy: advanced practice nursing issues and challenges—specialty association viewpoints. *Advanced Practice Nursing Quarterly, 3*(3), 31–35.

Brook, R.H. (1997). Managed care is not the problem, quality is. *Journal of the American Medical Association, 278*(19), 1612–1614.

Budson, R.D. (1994). Community residential and partial hospital care: low-cost alternative systems in the spectrum of care. *Psychiatric Quarterly, 65*(3), 209–220.

Carling, P.J. (1990). Major mental illness, housing, and supports: the promise of community integration. *American Psychologist, 45*(8), 969–975.

Carter Center. (1997). *Managing care in the public interest: The Eleventh Annual Rosalynn Carter Symposium on Mental Health Policy.* Atlanta: The Mental Health Program of the Carter Center.

Center for Mental Health Services, Substance Abuse, and Mental Health Services Administration. (1995). *Medicaid section 1115 waivers: mental health and substance abuse-related provisions of five state demonstrations.* Washington, DC: Author.

Fenton, W.S., Mosher, L.R., Herrell, J.M., & Blyler, C.R. (1998). Randomized trial of general hospital and residential alternative care for patients with severe and persistent mental illness. *American Journal of Psychiatry, 155*(4), 516–522.

Foundation for Accountability (FACCT). (1998). www.facct.org.

Goldman, W., McCulloch, J., & Sturm, R. (1998). Costs and use of mental health services before and after managed care. *Health Affairs, 17*(2), 40–52.

Goodwin, F., & Hill, E.D. (1997). *Power for performance breakthroughs: accelerators and inhibitors of innovation in behavioral healthcare.* Institute for Behavioral Healthcare, The Ninth Annual National Dialogue Conference on Mental Health Benefits and Practice in the Era of Managed Care. Tiburon, CA: IBH.

Grimes, D.E., & Garcia, M.K. (1997). Advanced practice nursing and work site primary care: challenges for outcomes evaluation. *Advanced Practice Nursing Quarterly, 3*(2), 19–28.

Group Health Cooperative of Puget Sound. The Center for Health Studies. (1998). *1997–1998 research activities:*

research in cost-effective management of common problems in primary care. www.ghc.org/chs/resprim.html#lias.

Health Care Financing Administration. (June 30, 1996). *National summary of Medicaid managed care programs and enrollment* www.hcfa.gov.medicaid.html.

Hart, S. (1995). *ANA managed care curriculum for baccalaureate nursing programs.* Washington, DC: American Nurses Publishing.

Joint Commission on Accreditation of Healthcare Organizations. (1997). *Comprehensive accreditation manual for managed behavioral healthcare.* Oakbrook Terrace, IL. Author.

Kertesz, L. (April, 1997). Psychological break: split on 'rights' highlights fight over managed care. *Modern Healthcare, 60,* 80.

Manderscheid, R.W., & Sonnenschein, M.A. (Eds.). (1997). *Mental health United States, 1996.* Rockville, MD: SAMHSA.

Manderscheid, R.W., & Henderson, M.J. (1997). The growth and direction of managed care. In Manderscheid, R.W., & Sonnenschein, M.A. (Eds.). (1996). *Mental health United States.* Rockville, MD: SAMHSA.

Mechanic, D.S. (1997). Key policy consideration for mental health in the managed care era. In Manderscheid, R.W., & Sonnenschein, M.A. (Eds.). (1996). *Mental health United States.* Rockville, MD: SAMHSA.

Munetz, M.R., & Geller, J.L. (1993). The least restrictive alternative in the post-institutional era. *Hospital and Community Psychiatry, 44*(10), 967–973.

National Advisory Mental Health Council. (1998). *Parity in coverage of mental health services in an era of managed care: an interim report to Congress by the National Advisory Mental Health Council.* www.nami.org.

National Alliance for the Mentally Ill. (1998). NAMI's mission and goals. www.nami.org/about/thing.htm#history.

National Committee for Quality Assurance. (1998). *Managed behavioral healthcare organization surveyor guidelines.* Washington, DC: Author.

Open Minds. (1998a). Largest specialty managed behavioral health programs by 1997 enrollment. Gettysburg, PA: Author. Personal communication.

Open Minds. (1998b). Press Release: 9% increase in managed behavioral health enrollment from 1997: survey identifies largest 12 programs in nation. Gettysburg, PA: Author.

Price, J.L. (1998). A reflective approach to career trajectory in advanced practice nursing. *Advanced Practice Nursing Quarterly, 3*(4), 35–39.

Psychiatric News. (1997). Sacks makes parity case to presidential commission. www.psych.org/pnews/97–10-17/parity.html.

Psychiatric Services. (1997). 75% of insured Americans now enrolled in managed care plans, *Psychiatric Services, 48*(8), 1094–1095.

Public Law 104–204. (September 26, 1996). Departments of Veterans Affairs and Housing and Urban Development, and Independent Agencies Appropriations Act, 1997. Title VII—Parity in the Application of Certain Limits in Mental Health Benefits.

Rogers, W.H., et al. (1993). Outcomes for adult outpatients with depression under prepaid or fee-for-service arrangements. *Archives of General Psychiatry, 50,* 517–525.

Rosenbaum, S., Silver, K., & Wehr, E. (1997). *An evaluation of contracts between state Medicaid agencies and managed care organizations for the prevention and treatment of mental illness and substance abuse disorders* (Vol. 2). Washington, DC: George Washington University.

Schwertz, D.W., et al. (1997). Teaching pharmacology to advanced practice nursing students: issues and strategies. *AACN Clinical Issues, 8*(1), 132–146.

Sing, M., et al. (1998). *The costs and effects of parity for mental health and substance abuse insurance benefits.* USDHHS Publication No. SMA 98–3205. Rockville, MD: Substance Abuse and Mental Health Services Administration, Center for Mental Health Services.

Smiddy, G. (1998). *Comprehensive health care reform demonstrations (4/30/98).* Personal Communication, Health Care Financing Administration.

Substance Abuse and Mental Health Services Administration. (1995). *Cost of addictive and mental disorders and effectiveness of treatment.* Washington, DC: USDHHS.

Stein, L.I., & Test, M.A. (1980). Alternative to mental hospital treatment. I. Conceptual model, treatment program, and clinical evaluation. *Archives of General Psychiatry, 37*(4), 392–397.

Stuart, G.W. (1998). Environmental context of psychiatric nursing care. In Stuart, G.W., & Laraia, M. (Eds.). *Principles and practice of psychiatric nursing* (ed. 6). St. Louis: Mosby.

Test, M.A. (1992). Training in community living delivering treatment and rehabilitation services through a continuous treatment team. In Lieberman, R.P. *Handbook of psychiatric rehabilitation.* New York: Macmillan Publishing Company.

U.S. Department of Health and Human Services. The President's Advisory Commission on Consumer Protection and Quality in the Health Care Industry. (1997). *Quality first: better health care for all Americans.* Washington, DC: Author.

Yurick, A., & Kobert, S. (1997). The psychiatric-primary care nurse practitioner: a futuristic model for advanced practice psychiatric-mental health nursing, *Archives of Psychiatric Nursing, 11*(1), 2–12.

chapter 3

Technology, Information, and Data Management

MARILYN P. VERHEY

■ INTRODUCTION

Advanced practice registered nurses (APRNs) in psychiatric-mental health nursing are practicing in the era of an information revolution brought about by the use of computers and other information technologies. The term *informatics* has been incorporated into the nursing vocabulary and is defined as "the specialty that integrates nursing science, computer science, and information science in identifying, collecting, processing, and managing data and information to support nursing practice, administration, education, research, and the expansion of nursing knowledge" (ANA, 1994b). Even the past 5 years have transformed the way in which nurses communicate, gather and evaluate information, and develop the knowledge

of advanced practice in psychiatric-mental health nursing. This chapter provides an overview of informatics for the APRN in advanced practice psychiatric-mental health nursing. It describes the management of information in four broad areas:
- Information for clinical decision making
- Information for systems management
- Information for evidence-based practice
- Information through electronic networking

INFORMATION FOR CLINICAL ■ DECISION MAKING

Clinical decision making in advanced practice psychiatric-mental health nursing relies on organized and systematic information and data for assessments, diagnoses, interventions, and evaluation of treatment outcomes. The extent to which this organized data is used by the individual APRN, and the extent to which APRNs contribute to the ongoing development and enhancement of existing classification schemes and databases, will determine the strength of the specialty in policy development, mental health outcomes research, and payment for services reform. This section describes the nursing and health care classification schemes, taxonomies, and databases that are relevant to the practice of advanced psychiatric-mental health nursing.

Nursing Minimum Data Set

The Nursing Minimum Data Set (NMDS) was designed by a national group of nursing and health care experts representing multiple specialties to provide a system for the ongoing collection of uniform, standardized nursing data elements for use by providers across multiple settings and patient populations (Werley et al., 1991). It was designed according to the principles of other health care minimum data sets, including the Uniform Hospital Discharge Data Set (UHDDS), which is mandated for use with all hospitalized Medicare patients. National implementation of the NMDS by nurses in all practice settings would provide an invaluable basis for nursing resource allocation, nursing research, and health policy decision-making (Werley, Ryan, & Zorn, 1995). The NMDS is composed of 16 elements grouped into three broad categories: 1) nursing care, 2) patient or client demographics, and 3) service elements (Box 3-1). Since the NMDS was designed to meet the basic data needs of the nursing profession, additional information to meet specific program information needs may be collected. Although published reports on use of the NMDS in psychiatric nursing settings do not exist, the use of this core database can facilitate the integration of psychiatric patient information into national, cross-specialty data sets. Inherent in the implementation of the NMDS in psychiatric settings is the need

---

box 3-1

ELEMENTS OF THE NURSING MINIMUM DATA SET

1. Nursing care elements
   a. Nursing diagnosis
   b. Nursing intervention
   c. Nursing outcome
   d. Intensity of nursing care
2. Patient or client demographic elements
   a. Personal identification*
   b. Date of birth*
   c. Sex*
   d. Race and ethnicity*
   e. Residence*
3. Service elements
   a. Unique facility or service agency number*
   b. Unique health record number of patient or client
   c. Unique number of principal registered nurse providers
   d. Episode admission or encounter date*
   f. Discharge or termination date*
   g. Disposition of patient or client*
   h. Expected payer for most of this bill (anticipated financial guarantor for services)*

*Elements comparable with those in the Uniform Hospital Discharge Data Set.
From Werley, Ryan, & Zorn, 1995.

---

for a common language to use in collecting information about the nursing care elements of patient diagnoses, interventions, and outcomes. The various initiatives used to develop these standardized nursing classification schemes are described in the next section.

Nursing Classification Systems

To provide national coordination of the development of a uniform nursing database system, the American Nurses Association (ANA) assigned responsibility for policy recommendations related to the development of database systems to the ANA Cabinet on Nursing Practice, which in turn formed the Steering Committee on Databases to Support Clinical Nursing Practice. The Steering Committee realized that no one vocabulary or classification system could be used consistently across all practice settings. The committee recommended that the profession work toward the development of a unified nursing language system (UNLS) that would allow linking or mapping of similar terms among diverse systems while allowing each classification system to remain a unique entity (McCormick et al, 1994). The Steering Committee developed criteria by which classification systems would be chosen for inclusion in a UNLS (Box 3-2). To date, five classification systems have been recognized by the Steering Committee: the North American Nursing Diagnosis Association (NANDA) taxonomy of nursing diagnoses, the Omaha Community Health Problem and Intervention Classification System (Omaha System), the Home Care Classification (HCC) system, the Nursing Interventions Classification (NIC) system, and the Nursing Outcomes Classification (NOC) system. Common elements among all five systems include their development and refinement through extensive nursing research efforts extending over a period of years, and their use of a numerical system of coding identifiers to facilitate computerization and mapping of the database elements.

North American Nursing Diagnosis Association. NANDA has been developing nursing diagnosis taxonomy for over two decades. This taxonomy is organized according to nine human response patterns: exchanging, communicating, relating, valuing, choosing, moving, perceiving, knowing, and feeling (Carroll-Johnson & Paquette, 1994). There are three types of nursing diagnoses: actual, risk, and wellness. *Actual diagnoses* describe human responses to health conditions or life processes that exist in an individual, family, or community. *Risk diagnoses* describe human responses that may develop in a vulnerable individual, family, or community, whereas *wellness diagnoses* describe human responses to levels of wellness in an individual, family, or community

---

box 3-2

CRITERIA FOR RECOGNIZING CLASSIFICATION SCHEMES: ANA STEERING COMMITTEE ON DATABASES TO SUPPORT CLINICAL NURSING PRACTICE

CLASSIFICATION SCHEMES USED FOR CLINICAL PRACTICE SHOULD HAVE THE FOLLOWING CHARACTERISTICS:

1. Clinically useful for making diagnostic, intervention, and outcome decisions
2. Stated clearly and unambiguously, with terms defined precisely
3. Tested for reliability of the vocabulary terms
4. Validated as useful for clinical purposes
5. Accompanied by documentation of the systematic methodology used to develop the scheme
6. Accompanied by evidence of a process for periodic review and provision for addition, revision, or deletion of terms
7. Terms that are associated with a unique identifier or code

CLASSIFICATION SCHEMES USED IN NURSING RESEARCH OR TO CLASSIFY NURSING LITERATURE SHOULD HAVE THE FOLLOWING CHARACTERISTICS:

1. Stated in clear and unambiguous terms, with terms defined precisely
2. Validated as useful for classifying its domain
3. A taxonomic structure that is conceptually coherent
4. Accompanied by documentation of the systematic methodology used to develop the scheme
5. Accompanied by evidence of a process for periodic review and provision for addition, revision, or deletion of terms
6. Terms that are associated with a unique identifier or code

From McCormick et al, 1994.

that have a potential for enhancement to a higher state. A NANDA website (www.nanda.org) is currently under construction.

NANDA's Diagnosis Review Committee (DRC) is responsible for overseeing of a four-stage process for developing new diagnoses that reflects the circular process of theory, practice, and research (Warren & Hoskins, 1995). Stage 1 involves an organized group submitting a diagnosis for consultation and education by the DRC about further development. During stage 2, authentication and substantiation, a comprehensive literature review is conducted, a definition and defining characteristics are developed, and content validity is established. During stage 3, the diagnosis is tested for clinical existence and usefulness through research. If it is clinically supported, the diagnosis is placed into the taxonomic structure. In stage 4, all diagnoses are carefully reevaluated for refinement or elimination.

In collaboration with NANDA, APRNs developed a comprehensive list of the phenomena of concern for psychiatric nursing (O'Toole & Loomis, 1989). Originally begun as the work of a Task Force of the ANA's Council on Psychiatric-Mental Health Nursing, the classification system has been refined and presented to the DRC for inclusion in the NANDA taxonomy. The use of NANDA diagnoses by psychiatric APRNs is not well documented in the literature. The limited use of NANDA diagnoses by APRNs may be related to the fact that reimbursement of APRN services is linked with the use of diagnoses from medical, rather than nursing, classification systems.

Nursing Interventions Classification. The Nursing Interventions Classification (NIC) was developed at the University of Iowa to provide a standardized language for nursing treatments performed by nurses in all specialties and all practice settings (McCloskey & Bulechek, 1996). Each of the interventions in the schema has a label name, a definition, a set of activities crucial to its performance, and background readings. The classification system includes both interventions initiated by a nurse in response to a nursing diagnosis and interventions carried out by a nurse in response to a physician's order. Interventions are grouped according to six major domains: physiologic (basic), physiologic (complex), behavioral, safety, family, and health system. Linkages between NANDA nursing diagnoses and NIC interventions have been developed and provide direction for diagnostic reasoning and integration of clinical nursing information system database structures. Further information about NIC can be found at its website (www.nursing.uiowa.edu/nic).

The behavioral domain of the NIC is relevant to APRNs' practice and includes interventions in the areas of behavior therapy, cognitive therapy, communication enhancement, coping assistance, patient education, and psychological comfort promotion. Pertinent classes are also found in the safety (crisis management), family (childbearing care, lifespan care), and health system (health system mediation, health system management, information management) domains. There are no reports in the literature of the use of NIC by psychiatric APRNs or in general psychiatric nursing settings. Psychiatric nursing knowledge could be enhanced by the clinical application of this standardized scheme for nursing interventions with populations of psychiatric-mental health patients. Systematized and aggregated data about psychiatric nursing interventions are crucial to the ongoing development of a psychiatric nursing research base.

Nursing Outcomes Classification. The Nursing Outcomes Classification (NOC), under development at the University of Iowa College of Nursing since 1991, is a comprehensive classification of patient outcomes that are responsive to nursing interventions (Johnson & Maas, 1997). The scheme contains 190 outcomes with specific indicators that are used to measure the effects of interventions according to a Likert scale. Each outcome includes between 5 and 20 measurable indicators. Linkages between NANDA diagnoses and NOC outcomes are provided. The classification system was developed through a rigorous process of extraction of outcome statements from multiple sources, grouping of the statements to develop nursing-sensitive outcome labels, concept analyses through focus groups, and content validation by master's-prepared nurse experts including representatives from the American Psychiatric Nurses Association (APNA). Field tests of the scheme are being conducted at two tertiary care hospitals, an acute-care community hospital, a long-term care facility, and a community health agency. Development of a coding system is in progress. The identification and development of additional outcomes is continuing and will include, in addition to the current individual patient or caregiver outcomes, family- and community-centered outcomes. Future research endeavors include psychometric evaluation; risk adjustment factors; evaluation of usefulness in clinical settings; and linkages between nursing diagnoses, nursing interventions, and nursing sensitive patient outcomes. Examples of outcomes of interest to APRNs in psychiatric-mental health nursing include abuse recovery, abusive behavior self-control, aggression control, cognitive orientation, distorted thought control, grief resolution, knowledge of disease process, knowledge of medication, psychosocial adjustment to life change, risk control of alcohol and drug use, self-esteem, self-mutilation restraint, and suicide self-restraint. Further information about NOC can be found at its website (www.nursing.uiowa.edu/noc).

The Omaha Community Health Problem and Intervention Classification System (Omaha System). The Omaha System, developed at the Visiting Nurses Association (VNA) of Omaha by Karen Martin and her colleagues, is a classification system that has been implemented in home care, public health, school health, clinic, ambulatory care, and other programs (Martin & Norris, 1996; Martin & Scheet, 1992). It has three components: a Problem Classification Scheme, an Intervention Scheme, and a Problem Rating Scale for Outcomes.

The *Problem Classification Scheme* is a taxonomy of 44 patient problems or nursing diagnoses representing four domains: environmental, psychosocial, physiological, and health-related behaviors.

The *Intervention Scheme* is organized according to four broad categories: health teaching, guidance, and counseling; treatment and procedures; case management; and surveillance. In the second level of the Intervention Scheme, 63 targets or objects of nursing action are defined. A third level provides for patient-specific information generated by the nurse. The Intervention Scheme is intended to be used with the Problem Classification Scheme and represents a research-based effort to link interventions with nursing diagnoses.

The *Problem Rating Scale for Outcomes* is a 5-point Likert scale for measuring patient progress in three conceptual areas: knowledge, behavior, and status of signs and symptoms. Suggested times for using the rating scale are upon admission to service, at interval points during service, and upon discharge. Data can be used to track individual patient progress or be aggregated to provide information about patient populations and agency operations. A website has been established to provide information about the Omaha System (con.ufl.edu/omaha/).

The use of the Omaha System in public health, home health, school health, and alternative community health delivery systems is well documented (Martin & Scheet, 1995). Specific reports of its implementation come from APRNs in state and county public health agencies, school-based clinics, community clinics, ambulatory care centers, and homeless clinics (Martin & Scheet, 1992). In these specialized examples, the system was used to assess and document psychiatric and mental health concerns. Use of the Omaha system in a focused psychiatric-mental health setting has not been documented in the literature.

Home Health Care Classification. Developed at Georgetown University by Virginia Saba and colleagues, the Home Health Care Classification (HHCC) of nursing diagnoses and nursing interventions provides a scheme for home health care nursing services (Saba, 1995). HHCC is organized according to 20 components of home care, which are used to classify the phases of the nursing process. NANDA-approved diagnoses were studied, expanded, and revised to include additional problems related to home health patients. The classification of nursing diagnoses includes a modifier of three possible expected outcome goals: improved, stabilized, or deteriorated. Outcomes are assessed upon admission, at specified intervals during care, and at discharge. The system includes 160 home health nursing interventions that are modified according to four nursing intervention services: assessment, direct care, teaching, and management. Each intervention requires one or more of the four intervention services to identify the specific type of care delivery. The system links the diagnostic and intervention components of the classification scheme. Relevant sections in the HHCC include adjustment impairment, decisional conflict, denial, emotional support, mental health care, mental health history, mental health screening, mental health treatment, and psychosocial analysis. Further information about HHCC can be found at its website (www.dml.georgetown.edu/research/hhcc). Again, no reports of the use of the HHCC in basic or advanced practice psychiatric-mental health nursing exist in the literature.

Use of nursing taxonomies and classification systems by APRNs. Although the nursing classification systems and taxonomies described previously include psychiatric and mental health domains and have been developed and tested through extensive research efforts, the journal literature does not present information about their use by psychiatric APRNs or their implementation in psychiatric-mental health care settings. Explanations for this may include the focus on medically oriented taxonomies for third-party reimbursement of APRN services and documentation of services within the managed care system. Additionally, the nursing taxonomies lend themselves to application within comprehensive, organized nursing delivery systems, whereas much of the work of psychiatric APRNs is within smaller clinics or private individual and group practices.

The current focus on the delivery of psychiatric nursing services in community settings may lead to an increased application of systems such as the Omaha System and the HHCC. Using standardized and uniform databases and taxonomies to contribute to the clinical information and knowledge base of nursing in general, and psychiatric-mental health nursing in particular, is vital to the nursing outcomes research that will enhance quality psychiatric and mental health care.

Other Taxonomies and Classification Systems

International Classification of Diseases. The *International Classification of Diseases (ICD)* is maintained and promulgated by the World Health Organization (WHO). The clinical modification of the ninth revision of the *ICD (ICD-9-CM)* was developed by the National Center for Health Statistics (NCHS) for use in the United States. NCHS is currently modifying *ICD 10* to create *ICD-10-CM*. The purposes of *ICD-9-CM* are to classify morbidity and mortality information for statistical purposes and to serve as a mechanism to report and compile health care data to assist in evaluating health care, planning delivery systems, determining patterns of care, analyzing payments for health services, and conducting epidemiologic and clinical research (National Center for Health Statistics, 1997). The classification is published in three volumes: a tabular list of diseases, an alphabetic index of diseases, and a volume of medical procedures in both tabular and index formats. The *ICD-9-CM* codes are used in several data sets and classification systems including the fourth edition of the *Diagnostic and Statistical Manual of Mental Disorders (DSM-IV)*, the Uniform Clinical Data Set (UCDS) and the Uniform Hospital Discharge Data Set (UHDDS). The UCDS was developed by the Health Care Financing Administration (HCFA) for use by state Peer Review Organizations to review hospital care and analyze data on patient characteristics and the processes of care. The

UHDDS is used for mandatory reporting to regulatory agencies and for Uniform Billing (UB) by most third-party payers.

Diagnostic and Statistical Manual of Mental Disorders. The *DSM-IV*, published by the American Psychiatric Association (APA, 1994a), is the primary taxonomy for the classification of mental disorders. The first edition of *DSM* was published in 1952, and as with subsequent editions, its development was coordinated with the publication of versions of the *ICD*. The purpose of *DSM-IV* is "to provide clear descriptions of diagnostic categories in order to enable clinicians and investigators to diagnose, communicate about, study, and treat people with various mental disorders" (APA, 1994b). *DSM-IV* was developed through the work of 13 work groups and included three stages: 1) comprehensive and systematic reviews of the published literature (published in *DSM-IV Sourcebooks*), 2) reanalysis of 40 existing research data sets, and 3) 12 field trials at more than 70 sites (APA, 1994a).

The diagnoses are clustered into categories and sub-categories, and each diagnosis is accompanied by a numerical *ICD-9-CM* code. Each diagnosis includes specific criteria that must be met for the diagnosis to be made. Modifiers indicating severity (mild, moderate, severe) and course (in partial remission, in full remission, history) may by applied to the diagnosis. Additionally, *DSM-IV* uses a multiaxial system that involves an assessment on five axes, each providing a different domain of information for clinical decision making, treatment planning, and outcome measurement. The five axes are as follows:

1. Clinical disorders and other conditions that may be a focus of clinical attention
2. Personality disorders and mental retardation
3. General medical conditions
4. Psychosocial and environmental problems
5. Global assessment of functioning

For further information about using *DSM-IV*, see the numerous educational guidelines and aids published by the APA. *DSM-IV* is available in an electronic version in DOS, Windows, and Macintosh formats. It is fully searchable, contains every word of *DSM-IV*, and can be installed on the hard drives of both desktop and laptop computers. A version of *DSM-IV* has been created specifically for use in primary care as a collaborative effort between the APA and primary care groups (APA, 1995). In addition, the American Academy of Pediatrics has developed *The Classification of Child and Adolescent Mental Diagnosis in Primary Care* to provide clinicians with a common language for describing the psychosocial aspects of childhood and adolescence (Woolrich, Felice, & Drotar, 1996).

Current procedural terminology. The Physician's Current Procedural Terminology (CPT) codes are published by the American Medical Association (1996). The system is used to code services and procedures for reimbursement by public and private third-party payers and is a basis for health policy discussions regarding payment systems. Although designed by physicians for physicians, APRNs and other providers also perform many of the procedures in the classification system. The codes are clustered under six major categories with subsections in each. Each procedure or service is identified with a five-digit code.

Studies have been conducted to assess the use of CPT codes by APRNs in a variety of specialties (ANA, 1994a; Griffith & Robinson, 1993). Currently, a coalition of organizations, including the APNA, the ANA, the APA, the National Association of Social Workers (NASW), and others, has been formed to collect data on 24 CPT codes used to report psychiatric services. Results of this study will have implications for federal legislation regulating Medicare payments to psychiatric clinical nurse specialists (CPT Code Project, 1997).

Systematized Nomenclature of Human and Veterinary Medicine. The Systematized Nomenclature of Human and Veterinary Medicine (SNOMED), developed and produced by the College of American Pathologists, is a multiaxial classification system created for the indexing of the entire patient record, including signs and symptoms, as well as diagnoses and procedures (http://snomed.org). The most recent version contains more than 150,000 terms and term codes in 11 separate modules.

Unified Medical Language System. The Unified Medical Language System (UMLS) is a project of the National Library of Medicine, in collaboration with several private sector organizations, government agencies, and university research groups, to integrate electronic biomedical information from a wide variety of sources (Lindberg & Humphries, 1995). The *UMLS Metathesaurus* contains concepts and terms from over 30 source vocabularies and classification systems and establishes relationships among terms from the source systems. It is intended to supply information that computer programs can use to interpret user inquiries, refine those inquiries, identify which databases contain information relevant to specific inquiries, and convert the user's terms into the vocabulary used by the relevant information source. All of the nursing, psychiatric, and health care classification systems and vocabularies described previously are included in the *UMLS Metathesaurus*. The Steering Committee on Databases to Support Clinical Nursing Practice is endorsing the concept of a Unified Nursing Language System (UNLS) as a subset of the UMLS.

INFORMATION FOR SYSTEMS
■ MANAGEMENT

The use of computer technology to manage clinical and administrative information in hospitals, ambulatory, and community-based service settings has the potential to greatly enhance the practice of advanced psychiatric-mental health nursing. Clinical information systems can streamline the maintenance of individual records as well as provide aggregated data for process and outcomes measurement, strategic planning, and clinical research. Administrative systems provide

mechanisms for billing, budget monitoring and financial planning, staffing, and other personnel functions.

The services provided by an APRN in a hospital or medical center may be supported by a house-wide hospital information system. Ideally, the clinical, financial, and other administrative components of the system are highly integrated. Clinical documentation and data retrieval may occur at the "point-of care" (e.g., at the bedside) while maintaining a centralized computer processor and database for all terminals. Hughes (1996) lists the possible components of a hospital information system as including applications to address acuity; admission, discharge, and transfer; budgeting; care planning and case management; case mix; decision support; managed care; medical records; order entry and results reporting; patient accounting; patient appointment scheduling; patient care documentation; pharmacy; quality management; and staff scheduling.

Individual "Stand-Alone" Systems

Other settings, such as a psychotherapy practice or community mental health agency, may use stand-alone systems such as *The Perfect Chart, Practice Manager (PM/2), Psych Access, Psych Advantage, Quick-Doc, Psych Office,* and *Easy Psychiatric Record Keeper.* For a brief description and contact information about these systems, refer to Box 3-3.

Integrated Information Management Systems

The UCLA Neuropsychiatric Institute and Hospital formed a working group to make recommendations for a clinical information system (Guze et al, 1996). The group developed the following criteria for a clinical database in psychiatry:

1. Client-server open system environment
2. Graphic user interface
3. Use of standard clinical formats and protocols

box 3-3

SOFTWARE PACKAGES FOR INFORMATION MANAGEMENT

THE PERFECT CHART

The Perfect Chart can record patient demographics, social history, biologic condition, and managed care and insurance information, as well as full diagnostic and session histories. It includes clinical templates with specialized diagnostic and treatment information, tests and tables to assist documentation, a special psychiatric-psychological dictionary, ready-made forms and letters, and standard prescribing templates for common psychotropic medications. It is available from Multi-Health Systems, Inc.

PRACTICE MANAGER (PM/2)

Practice Manager is designed to manage a psychiatric practice. Key features include inclusion of *DSM-IV*, patient bills and statements, insurance claim preparation, electronic claims submission, tracking of managed care approvals, treatment plan writer, progress notes, face sheets and other forms, and built-in reports. It is available from PM/2 Practice Management Systems, Inc.

PSYCH ACCESS

Psych Access is an on-line patient chart and communications network for behavioral care. Operating via Internet connections and using a Microsoft Windows 95 operating system,

box 3-3

SOFTWARE PACKAGES FOR INFORMATION MANAGEMENT—cont'd

Psych Access communicates between a psychiatric practice and managed care organizations for referrals, treatment authorization, and claims processing. Additional features include the ability to create and send dispositions, treatment plans, progress notes, and case mail in a standardized documentation format. It is available from Community Sector Systems, Inc.

PSYCH ADVANTAGE

Psych Advantage is designed to meet the needs of a psychiatric office and features systems for patient records, medical records, appointment scheduling, word processing, referral tracking, recalls, accounts payable, and reports. It is available from Compulink.

QUICK-DOC, PSYCH OFFICE, EASY PSYCHIATRIC RECORD KEEPER

Quick-Doc writes initial work-ups, progress notes, and treatment and discharge plans largely by picking from lists. It includes intakes, progress notes, treatment plans, discharge notes, outcome measures, forms and letters, and an appointment scheduler. Psych Office includes features for record keeping, prescriptions, and billing. Easy Psychiatric Record Keeper features a psychiatric text editor, *DSM-IV*, progress notes, lab results, and current medications. These and other software packages are available from Mental Health Connections, Inc.

4. Support for free-text notes and related customized templates
5. Support for entry and monitoring of treatment plans
6. Support for results reporting
7. Support for medication management
8. Support for entry of psychological instruments, assessments, and tools
9. Support for user development of instruments and tools
10. Support for entry and monitoring of *DSM* diagnoses
11. Support for appointment scheduling
12. Interfaces available for existing systems
13. Reasonable cost

The UCLA Neuropsychiatric Institute and Hospital is now a member of the PsychConsult Consortium, a group of nationally recognized academic departments of psychiatry, provider networks, community mental health centers, private group practices, public agencies, managed care organizations, and software developers. Under the aegis of the Askesis Development Group, Inc., the consortium has developed the PsychConsult

Behavioral Healthcare Management System designed to integrate administrative, financial, and clinical information management functions (Gerber, 1998). Through a graphical interface running on Windows 95 and Windows NT 4.0, the relational, distributed database is capable of aggregating financial and clinical data for up to four billion patients over an unlimited number of physical locations. PsychConsult has been designed to connect to and interact cooperatively with major medical center information systems, pharmacy and laboratory systems, third-party payers, managed care networks, and public agencies. A Consortium working group is refining the system to prepare for implementation in major psychiatric centers. The current features of the system for both providers and managed care are listed in Box 3-4.

INFORMATION FOR
■ EVIDENCE-BASED PRACTICE
Evidence-Based Practice

The rapid expansion of information and knowledge in psychiatric-mental health nursing and related areas is a now-familiar phenomenon. To address the "information explosion" and its effects on clinical practice, the paradigm of evidence-based practice has been evolving during the past decade (Evidence-Based Medicine Working Group, 1992; Geddes & Harrison, 1997; Sackett & Rosenberg, 1995; Sharpe et al, 1996). The application of the evidence-based paradigm consists of five steps:

1. Defining a patient problem and what information is needed to resolve the problem (i.e., converting information needs into answerable patient-focused questions)
2. Conducting a search of the literature
3. Selecting the most relevant literature and critically appraising the evidence for validity and clinical usefulness
4. Applying the results of the appraisal in clinical practice
5. Evaluating one's clinical performance

---

box 3-4

PSYCHCONSULT FUNCTIONALITY

PROVIDER

Patient accounting
Billing and electronic claims submission
Managed care and capitation management
Multi-location, centralized scheduling
Chart tracking and medical records management
Custom reports and graphs
Complete multimedia patient medical record
Intake and triage with smart decision support
Treatment planning with critical pathways
Medication management
Electronic outcome measures
Complete inpatient functionality
Financial applications: general ledger, accounts payable, payroll, human resources, and fixed assets

MANAGED CARE

Call center and triage line
Provider referrals
Mapping system
Care management
Outcomes and continuous quality improvement
Member services
Provider relations
Credentialing
Network management
Grievances
Claims adjudication
Financial applications: general ledger, accounts payable, payroll, human resources, and fixed assets

By engaging in evidence-based practice, the APRN in psychiatric-mental health nursing establishes a pattern of lifelong learning that continuously incorporates the most current clinical research and research-based clinical guidelines. Additional information about the evidence-based practice paradigm is available on the Internet:

- hiru.mcmaster.ca/ebm/default.htm
- cebm.jr2.ox.ac.uk/

The following section presents selected tools and strategies to support evidence-based practice, particularly in the areas of searching and evaluating relevant literature.

Bibliographic Databases

Conducting an electronic search of the health care literature is becoming a necessary and basic skill for clinical practitioners. Ideally, electronic bibliographic databases are available at a point-of-care workstation. However, even if point-of care technology is not available, the World Wide Web (WWW) has made electronic bibliographic databases easily accessible. The following databases are those most likely to be used by APRNs in psychiatric-mental health nursing.

Cumulative Index to Nursing and Allied Health Literature. The Cumulative Index to Nursing and Allied Health Literature (CINAHL) provides coverage of the professional literature in nursing and allied health disciplines, biomedicine, and consumer health. Virtually all English-language, as well as selected foreign-language nursing journals, are indexed along with publications from the ANA and the National League for Nursing (NLN). CINAHL also provides access to health care books, book chapters, pamphlets, nursing dissertations, selected conference proceedings, audiovisual materials, and educational software. Full text is available for selected nursing standards of practice, nurse practice acts, state nursing journals, and critical pathways. Other features include a citation index, research instrument descriptions, full-text research instruments, and

the indexing of the Cochrane Database of Systematic Reviews.

MEDLINE. The MEDLINE database is produced by the National Library of Medicine and indexes English and foreign language journals in the areas of medicine, allied health, and the basic life sciences. Free access is available through the Internet (see section on Information through Electronic Networking).

PsychINFO. Produced by the American Psychological Association, PsychINFO is a computerized database that indexes journals, technical reports, dissertations, and other materials in all areas of psychology and the behavioral sciences. PsychINFO is the computerized version of the print index *Psychological Abstracts,* but the PsychINFO database indexes more materials than its print counterpart. PsychLIT is a CD-ROM database that is a subset of PsychINFO. Another subset database is ClinPSYC, intended to meet the needs of practicing clinicians in mental health settings.

HealthSTAR. The HealthSTAR database is produced by the American Hospital Association and the National Library of Medicine. It comprehensively indexes materials in the nonclinical aspects of health care delivery. Subject coverage includes health policy; health insurance; administration and planning of health facilities; services and manpower; financial management; personnel administration; quality management; and regulation, licensure and accreditation that apply to health care delivery. Materials indexed include journals, books, theses, and technical reports.

GPO monthly catalog. The catalog indexes the publications of the U.S. Government Printing Office (GPO), which include reports of task forces, vital statistics, health care policy, epidemiology, and legislation.

Evaluating Information

Once information is retrieved, it must be evaluated for validity, usefulness, and relevance before it can be incorporated into clinical practice or become

box 3-5

USER'S GUIDES TO THE MEDICAL LITERATURE TOPIC AREAS*

I. How to Get Started (1993, v. 270, pp. 2093–2095)
II. How to Use an Article about Therapy or Prevention
   A. Are the Results of the Study Valid? (1993, v. 270, pp. 2598–2601)
   B. What Were the Results and Will They Help Me in Caring for My Patients? (1994, v. 271, pp. 59–63)
III. How to Use an Article About a Diagnostic Test
   A. Are the Results of the Study Valid? (1994, v. 271, pp. 389–391)
   B. What Were the Results and Will They Help Me in Caring for My Patients? (1994, v. 271, pp. 703–707)
IV. How to Use an Article About Harm (1994, v. 271, pp. 1615–1619)
V. How to Use an Article about Prognosis (1994, v. 272, pp. 234–237)
VI. How to Use an Overview (1994, v. 272, pp. 1376–1371)
VII. How to Use a Clinical Decision Analysis
   A. Are the Results of the Study Valid? (1995, v. 273, pp. 1292–1295)
   B. What Were the Results and Will They Help Me in Caring for My Patients? (1995, v. 273, pp. 1610–1613)
VIII. How to Use Clinical Practice Guidelines
   A. Are the Recommendations Valid? (1995, v. 274, pp. 570–574)
   B. What Are the Recommendations and Will They Help Me in Caring for My Patients? (1995, v. 274, pp. 1630–1632)
IX. A Method for Grading Health Care Recommendations (1995, v. 273, pp. 1800–1804)
X. How to Use an Article Reporting Variations in the Outcomes of Health Services (1996, v. 275, pp. 554–558)

box 3-5

USER'S GUIDES TO THE MEDICAL LITERATURE TOPIC AREAS*—cont'd

XI. How to Use an Article About a Clinical Utilization Review (1996, v. 275, pp. 1435–1439)
XII. How to Use Articles About Health-Related Quality of Life (1997, v. 277, pp. 1232–1237)
XIII. How to Use an Article on Economic Analysis of Clinical Practice
   A. Are the Results of the Study Valid? (1997, v. 277, pp. 1552–1557)
   B. What Were the Results and Will They Help Me in Caring for My Patients? (1997, v. 277, pp. 1802–1806)

*All published in *Journal of the American Medical Association (JAMA)* From Oxman, Sackett, & Guyatt, 1993.

part of the knowledge base of advanced practice. Several schema for evaluating clinical research have been developed, and two models are presented here as examples. Riegelman and Hirsch (1966) have developed a uniform framework for evaluating three basic types of clinical research studies found in the health care literature: case-control studies, cohort studies, and randomized or controlled clinical trials. The process begins by identifying the study design and study population. Then five components of the study are evaluated:

1. *Assignment.* The way in which individuals are assigned to study and control groups
2. *Assessment.* Evaluation of the investigation's results in the study and control groups
3. *Analysis.* Comparison of the results in the study and control groups
4. *Interpretation.* Evaluation of conclusions made about differences in results between the study and control groups
5. *Extrapolation.* Evaluation of conclusions made about the application of the findings to populations or situations not included in the study

Careful analysis of each step can help the APRN in psychiatric-mental health nursing identify the evidence that is valid and clinically useful and relevant.

Representatives of the Evidence-Based Medicine Working Group prepared and published a useful set of user's guides to the medical literature intended to help providers translate the results of research into clinical practice (Oxman, Sackett, & Guyatt, 1993). They based the guides on three basic questions intended to help the practitioner evaluate both primary research studies and integrative studies such as research reviews and practice guidelines:

1. Are the results of the study valid?
2. What are the results?
3. Will the results help me in caring for my patients?

The topics of the guides are listed in Box 3-5.

INFORMATION THROUGH ■ ELECTRONIC NETWORKING

Electronic networking is becoming a common method of communication and has dramatically changed the way APRNs can access information. Because of the Internet, both health care professionals and consumers can find information instantly. Examples include clinical and scholarly research; health care information from government agencies, professional associations, and ad-

box 3-6

DEFINITIONS FOR ELECTRONIC NETWORKING

Internet. A vast network of computers that exchange data using compatible telecommunications language. It is estimated that the Internet is used by more than one hundred million people. Electronic mail, or e-mail, is a commonly used feature of the Internet.

World Wide Web (WWW). An Internet service that allows users to browse, view, and transmit data files or programs in a graphic

box 3-6

DEFINITIONS FOR ELECTRONIC NETWORKING—cont'd

or other multimedia format, instead of strictly text files.

Browser. A computer interface program that allows the user to view and interact with WWW documents or pages. Examples include Netscape Navigator and Microsoft Internet Explorer.

Hypertext links. A mechanism that forms bridges or links between websites and allows the user to move from website to website. Hypertext links are usually underlined and highlighted on most web pages, or they may be represented by a picture or icon.

Uniform Resource Locator (URL). The WWW address that directs the browser to a particular WWW page. Most URLs start with "http" (hypertext transfer protocol) followed by punctuation ("://"), "www," and the information directing the browser to a particular web page. For example, the URL for the American Psychiatric Nurses Association is http://www.apna.org. The last three letters of the URL may indicate whether the web site represents an organization (org), an educational institution (edu), a government agency (gov), or a commercial venture (com).

Search engine. A database of websites where you can search, by typing in key words, for those sites that contain the information you are seeking. The name and URL address of commonly used Web search engines include the following:

General interest

Alta Vista	http://www.altavista.digital.com
InfoSeek	http://www.infoseek.com
Lycos Search	http://www.lycos.com
WebCrawler	http://www.webcrawler.com
Yahoo	http://yahoo.com

Health related

HealthAtoZ	http://www.healthatoz.com

vocacy groups; marketplaces; newspapers and other publications; and job-related information. The basic components of an electronic networking system are a computer, a modem, telecommunications software programs, and an account with an Internet Service Provider (ISP). Definitions of the most common terms used in electronic networking are found in Box 3-6. Most college and university campuses and many institutions have their own connection to the Internet and provide the service at no cost to students and employees, or the user can subscribe to a commercial service for a fee. Information about electronic networking is by its very nature obsolete very quickly since new technology and resources are being developed constantly. This section presents information about the potential of electronic networking for APRNs in psychiatric-mental health nursing practice that is as current as possible. However, readers are encouraged to update their knowledge in this area, possibly through the use of the Internet itself. Additional resources for accessing information electronically are found in Box 3-7.

Websites for APRNs

By the time these words are being read, vast numbers of new websites will have been developed, and the computer technology by which the WWW is accessed will have advanced enormously. The website of the APNA (http://www.apna.org) is an excellent starting point for electronic information searching. In addition to information about the organization, it includes information about professional resources, relevant legislation, and other items of interest to psychiatric APRNs. As an example, the APNA website has extensive links to other related websites. A list of these websites when this book went to press is found in Box 3-8. Among the many other relevant websites is that of the Psychiatric Society for Informatics, whose mission is to promote the understanding and use of informatics and information technology in psychiatry (http://www.psych.med. umich.edu/web/PSI/).

Box 3-7

RESOURCES FOR ACCESSING INFORMATION ELECTRONICALLY

1997 Healthcare guide to the Internet. Santa Barbara, CA: COR Healthcare Resources.

Grohol, J.M. (1997). *The insider's guide to mental health resources online.* New York: Guilford Publications.

Hancock, L. (Ed.). (1995). *Key guide to electronic resources: health sciences.* Medford, NJ: Learned Information, Inc.

Health care on the Internet: a journal of methods and applications. Hayworth Press. (1-800-HAWORTH; getinfo@haworth.com)

Hogarth, M., & Hutchinson, D. (1996). *An Internet guide for the health professional* (ed. 2). Sacramento, CA: New Wind Publishing.

Medicine on the Net. (A monthly magazine for health care professionals. anderson@cor-health. com, 805-564-2177)

Sparks, S.M., & Rizzolo, M.A. (1998). World Wide Web search tools. *Image: Journal of Nursing Scholarship, 30,* 167–171.

Other Opportunities for Electronic Networking

Electronic mailing lists. Often referred to as *listservs* after the software package that manages them, electronic mailing lists are discussion groups whereby messages on a particular topic are posted to a master e-mail list and then distributed as individual e-mail messages to the members of the listserv. By reading and posting e-mail messages on the topic, the user can share ideas, information, and research with others, nationally and internationally. There are listservs available on every topic imaginable, the size of the list is widely variable, and lists are created and closed down every day. Of particular interest to APRNs in psychiatric-mental health nursing is the listserv of the APNA, apnalist@nurse.org. Instructions for

box 3-8

APNA WEBPAGE-RELATED WEBSITES

INTERNATIONAL PSYCHIATRIC NURSING ORGANIZATIONS

Canadian Federation of Mental Health Nurses
Section of Psychiatric Nursing—United Kingdom
Australian and New Zealand College of Mental Health Nurses, Inc.

GOVERNMENT

Administration for Children and Families
Administration on Aging
Agency for Health Care Policy and Research
Americans with Disabilities Act
Centers for Disease Control and Prevention
Center for Mental Health Services
Decade of the Brain
Federal Food and Drug Administration
Fedstats
General Accounting Office
The Health Care Financing Administration (HCFA)
Healthfinder
Health Resources and Services Administration
Indian Health Service
National Center for Chronic Disease Prevention and Health Promotion
National Institute on Aging (NIA)
The National Institute on Drug Abuse
The National Institutes of Health (NIH)
National Institute of Mental Health
National Mental Health Services Knowledge Exchange Network (KEN)
NIH Guide to Grants and Contracts Database
Substance Abuse and Mental Health Services Administration
Thomas, the Online Service of the Library of Congress
Walk the Walk
The Zipper

HEALTH NEWS

The Association for Health Services Research (AHSR)
Creative Multimedia's Health Explorer

Health Care Information Resources: Alternative Medicine
Healthy People 2000: Mental Health and Mental Disorders Resource List
HealthWeb
Johns Hopkins AIDS Service
KidsHealth
Medical Tribune
ParentNews: A Unique Opportunity for Parent Information
Reuters Health Information Services
USA Today Health Index
The WholeFamily Center
Worldwide Healthcare Forums
Your Health Daily

MEDICAL

AIDS Treatment Data Network
Bioethics On-Line Service
Clinical Pharmacology Online
EthnoMed: Ethnic Medicine Guide
Home Care Nurse Page
Life Sciences Institute of Mind-Body Health: Self-Regulation of Mind and Body
Medical Decision Support
Medical Outcomes Trust
MEDLINE
Medscape
The Merck Manual
Neurosciences on the Internet
Pharmaceutical Companies on the Web
Rx List: The Internet Drug Index
WebSight News Digest
The World-Wide Web Virtual Library: AIDS

MENTAL HEALTH

Alzheimer's Disease Education and Referral (ADEAR) Center
American Self-Help Clearinghouse
At Health
Australian Transcultural Mental Health Network
Bazelon Center for Mental Health Law
Behavior Online

continued

3-8

box

APNA WEBPAGE-RELATED WEBSITES—cont'd

Beyond Stigma: ECT and Depression

Braincare

Center for the Study of Issues in Public Mental Health

CenterWatch Clinical Trials Listing Service

The Clifford Beers Foundation

Community Mental Health Management Information Systems Resource Center

Computers in Mental Health (CIMH)

Habit Smart

help! A Consumers' Guide to Mental Health Information

Depression Central

Dana BrainWeb

ERIC Clearinghouse on Assessment and Evaluation

Expert Consensus Guideline Series

Futurcom in Psychiatry

Georgia Mental Health Network

Institute for Brain Aging and Dementia

Internet Depression Resources List

Internet Mental Health

Laban's Addiction Specific Trainings

Mental Health Education Page: Removing the Stigma of Mental Illness

Mental Health InfoSource

Mental Health Matters

Mental Health Meetings

Mental Health Net

NPAD News: National Panic/Anxiety Disorder News

The National Center for Kids in Crisis

National Center for PTSD

National Coalition for the Homeless

National Foundation for Depressive Illness

National Resource Center on Homelessness

Personality Disorders

Practice Guidelines Coalition

Psychiatric Times

Psychlink

Psychopharmacology and Drug References on the Mental Health Net

Psychopharmacology TIPS

SafetyNet: Domestic Violence Information and Resources

Substance Abuse Guideline Exchange (SAGE)

UCLA Research Center for Severe Mental Illnesses

Wellness Reproductions & Publishing, Inc.

Western Psychiatric Institute and Clinical Library

Wing of Madness: General Mental Health Sources

MENTAL HEALTH ASSOCIATIONS

Academy of Eating Disorders

Academy of Psychosomatic Medicine

American Academy of Addiction Psychiatry

American Academy of Child and Adolescent Psychiatry

Alliance for the Mentally Ill/Friends and Advocates of the Mentally Ill

Alzheimer's Association

American Academy of Psychiatry and the Law

American Association for Geriatric Psychiatry

American Association of Suicidology

American Association for Marriage and Family Therapy

American Association on Mental Retardation

American College of Mental Health Administration

American Geriatrics Society

American Managed Behavioral Healthcare Association

American Occupational Therapy Association

American Professional Society on the Abuse of Children

American Psychiatric Association

American Psychological Association (PsychNET)

American Psychological Association Public Policy

American Public Health Association

Anorexia Nervosa and Bulimia Association

Anxiety Disorders Association of America

Association of Managed Care Providers

Children and Adults with Attention Deficit Disorders

Depression and Related Affective Disorders Association

APNA WEBPAGE-RELATED WEBSITES—cont'd

Family Caregiver Alliance
Institute for Behavioral Health Care
The International Association of Group Psycho-
therapy
Joint Commission on Accreditation of Health-
care Organizations
National Alliance for the Mentally Ill
National Alliance for Research on Schizophrenia
and Depression
National Association of Cognitive-Behavioral
Therapists
National Association of Psychiatric Health
Systems
National Association of State and Mental Health
Program Directors
National Council for Community Behavioral
Healthcare
National Council on Alcoholism and Drug Depen-
dence
National Depressive and Manic-Depressive Asso-
ciation
National Mental Health Association
Partnership for Behavioral Healthcare/Cen-
traLink
Professional Associations
Suicide Awareness/Voices of Education (SAVE)

NURSING ORGANIZATIONS

American Nurses Association
Association of Child and Adolescent Psychiatric
Nurses
Canadian Nurses' Association
Internet Technology Encouraging Research

Military Nurses
NursingNet
Telephone Nursing Service
US Department of Defense TriService

FOUNDATIONS

The Robert Wood Johnson Foundation
The W. K. Kellogg Foundation

COMMERCIAL PRODUCTS

AllHeart
Dinamap Critikon, Johnson & Johnson
On-Line Physician's Desk Reference (PDR)

OTHER LINKS

PsychLink
All-in-one search page
Electroconvulsive Therapy Information
Health A to Z
Internet Mental Health Resources
MedAccess
Medical Matrix
Mental Health Net: Psychopharmacology and
Drug References
MedWeb
National Child Care Information Center
Nursing Network Forum
Online Psych
Psyc Site
Yahoo Science: Psychology Search

Courtesy APNA website, http://www.apna.org/apnalink.htm.

using the APNA listserv are found on the APNA website, www.apna.org.

Bulletin boards. Bulletin boards are also referred to as *newsgroups,* or *Usenet groups.* Rather than the information being delivered to the user as an e-mail message, the user must go to the bulletin board to read or respond to the information on the topic.

Real-time interaction. Unlike using e-mail, listservs, or bulletin boards where there is a delay between the sending of and response to the sending of information, real-time interaction allows users to communicate synchronously, as with a two-person or conference telephone call. Various types of real-time communication are available, depending on the user's access to the Internet and computer system. This feature can be a low-cost method of timely communication among members of clinical or organizational work groups.

Telemedicine. Another application of electronic networking is a category of technology referred to as *telemedicine,* or *telehealth.* Clinical information is transmitted through a computer using voice, facsimile, pictures, video, and other specialized diagnostic equipment. Electronic communications networks can be used to convey clinical information between providers, or between the patient and the provider. One example of the latter application is the ComputerLink project of Case Western Reserve University whereby computer terminals were placed in the homes of Alzheimer's disease patients to allow their caregivers to access information and support through communication with the Information Network Services staff (Saba & McCormick, 1996). Another project is the Medical College of Georgia's Telemedicine Center's development of a neuropsychiatric multidisciplinary clinical Tele-mental health program for children and adolescents in a rural community in Georgia (McSwiggan-Hardin et al, 1997).

Ethics and Confidentiality

The computerization of information, especially patient records, raises a myriad of concerns about potential breaches in the confidentiality of information transmitted electronically. The following concerns, guidelines, and caveats can help ensure that electronic information is handled in a professional and ethical manner:

- When sending an e-mail message, remember that it can be printed or forwarded electronically to any number of individuals. Be careful and thoughtful about what is written in an e-mail message. A good rule of thumb is to decide whether you would be comfortable with what you have written in an e-mail message to be printed on the front page of a local newspaper. Common rules of correspondence etiquette apply to e-mail.

- Safeguards to protect the confidentiality of patient records are a vital element of computerized management information systems. The patient's right to privacy as delineated in the *Code for Nurses* (ANA, 1976) remains inalienable.

- Anyone can post information on the Internet. There is no peer review or mechanism to ensure the authenticity of what is found on the Internet. The need to evaluate information before applying it has never been greater.

- It is easy to download information from the Internet. However, the intellectual property rights of the person or organization putting the information on the Internet must be respected and protected.

IMPLICATIONS FOR ■ THE FUTURE

The future of advanced practice in psychiatric and mental health nursing is dependent on the demonstration of its ability to achieve clinically sound and cost-effective patient outcomes. The managed care environment has created an additional need for aggregate information and statistics about the costs, quality, and outcomes of nursing care activities (Jones, 1997). Standardized taxonomies and classification systems of diagnoses, interventions, and outcomes are crucial to the generation of computerized aggregate data for clinical decision making as well as health care policy development in psychiatry and mental health. APRNs must contribute to database and taxonomy initiatives that will describe and measure their effectiveness in assessment, treatment planning, interventions, and evaluation of outcomes. By the integration of information databases and vocabularies through the *UMLS Metathesaurus,* the future of advanced practice psychiatric-mental health nursing will be informed by computerized linkages among the biomedical literature; clinical records; diagnostic, intervention, and outcome taxonomies; and directories of information resources of various types.

Although computerized data systems have been developed in psychiatry for financial and other administrative purposes, the integration of these systems with computerized clinical data is in the early developmental stages in large psychiatric practice settings. The demonstration of cost-effective quality outcomes in mental health care will depend on linkages among all components of care in large aggregated data sets. Therefore APRNs should participate in decision-making groups as these clinical and administrative management information systems are being designed, implemented, and evaluated.

Two studies from the nursing literature illustrate the application of evidence-based practice to psychiatric-mental health settings. Dimmitt and Davila (1995) implemented a group psychotherapy intervention for battered women, based on previous research, that studied a survivor-group prototype and battered women's groups. The principles and findings of these studies were substantiated by the major process themes and evaluation results identified in the psychotherapy groups conducted by Dimmitt and Davila. Bergman, Ehrenfeld, and Golander (1995) describe the work of three clinical nurse specialists who implemented research-based practice on six geropsychiatric units. Mini-research groups were formed to study the research findings on several nursing interventions, including the use of dolls as a therapeutic influence on geropsychiatric patients, the impact of interpersonal relationships among patients, and the use of the Jacuzzi bath as a beneficial intervention. After examining existing research findings, interventions were modeled to reflect the evidence base. A 1-year follow up evaluation of the project indicated improved quality of care, increased family involvement, improved self-image and increased critical thinking of nursing personnel, and development of a model for cooperation and collaboration.

In addition to the use of research findings in developing and evaluating advanced practice nursing interventions, the ongoing development of evidence-based practice in psychiatric-mental health nursing relies on the use of evidence-based practice guidelines, such as the AHCPR Guidelines for the management of depression in primary care and metaanalyses of research findings, such as those of the Cochrane Collaboration. The use of practice guidelines is discussed at length in Chapter 12.

The Internet revolution has influenced communication in a way that is as significant as the invention of the telephone. As a specialty founded on basic communication skills, psychiatric-mental health nursing is participating in and benefiting from that revolution. APRNs can use electronic networking to share ideas and information with colleagues around the world and to maintain current knowledge of health care policy, legislation, and the latest government and regulatory agency information. They can easily access multiple databases of psychiatric and mental health information, including scientific literature databases, clinical guidelines, and educational materials. Given the wide range of resources available on-line, APRNs are challenged to sift through potentially relevant material and be aware of the differences in quality of the information found. Warren, Kramer, Hyler, and Kennedy (1997) compare trying to convey the potential of the Internet with "trying to describe what psychotherapy is. It really is something that needs to be experienced rather than described." What is clear is that the potential for the Internet to contribute to advanced practice in psychiatric-mental health nursing is both exciting and challenging. Electronic networking will continue to be an integral part of the experience of advanced practice psychiatric nursing.

RESOURCES AND CONNECTIONS

JOURNALS

Computers in Nursing
Evidence-Based Nursing
International Journal of Medical Informatics

Journal of the American Medical Informatics Association
Medical Library Association Journal

ORGANIZATIONS

American Medical Informatics Association (AMIA): AMIA Nursing Working Group www.gl.umbc.edu/~abbot/nurseinfo.html

American Nurses Association, Council on Nursing Services and Informatics www.nursingworld.org

American Nurses Association, Nursing Information and Data Set Evaluation Center www.nursingworld.org

American Nurses Association, Steering Committee on Databases to Support Clinical Nursing Practice www.nursingworld.org

Medical Library Association, Nursing and Allied Health Resources Section www.library.kent.edu/nahrs

National League for Nursing, Council on Nursing Informatics www.nln.org

References

American Nurses Association. (1976). *Code for nurses with interpretive statements*. Kansas City, MO: the Association.

American Nurses Association. (1994a). *ANA/NOLF CPT utilization survey summary*. Washington, D.C.: American Nurses Publishing.

American Nurses Association. (1994b). *The scope of practice for nursing informatics*. Washington, D.C.: American Nurses Publishing.

American Medical Association. (1996). *Physician's current procedural terminology*. Chicago, IL: the Association.

American Psychiatric Association. (1994a). *Diagnostic and statistical manual of mental disorders* (ed. 4). Washington, D.C.: the Association.

American Psychiatric Association. (1994b). *Quick reference to the diagnostic criteria from DSM-IV*. Washington, D.C.: the Association.

American Psychiatric Association. (1995). *Diagnostic and statistical manual of mental disorders, primary care version*. (ed. 4). Washington, D.C.: the Association.

Bergman, R., Ehrenfeld, M., & Golander, H. (1995). Stimulating research thinking: the case for mini-research. *Journal of Psychosocial Nursing, 33*(7), 34–39.

Carroll-Johnson, R.M., & Paquette, M. (Eds.). (1994). *Classification of nursing diagnoses: proceedings of the tenth conference*. Philadelphia: J.B. Lippincott.

CPT code project. (1997). *APNA News, 9*(6), 6.

Dimmitt, J, & Davila, Y.R. (1995). Group psychotherapy for abused women: a survivor-group prototype. *Applied Nursing Research, 8*, 3–7.

Evidence-Based Medicine Working Group. (1992). Evidence-based medicine: a new approach to teaching the practice of medicine. *JAMA, 268*(17), 2420–2425.

Geddes, J.R., & Harrison, P.J. (1997). Closing the gap between research and practice. *British Journal of Psychiatry, 171*, 220–225.

Gerber, B. (1998). Personal communication.

Griffith, H.M., & Robinson, K.R. (1993). Current Procedural Terminology (CPT) coded services provided by nurse specialists. *Image: Journal of Nursing Scholarship, 25*(3), 178–186.

Guze, B.H. et al. (1996). Databases for clinical psychiatry. *MD Computing, 13*(3), 210–215.

Hughes, S. (1996). Choices of nursing systems. In Mills, M.E.C., Romano, C.A., & Heller, B.R. *Information management in nursing and health care*. Springhouse, PA: Springhouse.

Johnson, M., & Maas, M. (Eds.). (1997). *Nursing outcomes classification (NOC)*. St. Louis: Mosby.

Jones, L.D. (1997). Building the information infrastructure required for managed care. *Image: Journal of Nursing Scholarship, 29*, 377–382.

Lindberg, D.A.B., & Humphreys, B.L. (1995). The UMLS knowledge sources: tools for building better user interfaces. In American Nurses Association. *Nursing data systems: the emerging framework*. Washington, D.C.: American Nurses Publishing.

Martin, K.S., & Norris, J. (1996). The Omaha system: a model for describing practice. *Holistic Nursing Practice, 11*(1), 75–73.

Martin, K.S., & Scheet, N.J. (1995). The Omaha system: nursing diagnoses, interventions and client outcomes. In American Nurses Association. *Nursing data systems: the emerging framework*. Washington, D.C.: American Nurses Publishing.

Martin, K.S., & Scheet, N.J. (1992). *The Omaha system: a pocket guide for community health nursing*. Philadelphia: W.B. Saunders.

McCloskey, J.C., & Bulechek, G.M. (1996). *Nursing interventions classification* (ed. 2). St. Louis: Mosby.

McCormick, K.A., et al. (1994). Toward standard classification schemes for nursing language: recommendations of the American Nurses Association Steering Committee on Databases to Support Clinical Nursing Practice. *Journal of the American Medical Informatics Association, 1*(6), 421–427.

McSwiggan-Hardin, et al. (1997). *The use of two-way interactive telecommunications in mental health care: approach to clinical research*. Paper presented at the annual national conference of the Society for Education and Research in Psychiatric-Mental Health Nursing, Washington, D.C.

National Center for Health Statistics. (1997). *International classification of diseases, ninth revision, clinical modifica-*

tion (ICD-9-CM). Washington, DC: US Government Printing Office.

O'Toole, A.W., & Loomis, M.E. (1989). Revision of the phenomena of concern for psychiatric mental health nursing. *Archives of Psychiatric Nursing, 3*(5), 288–299.

Oxman, A.D., Sackett, D.L., & Guyatt, G.H. (1993). User's guides to the medical literature. I. How to get started. *JAMA, 270*(17), 2093–2095.

Riegelman, R.K., & Hirsch. R.P. (1996). *Studying a study and testing a test: how to read the health science literature* (ed. 3). Boston: Little, Brown, and Co.

Saba, V.K. (1995). Home health care classifications (HHCCs): nursing diagnoses and nursing interventions. In American Nurses Association. *Nursing data systems: the emerging framework*. Washington, D.C.: American Nurses Publishing.

Saba, V.K., & McCormick, K.A. (1996). *Essentials of computers for nurses* (ed. 2). New York: McGraw Hill.

Sackett, D.L., & Rosenberg, W.M.C. (1995). The need for evidence based medicine. *Journal of the Royal Society of Medicine, 88*(11), 620–624.

Sharpe, M., et al. (1996). Psychosomatic medicine and evidence-based treatment. *Journal of Psychosomatic Research, 41*(2),101–107.

Warren, B., et al. (1997). Using the Internet. In Taintor, Z. (Ed.). *Computers, the patient and the psychiatrist: American Psychiatric Press Review of Psychiatry*. Washington, D.C.: American Psychiatric Press.

Warren, J.J., & Hoskins, L.M. (1995). NANDA's nursing diagnosis taxonomy: a nursing database. In American Nurses Association. *Nursing data systems: the emerging framework*. Washington, D.C.: American Nurses Publishing.

Werley, H.H., et al. (1991). The Nursing Minimum Data Set: abstraction tool for standardized, comparable, essential data. *American Journal of Public Health, 81*(4), 421–426.

Werley, H.H., Ryan, P., & Zorn, C.R. (1995). The Nursing Minimum Data Set (NMDS): a framework for the organization of nursing language. In American Nurses Association. *Nursing data systems: the emerging framework*. Washington, D.C.: American Nurses Publishing.

Woolrich, M.L., Felice, M.E., & Drotar, D. (1996). *The classification of child and adolescent mental diagnoses in primary care: diagnostic and statistical manual for primary care (DSM-PC) child and adolescent version*. Elk Grove Village, IL: American Academy of Pediatrics.

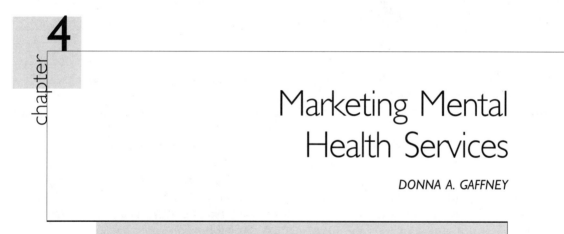

Marketing Mental Health Services

DONNA A. GAFFNEY

■ INTRODUCTION

"The main consideration is the strength of the leader, launch the attack on as narrow a front as possible, and the best defensive strategy is the courage to attack yourself," admonish Reis and Trout (1986). The history of marketing has its roots in the earliest skirmishes and battles of human civilization. Principles of defensive and offensive marketing are solidly grounded in the strategies and games of warfare. In their revolutionary book *Marketing Warfare*, Reis and Trout (1986) compare military strategies with product and service marketing. Their suggestions may seem somewhat intense for the helping professions, but in this time of fierce competition and

limited health care dollars, especially mental health dollars, there is a powerful message to be learned from the battlefields of Marathon, Hastings, and Bunker Hill.

This chapter provides the advanced practice registered nurse (APRN) in psychiatric-mental health care with the necessary tools for developing a marketing plan. Hanging a shingle and waiting for the first phone call is both unrealistic and naive. Although providers hope that the consumer will understand the well-meaning intent of mental health professionals, the reception may be anything but welcoming. In fact, because of the stigma still attached, few people think seeing a mental health professional is necessary, and mental health benefits are often the lowest priority of consumers and purchasers of health insurance plans. As mental health professionals in the era of managed care, the challenge for APRNs is to create the market for services.

The APRN must, therefore, have insight into his or her own practice and the needs of the consumer. The traditional *four Ps of marketing* (product, price, place, and promotion) will be expanded to include public relationships and networking, all of which are critical strategies for educating consumers in the next millennium.

UNDERSTANDING THE ■ PRINCIPLES OF MARKETING

The psychiatric field has long suffered from the stigma of mental illness and emotional distress. It is very difficult to sell the need for mental health services; the assumption is that people are all mentally well and will remain that way no matter what. Therefore effective marketing of mental health services needs an innovative approach combining traditional services with nontraditional outreach.

"Marketing today is not a function; it is a way of doing business. Marketing is not a new ad campaign or this month's promotion. Marketing has to be all-pervasive, part of everyone's job description. It is to integrate the customer into the design of the product and to design a systematic process for interaction that will create substance in the relationship" (McKenna, 1991).

To develop a workable marketing plan, the APRN must be comfortable with the concepts and terminology of the business world. *Marketing* is a business strategy that promotes information about a particular product or service. It combines demographic and sociologic research, strategic planning, product design, pricing policy, advertising, sales promotion, and actual selling (Cunningham, 1982). Perhaps the best known paradigm is the model of marketing as a dynamic process comprised of the four Ps (product, price, place, and promotion) (Kotler, 1976). Box 4-1 defines these principles. To understand the importance of each

box 4-1

THE FOUR Ps OF MARKETING

Product. An intangible service or material good that satisfies a need.
Price. The amount of money a product will cost the consumer.
Place. The location where services or goods can be secured by the consumer.
Promotion. Potentially influential communication of information regarding the goods or services by the seller to the consumer.

of the four Ps, the APRN needs an appreciation for general systems theory. These concepts help explain the success or failure of a marketing plan.

General systems theory is a logical, organized way of viewing various phenomena in the world. First applied to such sciences as mathematics, physics, and engineering in the late 1930s, it was not until the late 1960s that two authors, von Bertalanffy (1968) and Buckley (1967), applied general systems theory to the behavioral sciences. The tenets of general systems theory support the idea that there is a dynamic interaction within multivariable systems (von Bertalanffy, 1968). It is this interaction among the parts, not one singular part, that determines a specific outcome. Very simply put in marketing terms, it is not the product, price, place, or promotion that determines success but the dynamic process that occurs among these elements.

However, there are many challenges for APRNs. Mental health services marketing is severely hampered by the fact that satisfied customers rarely take a public position to promote their experience with psychiatric services. Service testimonials are almost nonexistent in the media, and the use of celebrity acknowledgments extolling the value of such services has only recently emerged in the past decade with testimonies from actors such as Rod Steiger and Patty Duke and the best sellers by Styron (1992) and Jamison (1997).

Barring a few regional differences (and Woody Allen), people do not usually talk openly about their therapists and psychiatrists; nor does the media. Therefore it is important to add another P to the dynamic marketing process: public relationships. This fifth component is more than public relations and service promotion. It includes personal, professional, and community networking and public service efforts that demonstrate the value of mental health services to various target populations.

It is essential for the APRN to clearly identify each area and the related objectives and strategies necessary for success. The marketing plan is the instrument that serves to organize the mental health provider and monitor the practice's progress.

BUILDING A
■ MARKETING PLAN

To understand the elements of a comprehensive marketing plan, it is useful to define the steps in the marketing process. Operationalizing a concept allows the APRN to see each component part as a separate entity, and it also allows visualization of the sequential steps in the process before the APRN executes them. Box 4-2 illustrates how APRNs can operationalize marketing within their practice context.

The steps of the operational definition reflect the elements of the marketing plan: the identification of the mental health service, goals of the practice, identification of the target, design of the service, promotion of the service, goal attainment, and ongoing evaluation of service and strategies. Kennedy (1991) describes the ultimate marketing plan as one that includes thorough research, planning, and sending the right message to the consumer. He also identifies the number one secret weapon called the *unique selling position* (USP). In short, the USP is the way of explaining the APRN's position against the competition (Kennedy, 1991). It identifies the most important benefit of the service to the consumer. The USP can

box 4-2

AN OPERATIONAL DEFINITION OF MARKETING

1. The APRN plans to offer service X.
2. The APRN wants to ensure financial success from the sales of service X.
3. The APRN performs demographic and sociologic research on target population T.
4. The APRN tailors product design and pricing of X to fit needs and preferences of T.
5. The APRN uses business strategies (advertising, networking, and promotion) to convince T to purchase service X.
6. A person in T becomes aware of a need or preference for service X and purchases it.
7. The APRN gains a profit from sales of service X to T.
8. The APRN regularly evaluates service and strategies to maintain and increase future profits from sales of service X.

From Barton, 1998.

address one narrow aspect or subspecialty within the APRN's practice or encompass all services offered. The goal of the USP is to find something unique about the practice that will be undeniably identified solely with the APRN and his or her practice. In Kennedy's book there are sample "think sheets" for developing the marketing plan. It is important to remember that a marketing plan is not a static document but one that changes over time and should be updated at least once a year. A sample page is presented in Box 4-3.

Philosophy of Care and Practice Mission

An APRN's philosophy and values become the foundation for the marketing plan. Professionals often do not consider the importance of this introspective process. It takes time and some journal-keeping to reeducate himself or herself to the goals and ideals of the profession learned in undergraduate and graduate programs. If the APRN is not

box 4-3

THINKING THROUGH THE PRESENTATION OF THE PRODUCT

1. Follow five steps to define your unique selling position:
   a. Explain the needs of your consumer.
   b. Explain the approach or service that fulfills that need.
   c. Explain why your service is the best approach, treatment, etc.
   d. Justify your price.
   e. Gives the reasons your consumer should act now.
2. How can you increase the consumer's interest in your service? List at least five ideas.
3. Set up a call to action.
4. What do you want the consumer to do?

From Kennedy, 1991.

clear in his or her own philosophy, then the consumer will not get the message. The APRN must be passionate about the philosophy, mission, values, and goals of the practice. A philosophy statement is not created or written for the sole purpose of setting up a practice but is inherent in the beliefs and values of the professional itself. Acknowledging the philosophy of the practice and writing a mission statement take time, and in the case of multi-partner practices, many hours where differences are addressed and commonalities are strenghthened. This must be done in the embryonic stages of developing the marketing plan. Elements, definitions, and example components of a marketing plan follow in Table 4-1.

There are general questions that APRNs need to ask themselves when developing the philosophy of the practice. The most important step is to evaluate and analyze their own philosophy of mental health care. How are the causes of mental illness viewed (e.g., from a systems perspective, an analytic approach, or through a psychobiologic lens)? What are the correlating factors of health and illness? How does the provider view treatment

approaches? This is the time for examining their theoretical framework and assessing how it fits with the practice goals the APRNs are trying to establish. The "soul searching" exercise draws upon early influences of people who have shaped their lives and continue to kindle the passion of their work.

Other areas to examine may include more specific mental health objectives. How are health promotion and disease prevention viewed by the APRN? There must be synchrony between values and beliefs of mental health services and measurable mental health objectives. If not, there is a strong possibility that the practice will fail because the goals do not meet the needs or the interests of the professionals. If an APRN is interested in treating illness and generating referrals from other professionals, then establishing a community wellness program will not serve this purpose. Instead this APRN should develop a strong network by meeting with workplace personnel, insurance providers, and primary care providers.

A philosophy of practice may change over time. Experience, education, and new findings shape the way a professional views the human condition. Certainly the biggest influence on mental health services in the past decade has been the psychopharmacology revolution. This has forced APRNs and other professionals to seek more education, redefine their practices, or set up collaborative relationships. Primary care has also gained much popularity among all health care providers. More primary care physicians are diagnosing and treating psychiatric illnesses. Several studies have cited the growing need to diagnose and treat mental illness within the primary care population (Kroenke et al, 1994). In fact, physical complaints are often somatoform in presentation and indicate that there may be psychiatric issues to consider as well as physical causes. Another question the mental health professional must address relates to prevention: Do people deserve support and guidance through life crises, and with such interventions are different outcomes achievable? Finally, the advent of alternative or complementary thera-

table 4-1

BUILDING THE FOUNDATION OF THE MARKETING PLAN

FOUNDATIONAL ELEMENT	DEFINITION	EXAMPLE
Statement of philosophy	A clear declaration of the practice's approach to mental health services (holistic, family, analytic, systems)	WellBeing Associates believes that mental health services are best delivered in a holistic manner, treating physical, psychosocial, and spiritual elements of the human experience within the context of the family.
Mission statement	A statement of how and what services the APRN intends to offer and to whom (the function of the practice)	WellBeing Associates will provide supportive as well as therapeutic services to all members of the family in a comprehensive and efficient manner.
Values held by the practice	A declaration by the practice that establishes its support of and belief in those aspects of the human experience deemed the most worthy, desirable, and important	WellBeing Associates believes that a family's emotional health is the foundation of family life and is critical to the well-being of each family member.
Purpose	A statement of intent by the APRN practice	WellBeing Associates will assist families as they deal with developmental milestones, situation crises, and relationship difficulties through comprehensive services focusing on improved communication, support, and education.
Goals	A specific aim of the practice (there is usually more than one goal)	WellBeing Associates will assist young women in transition from family to college life.
Objectives	Specific, measurable, identifiable courses of action that are necessary to achieve the stated goals (there may be 1 to 3 objectives for each goal)	WellBeing Associates will offer group sessions for young women entering first year of college.
Tasks	Distinct activities that are necessary to meet the objectives and will provide the criteria for the evaluation plan	WellBeing Associates will 1) identify critical issues and coping needed for this transition period, 2) recruit 12 women, 17 to 20 years old, 3) advertise through mail and newspapers, 4) hold eight sessions (attendance recorded), 5) evaluate group for content and effectiveness, and 6) revise the group treatment plan as needed.

pies and the focus on a holistic approach integrating mind and body is increasingly accepted by many health disciplines and will most likely merge with more traditional practices.

The mission statement tells the consumer what the APRN plans to do. It is based on the philosophies, values, and beliefs of every person in that practice or agency. Simply stated, the mission is the assignment to be carried out. Regardless of whether the practice will generate written materials for service promotion, defining the mission of the practice and publishing a mission statement is just as important for the professional as it is for the consumer. Writing the mission statement usually involves multiple brainstorming sessions and numerous drafts. Box 4-4 outlines several questions that the APRN can explore as the mission statement evolves.

---

box 4-4

DEVELOPMENT OF A COMPREHENSIVE MISSION STATEMENT

1. What motivates the APRN to provide this service?
2. Is the practice willing to let the mission evolve, grow over time, and change with the practice?
3. What are the goals of the practice? What does the practice or APRN want to do or provide?
4. What does the practice or APRN want to be to the consumer?

HINTS TO FACILITATE THE PROCESS

- Look to those who are admired in the mental health professions as well as other professions or businesses. Identify their philosophies.
- Read mission and goal statements of other provider groups, organizations (specifically non-profit organizations), hospitals, and clinics.

The values of the practice are those entities found worthy, important, and useful to the promotion, maintenance, and restoration of mental health. In addition, values can incorporate standards that are deemed desirable to the practice as well as the consumer. For example, the practice of the APRN may value an individual family's time, either at home or at work, and therefore arrange hours of operation to avoid any conflict with family activities. This evidences a consumer focus. However, this requires the APRNs to work hours that may not be conducive to their own family life. Keeping a balance between personal need and responsiveness to consumers and patients is a continuing struggle for many APRNs.

Goals and Objectives

The goals and objectives are the most specific elements of the marketing plan. The goals are broader and usually long-term in nature. The goal of a women's mental health practice may be to promote the mental health of postpartum women. The objectives are the means by which the practice will achieve the goals, the so-called "steps" to the long-term goal. Several objectives for this women's service may include 1) establishing contact with all new mothers in a hospital, 2) providing an opportunity for new mothers to meet each other, 3) identifying needs of new mothers, and 4) offering services based on the needs of new families. Goals are all-encompassing and are founded on the practice's philosophy that there are certain factors that influence the mental health of postpartum women. The objectives are measurable and observable. They also have specific tasks that are developed to measure the achievement of the objective. These tasks are critical to measuring quality and overall clinical effectiveness and overall outcomes.

■ MARKET RESEARCH

In health care, market research is often referred to as a *needs assessment* or *feasibility study* identifying what the consumer needs, how those services are best delivered, and in what form the service will be most used by the consumer. APRNs may assume that a consumer needs or desires a particular product or service without really researching the market to find out if this is true. Whether the product is mental health services or a new restaurant, most market data can be found in public, university, or hospital libraries, community and government offices, the census bureau, and on the Internet (Pinson & Jinnett, 1996).

Identifying the needs of a community may have a significant influence on the kinds of services a practice or agency decides to offer, whether they are new or already existing in the community. The APRN must identify the kinds of mental health services that will best support the target community. It is imperative to complete the assessment well in advance of selecting the office site.

Target Market

The target market provides information on the needs of prospective consumers. It also describes their characteristics and how they might use mental health services. At first this important research step is used to determine ideal office or agency location. Eventually, the assessment will facilitate service promotion as well as discovering new referral sources.

The most important assessment information is derived from collecting demographic data. Demographics include age (and age distribution in the population); gender; ethnic, cultural, and religious background; educational experiences; occupation; income; developmental or family status; and geographic location. All of this information can be obtained from census reports. It is also possible to approach local or community governments for real estate values and school district data. The best place to start is the public library where reference personnel can either provide the documents needed for the information or refer the market researcher to other sources. Developing the profile for the ideal consumer is a critical step in opening a practice or starting a specific program. For example, if a new postpartum depression-prevention program is going to be offered by a particular agency, locating the program at a site populated by senior citizens or young singles would not attract consumers who might benefit from such a program.

Schools and colleges are another source of prospective consumers. All schools should be identified, from preschool to college, in the geographic area to be served by the agency. Know the right questions to ask school administrators. Start at the library before querying anyone in person. The town hall in the community also has school information. School boards can provide details about schools as well. High schools publish reports that describe their students and the courses of study in their school. This information is traditionally sent to colleges with admission applications but is available to anyone who would like a copy. These documents also contain standardized scores, types of courses, and how the students compare with other schools in the state and in the country. However, it is critical to remember that it is not just the student body that may require mental health services but faculty members and families as well.

The developmental needs of the community are sometimes termed *family status* (Pinson & Jinnett, 1996). Each phase of individual growth and development and/or family stage requires different services and approaches to delivering those services. A family with young children is more likely to use mental health services if there is drop-in childcare and prevention programs addressing child development and parenting skills. Families in mid-life may be struggling with caring for older parents as well as dealing with adolescent or college-bound children. The geriatric population is more likely to be facing issues related to loss and retirement. It is necessary to understand the consumer and target a particular group for the APRN's services. A sample worksheet is presented in Box 4-5. It is a clear and simple means of describing the target market and identifying its needs.

box **4-5**

TARGET MARKET WORKSHEET

1. Who are the customers (patients/clients)?
   a. Economic level
   b. Lifestyle and psychological make-up
   c. Age range
   d. Gender
   e. Income level
   f. Buying habits
2. Where are the customers located?
   a. Where do they live?
   b. Where do they work?
   c. Where do they shop (obtain health care)?
3. What is the projected size of the market (patients/clients per year)?
4. What are the needs of the patients/clients?
5. How can this practice meet those needs?
6. What is unique about this practice?

Adapted from Pinson & Jinnett, 1996.

Sources of Referrals

Cultural, ethnic, and religious considerations can change a marketing strategy. APRNs need to understand the population and the community. They must learn as much as possible about the various ethnic or cultural groups, languages, habits, and religions and how the particular population perceives mental health and illness. If possible, the APRN should find someone in the community who can talk about traditions, health rituals, and taboos and cultivate an ongoing relationship with this person. The APRN can determine if counseling services are provided by clergy (ministers, rabbis, etc.). Pastoral counselors need formal mental health resources if issues escalate or crises develop.

Organizations and other agencies are also sources of referrals. Hospitals, clinics, and other primary health organizations will want to add the APRN's name to their list of referrals. Identifying the competition and locating other providers of mental health services are also important. Businesses may have workplace programs and refer their employees for services. Employee Assistance Program (EAP) personnel often recognize the need for additional mental health professional resources for brief psychotherapy referrals.

Other sources are less traditional but may be just as important as those listed previously. Women's resource centers have already found their own target market and may be valuable for services addressing women's issues. The Young Women's Christian Association (YWCA), Young Women's Hebrew Association (YWHA), Young Men's Christian Association (YMCA), and Young Men's Hebrew Association (YMHA) include virtually every segment of the population. In addition to being a source of referrals, the Ys are also potential program sites for public service offerings and physical advertising space. Community groups and clubs can provide additional access to consumers. All of this information can be found in the yellow pages of the local telephone book.

Law enforcement, the local and state police departments, children's services, and the judicial system (family court) may provide still more opportunities to define services and find potential consumers. Often there are court-mandated evaluations and treatment for juvenile offenders and their families. By contacting the department of social services in the community, the APRN may receive more information on becoming a referral source.

APRNs need to investigate hot lines, help lines, rape crisis centers, child abuse advocacy centers, and domestic violence safe houses. The best way to become acquainted with any of these crisis services is to meet with a director or board member. It is important to determine the rate of calls and referrals they receive each month and annually. Understanding seasonal variations is the key to the APRN's scheduling of services and programs. One rape crisis program was located in a community with five colleges and two junior colleges. During the summer when school was not in session, the rate of sexual assault and need for follow-up services was virtually nonexistent. However, with the first fraternity party in the fall semester, the incidence of reported rape soared. This is important information for two reasons: 1) outreach to crisis centers and hospital emergency departments; and 2) prevention programs in colleges and college health services. These sources are especially crucial during a student's freshman year.

Surveying potential consumers and community groups can be done by telephone or questionnaire or by reviewing annual reports. Telephone interviews with administrators in community institutions may be difficult to schedule. Mailed questionnaires generally take too long and have a low return rate. It might be possible to meet a representative from the organization who can offer background information. The APRN should keep a journal of important contacts during this survey process; it will be valuable later for networking. Keeping an electronic contact database will serve the APRN well in the long-term.

As a provider of mental health services, the APRN will want to know who pays for services in the area, the most popular plans used, and the types of coverage (benefits, annual and lifetime caps, etc.). If there is a large corporation in the community, a call to the personnel or human resources office will identify insurance coverage plans for employees.

Mental health professionals may decide to segment their total market. Engelberg and Neubrand (1997) define *market segmentation* as the process of dividing up a health care organization's total market into smaller groups based on similar needs and defining characteristics. Some forms of segmentation are based on demographics, regional or geographic variations, or behavioral or utilization factors. The organization then chooses to target each of those subgroups at a different time or in a different manner. Sometimes the APRN will be tempted to target the largest segment; however, it may be more prudent to start with a smaller segment and approach it as a "pilot" for the practice.

PLACE: ACCESS TO SERVICES ■ AND SERVICE DELIVERY

In real estate the familiar adage is "Location, location, location!" Consider where the agency, office, or program is situated in the community. Determine if the office or agency is in a residential, corporate, or commercial area. There is great value to a walking or driving tour of the area; the APRN can appreciate the community as an inhabitant instead of as a visitor. The image and reputation of the area, the physical appearance of the building itself, and its proximity to other services and facilities are critical to the ultimate success or failure of a practice. The physical plant's readiness for patients with disabilities (or "ADA compliance") may also be important.

In one study on adolescent depression, the researchers learned that teens referred for mental health services would not follow through if there was an office within the confines of the school building itself. In another community, mental health agencies requiring public transportation or a car ride were also underutilized by high school students. The most successful agency was located one block from the high school in a building with a variety of services and allowed students to come for information on their own, without a referral. It is not difficult to see the varying responses to these well-meaning programs. A school-based office that is used solely for mental health services will not attract students because they will try to avoid being noticed by their peers. One school in which the program failed made the mistake of painting a sign on the door, "Substance Abuse Counselor." However, school-based clinics are somewhat different; they usually offer a variety of health-related services. Students feel comfortable and develop relationships with the staff who can refer them to the in-house mental health provider.

Easy and accessible transportation, free or very reasonable parking, and an office hours schedule that has variety (customer-focused) will help make the practice flourish. The APRN should consider the characteristics of the target market: the location of their homes and workplace, the mode and length of their daily commute to and from work, and family status.

In addition to geographic location and accessibility factors, the APRN must consider the image of the office space and waiting area. The physical environment is the first thing the consumer will see and should evoke a positive response. Overcoming a negative physical space takes time. No matter how effective the APRN is in providing services, a negative space makes establishing a trusting relationship difficult.

The APRN assesses the impact of physical space on the senses:

- How does sound, both inside and outside of the space, enhance or distract the consumer? Sound can be a critical factor in how welcome the consumer feels. The use of white noise or other sound-producing machines is very popular. Such equipment can be purchased in a variety of stores for a very reasonable price. However, the APRN should not be tempted to install a television in the waiting room. This is the time for patients to focus on themselves, not to succumb to the distractions of game shows or all-news networks.
- Is there natural light or artificial lighting? Professionals can invest in full-spectrum lighting (bulbs are available for fixtures), which has been shown to promote a sense of well-being and act as natural sunlight. Fluorescent lighting is not an ideal choice because it is hard on the eyes, flickers, and may emit high frequency sounds.
- What is the smell or scent of the space? Should the APRN consider aromatherapy?
- Is the space comfortable, well maintained, and clean?
- Some colors are more comforting than others. What is the influence of color on the psyche?
- Comfortable furniture that is pleasing to the eye and the touch for both the professional and the consumer is important. Upholstered furniture sends a message of safety and allows the consumer to "settle in"; wooden or contemporary design chairs may appear cold and uncom-

fortable. If the APRN is offering a program or new service for a group of people, he or she must be sure there are enough chairs with extras readily available.

There are additions that the APRN can add to the physical setting of a practice. Often they are relatively inexpensive but perceived as extremely thoughtful on the part of the provider. The APRN should give consideration to the age and development of the consumers to be served. If there are children, placing child-oriented items, toys, games, and books in the waiting room as well as in the office will be appreciated. However, the APRN must think about the adults who bring the children for this service, and the environment must appeal to them as well. Current books and magazines (light reading as well as more serious publications) should be available for every age group. The most important point to remember about providing publications is to keep them current. Nothing should be more than 2 weeks old.

Symbols of growth, personal rejuvenation, and healing frequently come in the form of living things such as plants, flowers, and wildlife. In one practice the APRN brought a bouquet of fresh seasonal flowers to her office every week. She stated that the flowers were as much for her as for her patients; she enjoyed the colors and delicate fragrance they brought to her university office. Using plants and other greenery is also possible, but they must look healthy and flourishing. It is disconcerting for the patient to see dying plants starving for water and light. If artificial greens or flowers are used, the APRN should do so sparingly and with the best quality that the practice can afford. They should also be kept clean.

Market research is a rigorous, time-consuming process. However, upon completion of this intensive work, the APRN has focused on what is needed (the product or service), who needs it (the target market), and where it should be located (the place). The goal of market research is to answer the question, "Why will my mental health services fulfill a need or solve the problem?" Without adequate assessment information, the APRN is operating on a best-guess approach or meeting his or her own needs and not those of potential patients and the community.

■ PRICE: VALUE OF SERVICES

MacStravic (1997) reports that "while there is wide agreement on the importance of value, there are a wide variety of definitions." In the marketing arena, value is defined as quality for the cost of services. Value can also be understood as the net outcome of the positive versus negative effects consumers experience from using services. In health care the values of quality, peace of mind, reliability, access, breadth of service, and compassion are essential considerations for the consumer (MacStravic, 1997). "By looking for and finding ways to increase the value they offer, providers can avoid the all-too-obvious and self-defeating approach of reducing price" (MacStravic, 1997). When establishing fees for services, the APRN should keep MacStravic's words in mind. The price for service must be fair and consistent with the going rate in the community and in the geographic region. The APRN needs to find out what is customary and reasonable, then add value to his or her services. Readily accessible services and immediate appointment scheduling are two examples of how value can be added. For the consumer these benefits can translate into a savings of time, money, and effort. If the mental health professional is relocating from another region, he or she may take into account regional economic variations (e.g., APRNs may not be able to charge San Francisco fees in rural Idaho).

Extraordinary changes in health care financing and reimbursement have left both consumers and providers frustrated. Often mental health services are not reimbursable or are under-reimbursed. The new practice will have to find innovative strategies for its patients. The providers may consider as many third party payment options as possible. Credit cards and bank cards are an accepted way of life for many health care agencies. Flexible pay-

ment plans with a sliding scale based on income may also prove to be valuable. Another strategy is to consider creative packaging of sessions by organizing series payment plans (e.g., a series of five sessions at a 10% discount). Early payment incentives can also help the practice; that is, consumers who pay at the time of services or prepay will get a discount.

No matter how many options an APRN chooses to offer, all payment systems must be operational as soon as the doors open. Consider the case of one practice run by a nurse practitioner. They started to advertise and had many phone calls inquiring about their services. The practice intended to participate in ten plans, but only three were in place when they opened their doors for business. Potential clients were lost when they called for appointments and learned their health insurance was not yet accepted. Impatience will only lead to false starts, ultimately damaging the budding reputation of the agency or practice.

PROMOTION: COMMUNICATIONS ■ AND PUBLICITY

Getting the message out to potential patients is a necessary step in the marketing process. However, if the right product is not offered to the right target population, in the right place, and at the right price, the best promotional strategies will fail. Alward and Camunas (1990) identify eight categories of promotional strategies. Five of them specifically focus on communications: written materials, audio-visual material, corporate identity, media, and the news.

No matter what type of strategy is used, the message must be clear to the listener or reader. The most important goal is to identify the provider with the service. APRNs should use caution in choosing the name of the group or agency and try to avoid using clever or trendy names for the practice. For a group practice they may consider incorporating the name of the town, neighborhood, or street. Individual practices may use the name of the APRN.

Identification of the services' distinguishing qualities helps separate it from the competition and promote name recognition. APRNs must be aware of biases and stigma related to the mental health field and particularly how they may be interpreted by members of the community in which the practice is located. They should avoid words that may cause a negative response from the reader or viewer. There is a delicate balance between engaging the consumer with unbiased language that clearly describes the service and terminology more particular to psychiatry. In fact, more clinical vocabulary may drive the consumer away. The term *psychotherapy* may be perceived as a more intense, threatening word than *counseling*. Identifying specific issues and concerns or promoting mental wellness may be less provocative than listing treatment programs in some markets. APRNs should avoid assuming that the audience knows the value of mental health services. The message must clearly state why this service is important. At the same time, APRNs must be careful to not falsely advertise or exaggerate the benefits of their services.

Written Communication

Written communication and publications must have reader appeal. Letters and pamphlets should not have text only. The designer should consider a logo or a type font that will be identified with the service. Use of color, texture, and layout encourages the reader to take notice. A clear typeface that is easy to read conveys comfort, warmth, and support. When designing written materials the APRN should ask others for their reactions. One way is to invite a "focus group" to respond to the images they see. What is the message, feeling, or ambiance conveyed? The APRN cannot rely solely on professional designers, graphic artists, or printing companies. He or she should get feedback from other mental health professionals, referral sources, and consumers. It may help to examine the written communications of competitors, determining what is appealing or what represents the philosophy of practice.

Visual images, whether art or photography, convey the strongest, most powerful message. The use of a variety of materials (brochures, fold-over notes, postcards, business cards, and stationery) and the use of materials that carry the same images enhances the marketing campaign. However, the design should be classic and uncomplicated: solid figures or silhouettes should be used for artwork and black and white for photographs. (Color photography is prohibitively expensive.) When trying to sell mental health services, close-up facial expressions convey compassion and support in a much more sensitive fashion. For example, one agency was starting a new program for parents coping with sibling rivalry after the birth of a new child. The practice group used a black and white photograph of a young child holding an infant. It was a close-up shot allowing the audience to see both the smiling face of the older child, arms cradling the newborn, and the angelic look on the baby's face. The picture represented the wish for sibling harmony in every new parent.

The ink and the color of the paper should complement each other; light gray paper and off-white or cream colored paper are very effective with black ink. A second color ink should only be used for small accented areas in the material but will increase the cost. APRNs should avoid the use of trendy colors or gold or silver accents or logos that could appear to be a gimmick. The goal is to increase practice recognition. The APRN may want to consider a caption or brief statement to further define the message. Listing services on one side of a tri-fold brochure will tell the reader what is available in an easy-to-read format.

Language must be clear and brief. Reading levels are a significant factor in written materials when it is important to appeal to the broadest audience. In fact, most newspapers are written on a seventh grade reading level. Language that is too sophisticated may alienate important parts of the market. Personal success stories and quotes common in other product or service endorsements may be difficult to integrate into the body of an article without divulging confidentiality. Monthly newsletters and other periodical publications provide opportunities for service promotion. Mental health practices and agencies may want to develop their own newsletter for the public.

Distribution of written materials can be accomplished in several ways. Although mailing is the most expensive, it is also the most reliable. Placing written material in an envelope will help distinguish it from the daily "junk" mail that postal customers receive. When promoting a new service or program, consider using a postcard with a black and white photograph on one side and a brief message on the other side. The process of developing mailing lists and a professional resource guide is ongoing but may serve many market needs and will reinforce the establishment of the mental health practice within the community. When sending letters of introduction to other professionals and community organizations, the APRN must include a business card with name and services clearly identified. This allows the recipient to throw away the letter but file the business card. When referrals are made, the APRN should be sure to have the staff develop a system to recognize and thank all referral sources.

Written materials can also be distributed through other programs and agencies with similar goals that complement the practice. There is generally no charge for dropping brochures with these other organizations. For example, locations and related programs for distributing literature on parenting programs and services can include but are not limited to pediatric primary care services, children's specialty stores, gyms, daycare or child care centers, nursery schools, and church or synagogue newsletters.

Telecommunications

When setting up the practice's telecommunications system, the APRN must think very carefully about how telephone calls will be answered. The telephone call is the first contact the prospective consumer has with the service provider. It should be considered the practice's "front door," and as such, be attractive to the customer and easy to "open." Consumer preferences for reaching providers may vary from region to region, and the APRN should consider building questions addressing this area in the market research plan.

Most consumers do not like a menu-driven voice mail system. Often people try to bypass the options and speak to a "real person." In a profession where compassion, empathy, and personal relationships are the cornerstone of success, disembodied voices do not do much to promote the APRN's service. If a voice mail system is used, it must be the APRNs' own voice delivering the message, and it must always give an option for emergency contact through a pager or emergency telephone number. It is important for the staff to test the system before opening the practice and regularly to test system performance.

Communication "glitches" in the early stages of a therapeutic relationship will do much to undermine the establishment of trust. In addition, the APRN should be sure all calls are returned by the same evening. The system should be relatively simple, with only a few options. In a group practice the options should be for the different providers. Even if a receptionist is available during office hours, an answering system is necessary for times when the office is closed. Use of an answering service is not recommended because these tend to be groups of operators who receive batched calls from many different professional groups. When orienting new patients, the APRN should be sure to tell them how the office works so there will be no surprises. The practice may even want to develop a brochure or flyer detailing how to communicate with the APRNs.

Telephone accessibility is an important part of promoting the services available from a provider. Telephone numbers should be easy to remember. However, it may not be helpful to use the device of assigning a name or word to your number such as, 555-HELP. In addition to being somewhat unprofessional, the telephone "word," though easy to remember, is difficult to dial. The touchpad on a telephone has the letters printed in much smaller type than the numbers, and it is easy to dial a wrong number.

Toll-free numbers have been used for mail-order businesses for many years. The consumer relies on easy, cost-free accessibility of a toll-free number for many businesses and services. The APRN opening a practice or initiating a new service may want to consider adding a toll-free number. Most major telecommunications carriers offer very reasonable rates including a small monthly fee with additional charges for incoming calls. A toll-free number is assigned by the telephone company and then feeds into an already existing line in the office. Although most people use mental health services in their own local calling area, there have been many changes in telecommunications. Increased numbers of cellular phones, additional area codes (sometimes three in the same city), and practices that cross state and county lines may warrant installation of a toll-free number. The goal is to make it as easy as possible for the consumer to reach the APRN.

Electronic communications and the Internet are undoubtedly the wave of the future. Agencies and groups may want to explore creating their own website. The design and text of the website should reflect the philosophy and mission of the practice. Brief articles providing helpful information for Internet surfers and links to other sites will be very useful. Registering the domain name (the name of the website) is a relatively easy process that is not very expensive. Maintenance of the website is also reasonable averaging one or two dollars a day. However, the design and layout of the website can become expensive (anywhere from $1000 to $5000), especially if it is very complicated and has "moving" or interactive parts in the site. A chat room and an advice column are not recommended since there have been legal challenges with medical professionals prescribing and treating over the Internet.

APRNs may want to incorporate electronic mail (e-mail) and listservs into their practices. E-mail is becoming increasingly popular in all segments of society, but the professional may choose to use it for communicating with other colleagues only. A listserv is an electronic mailing list that can be updated and sent to recipients on a regular basis. In most cases the purpose of such a listing is to provide informational updates. For example, Kid Beat, offered by The Casey Center for Children and Families at the University of Maryland School of Journalism, is sent to recipients each week with national news on programs, policies, and the newest research developments related to all aspects of child and family welfare. Originally designed for journalists, increasing numbers of child and family professionals are subscribing to this service.

The agency or APRN may want to subscribe to these services as well as develop such an approach for organizations and community groups that are potential referral sources. Information could include citations of professional articles worth reading, governmental or reimbursement news, and policy changes. The message to other professionals and groups in the community is that this practice is a current and valuable resource. Once a listserv is established it can be maintained at a reasonable cost.

Television and radio advertising for mental health services is an expensive and high-risk venture. It is far better to receive publicity and television exposure about a new program or project.

■ PUBLIC RELATIONSHIPS

The fifth "P" of marketing, public relationships, builds upon two related concepts: community involvement and public service, the outreach strategies for building a practice. Mental health service marketing is hindered by public opinions of mental health and illness. In addition, consumers are less likely to rave about psychiatric-mental health treatment than they would about other less threatening, more acceptable and visible services. There is also a sense of the patient not wanting to divulge his or her own therapist because the patient may want to keep the therapist for himself or herself.

Professionals marketing mental health services must work to change these images and stereotypes. One very effective way to work toward this goal is to give the public a sample of the APRN's skills and approaches. In essence, the APRN is providing a sample of services. In one television news program, a nurse practitioner-based practice was featured. A nurse practitioner was featured talking to patients, performing assessments, and providing patient education. The audience was able to see her in action; they liked the sound of her voice and her mannerisms, the way she informed and educated the patient and never minimized any concern. This resulted in almost 100 telephone calls over the next week requesting that specific provider's services.

Professionals do not always need a television program to showcase their expertise. They can provide a sample of services on local, state, and national levels. One easy method is to offer a lecture, brief class, or presentation on an issue-focused topic. One APRN with years of experience advises that "when you do something for free, you will receive its benefits about 6 months later." The theory seems to be true. At the very least, word-of-mouth will follow. Professionals can easily provide educational programs in community, adult schools, resource centers, elementary and secondary schools, colleges, senior citizen housing, and workplace settings.

It is important for APRNs to get to know and participate in the community in which their practice is located. A good place to start is the Chamber of Commerce. The practice will be exposed to the goals of the community at large, as well as those who make their living as merchants or service providers. In addition to providing excellent contacts, membership in the Chamber of Commerce promotes a feeling of good will because the practice will be an interested and contributing member of the business community.

Meeting community leaders is necessary to understand and acknowledge their issues. Alward and Camunas (1990) suggest that good will is enhanced by giving time and money to good causes. The professionals in a practice or agency may not be able to financially support an organization, but they can donate time, effort, and expertise through a speaker's bureau or participate in development committees. The practice or agency must be a good citizen in the community. Although the benefits of these efforts may not pay off immediately, there will be long-term benefits and positive growth in the area of public relations.

■ NETWORKING

Building relationships and connections is essential to the growth and success of any business or practice. The old saying, "It is not what you know, but who you know" has a great deal of truth behind it. The concept that underlies that statement is *networking*. Michelli and Straw (1997) identify four different network types: personal, organizational, professional, and strategic. As the APRN begins the journey of establishing a practice and marketing services, there will be many individuals along the way who will provide information, support, guidance, and contacts. In addition some networks may be influential, providing access to a previously closed system and offering mentorship and advocacy along the way (Michelli & Straw, 1997). Individuals in these networks will be immensely helpful. They can help the APRN save time, avoid mistakes, and ensure long-term success. However, networks do not just appear; they take work and a conscious effort to cultivate and expand.

Michelli and Straw (1997) offer a five-step plan to use networking in every aspect of life:

1. *Recognizing and mapping networks.* The APRN identifies the people who inhabit each type of network (personal, organizational, etc.) and looks for overlap and links.
2. *Assessment of networking style.* These styles can be a conscious, goal directed approach; an intuitive approach where individuals seem to know people in every part of their lives; or an open approach dedicated to future development.
3. *Clarifying goals.* The APRN identifies which of the purposes is the most important goal. It is likely that the APRN will need individuals in

each of the areas of information, support, development, and influence.

4. *Development and enhancement of networking behaviors.* This step is crucial once the APRN has named those who will be most helpful in this new network. The "unwritten code of ethics" for good networking practice includes open-mindedness, keeping commitments, treating others as one wishes to be treated, freely asking questions and seeking advice, giving without exception, and expressing appreciation.

5. *Securing benefits.* The APRN ensures balance, creates visibility, and increases employability through network building.

EVALUATING THE
■ MARKETING PLAN

Evaluation is an ongoing process that should be integrated into every aspect of planning for services. The APRN must prepare a time frame for evaluation activities and stick to it. If necessary, a re-survey of the community may be required to update changing trends and target interests. Restructuring the service, pricing, location, and promotional strategies may result from new information learned during the evaluation process. When results are not as expected, the APRN should not view it as a failure but as an opportunity to change.

In addition to evaluating the marketing plan it is imperative to determine the quality and effectiveness of the services provided. It is far better to identify deficiencies in the practice before the patient population begins to diminish. Measuring clinical effectiveness can be accomplished through several mechanisms. However, the goals and objectives of the practice will provide the template upon which the evaluation program is based (Stuart, Reynolds, & Spencer, 1991). The first question to be raised asks whether the practice did what it set out to do by the dates established in the marketing plan. How satisfied were the patients? Did patients get better? How many complaints were recorded? Did the number of sessions remain constant given the same diagnosis? What were the utilization trends? What were the recidivism rates? What was the rate of referrals? Is the rate of referrals increasing or decreasing? APRNs should not be afraid to ask the patient population if they are satisfied. Brief patient surveys for individuals and families will not only inform the APRN if services are effective but may also provide new knowledge to guide and revise practice initiatives.

IMPLICATIONS FOR
■ THE FUTURE

With the ascendancy of the business orientation to the delivery of mental health services, APRNs will have to apply the principles and strategies of marketing in many aspects of their daily practice. They will have to learn more sophisticated ways of showcasing their distinctive niche in providing quality, cost-effective services in a field crowded with other mental health discipline competitors. Whether they work in a private group practice, community mental health center, or managed behavioral healthcare organization, APRNs will have to incorporate an entrepreneurial spirit into their approach to marketing their expertise to patient populations, providers, mental health organizations, and the community.

It may seem that the APRN needs to master an overwhelming amount of information to successfully market advanced practice services. The APRN might find it helpful to record what he or she is doing and learning at every step of establishing the practice. By keeping a journal and accurate records, it will be easier to retrace steps, find key information, and monitor progress. Other ways to develop the necessary skills include doing self-tutorials by reading professional and trade journals and books, accessing an experienced mentor, doing an internship in an innovative company, pursuing various educational programs, and conducting research.

Formal education and continuing education will become important sources of learning the latest developments in marketing and general business practices, as well as the skills and techniques related to good public relations and customer-friendly services. Graduate programs in nursing are connecting with MBA programs to offer courses and certificate programs to meet the needs of those now seeking master's degrees and those who are interested in post-master's study. Continuing education workshops and programs offered by professional organizations and companies that specialize in nursing, business, and other related fields are trying to capitalize on the need for knowledge and skills of health care professionals who are working in competitive health care markets. There are also fertile areas for market and clinical research. Studying the links between sound business practices and customer satisfaction and improved clinical outcomes will lead to best practices. Marketing is not only about developing and maintaining a practice; it is also about progress and growth for the patient, the provider, and the profession.

RESOURCES AND CONNECTIONS

BOOKS AND ARTICLES

Baber, A., & Waymon, L. (1994). *Great connections: small talk and networking for businesspeople.* Manassas, VA: Impact.

Bangs, D., Jr. (1992). *Creating customers.* Chicago: Upstart Publishing.

Bangs, D. (1995). *The market planning guide* (ed. 4). Chicago: Upstart Publishing Co.

Berk, R., & Rossi, P. (1990). *Thinking about program evaluation.* Newbury Park, CA: Sage Publications.

Blanchard, K., & Bowles, S. (1993). *Raving fans: a revolutionary approach to customer service.* New York: William Morrow, Inc.

Bly, R. (1991). *Selling your services.* New York: Henry Holt.

Husch, T., & Foust, L. (1987). *That's a great idea.* Berkeley, CA: Ten Speed Press.

Kelly, F., & Kelly, H. (1986). *What they really teach you at the Harvard Business School.* New York: Warner Books.

Sandhusen, R. (1987). *Marketing.* Happuage, NY: Barron's Educational Series.

Stubblefield, C. (1997). Persuasive communication: marketing health promotion. *Nursing Outlook, 45*(4), 173–177.

Young, W. (1988). *Copyright law: what you don't know can hurt you.* San Juan Capistrano, CA: Joy Publishing.

FEDERAL RESOURCES

U.S. Census Bureau
Public Information Office
US Department of Commerce
Washington, DC 20233
301-457-4100
Fax: 301-457-4714
www.census.gov

U.S. Copyright Office
Library of Congress
101 Independence Avenue, SE
Washington, DC 20559–6000
202-707-3000 (Information)
202-707-9100 (Forms and requests)
lcweb.loc.gov/copyright

U.S. Small Business Administration
Small Business Answer Desk
PO Box 46521
Denver, CO 80201-0030
800-827-5722
www.sbaonline.sba.gov

ASSOCIATIONS AND ORGANIZATIONS

American Management Association International
1601 Broadway
New York, NY 10019-7420
212-586-8100
Fax: 212-903-8168
www.amanet.org

American Marketing Association
250 Wacker Drive, Suite 200
Chicago, IL 60606
312-648-0536 or 800-AMA-1150
Fax: 312-993-7542
www.ama.org

The Direct Marketing Association
1120 Avenue of the Americas
New York, NY 10036
212-768-7277
www.the-dma.org

National Foundation for Women Business Owners
1010 Wayne Avenue, Suite 830
Silver Springs, MD 20910-5603
301-495-4975
Fax: 301-495-4979

LIBRARY RESOURCES

Bacon's Newspaper/Magazine Directory
City and County Data Book
Dun and Bradstreet Directories
Encyclopedia of Associations
Small Business Sourcebook
American Demographics

WEBSITES AND ELECTRONIC RESOURCES

Creative Eye Web Publishing
Small business resources: Legal information of all
kinds, searchable library of articles, finding a lawyer,
and much more.
(www.cyquest.com/design/resources.html)

The Casey Center for Children and Families
University of Maryland School of Journalism
A weekly listserv, KIDBEAT, compiling the latest re-
search, resources, and programs for and about chil-
dren and families.
Stacey Relkin, Research Director
8701-B Adelphi Road
Adelphi, MD 20783
Phone: 301-445-9534
Fax: 301-445-9659
E-mail: Stacey_Relkin@casey.umd.edu
(casey.umd.edu)

Small business resources

The Small Business Journal
Links to small business resources (organizations and
associations, tax-related resources, government resources, and how to locate businesses)
(www.tsbj.com/rsource.htm)

Small business information

Useful links to information on all aspects of starting
and running a small business: information on how
small businesses can obtain information and advice
from the government and deal with government
agencies. (safetynet.doleta.gov/text/smallbus.htm)

Prevention programs

Prevention First, Inc.
A clearinghouse of national programs, resources, and
conferences focusing on prevention
(www.prevention.org)

Join Together Online
A community-based website that addresses public policy. Links to over 50 policy sites and advocacy groups.
Includes legislators' email addresses and the Congressional Directory. (www.jointogether.org)

References

Alward, R., & Camunas, C. (1990). Public relations. Part
II. Strategies and tactics. *Journal of Nursing Administration, 20*(11), 31–41.

Barton, E. (1998). *An operational definition of marketing.*
Unpublished manuscript.

Buckley, W. (1967). *Sociology and modern systems theory.*
Englewood Cliffs, NJ: Prentice-Hall.

Cunningham, R. (1982). Hospital marketing is no cure.
Hospitals, 56(9), 73–75.

Engelberg, M., & Neubrand, S. (1997). Building sensible
segmentation strategies in managed care settings. *Marketing Health Services, 17*(2), 50–51.

Jamison, K.R. (1997). *An unquiet mind.* New York: Vin-
tage Press.

Kennedy, D. (1991). *The ultimate marketing plan.* Hol-
brook, MA: Bob Adams, Inc.

Kotler, P. (1976). *Marketing management* (ed. 3). Englewood Cliffs, NJ: Prentice-Hall.

Kroenke, K., et al. (1994). Physical symptoms in primary
care: predictors of psychiatric disorders and functional
impairment. *Archives of Family Medicine, 3*(9), 774–779.

MacStravic, S. (1997). Questions of value in health care.
Marketing Health Services, 17(4), 50–53.

McKenna, R. (1991). Marketing is everything. *Harvard
Business Review, 69*(1), 65–79.

Michelli, D., & Straw, A. (1997). *Successful networking.*
Happauge, NY: Barrons.

Pinson, L., & Jinnett, J. (1996). *Target marketing* (ed. 3).
Chicago, IL: Upstart Publishing.

Reis, A., & Trout, J. (1986). *Marketing warfare.* New York:
Penguin Books.

Stuart, G., Reynolds, R., & Spencer, M. (1991). Marketing
nursing in an academic psychiatric setting. In Alward,
R., & Camunas, C. (Eds.). *The nurses guide to marketing,*
New York: Delmar Publishers.

Styron, W. (1992). *Darkness visible.* New York: Random
House.

Von Bertalanffy, L. (1968). *General systems theory, foundations, development, applications.* New York: Braziller.

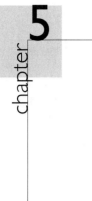

chapter 5

Cultural Diversity in Health Care Delivery

MARIA R. WARDA

■ INTRODUCTION

Culture pervades the lives of all people and forces an active interrelationship between the social milieu and the personality of each individual. Consequently roles, norms, and personal experiences are interpreted through a "cultural lens." Moreover, culture shapes the perception of reality and strongly influences societal forms of behavior. Different cultures reinforce different behaviors and provide acceptable ways for their expression. Culture also influences which behaviors are considered deviant and partially determines the types of adjustment for such problematic behavior.

This is not to say that culture is the single most significant variable in human psychology. It is one of the many factors that contribute to the complexities of psychological processes, and it is obviously important in the understanding of culturally diverse populations. Multiethnic societies may require from their members the learning of new skills for adaptation to cultural change and the subsequent development of bicultural identities. Cultural factors also play an important role in the behavior of mainstream individuals, although the greater uniformity of cultural elements makes it less obvious. Consequently, clinicians need to be attuned to the notion that mental health services to ethnically diverse populations must be delivered in a manner that is culturally relevant and linguistically appropriate.

Cross-cultural mental health research has focused on the reasons for underutilization of services by ethnic minorities and culturally relevant treatment approaches (Betancourt & Lopez, 1993). Less attention has been paid to the cultural aspect of the environments where mental health services are provided. The focus should be not only on serving people in culture-specific ways

113

but also in understanding institutions as cultural environments with their own unique care values, norms, and practices. Advanced practice registered nurses (APRNs), nurse administrators, researchers, and educators have an obligation to influence the development and implementation of structures and processes that reflect an understanding and appreciation for diversity within mental health settings.

Because culture is closely intertwined with concepts such as race, ethnicity, and social class, and because conceptual confusion has been an obstacle for progress in this area, it is important to define culture. After reviewing the elements found in the anthropology and cross-cultural psychology views of culture, Rohner (1984) proposed a conceptualization of *culture* in terms of "highly variable systems of meaning," which are "learned" and "shared by a people or an identifiable segment of a population." This concept is equivalent to that proposed by Herkovits (1948), who conceives culture as the human-made part of the environment. Culture is only one dimension of the nature of people. Depending on the clinician and/or researcher concerns, more biologic or social variables could also be assessed. The important point is that further specification will likely lead to a greater understanding of the roles of culture, race, ethnicity, and social class in psychological phenomena.

This chapter addresses the significance of culture to mental health care. Its underlying premise is that cultural values greatly determine the meaning of health, illness, or injury for individuals and families. Cultural differences in health care may create problems in communication, therapeutic alliance, the implementation of health care interventions, treatment compliance, and treatment outcomes. The focus is on the interaction among the culture of the client, the culture of the provider, and the characteristics of the health care setting in the delivery of culturally competent mental health care. This chapter provides clinical and managerial guidelines to APRNs who practice within a cross-cultural context. It suggests ways

to evaluate the effectiveness of a culturally responsive mental health delivery system. It is organized into two major sections that capture the essentials of what APRNs need to grasp in order to conceptualize fully how they care for an individual in the framework of that person's culture and within the context of the American mental health care system.

DIMENSIONS OF CULTURALLY ■ COMPETENT CARE

Although the literature abounds with discussions of the need for nurses to provide safe and optimal care to culturally diverse clients, little work has focused upon defining the dimensions of culturally competent care. Thus the purpose of this section is to identify and define the dimensions of culturally competent nursing care. Research to date gives evidence of five central dimensions of culturally competent care:

1. Awareness and sensitivity to cultural diversity
2. Knowledge of cultural concepts and patterns
3. Skills in the integration of cultural concepts into practice
4. Focus on the interaction among the patient's ethnic/cultural, biologic, psychological, sociologic, spiritual, and economic systems rather than the function of the isolated elements
5. Practice in a setting or environmental context where values, customs, and beliefs of individuals are respected

Although these dimensions are not well delineated in the literature, this section seeks to address them as distinct entities.

Awareness and Sensitivity to Cultural Diversity

Awareness and sensitivity are required for effective cross-cultural health care interaction. Awareness involves recognition of issues that relate to cultural diversity. Cues to the presence of issues occur on multiple levels, with many being subtle or covert (Kavanagh & Kennedy, 1992). Sensitivity implies understanding the implications and meanings of the processes from the points of view of those directly affected. Since intercultural sensitivity is not "natural" to people of any single cultural group, the development of this ability demands concern, time, energy, and flexibility in one's thinking. To overcome such ethnocentric biases requires that nurses take an honest look at their biases, values, and interpersonal style arising from their own cultural upbringing. Murphy and Macleod-Clark (1993) explored the experiences of nurses caring for ethnic minority clients. Some respondents in this study expressed negative feelings toward the ethnic minority patients for whom they cared. Although it is not known if these respondents were closed-minded, it could be one factor that contributed to the differences in establishing a good nurse-patient relationship.

Thus the first dimension, cultural awareness and sensitivity, is the beginning point for any person wishing to work effectively with ethnically diverse patient groups. It is necessary at this step to understand and accept the underlying premise: cultural differences exist, and culture is a valid and integral part of each person.

Knowledge of Cultural Concepts and Patterns

Awareness and sensitivity facilitate caring, whereas knowledge promotes understanding. Knowledge of patterned cultural characteristics and the symbolism and meaning attached to those characteristics are essential in understanding cross-cultural health care issues. Awareness and sensitivity to the role culture plays in health care needs to be broadened by the development of knowledge regarding the effect of cross-cultural education on patient care.

The level of educational preparation was significantly correlated with cultural knowledge and biases of nurses toward culturally different patients in an exploratory study of 274 randomly selected nurses (Rooda, 1993). Nurses in this sample with an associate degree or diploma had more knowledge of African-American cultural content than did nurses with a bachelor degree. A possible explanation for the findings of this study is that the majority of the ethnic minority nurses in the United States are educated at the Associate degree level. The multicultural nature of the learning environment can potentially lead to an increase in sensitivity toward and understanding of ethnically diverse clients.

A recent national survey attempted to ascertain how nursing programs were ensuring cultural competency in nursing education (Rodriguez, 1997). Most nursing programs responding to the survey indicated that cultural content is integrated throughout the curriculum. About 19% of the sample encouraged clinical experiences, but only 6% required students to complete cultural assessments. Only one program required evidence in the students' academic record that the program's cultural competence requirement had been met. Acquiring knowledge about cultural norms does not ensure sensitivity and/or application of cultural knowledge in practice. Nursing programs should be required to develop performance indicators and examinations that reflect multicultural emphasis. In addition, nurse administrators need to identify, implement, and evaluate organizational structures that guarantee the provision of culturally competent care to their patient population.

Skills in the Integration of Cultural Concepts in Practice

The third dimension of culturally competent care is a critical component that is probably the most difficult to incorporate. Awareness, sensitivity, and knowledge are not sufficient for successful cross-cultural intervention. Cross-cultural nursing therapeutic skills are also necessary. As identified by the American Academy of Nursing Expert Panel on Culturally Competent Nursing Care (Davis, et al. 1992), there are no well-tested models that can facilitate the provision of culturally competent care.

box **5-1**

RESEARCH EXAMPLE

This is an example of how an in-depth cultural assessment of individual or family's conceptualization of the mental illness experience can facilitate the identification of culturally congruent mental health care interventions. Warda and Matteoli (1993) used Kleinman's Explanatory Model of Illness (Kleinman, Eisenberg, & Good, 1978) to explore the perceptions of Chinese-American families regarding mental health care. Individual interviews with 10 Chinese-American families that had a mentally ill member indicated that these families were not aware of the cause of mental illness but readily identified somatic and psychological symptoms as being associated with mental illness. All families stated that health care professionals did not educate them about mental illness. These families said that they did not tell friends about their relative's mental illness. Violence and deterioration in the affected family member's condition were cited as the two main fears regarding mental illness. All families were able to identify medications as effective and expressed realistic expectations of treatment (e.g., improvement vs. cure). Two family coping mechanisms were identified: 1) role flexibility within the family system, and 2) utilization of the Chinese Alliance for the Mentally Ill as a source of family support. Suggestions offered by the families toward integration of culturally competent strategies in mental health care included 1) to recognize the use of Chinese herb treatments and integrate this in the plan of care, 2) to demonstrate respect for Chinese values of gender or sexual propriety when providing health care to Chinese patients, and 3) to offer occupational training as part of the mental health treatment. It is evident from these findings that differences in cultural values and language between patient or family and health care professional had an effect in these families' perceptions of mental health treatment.

A complex set of factors is likely to exist related to cultural knowledge and the integration of concepts into practice. Some general strategies for the implementation of culturally competent care have been identified in the nursing and related literature. First, a careful assessment of cultural background and individual factors can help identify patterns that may assist or interfere with a nursing intervention or treatment regimen. A second strategy is the use of cross-cultural communication, frequently the first challenge to be considered in health care that involves diversity. Verbal and nonverbal cross-cultural communication skills enable problem-solving processes that are acceptable and appropriate to the patient (i.e., culturally congruent) (Kavanagh & Kennedy, 1992). Finally, a cultural context approach has been suggested. This view assumes that patients are ethnically distinct based on their country of origin, historical point of entry, degree of acculturation, and language proficiency (Applewhite, Wong, & Daley, 1991). The strengths of various approaches must take into account the patient's opportunities to obtain favorable life conditions and to cope with stressful situations through cultural strengths. The absence of endemic or culturally specific models has often led to the adoption of traditional service models that may overlook differential needs but are generally amenable to high-risk patients. More research is needed to identify culturally specific strategies based on cultural concepts and to determine the subsequent utilization of services and efficacy of treatment. The example in Box 5-1 describes a study (Warda & Matteoli, 1993) that identifies culturally congruent mental health care interventions for a Chinese-American family.

The importance of shared meaning between the APRN and patient has been emphasized as the foundation for care that fosters health. The meaning of the illness experience cannot be the same for the patient and the health care professional because their contexts are different. However, the meanings for both can be made explicit, resulting in an understanding of each other's context.

Interaction of Ethnic/Cultural Systems and Other Systems

Supporting the patient's cultural beliefs as much as possible is an enabling strategy for successful coping. In addition, it is important to recognize that a complex interaction of cultural factors, life events, and socioeconomic status affects the health care behavior and attitude of ethnic minorities. Knowledge of these interactive processes is crucial to improving the delivery of health services to diverse ethnic groups. In the integrated approach, the existing knowledge regarding the specific elements is recognized (e.g., genetic predisposition to some illness). However, the primary emphasis is on arriving at clinical decisions that consider the potential consequence of change within one or more elements of the person on other related elements. The interaction of the ethnic/cultural system with other systems can perhaps be best seen in the consideration of the socioeconomic influences on health care.

Socioeconomic status. Access to health care is measured by the number of times a person uses health care services (Bodenheimer & Grumbach, 1995). Compared with insured people, the uninsured are less likely to have a regular source of health care and more likely to report delays in receiving health care. People without insurance are more likely than people who have private insurance to receive care in the emergency rooms or clinics of underbudgeted public hospitals, often enduring 7- to 8-hour waits before receiving service (Grumbach, Keane, & Bindman, 1993).

Poverty plays a role in almost every negative aspect of life in society, including violence, crime, mediocre education, and family fragmentation. Poverty also affects the management of medical and psychiatric illness and conditions. As a result, many general health and mental health services have been developed related to violence-connected behavior, substance abuse, prostitution-related HIV infections, perinatal illnesses caused by malnutrition and abuse, and suicide associated with unemployment (Ruiz, Venegas-Samuels, & Alarcon, 1995).

Data on the use of mental health services indicates that African-Americans and Hispanics have a lower probability of using outpatient mental health services than Caucasians. Conversely African-Americans and Hispanics have a greater probability of using inpatient mental health services than Caucasians (Schappert, 1993). These data certainly have a major bearing not only on the utilization of mental health services but on the quality of care and the type of access to mental health treatment as well. Outpatient mental health services permit patients to be treated while maintaining activities such as employment, recreation, and social and family ties. On the other hand, inpatient services keep patients away from the regular activities of daily life in their own cultural and social context. The need for inpatient care may be related to the fact that many ethnic minority patients only access the mental health system after their condition has reached an acute state. Seeking crisis-mode health care is in most instances related to low economic level and lack of health insurance. Another explanation for these differences could be the prejudicial and discriminatory attitudes that sometimes exist in the health care system as a whole. Mental health professionals referring patients to either inpatient or outpatient mental health services could be biased with regard to the effectiveness and appropriateness of outpatient services because of the ethnic origin of such patients.

Improving the utilization of mental health services, the access to mental health care, the rate of mental health insurance coverage, and the quality of mental health services among the ethnic minorities in the United States is a formidable task. It is compounded by factors such as language and cultural barriers, socioeconomic and educational levels, employment rates, type of employment, and ethnic or racial discrimination.

Biologic factors. Studies have revealed that race is related to being prone to certain illnesses and responses to treatments and medications. These tendencies may be hereditary, acquired, or both. Concurrent with a general consensus of the efficacy of psychopharmacology across ethnic groups, there also have been numerous reports of dramatic cross-ethnic variations in the dosing practices and side effect profiles in response to almost all classes of psychotropics (Rudorfer, 1993). Pharmacokinetics, the study of the fate and distribution of drugs in biologic organisms, has been most extensively investigated in terms of its contributions to cross-ethnic and interindividual variations in drug responses (Lin, Anderson, & Poland, 1995). Studies of ethnicity and psychotropic response to lithium and benzodiazepines will be used to illustrate the genetic mechanisms affecting drug responses.

Because body size and composition (percentage of fat) often vary significantly across ethnic groups, the volume of distribution of many psychotropic agents, especially those that are highly lipophilic (having an affinity for fat, absorbing fat), could vary. A significant ethnic difference in the distribution of lithium across cellular membranes exists between African-Americans and Caucasians. As a result of less active sodium-lithium countertransport system, African-Americans have a higher rate of central nervous system (CNS) related side effects, as demonstrated in a study by Strickland, Lin, and Fu (1995). According to these researchers, their findings require further examination.

A series of studies conducted in Japan, Taiwan, mainland China, and Hong Kong showed that the pharmacokinetic profiles of lithium were similar between Asians and Caucasians. These Chinese patients responded optimally, however, to significantly lower mean lithium concentrations (0.71 to 0.73 mEq/L). Thus it appears that compared with their Caucasian counterparts, Asian bipolar patients may require lower doses of lithium because of pharmacodynamic reasons (increased CNS responsivity) (Lin, Poland, & Nakasaki, 1993; Strickland, Lin, & Fu, 1995).

Four pharmacokinetic studies conducted in Asians residing in diverse areas of the world, including Los Angeles, St. Louis, Hong Kong, and Beijing, have confirmed earlier clinical and survey reports suggesting that Asians were more sensitive to benzodiazepines as compared with Caucasians. Three of the studies used diazepam as the drug, and one used alprazolam. These studies involved the administration of the test drugs by the oral or intravenous route or both. The consistent finding of a slower metabolism of benzodiazepines is quite remarkable, considering the diversity of sites and research methodology. Together they suggest that genetic factors may be more important than environmental factors in the control of benzodiazepine metabolism (Lin, Poland, & Nakasaki, 1993).

Psychological factors. The psychological system includes the mental and/or behavioral processes and characteristics of individuals and groups. It has long been recognized that certain unusual forms of psychopathology are restricted to specific areas or cultures (Levine & Gaw, 1995). The growing sophistication and increasing cultural sensitivity of modern psychiatry has led to a renewed interest in a set of phenomena known as *culture-bound syndromes* (CBSs). Yap (1967) defined the CBSs as a "form of psychopathology produced by certain systems of implicit values, social structure, and obviously shared beliefs indigenous to certain areas." Levine and Gaw (1995) proposed the use of a more precise term, *culture-specific,* for those syndromes that fulfill the following criteria:

1. The disorder must be a discrete, well-defined syndrome.
2. It must be recognized as a specific illness in the culture with which it is primarily associated.
3. The disorder must be expected, recognized, and to some degree sanctioned as a response to certain precipitants in the particular culture.
4. A higher incidence or prevalence of the disorder exists in societies in which the disorder is culturally recognized, compared with other societies.

Two examples from a group of CBSs related to anxiety are used to illustrate how, although anxiety is a universal phenomenon, the events precipitating it are highly influenced by culture. Lewis-Fernandez and Kleinman (1995) explained that it is the perception of a situation, or the cognitions associated with it, that determine the extent to which anxiety will be evoked. Because these cognitions are culturally mediated, clinicians may not recognize the similarities between the Western syndromes and their "culture-bound" counterparts.

The first example is *Ataque de Nervios*. This syndrome, seen in Latin American populations, includes symptoms of shaking, palpitations, flushing, and numbness (often accompanied by shouting or striking out), followed by falling, convulsive body movements, or amnesia (Guarnaccia, Canino, & Rubio-Stipec, 1993). An attack can resemble panic disorder with dissociative features. A typical Western patient will experience considerable anxiety after his or her first panic attack, fearing that it was due to a dangerous and unpredictable physical or mental defect. In contrast, a patient who experiences *ataque* can be presumed almost to expect these symptoms as the sequelae of psychosocial stress. Therefore the patient with *ataque* may not be susceptible to the same fears after an attack, yet the pathophysiology behind the two syndromes may be similar (Levine & Gaw, 1995).

The second example is *Taijin Kyofusho*. This syndrome, prevalent among the Japanese, is similar to social phobia. It is also referred to as *anthropophobia* (Simmons & Hughes, 1993). The afflicted are intensely anxious that their bodies, their body parts, or body functions may offend, embarrass, or displease others. Especially prevalent among youth, the pathology of this disorder may be the same as that of social phobia. The higher prevalence of the illness among Japanese is related to the values inherent in the culture that emphasize the importance of proper behavior in all social situations (Levine & Gaw, 1995).

Another issue related to the interaction of psychological factors and cultural values is the ongoing controversy over the effectiveness of psychotherapy services for ethnic minority groups. The criticisms have focused on prejudicial and discriminatory practices directed toward ethnic groups, therapist's lack of knowledge and understanding of sociocultural contexts of ethnic patients, inaccessibility or unavailability of services, and so on. The criticisms have stimulated studies examining ethnic and racial differences in the utilization of services, premature termination rates, patient preference for therapists, therapist prejudice, diagnosis and assessment, treatment strategies, and the process and outcome of treatment (Carter, 1995). Research to date has failed to systematically reveal outcome differences. Studies that integrate the patient's ethnic, biologic, spiritual, socioeconomic, and psychological systems are necessary in order to understand the concept of mental health in ethnic minority individuals and to test treatment effectiveness.

Spirituality. Some scholars of religion suggest that spiritual well-being can help people deal with health issues, partly because spiritual beliefs help people address issues of living. A spiritual outlook may place emphasis on the worth of each individual, the meaning of life, and the meaning of death. It may serve as the basis for the formation of values relating to the quality of life and to health. The term *religion* has been referred to as an adherence to the beliefs and practices of an organized church or religious institution. *Spirituality* is used to describe the transcendent relationship between the person and a higher being, a quality that goes beyond a specific religious affiliation (Shafranske & Malony, 1990). In this chapter, the term *spirituality* is used to represent a person's idiosyncratic "God representation."

Psychiatry's insensitivity toward spiritual issues is apparent in the research literature, which has largely ignored religious and spiritual variables. However, studies have shown that mental health professionals frequently are called upon to assess and treat spiritual issues (Lukoff, Lu, & Turner, 1995). In addition, more than 70% of the world's population relies on indigenous systems of care and the traditional healers who often conceptualize and treat patients' complaints as having spiritual causes (Jones, 1993).

In recent years, there have been a number of developments that have begun to address psychiatry's cultural insensitivity to the spiritual dimensions of life. In January, 1993 the Task Force on *DSM-IV* approved a diagnostic category titled "Religious or Spiritual Problem" (APA, 1994). For the first time in the *Diagnostic and Statistical Manual (DSM)* there is an acknowledgment that spiritual problems can be the focus of psychiatric consultation and treatment and that many of these problems are not attributable to a mental disorder.

It has been considered that the pathologic significance of religious language seldom can be determined by the immediate content alone, especially if differential diagnosis with psychotic disorders is being considered. Lukoff and colleagues (1995) discussed assessment methods for distinguishing religious and spiritual problems from psychopathology that presents with religious content. The *DSM-IV* specifically notes that clinicians assessing for schizophrenia in socioeconomic or cultural situations different from their own must take cultural differences into account:

Ideas that may appear to be delusional in one culture (e.g., sorcery and witchcraft) may be commonly held in another. In some cultures, visual or auditory hallucinations with religious content may be a normal part of religious experience (e.g., seeing the Virgin Mary or hearing God's voice) (APA, 1994).

The clinician's response to a person's religious or spiritual experience can determine whether the experience is integrated and used as a stimulus for personal growth, or repressed as a bizarre event that may be a sign of mental instability. Individuals undergoing powerful religious or spiritual experiences are sometimes at risk for being hospitalized as mentally ill. Agosin (1992) suggests using good prognostic indicators to help distinguish between psychopathology and authentic spiritual experiences, including 1) good pre-episode functioning, 2) acute onset of symptoms during a period of 3 months or less, 3) stressful precipitants to the psychotic episode, and 4) a positive exploratory attitude toward the experience.

Religion and spirituality are linked to psychological well-being, involve issues of love and relatedness, and provide a source of meaning and purpose in life, all of which are definite cultural notions. An exploratory study of Hispanic families' conceptions of serious mental illness in a family member focused on the role of religious institutions and religious healing as a source of solace (Guarnaccia et al., 1992). "Si Dios quiere" (if God wishes) or "Que Dios nos bendiga" (may God bless us) were common refrains when talking to Hispanic families about their expectations for the long-term prospect of their seriously ill family member. These expressions reflect Hispanic families' strong religious beliefs and, at the same time, the hopes and frustrations they experience in dealing with an illness that is deeply troubling and frequently defies explanation. Millit and colleagues (1996) used a sample of African-American and Caucasian college students to explore their views of the etiology and treatment of mental health problems. The participants responded to questions about vignettes describing individuals encountering a range of personal difficulties. African-Americans rated spiritual factors as more important in the etiology and treatment of the difficulties than did Caucasians.

The identified relationship between spirituality and cross-cultural health beliefs has implications for nursing. Helping patients and families find meaning in pain and suffering can be described as one of the goals of psychiatric nursing practice. The implications of ethnic/cultural identity, socioeconomic status, and biologic and psychological health on spiritual values and practices needs to be carefully examined by APRNs, clinicians, researchers, and educators.

Respect for Values, Customs, and Beliefs in the Practice Setting

There is a need for psychiatric nurses to maintain a focus on the environmental, cultural, and social experience of the individuals inhabiting the psychiatric treatment milieu. In the clinical setting of psychiatry where the therapeutic milieu is a major aspect of the treatment program, it is assumed that the behavior of an individual will always be a function of the total environment. Nursing administrators and clinical leaders are concerned with the environment in which nursing care takes place. Health care environments affect not only the patients who receive care but also the ways in which nursing care is provided. Modern health care settings struggling for organizational survival in today's turbulent environment mandate investigations aimed at understanding the social, symbolic, and reasoning properties of the environment.

Kavanagh (1991) analyzed institutionalized inequity and discrimination in the forms of sexism and racism within a psychiatric institution. In this study, despite an awareness of the roles that culture and gender play in the care of patients, mental health professionals tended to avoid critical examination of their own and coworkers' ethnicity and gender issues. Among staff members, an illusion of sameness discouraged acknowledgment of existing significant differences. This attitude implied that the effect of racism and sexism on those individuals not labeled as patients was of little consequence. Nurse leaders' commitment to the creation and maintenance of a culturally sensitive work environment entails a willingness to modify ineffective supervision and evaluation methods and to explore their own racial attitudes. This kind of search is painful because it increases self-awareness of values and behavior, forcing assessment of one's interpersonal contact and its effect on others.

Recruitment and retention of ethnic minority nurses is yet another complex task requiring innovative approaches. The minority nurse is interested in all the usual variables when seeking employment, such as quality nursing care, pay, benefits, part-time options, and a number of additional concerns:

- What is the attitude and receptiveness of the work setting toward ethnic minorities?
- What is their record of promotion of minority staff?
- What is the ethnic composition of the patient population, staff members, and managers?

- Is cultural competency a valued dimension of nursing practice?

Despite affirmative action efforts in the recruitment of ethnic minorities into nursing schools, their representation continues to be small. Data on enrollment in graduate nursing programs by race reveal that in 1995 only 5.9% were African-American, 3.1% were Asian, 2.8% were Hispanic, and 0.5% were Native American or Alaskan Native (AACN, 1996). Ethnic pluralism in nursing would provide minority nurses with a greater opportunity to communicate effectively with minority patients, make the professional life of the minority nurse less "lonely" and more fulfilling, and provide more role models for minority youths making career decisions and for those in nursing who have minimal experience in providing nursing care to ethnic minority patients. The challenge to the nursing profession, in addition to the provision of culturally competent care and assurance of minority representation within its ranks, is to develop new administrative structures, values, and processes that will support and enrich multicultural realities in nursing (Leininger, 1991).

The use of cultural-awareness, staff-development programs that include staff members of the dominant and various ethnic minority groups represented within the institution is one way to facilitate the development of cross-cultural nursing care practices. Seminars can cover topics such as work beliefs, values, cultural influences, and patterns of communication. Using examples of actual situations that are likely to be encountered in the process of providing nursing care and in working within a diverse environment can increase the active participation of all members of the organization. These workshops will increase the overall awareness of the psychodynamics of cross-cultural communications and understanding of the nature of discrimination and prejudice.

Psychiatric nurse leaders and scholars who are members of minority groups are needed to develop new corporate models that can accommodate different cultural values and to serve as role models and mentors of other minority nurses. This implies that a critical goal of nurse managers and clinical leaders is the mentoring and development of both majority and minority nurses to assume leadership roles. One function of a mentor is to provide opportunities for the nurse's professional socialization, such as in direct observation of the day-to-day performance of the APRN's role, by accompanying the mentor to interdepartmental meetings to acquire effective methods of communication, or to better understand the political workings of the organization. Some aspects of the leadership role may challenge the cultural beliefs and values of nurses. Learning the subtle differences between assertiveness and aggressiveness, or acquiring a new set of decision-making and problem-solving skills while maintaining one's own cultural identity, is a complex task. However, it is through the process of mentoring that nurses can receive encouragement and training as intellectual leaders who are skilled in clinical and administrative structures, functions, and processes that accommodate diversity. The mentoring process is described in greater detail in Chapter 20.

Culture is not something that is imposed upon a social setting. Rather, it develops during the course of social interaction and therefore is subject to change. Ignoring social stratification and inequality perpetuates race, gender, and class divisions and domination. In addition, institutionalized inequalities hinder potentially productive interpersonal and professional exchanges. Today's health care environment entails the management of a heterogeneous, culturally diverse employee group providing care to an equally dissimilar patient population.

Case Example

A study of the perceptions of Mexican-Americans regarding culturally competent care yielded data on the interaction of the ethnic/cultural, biologic, psychological, spiritual, and socioeconomic systems for one ethnic group. In addition, the context and characteristics of the health care system were important factors identified by the participants in the study. The Warda Culturally Competent Care Scale (Warda, 1997) is a method to obtain input from Mexican-American health care recipients for planning their culturally competent care. The availability of such information has implications for access and quality of care for this population. The literature has identified socioeconomic, cognitive, cultural, and system-related barriers to access to health care for Hispanics. In Warda's (1997) investigation the participants identified two cognitive barriers to health care utilization: inadequate knowledge of the health care system and monolingual fluency in Spanish. In addition, the study results indicate that the use of unprescribed medications, in particular antibiotics, is a common practice for this ethnic group. Nursing interventions cannot be culturally competent unless there is language concordance (particularly for Spanish monolingual patients) and patient education approaches that address orientation to the U.S. health care system and patients' views regarding the safety and efficacy of antibiotics.

The study findings also support a different perspective of spirituality and its role in matters of health and illness for Mexican-Americans. Mexican-Americans have strong and enduring spiritual beliefs, but those beliefs do not necessarily prevent them from acknowledging personal responsibility in matters of health and illness. Spirituality assumes a central role in the perception of, coping with, and management of health and illness for Mexican-Americans, but it is a shared control between the individual and his or her creator. The view that health is uniquely controlled by divine will, fate, or the environment was not supported in this study. This finding has implications for the planning and provision of nursing care to Mexican-Americans. Assuming that the concept of *fatalism* (the learned or generalized expectancy that the outcomes of situations are either contingent on one's behavior or controlled by external forces, such as fate, chance, or powerful others) should not be used solely to explain issues such as Mexican-Americans' failure to engage in preventive health care behaviors, lack of compliance with a treatment regimen, and underutilization of the health care system. The search for answers must then shift to other factors such as socioeconomic and system barriers. However, emphasis on the integration of spiritual factors in the planning and delivery of health care to Mexican-Americans should be a concern to nursing and an area of nursing action.

This study supported the notion that Mexican-Americans (among other sub-groups of Hispanics) have a preference for health care encounters that emphasize the patient's relationship with the individual provider in an atmosphere of trust and intimacy. Marin (1989) described that Hispanics have a preference for health care providers whom they have come to know through "pleasant conversation" or who are Hispanic with similar backgrounds. The distinguishing element between Hispanics' preference for positive, smooth, interpersonal relations in health care encounters, and similar values among other ethnics groups, is one of emphasis rather than substance. The establishment of an emotional rapport that will generate respect and understanding between the Mexican-American patient and the health care provider can have important effects on health care utilization and outcomes. Attention to cultural competency during the health care encounter will require that the health care provider 1) invest in acquiring knowledge and comfort with Hispanic verbal and nonverbal nuances of communication, 2) allocate sufficient time for listening attentively to patients and provide information in a courteous manner, 3) avoid confrontation and remain nonjudgmental when presenting health care information and recommending care regimens, and 4) incorporate and encourage the use of appropriate cultural health care practices.

Findings from this study suggest that for Mexican-Americans, the concept of *familism* remains a prominent cultural value. Individuals are expected to show loyalty and support and to fulfill role obligations in the family. Help and advice are usually sought from within the family system first, and important decisions are made as a group. Fam-

ilism is deeply ingrained in the Mexican-American culture and does not seem to change much in the process of acculturation. Health care providers can incorporate their understanding of the concept of familism in the care of Mexican-American clients by 1) facilitating the patient's access to family support, 2) using it to enhance the likelihood of patients' health care behavior changes, and 3) inquiring what information, in what manner, and with which family members the patient wishes that health care information to be communicated.

CULTURE AND THE MENTAL ■ HEALTH CARE SYSTEM

The current mental health care system needs the providers to be more attuned to the cultural values and life situations of their patients and to consider them when making health care decisions. Knowledge of culture-specific sociodemographic data that can be barriers to access to health care and diverse cultural beliefs and lifestyles, while appreciating individual variances, can form the basis for a culturally responsive health care system.

Just as individuals in a culture can have different personalities while sharing much in common, so do groups and organizations. Health care organizations have their own distinct cultures that are influenced by the characteristics of the patient or client, provider, and setting. Holzemer (1994) identified a system model (Fig. 5-1) for conceptualizing the effect of nursing care on the client, provider, and setting outcomes. The horizontal axis is a system axis of input and context, process,

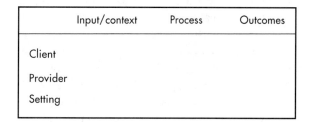

Figure 5-1 Holzemer's outcome model. From Holzemer, 1994.

and outcome. The vertical axis consists of the client, provider, and setting. In this model, outcome evaluation is conceptualized to be the interaction and linkages among the vertical axis of the client, provider, and setting with the horizontal axis of input, process, and outcome, with particular focus upon client outcomes.

Patient Outcomes

Recent reviews of psychiatric outcome research and utilization of outcome measures by APRNs in psychiatric nursing has revealed that there is a weak scientific base for evaluating outcomes of psychiatric care and that a significant number of APRNs do not use outcome measures (Barrell, Merwin, & Poster, 1997; Merwin & Mauck, 1995). In addition, there is a lack of knowledge in the area of culturally competent care outcome research.

When developing conceptual models of ethnically diverse patient outcomes, APRNs should consider the strengths, needs, and lifestyles of the patient and his or her family and community. For example, Tirado (1996) developed a patient satisfaction survey to be used for evaluating the degree to which health care organizations are providing culturally competent care to Hispanic and Chinese patients. This study used data from focus groups with Hispanic and Chinese patients and health care providers to develop a single instrument. Major cultural health care concepts relevant to both Chinese and Hispanic individuals guided the development of the instrument. Examples of cultural concepts for which items were developed are 1) access to linguistically competent care, 2) adequacy of health care provider communication style, 3) use of alternative sources of care, and 4) family role in care decisions. Because of its focus on patient-provider interaction and communication style, this tool is particularly well-suited to be used in outcome studies of Hispanic and Chinese patients' satisfaction with mental health care.

In another study of clinical outcomes, Glazer, Morgenstern, and Doucette (1994) examined psychological, clinical, treatment, medical, and racial variables of Caucasian and African-American patients and their correlation with higher incidents of tardive dyskinesia. None of the variables explained more than a minimal portion of the incidence of tardive dyskinesia. The findings indicated that the incidence of tardive dyskinesia was 1.83 times greater for African-Americans. African-Americans were more likely to have a diagnosis of schizophrenia and to receive higher doses of neuroleptic drugs primarily through depot medications. These results suggest the need for additional studies of differences in diagnostic and prescribing practices for African-American and Caucasian patients and of differences in the actions and side effects of neuroleptics.

Provider Outcomes

In reality, nursing care outcome evaluation would most likely focus on patient outcomes, but there are provider outcomes that are of particular interest in the area of culturally competent psychiatric nursing care. Types of provider outcomes important to measure include 1) effect of nurse-patient ethnicity or culture match on measures of process and outcome of culturally competent care, 2) level and type of cultural diversity education that demonstrates cultural competency in practice, 3) linkages between types and length of nursing experiences working with culturally diverse patients and nurse satisfaction, and 4) the relationship between nurses' personality attributes and cross-cultural nurse-patient relationship.

For example, Tirado (1996) developed the Provider Cultural Competence Self-Assessment questionnaire for use with health care providers as a guide in determining the degree to which they could benefit from further training or experience in providing culturally competent care. The investigator recommended that future studies explore the association of providers' responses to the questions with patients' adherence to prescribed medication regimens, the use of clinical services, and the clinical status outcomes. Evaluation of these associations may have implications for the hypotheses that cultural competence is predicated on issues such as 1) the providers' sharing their patients' ethnic or racial background, 2) the language match between provider and patient, and 3) providers' level of knowledge regarding their patients' cultural patterns.

Setting Outcomes

The dimension of setting has not received adequate analysis in the area of culturally competent care research. The characteristics of the organizational setting should be included as a variable in studies assessing the presence and effect of culturally competent care. Suggested areas of outcome evaluation within the dimension of the health care environment are assessment of the effect of cohorts of minority clinicians on health care organizational structures and behaviors, evaluation of the impact of mentoring on minority nurses' transition to leadership roles, and measuring the efficacy of cultural awareness workshops on cross-cultural staff relations.

Scheid and Greenley (1997) assessed institutional conformity by examining evaluations of effectiveness of 29 mental health services programs. Specialist programs responded to institutional demands by targeting services to those considered most in need: patients with severe mental illness. Generalist programs continued to provide care to diverse patient groups and to offer traditional services (such as psychotherapy). These factors resulted in lower evaluations of effectiveness for generalist programs. This research is important because it demonstrates that patient-congruent organizational processes and goal congruence (program objectives meet the expectations of the target patient population) are critical to a positive evaluation of effectiveness. These findings indicate the need for mental health programs to assess characteristics of their internal environment (e.g., culture, age, gender, mental health status, and socioeconomic status of patients; education, and providers' culture) and external environment (e.g., regulatory agencies) to establish congruence of treatment approach and increase program effectiveness.

IMPLICATIONS FOR
■ THE FUTURE

This chapter examines the relevance of cultural concepts to the provision and evaluation of quality, culturally competent mental health care. Culturally competent nursing care requires the nurse to have awareness and sensitivity to cultural diversity, knowledge, and skills in the integration of cultural concepts in practice; a holistic approach to the assessment, planning, and implementation of nursing therapeutics; and the opportunity to practice in an environment that values diversity. The relationship between the characteristics of the patient, the properties of the provider and setting, the provision of culturally competent care, and the outcomes of care has not been fully examined in the literature and merits further study.

The field of psychiatric nursing is challenged to contribute to the identification, empirical validation, and evaluation of relevant mental health cultural concepts. Measuring treatment efficacy of culturally competent mental health nursing care may require the use of methodologic triangulation to adequately address this broad and complex phenomenon. Training in research methods (both qualitative and quantitative) and instrument development may be crucial to the success of implementing psychiatric-mental health nursing research that can potentially demonstrate how nursing care changes diverse patient outcomes. Collaboration between APRN clinicians and nurse scientists will be necessary to fully describe and document culturally competent psychiatric nursing care.

RESOURCES AND CONNECTIONS

JOURNALS

Culture, Medicine, and Psychiatry
Journal of Cross-Cultural Psychology
Journal of Health Care for the Poor and Underserved
Transcultural Psychiatry

BOOKS

Ferguson, V.D. (1998). *Case studies in cultural diversity.* National League for Nursing Press.

Lipson, J.G., Dibble, S.L., & Minarik, P.A. (Eds.). (1996). *Culture and nursing care: a pocket book.* San Francisco, CA: UCSF Nursing Press.

WEBSITES FOR CULTURAL DIVERSITY ISSUES

The Hispanic Health Link: Connecting Communities and Creating Change

This site of the National Coalition of Hispanic and Human Services Organizations features news, calendar of events, job opportunities, and a comprehensive list of government, commercial, and nonprofit health-related sites.
www.cossmho.org

The University of Southern California's Center for Multilingual Multicultural Research

This site serves educators and minority students interested in multicultural issues. It offers links to scholarships and programs for minority faculty and students interested in becoming teachers.
www.rcf.usc.edu.cmmrl

The Office of Minority Health Resource Center

This site offers information, publications, mailing lists, database searches, and referrals on African American, Asian, Hispanic, American Indian/Alaska Native, and Pacific Islander populations.
www.omhrc.gov

The Immigrant Policy Project

This site provides information on culture and linguistic access to health care, upcoming legislation, and issues impacting diverse populations.
www.DiversityRx.org

References

Agosin, T. (1992). Psychosis, dreams, and mysticism in the clinical domain. In F. Halligan, & J. Shea (Eds.). *The fires of desire.* New York: Crossroad.

American Association of Colleges of Nursing. (1996). *1995–1996 enrollment and graduation in baccalaureate and graduate programs in nursing.* (Pub. No. 95–96-1). Washington, DC: the Association.

American Psychiatric Association. (1994). *Diagnostic and statistical manual* (ed. 4). Washington, DC: the Association.

Applewhite, S.R., Wong, P., & Daley, J.M. (1991). Service approaches and issues in Hispanic agencies. *Administration and Policy in Mental Health, 19*(1), 27–37.

Barrell, L.M., Merwin, E.I., & Poster, E.C. (1997). Patient outcomes used by advanced practice psychiatric nurses to evaluate effectiveness of practice. *Archives of Psychiatric Nursing, 11*(4), 184–197.

Betancourt, H., & Lopez, S.R. (1993). The study of culture, ethnicity, and race in American psychology. *American Psychologist, 43*(4), 301–308.

Bodenheimer, T.S., & Grumbach, K. (1995). *Understanding health policy: a clinical approach.* Connecticut: Appleton & Lange.

Carter, R. (1995). *The influence of race and racial identity in psychotherapy: toward a radically inclusive model.* New York: Wiley.

Davis, L.H., et al.(1992). AAN expert panel report: culturally competent health care. *Nursing Outlook, 40*(6), 277–283.

Glazer, W.M., Morgenstern, H., & Doucette, J. (1994). Race and tardive dyskinesia among outpatients at a CMHC. *Hospital and Community Psychiatry, 45*(1), 38–42.

Grumbach, K., Keane, D., & Bindman, A. (1993). Primary care and public emergency department overcrowding. *American Journal of Public Health, 83,* 372–376.

Guarnaccia, P.J., Canino, G.J., & Rubio-Stipec, M. (1993). The prevalence of ataque de nervios in the Puerto Rico Disaster Study: the role of culture in psychiatric epidemiology. *Journal of Nervous and Mental Disorders, 181,* 159–167.

Guarnaccia, P.J., et al. (1992). Si Dios quiere: Hispanic families experiences of caring for a seriously mentally ill family member. *Culture, Medicine and Psychiatry, 16,* 187–215.

Herkovitz, M. (1948). *Man and his works.* New York: Knopf.

Holzemer, W.L. (1994). The impact of nursing care in Latin America and the Caribbean: a focus on outcomes. *Journal of Advanced Nursing, 20,* 5–12.

Jones, J.W. (1993). Living on the boundary between psychology and religion. *Psychology of Religion Newsletter, 18*(1), 77–83.

Kavanagh, K.H. (1991). Invisibility and selective avoidance: gender and ethnicity in psychiatry and psychiatric nursing staff interaction. *Culture, Medicine, and Psychiatry, 15,* 245–274.

Kavanagh, K.H., & Kennedy, P.H. (1992). *Promoting cultural diversity.* Newbury Park: Sage.

Kleinman, A., Eisenberg, L., & Good, B. (1978). Culture, illness, and care. *Annals of Internal Medicine, 58,* 251–258.

Leininger, M. (1991). *Culture care diversity and universality: a theory of nursing.* Pub. No. 15–2402. New York: National League for Nursing Press.

Levine, R.E., & Gaw, A.C. (1995). Culture-bound syndromes. *The Psychiatric Clinics of North America, 18*(3), 523–236.

Lewis-Fernandez, R., & Kleinman, A. (1995). Cultural psychiatry. *The Psychiatric Clinics of North America, 18*(3), 433–448.

Lin, K.M., Anderson, D., & Poland, R.E. (1995). Ethnicity and psychopharmacology: bridging the gap. *The Psychiatric Clinics of North America, 18*(3), 635–647.

Lin, K.M., Poland, R., & Nakasaki, G. (1993). *Psychopharmacology and psychobiology of ethnicity.* Washington, DC: American Psychiatric Press.

Lukoff, D., Lu, F.G., & Turner, M. (1995). Cultural considerations in the assessment and treatment of religious and spiritual problems. *The Psychiatric Clinics of North America, 18*(93), 476–485.

Marin G. (1989). AIDS prevention among Hispanics: needs, risks behaviors and cultural values. *Public Health Report, 104,* 411–415.

Merwin, E., & Mauck, A. (1995). Psychiatric nursing outcome research: the state of the science. *Archives of Psychiatric Nursing, 9*(6), 311–331.

Millet, P.E., et al. (1996). Black Americans' and white Americans' views of the etiology and treatment of mental health problems. *Community Mental Health Journal, 32*(3), 235–242.

Murphy, K., & Macleod-Clark, J. (1993). Nurses' experiences of caring for ethnic-minority clients. *Journal of Advanced Nursing, 18,* 442–450.

Rodriguez, E.R. (1997). Cultural competency in nursing. *The Hispanic Nurse, 19*(4), 13.

Rohner, R.P. (1984). Toward a conception of culture for cross-cultural psychology. *Journal of Cross-Cultural Psychology, 15,* 11–138.

Rooda, L.A. (1993). Knowledge and attitudes of nurses toward culturally different patients: implications for nursing education. *Journal of Nursing Education, 32*(5), 209–213.

Rudorfer, M. (1993). Pharmacokinetics of psychotropic drugs in special populations. *Journal of Clinical Psychiatry, 54,* 50–54.

Ruiz, P., Venegas-Samuels, K., & Alarcon, R.D. (1995). The economics of pain: mental health care costs among minorities. *The Psychiatric Clinics of North America, 18*(3), 659–671.

Schappert, S.M. (1993). Office visits to psychiatrists: United States, 1989–1990. Centers for Disease Control and Prevention, *Advance Data 237,* 1–15.

Scheid, T.L, & Greenley, J.R. (1997). Evaluations of organizational effectiveness in mental health programs. *Journal of Health and Social Behavior, 38*(4), 403–426.

Shafranske, E., & Malony, H.N. (1990). Clinical psychologists religious and spiritual orientations and their practice of psychotherapy. *Psychotherapy, 27,* 72–78.

Simmons, R.C., & Hughes, C.C. (1993). Culture-bound syndromes. In A.C. Gaw (Ed.). *Culture, ethnicity, and mental illness.* Washington, DC: American Psychiatric Association.

Strickland, T., Lin, K., & Fu, P. (1995). Comparison of lithium ratio variations between African American and Caucasian bipolar patients. *Biological Psychiatry, 37,* 325–330.

Tirado, M.D. (1996). *Tools for monitoring cultural competence in health care.* San Francisco: Latino Coalition for a Healthy California.

Warda, M., & & Mateoli, R. (1993, October). *Chinese-American families perceptions of mental health services.* Paper presented at the meeting of the American Psychiatric Nurses Association Annual Convention, Chicago, IL.

Warda, M.R. (1997). Development of a measure of culturally competent care. (Doctoral dissertation. University of California, San Francisco, 1997). *Dissertation Abstracts International, 58*(6), 9738388.

Yap, P.M. (1967). Classification of the culture-bound reactive syndromes. *Australia and New Zealand Journal of Psychiatry, 1,* 172–179.

Collaboration and Partnership in Managed Care

SHARON MINDLIN STEINBERG, JUDITH GREGORIE D'AFFLITTI, and SUZANNE SAYLE JIMERSON

■ INTRODUCTION

Providing quality care often involves partnerships, negotiation, and collaboration. *Partnership* is a team based approach for a stated goal. *Negotiation* is setting up the terms and framework for the collaboration. *Collaboration* is the process of working together within the negotiated framework to achieve the goal of the partnership. The purpose of this chapter is to demonstrate how these concepts are applied to advanced practice psychiatric-mental health nursing. Advanced

practice registered nurses (APRNs) provide quality, cost-effective comprehensive services in many health care settings (APNA, 1997), and the processes of partnerships, negotiation, and collaboration outlined in this chapter are applicable to most teaching, research, administration, and clinical practice experiences.

Harvard Pilgrim Health Care (HPHC) is a nonprofit managed care organization (MCO) that provides care and coverage to more than 1.3 million members in Massachusetts, Rhode Island, Maine, and New Hampshire. HPHC is a complex hybrid organization with multiple service delivery models, including health maintenance organizations (HMOs), point-of-service organizations (POSs), and preferred provider organizations (PPOs). Harvard Vanguard Medical Associates, a closed-panel,

Acknowledgment: The authors thank Elizabeth P. Howard, PhD, APRN, Northeastern University School of Nursing, for her contribution to this chapter and the research study on clinical preceptorship experiences.

staff-model HMO (formerly called Harvard Community Health Plan) was part of HPHC but became a separate multispecialty group practice in 1997. Although many of the opportunities and experiences described in this chapter are unique to the particular structure of HPHC and Harvard Vanguard, they illustrate the effective use of the knowledge, skills, and competencies of APRNs. APRNs are working in changing, restructured health care delivery systems throughout the country. They have multiple opportunities to redefine their clinical practices, develop strategic partnerships, and negotiate and collaborate with other APRNs and health professions.

Integrated delivery systems and MCOs typically have nontraditional clinical and administrative structures. In the past, patient care was segregated among the separate professional groups. Furthermore, processes of care and financial components in hospitals and academic medical centers, outpatient departments, and community settings were kept separate. The current health care environment encourages reconnection of these separate entities into new partnerships to produce positive improvements in various health care systems. Nurses are in an excellent position to become essential to the emerging partnerships (O'Neil, 1998).

Partnering among health professionals implies developing relationships among parties, building trust, and establishing an atmosphere of candor in communication. It further involves shared decision making and working in multidisciplinary teams across health care delivery systems. Clinicians and administrators working in vertically integrated systems, as well as educators in health profession colleges and universities, can partner to make improvements and advances in clinical care, research, and educational endeavors. Nurses and other clinicians can help redesign the clinical environment. Their expertise and insights will also make a significant contribution to the teaching and learning experiences of future health professionals.

The American Nurses Association's Managed Care Working Group identified policies and posi-tions for the preferred characteristics of future health care delivery systems. Their publication, *Managed Care: Nursing's Blueprint for Action* (ANA, 1998) provides a clear direction for preparing the next generation of advanced practice nurses. Key principles include the following:

- The right of every individual to access health care services
- Consumer empowerment
- Interdisciplinary collaborative care that includes registered nurses
- Value-based health care services that maximize quality while controlling costs
- Systems that address the health needs of individuals, families, communities, and populations
- High standards of ethical behavior
- Accountability for quality, cost-effective health care shared by providers, plans, and health care systems
- A commitment to safeguard confidential patient information

APRNs have the skills and knowledge to be valuable partners in this changing environment. Interpersonal relationship skills, an understanding of systems, problem-solving abilities, flexible thinking, and an openness to new opportunities are essential attributes. Fig. 6-1 illustrates how partnerships, negotiation, and collaboration are

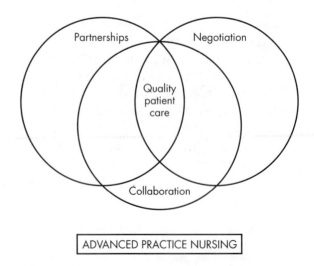

Figure 6-1 Dimensions of advanced practice nursing necessary for quality patient care.

central and interrelated for APRNs whose goal is to provide quality patient care.

PARTNERSHIPS IN THE ■ TEACHING HMO MODEL

The "teaching HMO" can create vibrant research and clinical teaching practice settings and has the potential to transform health professions education in the next century just as the teaching hospital transformed it in this century. The role of an APRN in a joint HMO/academic medical school department highlights the possibilities for forging unique partnerships. The APRN's role interfaces with physicians, nurses, psychologists, social workers, physician assistants, health policy researchers, and other clinicians and administrators in the managed care setting. It further links nursing and nurses in the HMO to colleges and schools of nursing and the larger health care community. Underpinning the role is the concept of the teaching HMO (Moore et al., 1994) and the opportunities that newer delivery systems offer for teaching, research, and clinical practice. Fig. 6-2 illustrates the multiple linkages that can develop between the HMO and other partners. A description of the Department of Ambulatory Care and Prevention (DACP), in HPHC, as well as several key interdisciplinary and nursing partnerships coordinated within the DACP, demonstrate this concept in practice.

The DACP was created in 1992 as a joint partnership between Harvard Medical School (HMS) and HPHC and is funded by HMS and the HPHC

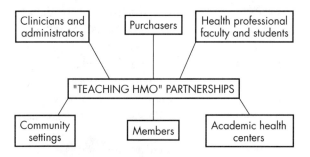

Figure 6-2 Opportunities for multiple partnerships in a "Teaching HMO."

Foundation. It was the nation's first medical school department to be based in a freestanding HMO. The DACP is committed to providing health profession students and researchers with access to the ambulatory managed care setting and to paying attention to three dimensions of health care simultaneously: 1) the needs of the individual, 2) the needs of the population, and 3) the improvement of the health care system (DACP, 1995). One of the educational goals of the DACP is to train clinicians in the wide range of interdisciplinary skills they will need to practice in the rapidly changing health care environment. The DACP's multidisciplinary staff teaches medical students and residents, nursing students, physician assistants, mental health fellows, and others. In particular, a mental health fellowship, the nursing teaching program, and selected examples of research initiatives illustrate the opportunities for APRNs, nursing educators, and students to participate with other health professionals in existing and emerging collaborative partnerships.

The Mental Health Fellowship

The Mental Health Fellowship at HPHC is sponsored by the DACP and coordinated by two DACP faculty members—a psychiatric clinical nurse specialist (CNS) and a psychologist. The fellowship aims to prepare mental health clinicians from different disciplines to work in integrated managed care systems and to partner with a variety of health professionals to provide services to individuals and populations. The HMO provides an excellent site for teaching mental health professionals the skills and competencies required to work within managed care systems (Donovan, Steinberg, & Sabin, 1991, 1994).

This interdisciplinary program is open to master's-prepared psychiatric APRNs, psychiatric social workers, postdoctoral psychologists, and senior psychiatric residents. The fellowship is 1 year in length, usually on a half-time basis. The 20 hour/week program has two key components: a $17\frac{1}{2}$ hour clinical placement at a health center and a $2\frac{1}{2}$ hour central academic seminar designed to support the learning at the clinical site. The program is clinically based and strives to help fellows develop a creative "innovativeness" to practice, work collaboratively with other mental health professionals as well as other primary and specialty care specialists within the HMO, and learn models of quality time-effective treatment, while being mindful of access and resource allocation issues.

The mental health fellowship program is successful because of the partnership of the CNS and the psychologist. They have developed this program over 15 years and have mutual trust and respect for each other's skills and abilities. Their work together builds on this relationship. They share the work of the program by developing the curricula; relating to the clinical supervisors, preceptors, and training coordinators; preparing the central seminar curricula; evaluating and improving the program; developing faculty; recruiting new fellows from colleges and universities and mental health facilities; teaching classes; and writing papers.

Given the interdisciplinary nature of the fellowship and the clear expectation that each fellow will work collaboratively within the seminar and within the clinical setting, it is extremely important that the leadership and structure of the program support nonhierarchical learning experiences. Discussions in the seminar attempt to draw out each fellow. Inclusionary language (e.g., mental health clinicians) is most often used. One of the primary challenges for the fellowship directors is to identify the learning needs of the multidisciplinary group of fellows and to respond with innovative, flexible, helpful teaching strategies that enable the fellows to translate their existing clinical skills, theoretical orientations, and the unique qualities of their professional discipline into the realities of working in a managed care setting. Invited speakers include professionals from each of the mental health disciplines. The multidisciplinary mix of course leaders, guest speakers, and fellows creates rich discussion. The fellowship directors also highlight the unique contributions of each fellow's professional education and clinical background to facilitate an appreciation among the various professions and encourage the development of clinical partnerships.

Multiple partnerships are central to the success of the fellowship. The fellowship directors have developed partnerships with 1) clinicians and administrators at the various clinical sites; 2) faculty at local colleges, institutions, and training programs that prepare candidates for the fellowship year; 3) the multidisciplinary group of fellows; 4) clinical supervisors and preceptors; 5) other faculty in the DACP; 6) a talented group of clinicians who teach every year in the central seminar; and 7) the mental health departments who have hired more than 60 graduates of the program to work at HPHC. As many as a dozen different clinical sites have had fellows. The fellowship directors work to ensure that the clinical sites take fellows from different disciplines in different years to ensure the multidisciplinary nature of the program and to engage numerous clinical faculty and supervisors in the program.

Nursing Teaching Partnerships

The CNS who codirects the mental health fellowship in the DACP also coordinates the teaching activities, at the 14 Harvard Vanguard clinical health centers, of more than 80 APRNs who precept graduate APRN students. APRN students are placed in primary and specialty ambulatory care areas as well as mental health departments with skilled nurse practitioners (NPs), CNSs, and certified nurse midwives (CNMs). Every health center has APRN students who represent more than a dozen academic nursing programs. APRN students quickly learn that teamwork through partnerships is key to meeting the physical and mental health needs of a panel of patients. APRN students diagnose and treat patients with complex problems; consult with APRNs and physicians; and negotiate with administrators, family members, and other clinicians to ensure that necessary services are provided. Sophisticated information systems, quality improvement innovations, and protocols are essential tools.

The nursing teaching program further illustrates the teaching HMO model and demonstrates the future potential and value of partnerships between academic nursing programs and HMO delivery systems. Nursing faculty, both in the HMO setting and from colleges of nursing, are increasingly recognizing the need to identify and teach the skills and competencies required to function in managed care settings. Students have the opportunity to work side by side with other clinicians and understand that the APRN role is essential to the health care team. Harvard Vanguard and other HMOs need to build on the opportunities to develop cross-training and multidisciplinary experiences for health profession students, both in the classroom and in the clinical ambulatory setting, and to augment existing partnerships between MCOs and academic health professional schools. The skills learned in the HMO setting are readily transferable to the variety of settings that require cost containment and rapid assessment and treatment planning. Like the mental health fellows, APRNs are learning first-hand how organizational context and economic constraints influence the delivery of health care.

Research Partnerships

The research agenda of the DACP is to identify health promotion issues that are amenable to thoughtful inquiry and to advance an understanding of these issues. Research that capitalizes on the special features of the managed care environment, available through affiliations with HPHC and Harvard Vanguard, is of primary focus. This research includes asking questions about defined populations and studying the delivery of comprehensive care. There are countless opportunities for nurse researchers to pursue a nursing research agenda in the MCO.

The APRN in the DACP is an active participant in research studies. For example, an experienced APRN partnered with a physician faculty member to do a qualitative study of end-of-life care in managed care (Steinberg & Block, 1998). Together they met with clinicians, administrators, and family members whose loved ones had recently died and asked about the processes and experiences of care at the end of life. Data analysis highlighted the strengths and weaknesses of the existing system and led to substantive changes in the delivery of end-of-life care services. The HPHC insurance benefit for at-home nursing care at the end of life was improved, a multidisciplinary palliative care team was established in the HMO, guidelines for bereavement care were established, and quality improvement projects have been initiated. This research partnership highlights the possibilities for APRNs to pursue research ideas within the HMO, the opportunities for translating research into action and change within a responsive system, and the satisfaction of improving care for the more than one million members in the MCO.

Another example of an ongoing research partnership is between the nursing faculty in the DACP and a faculty member from a local school of nursing that sends APRN students to Harvard Vanguard for clinical preceptorship experiences. The principle investigators are examining and evaluating the HMO ambulatory care teaching and learning experiences of APRN students, faculty, and preceptors in relation to the knowledge, skills, and competencies identified in *Essentials for Master's Education for Advanced Practice Nursing* (AACN, 1996) and the resource paper, *Preparing Learners for Practice in a Managed Care Environment* (Council on Graduate Medical Education, 1997).

The results of this study will be useful in informing faculty, changing curricula, and establishing collaborative educational programs with other health profession students. The partnership between the nursing professor and the DACP nurse faculty member capitalized on the nursing professor's research expertise in evaluating nursing education and the DACP faculty member's understanding of the managed care environment and the clinical learning experiences. The desired outcome of the study is to establish significant partnerships among academic nursing, the HMO, and other health professional disciplines.

In the DACP, the nursing faculty evaluate and work with the educational materials prepared by other health professions, including medicine. For example, the skills and competencies identified in the Council on Graduate Medical Education report seem relevant to the ambulatory care practices of APRNs and compatible with a nursing perspective. Ideally, health professional groups will 1) work together to articulate a shared vision; 2) collaboratively identify the knowledge, skills, and competencies necessary for an interdisciplinary group of health care clinicians to provide quality care; and 3) continue to recognize and value the unique contributions of each professional group.

Clearly promising partnerships can develop in a teaching HMO between APRNs, faculty, students, and other health professionals. If nursing is to be a prominent player in the changing health care environment, nurses need to actively seek such partnerships. Changing health care settings and integrated delivery systems offer many opportunities to expand and explore innovative programs.

■ NEGOTIATION

Negotiation is the mutual discussion and arrangement of the terms of a transaction or agreement (Flexner, 1993). The word *mutual* in this formal definition should be familiar to all APRNs because they are taught the principles of mutual decision making early in their careers. Negotiation is a process in which the APRN is highly skilled. In addition to mutuality, negotiation involves the basic steps of the nursing process as listed in Box 6-1.

Facilitating negotiation involves knowing how to communicate with people (Snyder-Halpern & Cannon, 1993). There are three areas that a skilled negotiator needs to grasp firmly:

---

box 6-1

NURSING PROCESS AND NEGOTIATION ACTIVITIES

Analysis of the problem. Diagnosing the situation through gathering information and organizing it.

Planning. Generating ideas and actions based on facts that will solve the problem mutually.

Implementation. Understanding the role that each side will play and acting on that understanding.

Evaluation. Using criteria to measure or decide and measure successful outcomes.

- How to reflect another person's perception of the problem
- How to deal with highly charged emotions
- How to handle misunderstandings

The APRN knows how to be empathic. He or she tries to understand the patient's perceptions by listening carefully and communicating an understanding of the patient's feelings and the experiences underlying those feelings (Egan, 1997). Dealing with highly charged emotions is also part of the APRNs work, and using stress management to defuse situations becomes second nature to the experienced APRN. The pathway to handling misunderstandings is through good communication techniques that the effective APRN has mastered.

Negotiation involves knowing that behind each party's interests are basic human needs: security, economic well-being, a sense of belonging, recognition, and control over one's life (Fisher, Ury, & Patton, 1991). These needs are basically the same as Maslow's (1968) hierarchy of needs, which should be familiar to all nurses. Maslow's hierarchy is a foundation for planning holistic nursing care. Fig. 6-3 illustrates the multiple stages and skills that facilitate the negotiation process.

Negotiation in a Group Practice

Approximately 200 APRNs work for Harvard Vanguard. Harvard Vanguard contains 14 health cen-

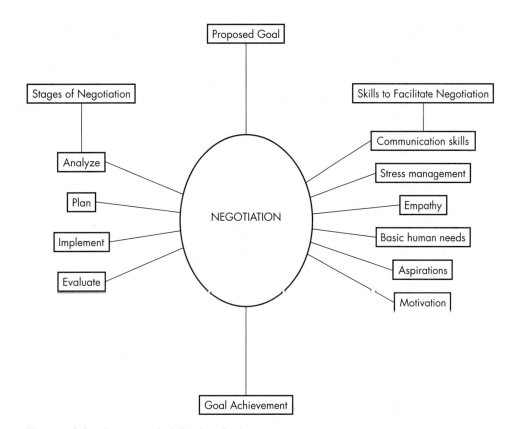

Figure 6-3 Stages and skills that facilitate negotiation.

ters, each with primary care, medical specialties, and mental health departments. Communication among clinicians to enhance good patient care and "collaboration to achieve collective responsibility" (Wocial, 1996) for good patient outcomes are high priorities at Harvard Vanguard.

From its beginning in 1968 as Harvard Community Health Plan, the Harvard Vanguard appreciated the skills of APRNs. The breadth and depth of APRN skills have contributed to the growth and reputation of the group, and the APRNs are important practice partners with their physician colleagues. Introducing prescription writing into the APRNs' practices went smoothly as physicians valued this role enhancement as a benefit to patient services. APRNs at Harvard Vanguard practice in the expanded role with a high degree of autonomy.

However, the APRNs in the Harvard Community Health Plan health centers rarely had influence in the management of the HMO, and the APRNs benefit structure was set up very differently from that of the physicians. When the economics of health care began to shift in the 1990s, the HMO merged with a large preferred provider organization (PPO) to guarantee financial survival. This newly merged organization (HPHC) now consisted of many private physicians' practices that did not employ APRNs.

In the few years after the merger, it became clear to the APRNs and other health professionals working in the HMO that it was hard for HPHC to differentiate and market the unique collaborative multispecialty group practice delivery system from other parts of the large MCO. The resources of the larger merged MCO were not being used to highlight, enhance, and grow the health center practices. Clinicians and administrators in the health centers began to suffer an identity crisis. The decision was made by the chief executive officer (CEO) that the health centers division needed to become again an independent group practice. To formulate such a plan, the CEO called together an assembly to make decisions about the future of the health centers. The leadership, which was composed of 40 clinicians who were elected by their colleagues to represent them in establishing a new group practice, established a group practice culture of decision making. The group practice at this point consisted of approximately 800 physicians and psychologists, 200 APRNs, 60 physician assistants, 400 RNs, 70 social workers, as well as support staff and administrative managers. Given the large number of physicians versus other practitioners, the APRNs recognized they would need to begin actively negotiating to ensure a recognized role in the new group practice.

Firmly believing in the multidisciplinary collaborative model of care, APRNs ran for election for the assembly to represent the interests of all APRNs as well as other advanced practice clinicians (e.g., social workers and physician assistants). Because the group was physician-dominated in terms of numbers and historically in terms of decision making, APRNs knew that a high level of empathy toward physician colleagues would be needed to be successful in negotiating nursing's interests in the new group practice. The APRNs' election campaigns promised to 1) promote the importance of nursing roles by bringing to the assembly numbers showing contributions to patient care (data and analysis), 2) show how advanced practice clinicians improve patient care outcomes (planning), and 3) define future roles in the new group practice as plans moved forward (implementation). For the most part, the APRNs promised good communication and an openness to all ideas. All clinicians were invited to discuss their perceptions of the assembly process, and misunderstandings were clarified. After each assembly meeting a memo was sent to all advanced practice clinicians describing what decisions were being made and inviting feedback to help promote good decision making.

The most heated issue before the assembly was how to financially support the new group practice. The concept that emerged early in the dialogue was that physicians would "set aside" a certain percentage of their salaries to ensure the organization's solvency. This percentage would be returned if budget targets were favorable. It quickly became clear that with financial responsibility, the governance structure or ongoing decision-making structure would also be a physician responsibility. This was an outcome that advanced practice clinicians participating in the assembly wanted to avoid, because they firmly believed that shared governance with the physicians would lead to the best health care practice. This belief was rooted in the idea that "an integrated whole rather than a combination of separate professional fields is important to patient outcome" (Mariano, 1989).

Thus the advanced practice clinicians proposed that the same percentage of advanced practice clinicians' salaries be set aside, pointing out their contributions to the group practice and their commitment to the new group. Additionally, the advanced practice clinicians strongly noted that the total amount set aside, or financial risk by the physicians, would drop approximately 5% with the contribution of advanced practice clinicians, an obvious inducement to the physicians.

Looking back at Maslow's hierarchy it may seem that this proposal violated one of the basic tenets of the interests of the advanced practice clinicians, namely economic well-being. They proposed the same set aside percentage as the physicians to emphasize their wish to be equal partners in the new group practice. Equal partners means equal participation in the governance of the new group, equal participation in the benefit structure, and equal ownership of the newly restructured group practice. The advanced practice clinicians and physicians would become voting members of the corporation (VMOCs). The advanced practice clinicians believed that this equality would increase their sense of belonging, recognition, and control over their practice, thus strengthening their interests according to Maslow. They believed that they could be better patient advocates from inside the governing framework. They also recognized that economic well-being might not be affected adversely if the group made responsible decisions in its budget process—decisions in which they wanted to be involved. The assembly agreed and voted to include advanced practice clinicians as VMOCs.

Negotiations with Nurses and Other Advanced Practice Clinicians

The APRNs had three further important negotiations. The first negotiation was with advanced practice colleagues, some of whom were not so sure that such equality was worth the financial risk. The second negotiation was with the union, which represented both the RNs and the APRNs (all nurses voted as a group). Union members were not clear that becoming VMOCs represented appropriate progress in their roles in the new group practice. In addition, the union would lose some negotiating power as the set aside percentages would not be part of their contract with the new group. The third negotiation was with the RNs who would not be VMOCs but who were concerned about lessening the union's negotiating power.

To accomplish these negotiations, the APRNs needed help from many different people. Studies of negotiation consistently show strong correlation between aspiration and result (Fisher, Ury, & Patton, 1991), so support was sought from like-minded APRNs. The APRN negotiating group recognized that they needed to seek more information on the implications of VMOC status. Memorandums were sent to all APRNs requesting donations to hire a lawyer familiar with both health care and union representation from whom they sought important guidance. The APRNs recognized that they needed to be prepared and educated not only in the business of health care, but also in the

business of union representation (analysis of the problem). Meetings were held with more memoranda sent, sharing with all APRNs the information that they had gathered from counsel and offering to answer the concerns of all (planning). The union was included in the information loop, and its representatives were invited to all of the meetings. With the help of all those involved and excited about the VMOC opportunity, the APRNs began talking to their RN colleagues to assure them that all nursing would benefit from APRN involvement because nurses' voices would help shape patient care decisions. The APRN negotiating group asked for and received support from the other advanced practice clinicians. The other advanced practice clinicians shared their enthusiasm for being part of a unique health care group where clinicians would create policies and develop strategies to promote patient care, and they encouraged the APRNs to be equal partners with them as the organization changed.

With as much information as any other practice group about what being a VMOC in the changing group meant, the APRN negotiators found that their biggest challenge was handling the emotional aspects of the decision. As the night approached for the union membership to vote, anxiety climbed and the feelings of insecurity festered. Phone calls were accepted at all hours from nurses who had been involved in the beginning of the process and nurses who were now just becoming involved. As the APRN negotiators tried to give information, they recognized that change brings fear and, with that, a certain amount of distorted thinking because people's listening skills are blunted by their fear. The group of APRNs supporting VMOC membership realized that their colleagues needed to have their fears heard in order to consider other aspects of the issue. The APRN negotiators patiently used stress management techniques and communication skills as they responded to every negative argument about becoming a VMOC, with the positive argument in a way that was supportive and respectful of their nursing colleagues. They expressed excitement for the future while acknowledging that change does involve risk. They wanted people who called to feel heard, have their fear allayed, hear the arguments, and be persuaded that being a VMOC was the correct decision.

The night of the meeting immediately preceding the vote, APRNs in favor of VMOC status spoke of the opportunity that lay before the nurses and repeated every fact and option available. They wanted to create a health care organization where equality of effort would exist among all levels of advanced practice clinicians and physicians. They asked the CEO (a non-physician) to speak about his firm belief in the rightness of inclusion of APRNs in the core of the group. Those not favoring VMOC status used emotional arguments highlighting lack of trust in the new organization and the possible financial risk. When the votes were counted, VMOC status was resoundingly confirmed and APRNs became partners in a new multispecialty group practice.

■ COLLABORATION

Rapid advances in health care information and technology make collaboration essential for complete and effective patient care. No one discipline can provide all of what is needed to maintain health and treat disease (McCloskey & Maas, 1998). *Collaboration* is the process of working together, as its Latin root implies. In collaboration there is a common goal. The process to achieve that goal is agreed upon. Values are shared and respect is mutual. There is power equality in effecting action. Relationship building and shared decision making are two salient features of collaboration, and decisions are made through negotiations, consensus, cooperation, and assertiveness (Sullivan, 1998).

Trust is an essential attribute of the collaborative relationship. Trust can exist only if there is competence on the part of the collaborators to achieve their common goal (Sullivan, 1998). Competence engenders trust. APRNs are competent to make independent clinical assessments, provide independent clinical treatment, create and evaluate clinical programs, teach patients and other health care providers, and understand and use basic group skills in clinical and collaborative work. They are competent to collaborate in direct service, education, research, and management.

In addition to competence and trust, collaboration requires support from people and the system surrounding the people. A committed administration, supportive leadership, stable work force, and sufficient resources are also necessary (Sullivan, 1998). Equality in power is needed—not the informal power nurses are used to, but formal recognized power sharing. Barriers to collaboration include competition, defensiveness, aggressiveness, territoriality, and close-mindedness (Valentine et al., 1990).

Example of Collaborative Practice

At Harvard Vanguard, the Mental Health Department is integrated with all other clinical departments. APRNs attempt to work closely with primary and specialty care areas to provide total care for a patient's health. The obstetrics and gynecology (ob/gyn) department had many patients needing mental health referrals for timely and specialized intervention. The patients and ob/gyn clinicians were feeling ineffectively served by the mental health department. The chief of the mental health department asked for a staff member to collaborate with the ob/gyn staff to improve services to patients and colleagues. An APRN in psychiatric mental health nursing expressed interest and provided 5 hours a week of her mental health clinical time to design and implement a responsive program.

The multispecialty group practice in the health centers fosters and supports collaboration. Harvard Community Health Plan was founded on the premise that effective and efficient care in an increasingly complicated clinical world could only be given by the joint effort of many health profession disciplines with the same goal: quality, cost-efficient health care for the community. All disciplines are perceived as necessary and competent, so there is trust in the working relationships. Clinical decision making is processed and shared, and power in decisions is given to the most appropriate clinician. Clinicians are supported by the administration and the system to negotiate whatever works with each other to provide for patient needs. The APRN in this case felt supported administratively and collegially to work with the ob/gyn department for the benefit of patients' needs.

The APRN spoke first with the chiefs of both the mental health and ob/gyn departments about the perceived needs of their departments. She then spoke to all ob/gyn clinicians to learn about their needs for interdisciplinary support and care of their patients. She researched the mental health problems related to obstetrics and gynecology and used her knowledge and skills for effective consultation.

The APRN asked for and readily received office space to see patients in the ob/gyn department, rather than requiring people to come to the mental health department. This was done to enhance collegiality and communication between the clinicians and to facilitate the ease with which all patients, even those who might be reticent to be seen in the mental health department, could have access to mental health care. Creating office space and administrative support for the APRN's clinical practice in the ob/gyn department took flexibility and commitment on the part of that department and spoke to the shared goal of integrated patient care.

The APRN then negotiated a mutually convenient monthly time when she could be available to all clinicians to discuss cases and problems. All clinicians were enthusiastic about this opportunity for communication and education, but in reality it was usually the ob/gyn nurses who came to the meetings. Physicians' schedules were more variable and the APRN needed to seek them out individually. They were, however, receptive to contact and initiated it readily themselves when appropriate.

Additional collaborative and consultative initiatives followed. The APRN designed and taught inservice sessions at some monthly ob/gyn department meetings on subjects of interest and need, especially postpartum depression. Subsequently, the psychiatric APRN and the ob/gyn staff designed preventive and early interventions for postpartum disorders and pregnancy loss. The APRN and an APRN nurse colleague in the central infertility department were concerned about the stress of infertility on couples. They collaborated to design and implement an interdepartmental couples group to support infertile couples to move on constructively in their infertility process. In addition, a collaborative research project with a DACP nurse researcher colleague aimed to improve treatment interventions for the support of families with premature infants. The APRN also consulted with a physician-nurse team developing a practice for patients with vulvar disease to address the emotional needs of these women.

Since the 1963 Surgeon General's Report recommended that nurses do primary care in collaboration with physicians, collaboration has been most often written about in the context of nurses and physicians (Sullivan, 1998). Major considerations for this then innovative idea about nurses and doctors collaborating for patient care included nursing competence for the expanded role, legal limitations on scope of practice, the nurse's willingness to assume clinical responsibility, assertive versus aggressive behavior on the part of nurses, and content of the appropriate nursing role (Devereux, 1981). Nursing should now be beyond the need to justify the usefulness and competence of APRNs and move directly to the task of providing advanced practice collaborative care. The APRN in today's reengineered health care settings collaborates with many professionals and the focus can certainly be expanded to include much more than nurse-physician collaboration.

In the preceding model of clinical practice collaboration the APRN collaborated with many health professionals. She worked together with other nurses, physicians, lactation consultants, social workers, and support staff. She negotiated her role with clinicians and administrators. The end point of collaboration, of course, is with the patient, but initially, successful working relationships were established with the many others whose roles were affected by the APRN's work.

Collaboration starts with two or more people with shared values agreeing to work together for a common goal. In this case the APRN and the staff of the ob/gyn department agreed to collaborate to improve the mental health care of all ob/gyn patients. Because they believed in their mutual competence, they trusted each other to work together on the special problems of these patients. The APRN took the risk of asking for practice space in the ob/gyn department and asking for time in departmental meetings to share knowledge and plan interventions. She asserted her knowledge of psychiatric problems so that decisions could be made jointly about the treatment of patients with both ob/gyn and mental health needs. There was open and honest sharing of information and needs, and no one clinician's input and treatment plan was valued or acted upon to the detriment of another's. All clinicians felt equally empowered. The collaboration in this example of practice is effective because all essential aspects of collaboration are present as illustrated in Fig. 6-4.

Nursing Perspective in Collaboration

A nursing perspective and unique skill are also essential to the success of this example of collaborative practice. The patient's needs are always considered, including the patient's demographics and environment, financial, and social situations. This information informs the clinical evaluation and treatment plans generated for the specific ob/gyn and mental health problems.

The integration of the total person with his or her illness and treatment planning for that illness are unique aspects of nursing care. Collaboration among disciplines does not mean ignoring the unique contribution of each discipline involved. On the contrary, collaboration requires at least

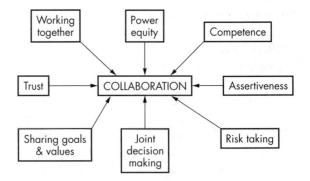

Figure 6-4 Elements of a successful collaboration.

two perspectives and knowledge bases or there would be no need to work together for a common goal. Harvard Vanguard, like many other health organizations, attempts to blend disciplines for the sake of management efficiency. For example, nurses, physician assistants, and social workers are often called *mid-level providers*. They are lumped together for administrative purposes and not recognized for their unique skills and contributions. This approach can undermine the power that comes from strong professional identity and the value that comes from having a unique body of knowledge. Power is essential for effective collaboration (McCloskey & Maas, 1998). To have power, nursing must insist on being valued and recognized for its contributions to have power.

IMPLICATIONS FOR
■ THE FUTURE

This chapter highlights the possibilities that can develop for advanced practice psychiatric-mental health nurses when they seize new opportunities and are open to developing their skills. APRNs have the core knowledge, skills, and competencies that are essential for effective practice. Newer delivery systems demand a refocusing of undergraduate and graduate nursing education. Roles are developing for nurses that are nontraditional and certainly more collaborative. Innovations in teaching, research, clinical practice, and administration will be the cornerstone for the future.

Interdisciplinary partnerships are essential to provide health care over the health care continuum. Nonhierarchical settings are becoming more commonplace. The APRN is well positioned for assuming greater responsibility in evolving health care systems. Skillful use of partnerships, negotiation, and collaboration will allow APRNs to provide quality health care to their patients. Rather than be fearful of the changes that are rapidly transforming familiar institutions, APRNs can embrace their competencies with confidence and enthusiasm and take their rightful place in the health care delivery systems of the future.

RESOURCES AND CONNECTIONS

RELATED BOOKS

Bauer, J.C. (1998). *Not what the doctor ordered* (ed. 2). New York: McGraw Hill.

Hesselbein, F., Goldsmith, M., & Beckhard, R. (Eds.). (1997). *The organization of the future*. San Francisco: Jossey-Bass Publishers.

Seaburn, D.B., et al. (1996). *Models of collaboration: a guide for mental health professionals working with health care practitioners*. New York: Basic Books.

INTERNET SITES

Robert Wood Johnson Foundation www.rwjf.org
Muskegon Community Health Project mchp.org
W.K. Kellogg Foundation www.wkkf.org
Harvard Pilgrim Health Plan www.harvardpilgrim.org
Group Health Cooperative of Puget Sound www.ghc.org
Collaborative Family Healthcare Coalition www.cfhcc.org

References

American Association of Colleges of Nursing. (1996). *The essentials of master's education for advanced practice nursing*. Washington, DC: Author.

American Nurses Association. (1998). *Managed care: nursing's blueprint for action*. Washington, DC: Author.

American Psychiatric Nurses Association. (1997). *Report of the APNA Congress on advanced practice in psychiatric nursing*. Washington, DC: Author.

Council on Graduate Medical Education. (1997, September). *Preparing learners for practice in a managed care environment*. (Resource paper). Washington, DC: Author.

Department of Ambulatory Care and Prevention. (1995, December). *Annual report*. Boston: Harvard Medical School and Harvard Pilgrim Health Care.

Devereux, P.M. (1981). Nurse/physician collaboration: nursing practice considerations. *The Journal of Nursing Administration, 11*(9), 37–46.

Donovan, J.M., Steinberg, S.M., & Sabin, J.E. (1991). A mental health fellowship program in an HMO setting. *Hospital and Community Psychiatry, 42*, 952–953.

Donovan, J.M., Steinberg, S.M., & Sabin, J.E. (1994). Managed mental health care: an academic seminar, *Psychotherapy, 1*, 201–207.

Egan, G. (1997). *The skilled helper: a problem-management approach to helping*. Pacific Grove, CA: Brooks/Cole.

Fisher, R., Ury, W., & Patton, B. (1991). *Getting to yes: negotiating agreement without giving in*. New York: Penguin Books.

Flexner, S. (Ed.). (1993). *Random house unabridged dictionary* (ed. 2). New York: Random House.

Mariano, C. (1989). The case for interdisciplinary collaboration. *Nursing Outlook, 37*(6), 285–288.

Maslow, A.H. (1968). *Toward a psychology of being*. New York: John Wiley & Sons.

McCloskey, J.C., & Maas, M. (1998). Interdisciplinary team: the nursing perspective is essential. *Nursing Outlook, 46*(4), 157–63.

Moore, G.T., et al. (1994). The "teaching HMO": a new academic partner. *Academic Medicine, 69*, 983–989.

O'Neil, E. (1998). Nursing in the next century. In O'Neil, E., & Coffman, J. (Eds.). *Strategies for the future of nursing: changing roles, responsibilities, and employment patterns of registered nurses*. San Francisco, CA: Jossey-Bass.

Snyder-Halpern, R., & Cannon, M. (1993). A framework for the development of nurse manager negotiation skills. *Journal of Nursing Staff Development, 9*(1), 14–19.

Steinberg, S.M., & Block, S. B. (1998). Caring for patients at the end of life in an HMO. *Journal of Palliative Medicine, 1*(4), 387–399.

Sullivan, T.J. (1998). *Collaboration: a health care imperative*. New York: McGraw-Hill.

Valentine, et al. (1990). A collaborative approach to clinical standards development. *Psychiatric Clinics of North America, 13*(1), 171–185.

Wocial, L. (1996). Achieving collaboration in ethical decision making: strategies for nurses in clinical practice. *Dimensions of Critical Care Nursing, 15*(3), 150–152.

Health Policy, Politics, and Advanced Practice Nursing

JUDITH HABER and MAUREEN BEIRNE STREFF

■ INTRODUCTION

To participate in the shaping of health and mental health care delivery, advanced practice registered nurses (APRNs) in psychiatric-mental health must think about politics as a means and policy as an outcome. They can then act to influence change in federal, state, and local arenas. As nursing leaders, APRNs are challenged to participate more fully in politics and policymaking within and outside their workplaces to shape policy for the benefit of the consumers of mental health services. A critical mass of APRNs needs to be politicized if the mental health voice is to be brought to the policy tables in meaningful ways. This chapter provides a framework for linking policy and politics to advanced psychiatric nursing practice.

POLICY, POLITICS, ■ AND POWER

Policy: What Exactly Is It?

Policy is defined as "the principles that govern action directed towards given ends" (Titmus, 1974). Policy involves the application of reason, conscious decision-making, and problem-solving. Embedded in the policymaking process are the choices that society, a segment of society, or an organization makes regarding its goals, priorities, and allocation of resources.

As described in Table 7-1, several types of policy are commonly encountered in policymaking arenas which include either the public or private sector (Mason & Leavitt, 1993). Policy includes a broad range of activities that involve the estab-

table 7-1

COMMON TYPES OF POLICY

TYPES	DEFINITION	EXAMPLE
Public policy	Policy formed by governmental bodies such as the Congress	Law passed by Congress mandating direct Medicare reimbursement for APRNs regardless of geographic or practice setting. This law could be regarded as a policy that promotes increased choice and access to mental health care delivered by nonphysician providers.
Social policy	Directives that promote the welfare of the public or a segment of the population	The state legislature writes regulations that deal with job training programs for women on public assistance that mandate content on how to deal with sexual harassment in the workplace. This law could be regarded as a policy that promotes the mental health of women.
Health policy	Directives that promote the health of the citizens of a community	The Board of Representatives of city X believes that all victims of rape should be provided with counselling services to assist them in coping with the experience. The Board passes legislation authorizing a funding stream for a rape crisis counselling center, which can be regarded as a policy that establishes crisis intervention as a required service for trauma victims.
Institutional policy	Policies that govern the workplace and the accomplishment of its goals	As a reflection of the institutional policies related to how health system ABC will treat its employees, the hospital's governing council develops and implements a policy that prohibits sexual harassment in the institution and includes a grievance process for reporting and handling sexual harassment claims.
Organizational policy	Rules governing and the positions taken by organizations	The American Nurses Association passes a resolution that opposes the registered nurse's participation in assisted suicide. This can be regarded as a policy that affirms the organization's beliefs and values.

lishment of authoritative guidelines in the form of laws or other official rules and regulations, position statements, or documents that deal with an issue of public concern and affect the conduct of public affairs. In essence, a policy refers to a specific organizational decision to take action or not take action with regard to a specific issue.

In the private sector, policy decisions are made by social service agencies, health care organizations, insurers, and managed care organizations. These include directives regarding conditions of employment, health care coverage parameters, and the delivery of health care services. In the public sector, policy refers to local, state, and federal legislation and its accompanying rules and regulations, as well as court rulings that affect individual and institutional behavior under the

particular government's jurisdiction (Hanley, 1993). Policy can also refer to administrative decisions in interagency and intraagency activities, including interpretive guidelines for rules and regulations and judicial decisions that interpret the law. Examples of public sector policymaking include state licensure for professional practice and recent revisions in the federal Medicare legislation authorizing direct reimbursement to APRNs, which resulted in the development and interpretation of rules and regulations by the Health Care Financing Administration (HCFA).

Numerous opportunities exist for all APRNs to influence the shaping of policy, particularly health policy. One example of this is described in Box 7-1. Knowledge of the policy stakeholders, the elected or appointed officials, interest group repre

box 7-1

HEALTH POLICY DEVELOPMENT IN ACTION

Violence is a major physical and mental health care problem, costing the United States thousands of lives, millions of dollars, and untold physical and psychological morbidity. Only in the last decade has the role of the health care system been considered as important as the judicial system in dealing with violence (USDHHS, 1990). Dr. Ann Burgess, a psychiatric nurse, was instrumental in influencing that health policy shift through her early and influential program of nursing research in the area of violence. Burgess' initial article on the rape trauma syndrome (Burgess & Holstrum, 1974) is considered a classic in rape research and is cited in many articles on the subject. Her program of research has established a model of how children respond emotionally to sexual abuse that explains their ongoing and delayed symptoms (Hartman & Burgess, 1988). She is frequently an advocate for child victims of sexual assault as an expert witness in courts and works regularly with the Federal Bureau of Investigation (FBI) to formulate policy related to violence. The most influential policy component of Burgess' work was her participation as one of only nine national experts on violence on the Department of Justice Task Force on Family Violence formed in 1983. The report from that commission clearly indicated that the health care system needs to be involved in national efforts to address the problem of violence.

Shortly after that report was issued, then Surgeon General C. Everett Koop organized a workshop to formulate the responsibilities of the health care system in relation to violence. Dr. Burgess and her colleague Dr. Carol Hartman wrote the background paper on rape and sexual assault for that conference (American Academy of Nursing Expert Panel on Violence, 1993). Twenty other nurses joined Burgess, among the 150 invited national experts on violence from all disciplines, at the workshop. She held an informal caucus to make sure that nursing's voice would be heard in the resulting policy initiatives.

As an outgrowth of the Surgeon General's conference, official health care policy for the U.S. Public Health Services has been to consider violence as a critical health problem. The change in policy was formalized by inclusion of a set of objectives on Violence and Abusive Behavior in the original *Healthy People 2000* (USDHHS, 1990) guidelines for national health care in the next decade, which remain included in the revised *Healthy People 2000* (USDHHS, 1995) document.

sentatives, or individuals who are directly involved in shaping a particular policy and who may be directly affected by its outcome is particularly important (Hanley, 1993). This was evident in the grassroots campaign by APRNs to include clinical nurse specialists (CNSs) in the 1997 revision of the Medicare reimbursement legislation. At stake was elimination of a barrier to practice, increased access to health care services, and expanded provider choice for consumers.

Politics: The Nuts and Bolts of It

"Politics is a domain of activity in which participants attempt to influence organizational decisions and activities in such ways that are not sanctioned by either the formal authority system of an organization, its accepted ideology or certified expertise" (Shortrell & Kaluzney, 1994). Embedded in the definition of politics is the idea of influence, specifically, influence related to the allocation of scarce resources. In fact, politics is a process by which a person or group of people influences the decisions of others and exerts control over situations and events (Mason, 1990).

The term *politician* has historically connoted the ability to deal with people and accomplish good things for the good of the people and the country (Thorndike & Barnhart, 1979). Nurses have demonstrated that they can be and are politicians in the historic sense of the word. For some people, however, the terms *politics* and *politician* connote negativity. *Politician* often is used slightingly or contemptuously to suggest a person without principles scheming for one's own or one's party's good, to make deals using bribes, unethical compromises, or payoffs. The positive connotation increasingly has been more applicable to the political image of professional nurses astutely using political skills: "knowing how to be persuasive, how to garner and use power effectively, how to analyze problems impeding goals, and how to mobilize people to work collectively" (Leavitt & Barry, 1993). Former Speaker of the House of Representatives Tip O'Neil, in his book, *All Politics is Local and Other Rules of the Game* (O'Neil & Hymel, 1994), offered a guideline to manage both the positive and negative connotations of the political process: "For me politics is always about values combined with instincts. Put those together and you get a rule" (O'Neil & Hymel, 1994). As the title of his book suggests, Mr. O'Neil based his career on the maxim, "all politics is local." Sharp (1994) proposes that O'Neil's rise to power rested primarily on personal relationships, party loyalty, and favors that he did for constituents and colleagues. APRNs should discuss how the same principles could help psychiatric nurses "work the system," whether it be the health care system or the political system.

Although the 2,500,000 registered nurses outnumber physicians, dentists, and every other group of health professionals in the United States (Lee & Estes, 1997), they have been slow to understand the political nature of the world, and the need for nurses to participate proactively in the political arena and exercise leadership to influence the political process and effect policy change. Economic oppression led to engagement in political activity to remove barriers to practice as far back as 1948. At that time the American Nurses Association (ANA) identified third-party reimbursement for nursing services as a priority in the association platform. Fifty years later some states still do not have mandatory third-party reimbursement for services provided by APRNs.

Power: An Essential Component of Creating Change

Power can be defined as that which enables a person to accomplish goals. Box 7-2 highlights seven common types of power that can be used to support effective leadership. The concept of power is generally not associated with the nursing profession (Roberts & Chandler, 1996). The media, the public at large, and other opinionmakers refer to the power of health related corporations (e.g., pharmaceutical companies, trade associations such as the American Hospital Association

TYPES OF POWER

1. *Reward power.* Power obtained by the ability to grant favors or reward others with whatever they value.
2. *Coercive power.* Power based on a person's real or perceived fear of punishment by another person.
3. *Legitimate power.* Power derived from a person's organizational title or position rather than from a personal quality.
4. *Expert power.* Power gained through knowledge, expertise, or experience.
5. *Referent power.* Power given to others by association with the powerful leader or because they are perceived as powerful.
6. *Information power.* Power that results when one person has, or is perceived to have, special information that another desires.

From Marquis & Huston, 1992.

TOP TEN LOBBIES IN THE UNITED STATES

1. American Association of Retired Persons (AARP)
2. American Israel Public Affairs Committee (AIPAC)
3. American Federation of Labor–Congress of Industrial Organizations (AFL-CIO)
4. National Federation of Independent Business (NFIB)
5. Association of Trial Lawyers of America (ATLA)
6. National Rifle Association of America (NRA)
7. Christian Coalition
8. American Medical Association (AMA)
9. National Education Association (NEA)
10. National Right to Life Committee

From Birnbaum, 1997.

[AHA], professional organizations such as the American Medical Association [AMA], and trade unions such as Local 1199), but seldom are nurses and nursing automatically considered powerful. However, a 1997 survey conducted by *Fortune Magazine* (Birnbaum, 1997) indicates that the ANA is now the seventy-eighth most powerful lobby in the United States, closely positioned to the National Cattlemen's Beef Association. As indicated in Box 7-3, the AMA ranks eighth, whereas the AHA ranks twenty-first. Neither the American Psychiatric Association, American Psychological Association, nor the National Association of Social Workers is listed in the ranking of the top 100 lobbying groups.

Too often, psychiatric nurses have failed to exercise the power of their knowledge and competence in providing patient care, thereby demonstrating how their practice makes a difference (Buerhaus, 1996). In most health care settings, psychiatric or otherwise, the closer the nurse is to direct patient care, the less powerful he or she

is, and the less likely he or she is to track data that document how nursing interventions influence clinical outcomes. Moreover, most nurses have not understood, mastered, or used political skills consistently in their work, nor do they understand that there is a constructive relationship between power, politics, and influencing change in policy. Sharp (1995) suggests that, all too often, nurses question why they should care or get involved. Content with going to work and not rocking the boat, they do not understand that political savvy is now a nursing skill, one that affects the nurses' ability to influence the development of and changes in policy that have a direct impact on patient care.

Psychiatric nurses, as long-standing participants in the workforce, have spent considerable time nurturing, sustaining, and supporting their colleagues in psychology, psychiatry, and social work, often as silent partners with little tangible recognition in job status or salary. Their absence or limited presence in major deliberative bodies in their workplace organizations is an issue of concern and calls for concerted action. For example, nursing representation on powerful workplace committees where organizational policies are determined and financial or other resources are allocated is not regarded as a high priority by most psychiatric nurses. Therefore it is not surprising that the membership of these committees is comprised of those, primarily men, in the higher echelons of the organizations.

For women, such as nurses, there is often a negative connotation when the same drive is evident. However, Ferguson (1993) comments that "one need only ask or observe who shapes policy versus who carries it out; who has sign-off authority for major decisions in the workplace; or how many women and nurses sit on the boards of for-profit and non-profit corporations or are chief executive officers or chief operating officers of hospitals or community-based health agencies" or are elected or appointed legislators or government officials. One can conclude that, as a largely female profession, nurses will not be readily invited to join key committees or apply for corporate leadership positions. Rather, they must be proactive in using their power tools and political skills to seek such opportunities.

If nurses stay as reactive (or even worse, inactive) stakeholders, they set themselves up to miss out on important policymaking opportunities that affect their practice and the health of their patient constituency. To effect change in policy arenas, nurses must be "players with seats at the political and policy tables." Contributing expertise through workplace, community, and/or professional organizational involvement is a key vehicle for increasing the profession's visibility profile, thereby becoming recognized as a powerful player and sought for influential leadership positions (Helms, Anderson, & Hanson, 1996).

Over the years, numerous psychiatric nurses have held leadership positions in prestigious organizations. Dr. Hildegard Peplau, the mother of psychiatric nursing, is the only nurse who was both Executive Director and President of the ANA. Dr. Claire Fagin, former Dean of the School of Nursing at the University of Pennsylvania and a well known psychiatric APRN, served as Interim President of the University of Pennsylvania, the first nurse to serve as a President of an Ivy League institution. Dr. Rhetaugh Dumas, another highly visible psychiatric nurse, is a former Dean of the School of Nursing at the University of Michigan and has been President of the National League for Nursing, a nursing organization that plays a major policy role through its educational accreditation programs. Past President of APNA, Nancy Valentine, was Assistant Chief Medical Director for Nursing Programs at the Department of Veterans Affairs in Washington. In her role as Chief Nursing Officer (CNO), Valentine provided leadership for the development of policy about the delivery of patient care by the 76,000 RNs and APRNs employed by this federal organization throughout the United States.

Recent accomplishments of APRNs signal that the national leadership role played by and scope of influence of psychiatric nurses has begun to accelerate. For example, as President of the ANA from 1992 to 1996, Virginia Trotter Betts, an attorney and APRN, was instrumental in substantially increasing the ANA's role in political activism and public policymaking. She played a key role in the historic implementation of *Nursing's Agenda for Health Care Reform* (ANA, 1991) and through use of political activism advanced the visibility and influence of professional nursing in Washington, D.C. In 1998 she was appointed to the post of Senior Advisor on Nursing Policy and Senior Health Policy Advisor of the United States Department of Health and Human Services (USDHHS). In that role she monitored and participated in all USDHHS policy work that involves the nursing profession. Issues include nursing education, licensure, scope of practice, nursing research, nursing workforce concerns, and nursing reimbursement and practice arrangements. The ANA President, Beverly Malone, also a psychiatric APRN, commented that Betts' appointment showed "that registered nurses continue to take their rightful place at the highest levels of health care decisionmaking" (ANA, 1998). In addition,

President Malone and three other nurses were appointed members of the President's Advisory Commission on Consumer Protection and Quality.

Paths to Power

Ferguson (1993) has named four paths to achieving a more visible and powerful presence that include the following:

1. *Power through knowledge.* First, knowledge is a significant resource that confers authority on its possessor. Knowledge can be used strategically and effectively to inform, educate, and influence decisions made by policymakers, legislators, and other key leaders who control allocation of resources. For example, APRNs have expert knowledge about the delivery of psychiatric-mental health care by APRNs and its effect on clinical outcomes. This knowledge was used to inform and influence legislators about including CNSs in the 1997 Medicare reimbursement legislation. Similarly, this expert knowledge has been used to educate and influence managed care companies and managed behavioral healthcare organizations to credential and employ APRNs as providers.

2. *Power through competence.* Power is accumulated and expanded as APRNs address their expertise in practice, education for practice, research base that improves and validates practice, and administrative activity to enable practice (Ferguson, 1993). In an era of dramatically increased accountability, consumers, policymakers, and legislators are demanding that reimbursable health care services demonstrate their effectiveness from a quality perspective, as well as their cost-effectiveness. As APRNs compete for increased participation in management, governance, planning, and policy development in the health care system, they must value scholarship in the form of research and continually apply it to the evaluation of their practice. Outcome data about the delivery of advanced practice psychiatric nursing services must demonstrate how these services make a

difference in the lives of consumers of mental health care, their primary patients. Such "hard evidence" of competence can be presented to consumers, employers who purchase health insurance for their employees, and public and private third-party payers, including managed care companies, policymakers, and legislators (Haber, 1997a). Data that validate competence can be used to establish and maintain an APRN power base in mental health care. In one of the few outcome research studies in the specialty, Baradell (1995) reports findings of outcome studies that examined the treatment efficacy of psychiatric-mental health CNSs in community-based private practice settings. Retrospective patient data revealed significant improvement in clinical symptoms, improvement in perceived quality of life, and high satisfaction with mental health care provided by CNSs who, Baradell (1994) demonstrated, are more cost-effective providers of mental health services than psychiatrists or clinical psychologists.

3. *Power through affiliation.* Nursing is only beginning to understand the benefits of collective action, mutual support, and coalition building as vehicles for expanding nursing's power base. APRNs who participate in interdisciplinary organizations, boards, and associations; forge alliances with consumer groups; and build coalitions within and among diverse professional and consumer organizations maximize the potential for successfully tackling today's complex mental health legislative and policy issues. With cost-cutting, restructuring, competing values, turf issues, and lack of resources (including time), individuals and organizations must work together. Professional organizations and community groups increase their numbers, voice, and power when they forge partnerships to influence legislative and policy change. The Robert Wood Johnson Foundation (1995) has identified the coalition as one of the most effective ways to initiate and sustain social change.

   On the state level, the Council of Connecticut Mental Health Providers (CCMHP) is an example of an effective interdisciplinary coalition. The CCMHP has representation from the five state-wide mental health provider organizations that affiliated in 1993 to support the enactment of responsible health care reform, which included comprehensive mental health benefits. As the representative from the Connecticut Society of Nurse Psychotherapists, Judith Haber chaired CCMHP in 1995 and 1996 when the coalition worked effectively to have the Professional Corporation (PC) and Limited Liability Company (LLC) laws in Connecticut changed to allow for the creation of multidiscipline versus single discipline PCs and LLCs. This enables clinicians from more than one professional mental health discipline to have an ownership position in these entities. The successful legislative outcome was the result of 2 years of building trust, setting aside turf issues, making legislative friends, and building collaborative relationships among the respective lobbyists, thereby expanding nursing's scope of power and influence through the forging of alliances (Haber, 1996a).

Previously this interdisciplinary model had been effective in California. In the early 1980s, Jane Ryan (American Psychiatric Nursing Association's ninth President) forged the way for nursing to be represented in a multidisciplinary coalition, the California Council on Psychiatry, Psychology, Social Work, and Nursing. This group tackled issues of mutual concern representing 40,000 mental health providers (Pelletier & Pothier, 1988).

4. *Power through caring.* APRNs have, throughout their history, been perceived as altruistic and caring. In this era, where the showcasing of power exists side by side with the values of humanism, caring, and focused performance, APRNs are positioned well to exert greater influence. They need to acknowledge to themselves and to each other the power inherent in caring (Benner, 1984). Findings from Benner's phenomenologic research study indicate that respect for, acceptance of, confidence in, and hope for the person's future constitute dimen-

sions of caring for psychiatric patients. These data are also congruent with mental health agendas pursued by consumer advocacy organizations such as the National Alliance for the Mentally Ill (NAMI). Numerous psychiatric nurses to whom these caring dimensions are of vital importance have played national leadership roles in NAMI and other mental health advocacy groups.

Connections: Policy, Politics, and Values

Mason and Leavitt (1993) state that "contemporary policy development is a complex, dynamic, multidimensional process that reflects the values of those who are setting the policy agenda, determining policy goals and alternatives, formulating policy, and implementing and evaluating it." Values of stakeholders involved in policy development, implementation, and evaluation may conflict, as is often the case in policy arenas with diverse constituencies. In such cases, politics necessarily comes into play as stakeholders jockey for position to influence the outcome. For example, when the APRN coalition in Connecticut made a decision to initiate legislation to amend the state Nurse Practice Act in order to eliminate physician direction and prescriptive protocol requirements from the statute, the conflicting of APRNs' and MDs' values initiated a political war in which both stakeholders exercised their political influence to achieve the outcome to which their stakeholder group was committed (Haber, 1997b). Despite the significant amount of legislator education regarding plenary prescriptive authority for APRNs conducted by the coalition, the physicians' longevity as key players at the policy table maximized the effect of their lobbying campaign designed to discredit APRN competence to have plenary prescriptive authority. This is consistent with the tendency of the health care delivery system to not recognize nurses as professionals with expert knowledge who create solutions to complex health care problems (Murphy, 1992). When nurses are not at the policy tables in significant numbers for long periods of time, the policies that result often reflect the dominant values of society. These values are based on competition, individuality, and power and often do not support the health and development of women, families, and communities.

Public policy is about choices that are based on values that come into play in the political dynamics of policymaking. When individuals or groups with differing values, like APRNs and MDs, enter into the policy process, politics often shapes the process of developing policy rather than substantive issues like expanding consumer access to comprehensive mental health services.

POLICY DEVELOPMENT
■ AND ANALYSIS

The *policy development process* refers specifically to the purposive course of government action through which a policy moves from its emergence as an idea or area of public concern, to a successfully enacted legislative bill, and finally to a working program that acts in the public's interest. These actions occur at many different levels of the public hierarchy—national, state, county, city, district—with some form of public participation, either direct or indirect, through elected or appointed officials. This process involves four steps: 1) shaping the idea, 2) building a base of support, 3) moving the idea, and 4) taking the idea to the wire (Sochalski, 1993). Each of these steps is presented using the Medicare reimbursement for APRNs initiative as an example (Haber, 1998).

Shaping the Idea

Translating an issue of professional or public concern into policy requires an organized and committed planning group. The process of involving others to shape the idea and build a broad base of support is crucial to launching a successful policy initiative. The more an idea is discussed with key stakeholders, the more evident its strengths and weaknesses become. The goal is to

design a successful plan by obtaining va... tions and addressing potential pitfalls.

Example. In 1990 the ANA provided the init. leadership in successfully lobbying for legislation that provided direct Medicare reimbursement for CNSs and nurse practitioners (NPs) practicing in designated rural areas. Subsequent lobbying efforts had been successful in getting legislation introduced in the U.S. Senate and the House of Representatives to provide direct Medicare reimbursement in all geographic areas, regardless of practice setting and minus physician supervision. However, the legislation ground to a halt in 1993 when national health care reform failed, as well as in 1995 when budget battles over Medicare and Medicaid cuts prevailed.

However, as the 105th Congress convened in 1997, several issues of public concern emerged that made the policy and legislative climate more favorable to this legislation. The data revealed that Medicare enrollment had grown from 19.1 million persons in 1966 to 37.8 million in 1996, with the elderly Medicare population having grown from 19.1 million to 33.3 million over that same period. The Medicare program had begun to cover those with a disability in 1973 (including persons with serious and persistent mental disorders); that population had grown from 2.2 million in 1975 to 4.6 million in 1996 (Congressional Record Service, 1997). In addition, one of the lowest disease categories receiving treatment was mental disorders, noted at 3%, a reflection of the underserved status of this population compared with population prevalence of major psychiatric disorders regardless of age. Moreover, the *Medicare and Health Care Chartbook* (Congressional Record Service, 1997) predicted that because of the baby boom and increased longevity, Medicare enrollment was expected to grow and that by 2015 the elderly population was projected to increase to 43.7 million. Coupled with these demographic trends were changes in health care delivery (e.g., shift to community-based primary care, decreased length of hospital stay, increase in ambulatory and home health care) that highlighted issues related to consumer access to health care services, provider diversity, and cost-effective, quality health care.

In light of these data, it seemed as though the moment was right for APRNs to once again launch the direct Medicare reimbursement initiative in the U.S. government.

Building a Broad Base of Support

The planning committee becomes the foundation upon which an extensive network of support is built. Whether the initiative is a statewide legislative project or enactment of a law in Congress, carefully identifying advocates is essential. Each person or group contacted has the potential to become an ally and the source of more allies. Forming a coalition of vested stakeholders becomes a priority for maximizing success (Haber, 1996a). Translating the idea into language that is meaningful to a specific constituency is an essential ingredient in a successful campaign. Preparation of "talking points" that frame the issue specifically to the context of a particular constituency is an effective strategy. When soliciting support, both allies and opponents as well as the reasons for their positions should be identified. This will sharpen the arguments needed when the opposition begins to assert its position.

Example. The Report of the APNA Congress on Advanced Practice in Psychiatric Nursing (APNA, 1997) and the ANA Legislative and Regulatory Initiatives for the 105th Congress (ANA, 1997) reflect unanimous support in relation to removing barriers to nursing practice and acknowledging the need to use the combined power of organizational partnerships to effect legislative change. The outcome of the 1996 APNA Advanced Practice Congress was a mandate to 1) develop a legislative agenda, 2) develop a legislative office within the APNA headquarters to ensure a psychiatric nursing voice in the U.S. government, 3) partner with other nursing organizations to increase the base of support and influence with policymakers and legislators, and 4) establish the Legislative Task Force to address the legislative agenda of the Association.

The Legislative Task Force was composed of ten members, each of whom coordinated the legislative activity in five or six states, thereby providing grassroots support for the entire United States and Puerto Rico. The regional coordinator identified APNA members in each state for which they were responsible, ideally at least one in each Congressional District, to serve in the capacity of a State Legislative Affiliate (SLA). Each SLA worked with the APNA membership in his or her state to develop a grassroots response team to accomplish the legislative goal of amending the Medicare statute to provide direct Medicare reimbursement to APRNs regardless of geographic area or practice setting and without physician supervision.

This infrastructure was in place when the APNA appointed a director of government affairs in 1996, thus establishing a legislative office. The director mentored the Legislative Task Force members and SLAs in relation to building a broad base of support and developing or expanding their advocacy skills. Legislative partnerships were developed with the ANA, other psychiatric nursing organizations (e.g., the Society for Research and Education in Psychiatric Nursing, the International Society of Consultation Liaison Nurses, and Association for Child and Adolescent Psychiatric Nursing), nurse practitioner organizations, and consumer groups such as the NAMI and the American Association of Retired Persons (AARP). A critical source of support was obtained when President Bill Clinton included expanded Medicare reimbursement for APRNs as an item in his FY97 budget to Congress. The major opposition to the legislation was anticipated to come from physician organizations who allege that APRNs are not educationally or clinically qualified to practice autonomously. Opposition was also anticipated from legislators who still thought that the addition of the CNS provider category would add a significant expense to the Medicare budget rather than representing a budget-neutral item.

Moving the Idea

Once an idea has been carefully crafted, tested out on a select group of supporters, refined, and given support from a diverse set of groups, the initiative is ready to be launched. As this phase begins, overt and covert forces emerge that can derail the best efforts to move the idea forward (Sochalski, 1993). Five important forces that act as barriers to change are rhetoric, inertia, precedent setting, opposing forces, and timing.

Rhetoric, the art of persuasive arguments, can be used as a powerful tool to control discussion, influence opinions, and prevent action by speaking to the core prejudice of an issue, while basing that argument only loosely, if at all, on fact. Physicians have historically used the rhetoric of "second class care" when opposing the expanded role of APRNs, although many outcome studies have been conducted to refute their arguments (Aiken, Smith, & Lake, 1994; Office of Technology Assessment, 1986).

Inertia becomes an important barrier to change because there are always more forces that support inaction than those that promote change. Similar to rhetoric, inertia is often deliberate; slowing the pace of change can provide windows of opportunity to derail legislation or for the opposition to develop responses. Inertia may mean that those in decision-making positions are unsure about the path to be taken, weighing the familiar, less controversial position against the blazing of a new, uncharted path. It may also be a signal that the issue has come up against a barrier. This does not mean that a course of action needs to be abandoned; however, an adjustment in the strategy may be required.

Precedent-setting legislation is often accompanied by red flags like rhetoric and inertia. In general, change in the status quo is regarded cautiously, and barriers to change that can derail a plan can be erected quickly. Success in moving an idea is proportional to how effectively the opposition is neutralized.

Opposing forces can come from almost anywhere. Anticipating the opposing forces and the messages they convey will help in preparing to neutralize their arguments. At some point there may be a showdown, and the people best positioned will prevail.

Timing plays an important role in maximizing the likelihood of success. Sometimes opposing forces emerge late in the game, and there is not sufficient time to assemble arguments to neutralize their opposition. In some cases the window of opportunity for introduction or passage of legislation is small, and a legislative or policy opportunity is lost forever. However, in many cases the initiative can be introduced again, and with a greater chance of success, in another legislative session.

Example. The APNA and ANA were key organizations in securing Congressional leadership to introduce the "Primary Care Health Practitioner Incentive Act of 1997," which was filed by Senators Grassley (R-IA) and Conrad (D-ND) and Representatives Johnson (R-CT) and Towns (D-NY), all of whom had sponsored the 1993 and 1995 versions of this legislation. On February 27, 1997, Senators Grassley and Conrad were joined by Senator Ernest Hollings (D-SC) as they introduced S370, the bill that would amend Title VIII of the Social Security Act to provide Medicare reimbursement for NPs and CNSs. In the House, Congresswoman Johnson and Congressman Towns introduced the same bill, HR 893.

Almost immediately, overt forces from the physician lobby sought to discredit the APRNs effort to obtain expanded Medicare reimbursement, especially the phrase that would eliminate the need for physician supervision. Standard rhetoric about inconsistent and inadequate educational preparation, encroachment on physician scope of practice, and consumer endangerment was used to control discussion, influence opinions, and decrease support for the legislation. When Senators Grassley and Conrad considered eliminating CNSs from the legislation, arguing that the cost of including another APRN provider group would be too expensive, covert forces from within the NP constituency supported this position, thereby advancing the cause of NPs at the expense of all APRNs.

This argument had been effective in eliminating mention of CNSs in the 1993 and 1995 versions of this legislation because the CNS constituency had not anticipated this argument and did not have, until too late, outcome data to refute allegations about the purported expense of including the CNS provider group in that legislation. However, by 1997 the CNSs, especially the psychiatric CNSs, were prepared from the start with sufficient cost-effectiveness and quality outcome data validating the efficacy of their services to neutralize similar arguments from opposing forces.

The Chair of the APNA Legislative Task Force in collaboration with the APNA director of government affairs launched a grassroots lobbying effort coordinated by the SLAs in each geographic region. Using the booklet entitled *Grassroots Guide to Advocacy* (APNA, 1997), APNA members nationwide responded to a series of APNA ACTION ALERTS, with letters, e-mails, faxes, and phone calls to Senators Grassley and Conrad voicing their opposition to a bill that would only include NPs. In addition, numerous consumer letters were also received. Members of the APNA knew that they had been successful when the director of government affairs was told by staff members in the Senators offices to "call off the nurses; we get the message."

To ensure that both the Senate and House versions of the bill would be taken up for action in committee instead of being left to languish and die, it was crucial for APNA members to alert their own Senators and Representatives to sign on as cosponsors, or at least offer their names as being supportive of this legislation should it be challenged in committee or debated on the floor of the Senate or House as the legislative process continued. Another round of APNA ACTION ALERTS, followed by more letters, phone calls, and visits to the state or Washington offices of

legislators, created a groundswell of cosponsors for and supporters of these bills, a key step in accruing a critical mass of support to neutralize remaining opposition. Behind the scenes, the ANA and APNA Governmental Affairs offices were lobbying on behalf of APRNs on an ongoing basis; they had their finger on the pulse of the legislative momentum and alerted the membership whenever an intervention was required.

These efforts were successful. The bills, S370 and HR893, were considered by the Senate Finance Committee and the House Ways and Means Committee on Health for the "mark-up," the process by which the Congressional Budget Office (CBO) estimates the cost of a particular bill in the budget and assigns a score that is very influential in the committee's decision making. It was time for another round of intensive lobbying since this was the juncture at which the CNSs had been eliminated from the 1995 Medicare legislation. By mid-June, 1997, both houses had approved minor changes in the overall legislation. With the essential portions of the legislation still intact, the bills were sent to the Conference Committee (composed of members of the Senate and House), whose task it was to combine both chambers' versions for inclusion in the overall FY97 budget bill.

Taking It to the Wire

The creation of public policy and enactment of legislation requires hard work, perseverance, and endurance. Many skills and talents are required to orchestrate successful passage of legislation that brings about changes in public policy. Legislative victories are often not accomplished in one legislative session. It may take several days of legislative relationship building and education coupled with timing in relation to the political and policy climate for the maximum number of forces to be in optimum alignment for a successful outcome (Haber, 1996c). As the final days before a vote approach, anxiety and excitement abound. The final flurry of lobbying activity telescopes into an intense series of maneuvers designed to ensure victory.

Example. Always a critical element, timing became increasingly important when, on July 28th, 1997, five business days away from the August Congressional recess, the budget bill still was not signed. Competing forces lobbying against the Conference Committee version of the bill were ever present and could, at a moment's notice, convince one of the Conference Committee members to change any of the required language necessary to keep the proposed expanded Medicare legislation intact within the overall budget bill. Moreover, if the entire budget bill was not addressed until after the August recess, the APNA and ANA were aware that there was no chance of finishing the budget bill in 1997, thereby losing another window of opportunity to eliminate discrepancies in Title VIII of the Social Security Act, which restrict access to health care for the Medicare population.

Fueled with continued energy by their collective power, the final lobbying efforts brought the membership of the APNA, ANA, and NP organizations to the White House via e-mail, telephone, and fax machines, contacting the President's aides in an effort to communicate how essential it was for the President to work with the Congress to pass a budget bill before the August recess. On July 31, the Senate and the House both passed tax cut packages and sent the first balanced budget agreement in 30 years to President Clinton's desk. The President signed into law on August 5 the new budget bill, Public Law 105–33. This amended in Section 4511, Title XVIII of the Social Security Act by expanding direct Medicare reimbursement for CNSs and NPs in all geographic locations and practice settings, effective January 1, 1998. Medicare recipients now had a choice about accessing the APRN provider group. This victory, which took 10 years to accomplish and thousands of staff and volunteer hours, has resulted in a change in public policy that would not have been possible without the organizational partnerships that were forged during this legislative journey. Another partnership was forged with the Health Care Financing Administration (HCFA), which is responsible for writing the rules and regulations that act as the directive to Medicare carriers in each state to implement this provision (Haber, 1998). The latest HCFA rules and regulations for third party reimbursement of APRNs can be found on the HCFA's website (www.hcfa.gov/pubforms/transmit). The regulations change often, and APRNs should check the HCFA website frequently to apprise themselves of the most recent regulations for Medicare reimbursement.

■ POLITICAL ACTION TOOL KIT

Health care policy and/or legislation at the federal or state level will affect APRNs. As in any legislative battle, there will be winners and losers. With the active participation of APRNs and the consumers of mental health care, both constituencies can be winners. It has been said that a 1000 mile journey begins with the first step. APRNs took that first step when they gave voice to the value of their practice by committing themselves to having that voice heard by policymakers at the state and national levels through grassroots political action. The Medicare reimbursement victory provided APRNs with several valuable lessons about effecting change in the policy and politics arena.

One of the most effective methods for getting the voice of APRNs heard by those who make decisions about health policy and health related legislation is to develop a relationship with state and federal legislators. APRNs are experts in the delivery of mental health care, particularly for a patient population that has a high use of mental health services, those with serious and persistent neurobiologic disorders. This expertise can be used as a vehicle for developing a relationship with a legislator. For example, legislators need to be educated about mental health policy and legislative issues and about how APRNs make a difference in terms of cost and quality. APRNs want to become their legislator's resource on mental health issues, someone they can call when they need important and reliable information. Consider the fact that there is strength in numbers; numbers provide political clout. Decisions are usually based on power (money and voting blocks). The nursing profession has realized increasingly the importance of financially supporting candidates who support issues of interest to the nursing profession. However, groups such as medicine, the hospital industry, labor, the nursing home industry, and the insurance industry are bigger players with much more financial capital. Therefore highly organized grassroots voter blocks, such as approximately 75,000 psychiatric nurses nationwide, take on increasing importance and can be used to influence policymaking and the political process, especially regarding mental health issues.

On the surface an issue or decision may be philosophically debated on its values and ideals, but the final decision is really based on power (Haber, 1996b). The political action tools identified in Box 7-4 will assist APRNs in increasing grassroots political power through development

---

box 7-4

POLITICAL ACTION TOOL KIT

1. Make an appointment by calling or writing your legislators at their local, state, or federal office.
2. Clearly identify the issue (e.g., parity, Medicaid reimbursement) you want to discuss, and rehearse what you plan to say. Decide how large a contingent will join you and would be most effective; determine its composition.
3. Set a definite agenda; prepare examples and facts to illustrate your position.
4. Use facts, figures (e.g., supply and demand data, prevalence statistics, outcome data), and consumer-driven vignettes to support the desired change. The Internet resources in this chapter provide an array of online resources to assist you in collecting data about health policy and legislative issues.
5. Arrive on time and identify yourself as a constituent and a nurse, in this case as an APRN.
6. Meet with the staff person for health care issues if the legislator is busy. Key staff members are extremely influential in shaping the positions the legislator ultimately adopts. They are important friends to make.
7. Be prepared to discuss the issues. Familiarize yourself with your legislator's previous position on this issue.
8. Keep the atmosphere open and friendly. You are there to educate your legislator, exchange ideas, and gain his or her support. If that is not possible, keep the lines of communication open.
9. If you do not know an answer to a question that the legislator asks, say so. Explain that you will get more information, and then be sure to follow through. That provides an opportunity for another contact.
10. Leave a folder of literature on the subject and your business card with your legislator or the staff member.
11. Follow up your visit with a thank you note and perhaps more information on the issues discussed or an invitation to spend a day with you at your agency to illustrate the effects of a psychiatric APRN on the lives of consumers of mental health services.
12. Consider working on your legislator's campaign if election time is close at hand. This is an excellent way to get to know the legislator and his or her staff and have another opportunity to promote your issue.
13. Consult with the director of government affairs at the APNA to decide what the next strategy needs to be in terms of moving the issue forward.
14. Check APNA and ANA websites regularly for legislative updates.

of legislative relationships with senators, congresspersons, or their key staff members (Haber, 1996b).

IMPLICATIONS FOR ■ THE FUTURE

It is evident that the time is ripe for all nurses to become active in the policymaking and legislative arenas. APRNs can make a difference in shaping the nature and direction of the national mental health system. It is essential that APRNs seize the window of opportunity to become key players who shape the nature and direction of access to and quality of the delivery of mental health services. APRNs must take an active role through knowledgeable participation in health policy and legislative initiatives, and skilled interaction with political parties, campaigns, and grass roots efforts of professional organizations, as well as the pursuit of political office at the local, state, and federal levels.

RESOURCES AND CONNECTIONS

Agency for Health Care Policy and Research
www.ahcpr.gov
American Public Health Association
www.apha.org
Centers for Disease Control and Prevention (CDC) www.cdc.gov
Fedstats www.fedstats.gov
For information about Medicare coverage for NPs, PAs, and CNSs, go online to:
www.hcfa.gov/pubforms/transmit/ab981560.htm
and www.access.gpo.gov/nara/110298/2fr02no98.txt
General Accounting Office www.gao.gov
Health Association of New York State
www.hanys.org
Health Care Financing Administration (HCFA) www.hcfa.gov
Idea Central: Electronic Policy Network
www.epn.org/idea/health.html
National Institute of Mental Health
www.nimh.nih.gov

New York State Department of Health
www.health.state.ny.us
New York Temporary Commission on Lobbying www.nylobby.state.ny.us
Public Interest Groups Hub www.essential.org
R.W. Johnson Foundation on State Health Policy www2.umdnj.edu/shpp/homepage.htm
State News: Council of State Governments
www.statenews.org
Thomas, the Online Service of the Library of Congress ww.lcweb.loc.gov
To obtain the address of your Medicare carrier, go online to: www.hcfa.gov/regions/default.htm

References

Aiken, L.H., Smith, H.L., & Lake, E.T. (1994). Lower Medicare mortality among a set of hospitals known for good nursing care. *Medical Care, 32,* 771–787.

American Academy of Nursing Expert Panel on Violence. (1993). Violence as a nursing priority: policy implications. *Nursing Outlook, 41*(2) 83–92.

American Nurses Association. (1991). *Nursing's agenda for health care reform.* Washington, DC: Author.

American Nurses Association. (1997). *Legislative and regulatory initiatives for the 105th Congress.* Washington, DC: Author.

American Nurses Association. (1998). *Capitol Update, 16*(4), 1.

American Psychiatric Nurses Association. (1997). *Report of the APNA Congress on Advanced Practice in Psychiatric Nursing.* Washington, DC: Author.

American Psychiatric Nurses Association Legislative Task Force. (1997). *The American Psychiatric Nurses Association grassroots guide to advocacy.* Washington, DC: Author.

Baradell, J. (1995). Clinical outcomes and satisfaction of patients of clinical nurse specialists in psychiatric-mental health nursing. *Archives of Psychiatric Nursing, 9*(4), 240–250.

Baradell, J. (1994). Cost-effectiveness and quality of care provided by clinical nurse specialists. *Journal of Psychosocial Nursing, 32*(3), 21–24.

Benner, P. (1984). *From novice to expert: excellence and power in clinical nursing practice.* Menlo Park, CA: Addison-Wesley.

Birnbaum, J.H. (1997). Washington's power 25. *Fortune,* December 8, 1997.

Buerhaus, P.I. (1996). Quality and cost: the value of consumer and nurse partnerships. *Nursing Policy Forum, 2*(2), 12–16.

Burgess, A.W. & Holstrum, L.L. (1974). Rape trauma syndrome. *American Journal of Psychiatry, 131,* 981–986.

Congressional Record Service. (1997). *Medicare and health care chartbook.* Washington, DC: Government Printing Office.

Ferguson, V.D. (1993). Perspectives on power. In Mason, D.J., Talbot, S., & Leavitt, J.K. (Eds.). *Policy and politics for nurses* (ed. 2). Philadelphia: W.B. Saunders.

Haber, J. (1996a). Coalition building: an effective vehicle for achieving legislative change. *Journal of the American Psychiatric Nurses Association,* 2(4), 127–128.

Haber, J. (1996b). Cultivating grassroots political savvy. *Journal of the American Psychiatric Nurses Association,* 2(2), 58–60.

Haber, J. (1996c). The Medicare reimbursement journey. *Journal of the American Psychiatric Nurses Association,* 2(5), 167–168.

Haber, J. (1997a). Mental health parity: victory on the horizon. *Journal of the American Psychiatric Nurses Association,* 3(1), 22–23.

Haber, J. (1997b). The risk-reward ratio of amending a state nurse practice act. *Journal of the American Psychiatric Nurses Association,* 3(5), 166–168.

Haber, J. (1998). Making sense of the new Medicare reimbursement laws. *Journal of the Psychiatric Nurses Association,* 4(2), 67–68.

Hanley, B.E. (1993). Policy development and analysis. In Mason, D.J., Talbot, S., & Leavitt, J.K. (Eds.). *Policy and politics for nurses* (ed. 2). Philadelphia: W.B. Saunders.

Hartman, C.R., & Burgess, A.W. (1988). Information processing of trauma. *Journal of Interpersonal Violence, 3,* 443–457.

Helms, L.B., Anderson, M.A., & Hanson, K. (1996) "Doin' politics": linking policy and politics in nursing. *Nursing Administration Quarterly, 20*(3), 32–41.

Leavitt, J.K., & Barry, C.T. (1993). Learning the ropes. In Mason, D.J., Talbot, S., & Leavitt, J.K. (Eds.). *Policy and politics for nurses* (ed. 2). Philadelphia: W.B. Saunders.

Lee, P.R., & Estes, C.L. (1997). *The nation's health.* Sudbury, MA: Jones and Bartlett.

Marquis, B.L., & Huston, C.J. (1992). *Leadership roles and management functions in nursing.* Philadelphia: J.B. Lippincott.

Mason, D. J. (1990). Nursing and politics: nursing comes of age. *Orthopaedic Nursing, 9*(5), 11–17.

Mason, D. J., & Leavitt, J.K. (1993). Policy and politics: a framework for action. In Mason, D.J., Talbott, S., & Leavitt, J.K. (Eds.). *Policy and politics for nurses* (ed. 2). Philadelphia: W.B. Saunders.

Murphy, N.J. (1992). Nursing leadership in health policy decision making. *Nursing Outlook, 40*(4), 158–161.

O'Neil, T., & Hymel, G. (1994). *All politics is local and other rules of the game.* New York: Time Books.

Office of Technology Assessment. (1986). *Nurse practitioners, physician assistants, and certified nurse-midwives: a policy analysis, health technology case study No. 37.* Washington, DC: US Government Printing Office.

Pelletier, L.R., & Pothier, P.C. (1988). Promoting interprofessional collegiality: national and state models. *Archives of Psychiatric Nursing, 2*(5), 307–311.

Robert Wood Johnson Foundation (Spring, 1995). Coalitions: effective agents for social change. *The Newsletter of the Robert Wood Johnson Foundation, 8*(2), 1–2.

Roberts, S.J., & Chandler, C. (1996). Empowerment of graduate students: a dialogue toward change. *Journal of Professional Nursing, 12*(4), 233–239.

Sharp, N. (1994). All politics is local: and other rules. *Nursing Management, 25*(3), 22–25.

Sharp, N. (1995). *The nurses' directory of capital connections.* Washington, DC: Capitol Associates.

Shortrell, S., & Kaluzney, A. (1994). *Health care management* (ed. 3). Albany, NY: Del Mar Publishers.

Sochalski, J. (1993). The dynamics of public policy: a walk through the process. In Mason, D., Talbott, S., & Leavitt, J. (Eds.). *Policy and politics for nurses* (ed. 2). Philadelphia: W.B. Saunders.

Titmus, R.M. (1974). *Social policy: an introduction.* New York: Pantheon Books.

Thorndike, E.L., & Barnhart, C.L. (1979). *Scott Foresman advanced dictionary.* New York: Doubleday & Co.

United States Department of Health and Human Services, Public Health Service. (1990). *Healthy People 2000: national health promotion and disease prevention objectives* (DHHS Pub. No. 91–50212). Washington, DC: US Government Printing Office.

United States Department of Health and Human Services, Public Health Service. (1995). *Healthy People 2000 review 1994* (DHHS Pub. No. 95–1256-1).Washington, DC: US Government Printing Office.

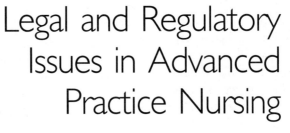

Legal and Regulatory Issues in Advanced Practice Nursing

LINDA M.E. AUTON

■ INTRODUCTION

This chapter covers the general aspects of the law and its effects on the advanced practice registered nurse (APRN) in psychiatric-mental health nursing. It is important to be aware that state laws may vary; the astute nurse should always review issues with a local lawyer knowledgeable in the area of law in which the issue arises.

■ TORTS

The term *tort* comes from Latin, meaning 'to twist, twisted, wrested aside.' It is a private or civil wrong or injury, other than breach of contract, for which the court will provide a remedy in the form of an action for damages. There must always be a violation of some duty owing to the plaintiff, and generally such duty must arise by operation of law and not by mere agreement of the parties.

Unintentional Torts

Unintentional torts are wrongful acts, damage or injury done as a result of negligence or malpractice. These torts are the most common suits brought against APRNs. They do not require that a specific intent to cause injury or damage be present.

Negligence. Negligence is an unintentional act, or failure to act when the act was required, that causes harm. The burden is on the plaintiff to prove four elements:
1. There was a duty of due care owed by the defendant to the plaintiff.
2. The defendant breached the duty of due care owed.
3. The breach of the duty was the direct cause of harm to the plaintiff.
4. The breach of the duty was the indirect cause of harm to the plaintiff.

If any one of the elements is not proven, then that claim is defeated.

The *duty of due care,* as it pertains to nurses and nursing, is owed to anyone to whom a reasonable person could foresee injury occurring as a result of a nurse's actions. No duty is owed to unexpectedly injured persons or patients. Courts differ about when the defendant nurse could have reasonably foreseen danger. Some courts impose a duty of due care owed to anyone injured as a direct result of negligence. Other courts impose a duty owed only to the foreseeable plaintiff or class of persons in the zone of danger.

The due care owed, or *standard of care,* is that of a reasonable nurse under the same or similar circumstances. The defendant nurse's good faith is immaterial. The circumstances dictate the standard of care required. The standard of care is established by custom, although it is not conclusive. Complying with a statute is not usually conclusive, but a violation of the statute may be negligence per se (duty and breach do not have to be proven). An APRN is held to the standard of an advanced practice nurse with the same or similar education, training, and experience. Physicians and nurses used to be held to the standard of the doctors and nurses in the same community, but courts are now imposing a similar community standard. Where there is national certification, a national standard is imposed.

One of the most contested areas in proving negligence is the foreseeability of the harm caused by the negligent act. This is a policy decision regarding who should bear the loss for unexpected injuries or expected injuries caused in unexpected ways. Causation must be either a direct cause (proximate) or an indirect cause. A *direct cause* is one in which no harm would have occurred if not for the act. Direct cause is rarely in issue.

The liability extends to foreseeable results. For example, a direct cause could be the failure to place someone on suicide precautions when all the signs and symptoms are present and there is a physician's order present for implementing suicide precautions. The patient's resultant suicide is therefore foreseeable. The courts are divided when direct causation leads to unexpected types of injury, but all courts hold the defendant liable when unforeseeability only goes to the extent of the injury. The courts require that the plaintiff be taken as is. If the patient has a thin skull, and in an attempted suicide (even with suicide precautions present) the defendant jumps off a bed and death ensues resulting from brain injury, that would be considered foreseeable.

Indirect cause means that an intervening force extended the result of the defendant's negligence or combined with the defendant's act to produce the injury. The court considers two aspects of indirect cause:
1. The nature of the intervening act
2. The results of the negligent act

A dependent intervening act is a normal response to a situation created by the defendant's negligent act. For example, negligent medical treatment for a suicide attempt caused by the failure to implement suicide precautions would be foreseeable, and the defendant nurse would be held liable for the resulting injuries. If an injury is inflicted or aggravated by a rescuer, that is deemed foreseeable, as is injury or aggravation of an injury resulting from an escape attempt. An intervening criminal act or tort terminates liability if the acts are unforeseeable.

If foreseeable results are produced by unforeseeable intervening forces, liability is usually imposed. However, some courts do not impose liability when the intervening act is intentional or reckless conduct by a third party. If the result is what was threatened by the defendant's negligence, then intervening acts of God, abnormal rescue attempts, and criminal acts would not relieve the defendant of liability. If the results are unforeseeable, then these intervening causes *would* relieve the defendant from liability.

For a plaintiff's case to be successful, the patient must have been injured by the negligent act. Injury is not usually contested unless the cause is obscure or not related to the act or injury. The jury can only award monetary damages, so the plaintiff must show not only the money lost from work or opportunities but also how the injury caused pain and suffering. A good plaintiff's attorney will instruct the plaintiff to keep a journal and document the type of pain, its effects, and medical costs related to alleviating pain and injury.

Certain defenses apply to negligence claims. These include contributory negligence, assumption of the risk, and comparative negligence. *Contributory negligence* is conduct on the part of the plaintiff that contributes to his or her own injuries and that falls below the standard of care to which he or she is required to conform for his or her own protection. The plaintiff is prevented from receiving damages (barred from recovery of damages) because the injury was as much the plaintiff's fault as it was the defendant nurse's fault. The court says that the plaintiff owes a duty to himself or herself. For example, if the plaintiff, without excuse, fails to follow medical discharge instructions, then the defense of contributory negligence may be claimed by the defendant nurse.

Assumption of the risk occurs when the plaintiff consents to confront harm from a particular risk. The plaintiff may not recover demages for an injury to which he or she assents if the plaintiff:
1. Recognized and understood the risk
2. Voluntarily chose to encounter the risk

Assumption of the risk may be implied by the conduct of the defendant. However, the defendant must prove that the plaintiff knew of the specific risk and voluntarily chose to encounter the risk.

Comparative negligence is followed by more than 40 states that reject the rule that contributory negligence is a complete bar to recovery of damages. These states base liability on the comparative fault of the plaintiff and defendant. There are two forms of comparative negligence:
1. Pure comparative negligence, which allows the plaintiff to recover a percentage of damages even if the plaintiff's negligence exceeds the defendants.
2. Partial comparative negligence, in which the plaintiff may recover a percentage of damages only if the plaintiff's own negligence is less than the defendant's. Some states allow recovery if the plaintiff's negligence is equal to the defendant's.

Nursing malpractice. *Nursing malpractice* is a distinct subset of negligence in which the standard of care is that of a reasonable nurse with the same or similar credentials and experience in the same or similar circumstances. The standard of care is developed from many sources; the most crucial is the testimony of the expert nurse. The other sources include but are not limited to the Joint Commission on Accreditation of Healthcare Organizations (JCAHO) requirements; state statutes and regulations; the American Nurses Association (ANA) treatises and publications, bylaws, rules, and regulations; and policies and procedures of the facility in which the defendant is employed.

There are two defenses used in nursing malpractice that relate to the standard of care and may not be used in other negligence cases. These are the *error in judgment rule* and the *two schools of thought doctrine*. The *error in judgment rule* may be used successfully to defend a claim by arguing that the standard of care was met even though a mistake was made. An error in judgment does not prove malpractice if the standard of care was followed by the nurse using the skill, knowledge, and care routinely used by nurses with the same background and experience.

The *two schools of thought doctrine* may be a good defense when there is more than one method of treatment recognized by nurses as being proper. A nurse is not negligent in choosing one treatment over the other as long as the nurse treats the plaintiff according to the method deemed appropriate by a considerable number of nurses.

Intentional Torts

An *intentional tort* is an act performed with the intent to cause harm to someone's person or property. An *act* is the external manifestation of the actor's will; it is a volitional movement by the actor of some part of his or her body. For example, if the defendant intentionally rams the medication cart into the plaintiff, the act would not be the moving of the cart but the movement of the defen-

dant's arms and legs in setting the cart in motion and directing it at the plaintiff. Because the act must be volitional, it can not be intentional if it occurred while the person is having a seizure, asleep, or under the influence of drugs. A reflex is not volitional either. However, persons who are not legally competent are still capable of volitional conduct (minors and insane persons may be liable for their acts).

As well as the act, there must be the intent to cause harm to another. The intent is measured by whether the defendant acted with the desire to cause harm or believed that harm was substantially certain to occur. The desire and belief are based on the subjective consideration of what was in the defendant's mind when the act occurred. The basic question is not what a reasonable person would have desired or believed, but what the *defendant* desired or believed.

Under the doctrine of transferred intent, if the defendant acts with intent to cause harm to the person or the person's property, the defendant will be liable on an intentional tort if any harm occurs to that person or even to an unexpected person or unexpected harm. For example, if a nurse tries to hit someone who ducks and actually strikes another person, the nurse is liable to that other person.

There are many intentional torts. Those most likely to be involved with nursing are assault, battery, false imprisonment, intentional infliction of emotional distress, defamation, abandonment, and conversion. As with negligence, the definition of each tort consists of the elements. The plaintiff must prove each element to win the case.

Assault. An *assault* is an act by the defendant to threaten to cause a harmful or offensive touching of the plaintiff or to put the plaintiff in apprehension of an immediate harmful or offensive touching of his or her person. This cannot be done by words alone, and the threatened harm must be imminent.

Battery. *Battery* requires the same elements as assault, but an offensive or harmful touching must occur. The person does not need to be aware or have knowledge of the offensive touching at the time it occurs.

False imprisonment. *False imprisonment* is an act by the defendant to confine the plaintiff to a specific area, an actual confinement, and causation. The act must be volitional, but words alone may be sufficient. The plaintiff must be restricted to a limited area without the knowledge of reasonable means of escape, and the plaintiff must be aware of the confinement at the time. The cause of the confinement may be by physical forces against the plaintiff or a member of the plaintiff's family, threats of immediate harm to the plaintiff or the family, or actual or apparent physical barriers. This includes refusing to release the plaintiff when under a duty to do so, or assertion of legal authority and the plaintiff's submission to it.

It is important when considering a defense to this charge to remember that the principles of commitment of mental patients provides apparent authority to detain and confine people. However, even when these principles are properly followed, confining a patient against his or her will has been ruled to be false imprisonment. For example, in Cook vs. Highland Hospital (1915), Ms. Cook was admitted to a private hospital for rehabilitation, and she signed an agreement to follow the rules of the Highland Hospital. The rules of confinement were not explained to her, and she believed she could leave anytime she wanted. When Ms. Cook had a disagreement with hospital authorities and wanted to leave, she was confined against her will for 32 days. The court ruled that even though she agreed "to abide by the rules," this agreement did not justify detaining her against her will.

Patients who are mentally ill or a danger to themselves or others may be subjected to involuntary confinement. This aspect is highly regulated, usually by statutes that vary from state to state, so APRNs of established facilities are not required to guess at the conditions under which confinement is proper. APRNs should be very familiar

with the statute in effect in their state and understand the implications for their practice.

Intentional infliction of emotional distress. Intentional infliction of emotional distress involves an extreme and outrageous act by the defendant with an intent to cause severe emotional distress. An *extreme and outrageous act* must exceed all bounds of decent behavior. Words alone may suffice, but simple insults do not. Intent is inferred when the defendant knows that the plaintiff is particularly sensitive to emotional distress. No demonstrable harm is required. A family member may recover damages if the defendant knew of the intent.

A recent case identifies outrageous behavior in a psychiatric setting (Adams vs. Murakami, personal communication). A woman of low intelligence with chronic schizophrenia gave birth to an autistic child. She had been under a doctor's care in a convalescent hospital and alleged that the doctor knew that she was of childbearing age, had been sexually active, and was in an environment where sexual relations frequently occurred. Further, she alleged that despite her request, the doctor refused to prescribe birth control pills and failed to examine her when she began showing signs of being pregnant. He failed to counsel her that her mental condition was genetically linked and could be passed on to the child, and he failed to discuss abortion or inform her that the stress of childbearing frequently exacerbates the mental problems of schizophrenia. He further failed to discontinue her strong psychotropic medications and failed to inform her that they were contraindicated for pregnancy and could seriously harm the fetus. The jury found this evidence proof of medical negligence and intentional infliction of emotional distress and awarded the patient over one million dollars.

Defamation. *Defamation* occurs when the defendant has published or communicated, to a third party, a statement regarding the plaintiff that injures the plaintiff's reputation or will diminish the esteem, respect, goodwill, or confidence in which the plaintiff is held. Language uttered only to the plaintiff does not merit legal action. However, publication to any third person is sufficient. Publication includes speaking, writing, or in any way communicating to someone else. The publication must be intentional or negligent. The defendant must have reason to foresee that a third party would overhear or see. Anyone who republishes or disseminates the defamation is also liable in damages and must have his or her own specific defense.

There are three specific defenses to defamation:
1. Consent
2. If the statement is true
3. Certain privileges; an absolute privilege exists when the defamation is uttered during participation in processes of government

The First Amendment of the Constitution protects free speech and is held to outweigh the interest in protecting the reputation of public officials and public figures. The defamation is privileged if it is a public person, unless it was published with knowledge of falsehood or reckless disregard for the truth. The public person must prove the case with convincing clarity, a higher standard than a private person.

Abandonment. *Abandonment* in medical issues refers to a unilateral, premature termination of the medical treatment of a patient, with neither consent obtained nor adequate notice. This can occur in emergency rooms when a patient may be triaged, placed on a gurney, put in the hall, and not seen again until someone notices that the patient is not breathing. Transporting patients for testing can also lead to situations in which the patient is left alone. To prevent abandonment, appropriately transferring the case to another practitioner of the same or similar expertise is vital.

Conversion. *Conversion* is an interference with the plaintiff's possession of his or her personal property (essentially theft). The APRN should ensure that all valuable items of the patient are secured or returned home. Any items retained by the patient should be logged in the medical record,

and the patient should sign an acknowledgment that the facility waives responsibility for those retained items.

■ DEFENSES TO TORTS

The principles of the intentional torts also include certain defenses that apply to APRNs. Self-defense is a common defense as long as the APRN uses reasonable acts to avoid or prevent the threatened contact. Informed consent provisions may apply as a defense to the tort of false imprisonment. The best defense is the defense of fact (i.e., clear and effective testimony based on adequate records). The great majority of lawsuits against nurses that end in victory for nurses occur because the nurse was not guilty of the alleged tort or malpractice and can prove it with records and witnesses.

There are other general legal defenses that may be used by nurses to protect themselves within the legal system if they are one of the defendants in a malpractice or tort lawsuit. Seven general defenses applicable to negligence, nursing malpractice, battery, and the other specific torts are defined in Box 8-1.

The importance of adequate and accurate records is critical. Many malpractice and tort lawsuits are based on events long past. These records are essential to refresh the APRN's memory of events, convince the court of the validity of the defense, and rebut the plaintiff's allegations.

It is important to adequately record in every patient's medical record all treatment contemporaneously and in chronologic sequence and record the informed consent of the patient to treatment. All accidents and incidents during the course of patient care must be recorded and filed with the appropriate office in the facility. Failure to file these with the appropriate office may make them available to the plaintiff's attorney, even when they are clearly peer review documents. Adequate records can mean the difference between success and failure in a malpractice lawsuit.

box 8-1

GENERAL DEFENSES APPLICABLE TO NEGLIGENCE, NURSING MALPRACTICE, BATTERY, AND THE OTHER SPECIFIC TORTS

1. *Statute of limitations.* The case must be brought to court within the time allowed by state statute. The usual requirement is that the case must be brought to court within 1 to 3 years from the act or discovery of malpractice.
2. *Release and satisfaction.* Before a case is filed, the plaintiff and defendant enter into an agreement that the defendant pays a certain sum to the plaintiff and no case will be filed.
3. *Respondeat superior.* The employer is responsible for the negligent acts of the employee.
4. *Good Samaritan law.* This law protects those who provide health care for an emergency or disaster without reimbursement.
5. *Unavoidable accident.* The facts indicate that the injury was not a product of the APRN's negligence, but simply an accident.
6. *Sovereign immunity.* If the APRN is a federal or state employee, this defense protects the APRN from liability when acting within the scope of employment. The trend is to erode this defense.
7. *Defense of fact.* The defendant cannot prove each element because the APRN has adequate documents and witnesses to disprove the allegations.

Statute of Limitations

Each state has a statute of limitations that specifies a deadline by which a lawsuit must be filed. When the filing of the tort or malpractice suit does not satisfy the requirements of the statute of limitations, the plaintiff loses the right to sue the defendants. This defense is listed first because it is the easiest to establish and may eliminate the lawsuit entirely, regardless of the merit of the claims.

The time for filing a lawsuit generally begins when all of the elements for the cause of action have accrued. The deadline varies from state to state, and the time from which the deadline's clock begins to run also varies. Generally, the three most common times in which a medical malpractice action has accrued are at the time the malpractice, negligence, or intentional tort was committed; at the time the harm to the plaintiff was discovered or should have been discovered; and at the time the medical relationship between the plaintiff and defendant ended.

Every state has different time limits (1 to 3 years is common) and different guidelines that determine the time during which the lawsuit must be filed. Certain states have a *statute of repose* that limits any lawsuits at all if not filed within the time provided by the statute. If the lawsuit is filed beyond the statute of limitations or the statute of repose, it should be dismissed regardless of the merits of the case.

Release and Satisfaction

A *release* is an executed agreement by a claimant to a potential defendant in which, in exchange for consideration (money), the claimant releases the potential defendant from any further liability. In nursing malpractice this means a negotiated settlement payment out of court and before legal proceedings. If the agreement is appropriately worded, no further liability will be enforced by the court.

Respondeat Superior

Respondeat superior is a latin term handed down from English common law that means 'let the master answer.' In the case of malpractice, the "master" is usually the employer. When nurses are hired, they owe a duty of care to the employer's patients while they are on duty and acting within the scope of employment. They must be performing the tasks required to accomplish the employer's goals. If a nurse breaches that duty or standard of care and causes the patient harm, the hospital or employer may be held liable under respondeat superior. The nursing act must occur while the nurse is on the premises of the employer (or while engaged in the employer's work), during the time of the employment, and while performing duties required by the employer for the action to he considered within the nurse-employer relationship. In Pisel v Stanford Hospital (1980), a nurse-manager changed a patient's medical records. The hospital was held liable for her actions since she was working within the scope of employment.

When the nurse is a defendant of a malpractice lawsuit, the principle of respondeat superior can allocate all or part of the liability to the employer. The elements for respondeat superior are as follows:

1. An act of an employee
2. During an employment relationship
3. Negligent act occurring
4. Within the scope of employment

To establish if the act was within the scope of employment, the court must consider the following:

1. The time, place, and purpose of the act
2. Its similarity to what was authorized
3. The extent of departure from normal methods
4. Past dealings between the employer and the employee
5. Whether the employer had reason to expect that such an act would be done

An employer is vicariously liable for all tortious acts committed by an employee within the scope of the employment. The defense does not apply when the tort is committed outside the scope of the employment (e.g., a criminal battery by an employee is not part of the job).

In contrast, employers of independent contractors are not held vicariously liable for negligent conduct. The APRN's status as an employee or independent contractor may be resolved within the employment contract or factually by the amount of control exercised over the APRN with respect to the performance of job duties. The more control is exercised, the more likely the APRN is considered to be an employee, and liability may be imputed to the employer. If the employer is liable under respondeat superior, this may or may not relieve the APRN from liability. By law, the person who commits the tort is almost always liable, even when there is an employment relationship. However, respondeat superior may relieve some of the liability that the APRN faces and will provide a "deep pocket" for the plaintiff's lawsuit for monetary damages.

Good Samaritan Laws

Good Samaritan laws are statutes that vary state by state. They protect those who provide health care for an emergency or disaster without reimbursement. This protects nurses from liability when they help victims of accidents but does not apply if the nurse receives a fee (e.g., the nurse is an employee in an emergency room). These statutes generally do not protect an APRN if the nurse commits an intentional tort or gross negligence but do protect against mistakes that constitute general negligence. The reason for such laws is to encourage "good Samaritans" to help in emergencies.

Unavoidable Accident

When the facts indicate that the plaintiff's injury was not a product of the defendant's negligence but simply an accident, the defense of *unavoidable accident* protects the APRN from any liability. For example, a psychiatric-liaison nurse sees a patient walking along a hospital corridor who falls, breaks his ankle, and sues. If no one was at fault, and no condition of the floor caused the accident, the psychiatric-liaison nurse defendant can be absolved of any liability. This also illustrates how the documentation and accurate reporting of all incidents and accidents is important. In this case, a description of the floor condition in a report of the incident may make a difference years later when the lawsuit is filed.

Sovereign Immunity

Some states prevent lawsuits against the state or agencies of the state under sovereign immunity. This defense protects an employee from liability when acting within the scope of employment. If the APRN is a state or federal employee, the requirements of the Federal Torts Claim Act, or similar provisions of a state torts claim act, may prevent lawsuits from establishing any liability for both the employer and employee.

The trend in the statutes is to erode this as a defense for negligence. The Federal Torts Claim Act now allows the federal government to be sued, and the provisions of the state statutes vary and should be checked.

Vicarious Liability

Defenses may also be mounted against cases in which vicarious liability is asserted. *Vicarious liability* occurs when the law imposes liability for the acts of another. This includes respondeat superior, ostensible authority, and corporate liability. APRNs are assuming more responsibility for supervision of staff and employees and may be the employers of others when managing nursing clinics outside of the auspices of hospitals and other facilities. Understanding the potential liability for their actions as it affects the APRN and the APRN's business enterprise is vital as nurses become autonomous and control their own practices.

Corporate Liability

Unlike respondeat surerior, which requires an employer-employee relationship, a hospital may be liable for independent contractors under the doctrine of *ostensible authority*. The issue of ostensible authority arises when a patient has a rational basis to believe that the independent contractor is a hospital employee. The independent contractor may be a physician or an APRN with privileges. Most frequently, this arises in the emergency room where patients come for evaluation and treatment.

The court reviews four factors:

1. *Subjective.* Whether the patient at the time of the admission looked to the hospital for treatment or merely viewed the hospital as a place where his or her physician would treat him or her.
2. *Inherent function.* Whether the inherent function exists in and is inseparable from the hospital (for example an emergency room APRN).
3. *Reliance.* The patient relies on the hospital's judgment (e.g., by choosing one hospital over another for elective surgery), and the patient is injured because of something the hospital did or failed to do.
4. *Control.* Similar to control establishing an employment relationship, if the hospital exercises a specific degree of control over the independent contractor (e.g., dictating the hours worked, providing all equipment, and specifying the functions of the practice of the independent contractor), the hospital may be liable for the independent contractor's actions.

Corporate Negligence

There are two separate responsibilities of a hospital that the court has considered under the doctrine of corporate negligence.

1. The hospital is responsible to monitor and supervise all medical and nursing personnel within the facility, whether the personnel are employees or independent contractors. This includes the quality of care rendered by the personnel and requires periodic review of the staff members' competency. If a patient suffers an injury because the hospital fails to monitor or supervise staff or contractors, then the hospital is liable.
2. A hospital is liable for failing to investigate an APRN's credentials before granting hospital privileges. This requires the hospital to review the APRN's record in the National Practitioner

Data Bank (a central repository for all actions taken by a state regarding a licensed health care practitioner) and report to the National Practitioner Data Bank any action taken regarding the licensee.

In Bost v. Riley (1980), the Court held that a hospital could be held negligent for "failing to have a sufficient number of trained nurses attending the plaintiff, failing to require a consultation or examination by members of the hospital staff, and failing to review the treatment rendered to the plaintiff." The hospital had a duty to make a reasonable effort to monitor and oversee treatment prescribed and administered by physicians and nurses in the facility.

■ TESTIFYING IN COURT

APRN as Expert Witness

Expert witnesses are people with special professional qualifications who are called to testify in court. APRNs have served very effectively in this capacity. For nursing malpractice, such witnesses are not defendants or parties to the case. They are simply experts whose role is to assist the court and jury in determining what "reasonable" care was required under the circumstances.

The ideal expert is an APRN with an active practice for 5 to 10 years and who has a professorship at a top level university. This assures the lawyer that the person is familiar with the actual practice and can teach effectively. Frequently, the publications of the expert may be used to assist in establishing the standard of care in a particular instance.

Another area about which the lawyer will be inquiring is whether the APRN has testified in a deposition or trial in the past, and if so, whether it was for the defendant or the plaintiff. An expert who solely testifies for one side or the other over time will lose credibility and will not be as effective as an expert.

An expert is usually hired by the plaintiff's attorney to review the medical record and other

---

box 8-2

GUIDELINES FOR TESTIFYING IN COURT OR GIVING A DEPOSITION

1. Do not hide the facts for which you are asked specific questions.
2. Be sure you understand the question.
3. Do not volunteer information at any time.
4. When your attorney objects, stop speaking.
5. Answer every question, if you know the answer, unless your attorney instructs you not to answer.
6. Check factual questions against the record, even if you are sure of the answer.
7. There is nothing wrong with not knowing or not remembering. Simply state "I don't know" or "I don't remember." Be aware of the difference between the two.
8. Dress neatly.
9. Be courteous and use good manners.
10. Do not argue or become hostile.
11. Tell your attorney if you need to take a break.

---

documents and form an opinion of the case. The wise defense attorney obtains similar reviews and uses nursing experts. If the expert's opinion supports the party requesting the review, the expert should not automatically accept the case. The expert must firmly agree with the party's point of view, be extremely conversant with the standards of care and authoritative texts of the field, be able to devote adequate time to the case, be comfortable with the attorney, and be fairly compensated. See Box 8-2 for guidelines for being an expert witness.

Nurse as Defendant

After a lawyer has had a case reviewed by an expert, a lawsuit may be initiated with a complaint. In certain instances, particularly where causation and damages are very clear, the lawyer may notify the defendant by mail of the potential suit and open up negotiations to settle it before filing. If this occurs, a defendant *must immediately* notify his or her insurance carrier and, if covered by the facility's insurance policy, the risk manager. The insurance companies may refuse to defend or pay damages if they do not get timely notice of the case. At this stage a release and satisfaction may be entered into that settles the matter completely.

If not settled, or if the attorney elects to initiate the suit, the defendant may be served with the complaint and a summons. These must be given immediately to the insurance company. The company will appoint a lawyer to represent the defendant, file an answer to the complaint in a timely fashion, and guide the case through the legal process. Once an answer is filed, the case will frequently have to go before a prelitigation panel, medical tribunal, medical review panel, or arbitration panel. The type of review is specified by the individual state, and in certain states, the case must be presented to the prelitigation panel before it is filed.

Because APRNs are nurses 24 hours a day and can seldom prevent others from asking for their assistance when off duty, it is good practice for the APRN to have individual professional liability insurance. Some practitioners believe that if they "go bare" they will be less of a target. Practically, a lawyer never knows what insurance, if any, a defendant may have until after the lawsuit is filed. Therefore failing to have insurance does not ensure that the APRN will not be sued. If the defendant has personal malpractice insurance and is covered by the facility, notice should be given to both immediately. Any issue as to which company will pay for what can be resolved between the companies, and the defendant should not be concerned.

Upon receiving the complaint, the defendant nurse should not speak to anyone about the case except the insurance company and his or her lawyer. Under no circumstances should the defendant speak to the plaintiff, the plaintiff's attorney, or staff members. The defendant should obtain guidance from his or her lawyer regarding speaking

box 8-3
LEGAL TERMS
Interrogatories. Written questions that must be answered in writing within a specified amount of time.
Request for production of documents. A request for documents in the opposing party's possession, custody, or control that may lead to discoverable information.
Admission of facts. Presentation of the opposing party of written statements that must be admitted or denied. If no answer is given, the statements are deemed admitted.
Examinations. Medical or psychiatric examination may be appropriate if the plaintiff has put his or her physical or mental status at issue. The defendant has a right to request an examination by an expert in the field.
Depositions. A structured interview, under oath, before a notary public or someone able to accept the oath.

to hospital or facility supervisors, the risk manager, or the hospital attorney.

After the complaint is answered, the case then enters the discovery phase. All information, facts and circumstances surrounding the alleged malpractice, are "discovered" by the plaintiff's and defendant's legal counsels. Techniques used include interrogatories, requests for production of documents, admissions of facts, physical and mental examinations, and depositions. This is the most time-consuming part of the litigation and may take several years to complete. These legal terms are defined in Box 8-3.

Depositions are the most significant tool used in discovery. The purposes of a deposition are as follows:
1. Gather all discoverable information.
2. Assess the credibility, demeanor, knowledge, and appearance of the witness.
3. Assist the attorneys in assessing the strengths and weakness of the case.

4. Help the attorneys to formulate settlement and trial strategies.
5. Determine the availability and limits of insurance coverage.
6. Preserve the testimony of a witness who may not be available at trial because of death or relocation.
7. Determine the cause, extent, and types of injuries.
8. Determine the facts and circumstances of the alleged malpractice and the breaches of the standard of care.
9. Use during the trial to refresh the memory of the witness or to impeach the witness's credibility.

During the deposition or when an APRN is testifying in court as a defendant, the guidelines in Box 8-2 should be followed.

Once discovery is completed, a pretrial hearing may be set. This is to try to narrow the issues, see which elements do not need to be tried but are agreed upon, and decide on the qualifications of witnesses, what evidence should be allowed, and whether an expert is qualified to testify.

On the day of trial, there may be several motions heard before the case begins. These motions usually are to try to limit the testimony in certain areas. The next step is to select a jury. The attorneys or the judge asks questions (i.e., conducts a *voir dire*) of the potential jurors to identify whether there are any biases, prejudices, or relationships between the jurors and the plaintiffs, attorneys, defendants, or significant others. Each side has a specified number of challenges for cause or preemptory challenges. A preemptory challenge does not require a lawyer to give a reason or cause for the removal of the juror. If there is a challenge for cause, then the attorney alleges that the juror has a bias or prejudice.

Once the jury is selected, the opening statements are presented by the opposing counsel. The opening statements are a summary of what the parties intend to prove. They are not evidence themselves. The plaintiff then presents evidence to prove the four elements of negligence. Evidence will be from witnesses, expert testimony, documents including the medical record, policies, procedures, and treatises. The plaintiff's attorney conducts a direct examination, using open-ended questions, and is prohibited from asking questions that are leading or require a yes or no reply. The defendant's attorney may then cross-examine the witnesses, trying to discredit the witness and testimony. Usually the plaintiff may then do a redirect examination and the defendant may recross-examine. After the plaintiff has presented all the evidence and witnesses, the defense will plead its case to refute the testimony, exhibits, and witnesses. Now, the defendant must use direct examination, and the plaintiff will use cross-examination.

After all the evidence has been presented, the defense rests. The defense may then move for a directed verdict against the plaintiff by arguing that that plaintiff has not met the burden of proof (e.g., the plaintiff has failed to prove one of the required elements). If the judge agrees, the trial ends in favor of the defendant. If not, the motion is denied and the closing arguments are given. During closing arguments, each attorney summarizes the evidence presented putting it in the light most favorable for the client. Again, closing arguments are not testimony, but merely a summary.

The judge will then instruct the jury as to the law to be applied. Once that is completed, the jury retires to deliberate. The jury is required to decide whether there was malpractice. If the jury decides that there was malpractice, they must also award damages.

If one of the parties disagrees with the verdict, the case may be appealed. The facts as found by the jury can not be challenged. The case can be appealed only on an issue of law. An appeal can take several years, particularly if it goes to the appeals court, then to the supreme court. Frequently, the case will be settled for a lesser amount of damages during the appeal process.

■ SPECIAL ISSUES

Competency

Generally, a person is competent to make all decisions on his or her behalf until a court states otherwise. Before a guardian may be appointed for reasons other than minor status, the potential ward must be determined to be an "incapacitated person" under the appropriate state law. Most states follow the Uniform Guardianship and Protective Proceedings Act (UGPPA, 1982) in some form. Usually, the respondent (potential ward) must meet both criteria of a two-prong test:

1. The respondent must have a disabling condition, such as mental illness, mental deficiency, physical illness, or substance abuse, *and*
2. The disabling condition must have led to a lack of sufficient understanding to make or communicate responsible decisions.

The UGPPA of 1997 addresses the many justified criticisms of the UGPPA of 1982. The 1997 Act restructures the definition in terms of functional abilities, which identifies that a person may have the capacity to do certain things and not others. It also identifies that there are varying levels of competency in the law depending on what is to be done, just as there are varying levels of actual ability. The nature of the disability is now irrelevant. The court must now find that the respondent is "unable to receive and evaluate information or make or communicate decisions to such an extent that the individual lacks the ability to meet essential requirements for physical health, safety, or self-care, even with appropriate technological assistance."

Each state may enact the UGPPA as it sees fit. Therefore each state's statute dealing with guardianship must be reviewed for the actual, current definition in that state.

Incompetency

A patient committed to a mental institution is competent to make treatment decisions until adjudicated incompetent by a judge. Therefore, until there is an adjudication of incompetency, the patient must be provided all the appropriate information to make informed decisions about his or her care and afforded all the rights and privileges anyone may exercise.

The medical records and treatment team are the best source of information to identify the capacity of a patient to make informed decisions. If it appears that someone does not have the ability to make reasoned decisions, that information must be communicated to the treatment team and documented in the patient's medical record. Once this is documented, the team should proceed promptly to obtain a guardianship from the court with some suitable person serving as guardian, usually a family member. However, frequently a family member is not available and may not be appropriate to serve as guardian. Some families are overburdened by their incapacitated relative and may prefer that an outside person serve as guardian. Having an outside person as guardian relieves the burden from the family and allows them to be supportive of their family member. Other times the family may be unable to provide any assistance, and it is in the best interests of the respondent for an outside individual to become the guardian.

Guardianship

Once appointed, the guardian has several duties and responsibilities, depending on the structure of the guardianship. Since a person may demonstrate differing capacities in different areas, a guardianship may be structured to reflect those capacities. The 1997 UGPPA specifically encourages use of less restrictive alternatives to guardianship, and when those do not suffice, a limited guardianship is preferred.

Generally, a guardianship includes both the person and his or her estate, and unless specified, most petitions for guardianship assume that the guardianship is plenary. The guardian makes all the personal decisions, including medical and psychiatric treatment, and controls the money and property of the individual. However, the guardianship may be limited to just the person or just the money and property (sometimes referred to as a conservatorship). It may also be limited to specific acts and powers as specified by the individual judge or court.

Temporary guardianship is an expedited process to provide for an individual in an emergency or where a delay would be detrimental to the patient's health, safety, and welfare. It is usually limited to 3 months. Once the time is complete, a further hearing must be held for a permanent guardianship. If no hearing occurs, the guardianship lapses, and the temporary guardian's powers lapse.

Once a guardian is in place, the guardian must be given all the rights of the ward. Access to medical records, including psychiatric records, should be provided as well as access to the treatment team. It is vital to keep the guardian involved with the treatment team and apprised of the treatment plan so appropriate actions can be undertaken. The guardian is the person who can give informed consent on behalf of the ward, and all treatment changes and choices should be discussed with the guardian, just as the team or primary provider would with the patient.

The guardian should take into consideration the preferences and views of the ward in making decisions both before and during the guardianship. The guardian must maintain enough contact with the ward to know of the ward's abilities, limitations, needs, and opportunities. Where reasonable, the guardian should encourage the ward to participate in decision making, to act on his or her behalf, and to work toward learning or regaining the ability to manage financial and personal affairs.

Minor

When the patient is a minor (under 18 years of age), the patient does not have the legal capacity to consent to treatment, except in specific and limited instances. A minor may be considered emancipated and able to make all decisions when the minor is married or has been found emancipated by the court. For treatment of venereal diseases, pregnancy, and certain other instances, the minor may give consent for treatment. However, these instances may vary from state to state.

Extraordinary Treatment

Do not resuscitate (DNR) orders, artificial maintenance or removal of hydration and nutrition, sterilization, abortion, antipsychotic medication, electroconvulsive therapy, and psychosurgery are some of the extraordinary treatment issues dealt with by the courts for incompetent patients and their guardians. In these instances, the courts have determined that the guardian does not have the authority to consent to these procedures without the intervention of the court. The court must balance the individual's interests and preferences against specific state interests. The state's specific interests are as follows:

1. Preservation of life
2. Protection of innocent third parties
3. Prevention of suicide
4. Maintenance of the ethical integrity of the medical profession
5. Preservation of order in penal institutions

The underlying principle in all of these cases is the constitutional right of an individual to privacy, a guarantee that encompasses the choice to accept or refuse medical treatment. This right extends to competent patients and to incompetent patients because the value of human dignity extends to both.

Procedures and legal standards may vary, but many courts require a judicial hearing to determine the competence of a patient and to make treatment decisions before the nonemergency administration of antipsychotic medications against a person's will. The factors are the same or similar to those used in extraordinary treatment cases.

The factors include the express preference of the ward, the ward's religious beliefs, the effects on the ward's family, the probability of adverse side effects, the consequences if the treatment is refused, and the prognosis with treatment.

In the widely known Rogers (1983) decision, the Massachusetts Supreme Judicial Court held the following:

1. A person with a diagnosis of mental illness, whether institutionalized or not, has a right to refuse treatment with antipsychotic medications.
2. The right to refuse is not absolute and may be overcome in emergency situations:
   a. If institutionalized, the individual, whether competent or not, may be medicated to restrain only if the individual poses an imminent threat of harm to himself or others and only if there is no less restrictive alternative.
   b. If noninstitutionalized, the individual, whether competent or not, may be medicated under the same circumstances, except that involuntary hospitalization must be considered as an alternative.
3. A person who is incompetent has the same right to refuse treatment with antipsychotic medications as does a competent person. Only when even the smallest delay would cause immediate, substantial, and irreversible deterioration of a serious mental illness will a person, whom a physician in the exercise of professional judgment believes to be incompetent, be treated over his or her objections on an interim basis while a petition to the court is pursued.
4. A person's competency is a legal determination that may only be made by a court. Therefore, when a physician believes that a person who is refusing treatment is incompetent, there must be a judicial determination of incompetence and substituted judgment before the person may be medicated with antipsychotic medications.
5. If the person is competent or the court's substituted judgment is that the person would refuse treatment, then that refusal must be respected except in an emergency or when there are countervailing state interests that are sufficiently compelling to override the decision.

APRNs should understand and apply the factors in their decision making regarding antipsychotic medication use in patients, whether or not they are hospitalized at the time. The APRN can explore the likely outcome of a court hearing, address differences of opinion within the family and treatment team, and assist in a resolution that may not need to include the court. If a guardian is involved, however, the issue must be presented to the court for resolution. Input from the family and treatment team regarding what the patient has said and done in the past will be helpful for the court to make the appropriate decision.

Informed Consent

The basic principle behind informed consent is that competent adult patients have a right to self-determination. The result of the application of this principle is that the plaintiff, when he or she agrees to have a procedure or treatment performed by an APRN knowing the risks and alternatives, assumes the express and implied risks and consequences of the treatment and consequential liability.

Informed consent involves giving the patient sufficient information to make an intelligent choice to accept or reject the treatment based on a full disclosure of the facts. This information must be given by the APRN who is responsible for performing the procedure. If a physician or another health care provider will actually perform the procedure, the APRN should not be required to provide the information. The patient must be informed of the following:

1. Nature of his or her medical condition
2. Benefits of the proposed treatment or procedure
3. Risks involved with the proposed treatment
4. Alternatives to the treatment with their risks and benefits

5. Consequences if no treatment is performed

Although the elements of informed consent are relatively similar from state to state, what the court requires the plaintiff to prove may be very different. Some courts apply the "subjective" standard—what that patient would or would not do under the circumstances. Most courts apply the "objective" standard—what a reasonable patient would do under the same or similar circumstances.

Confidentiality

With the advent of TeleMedicine, the issue of confidentiality and privacy has been given great attention. Medical information is now transmitted by video and computer. Every safeguard possible should be used consistently to protect the patient's privacy. It is no longer appropriate to only be cautious of the person to whom you are speaking and who may overhear a conversation. Any transmitted information must be carefully protected from the public.

The general rule in most states is that "unauthorized revelation of any confidential communication given in the course of treatment is tortious conduct which may be the basis for an action in damages." As a federal district court stated in Hammons v. Aetna Casualty (1965), "When a patient seeks out a doctor and retains him, he must admit him to the most private part of the material domain to man. To promote full disclosure, the medical profession extends the promise of secrecy referred to above. The candor which this promise elicits is necessary to the effective pursuit of health; there can be no reticence, no reservation, no reluctance when patients discuss their problems."

Despite the defense of "truth" described with respect to defamation, the tort of invasion of privacy is deemed to be committed by those who disclose confidential information without authorization of the patient. The holder of the privilege is the patient, the guardian, or if the patient is dead, the personal representative of the patient.

The therapist is required to claim the privilege whenever the therapist is present when the communication is sought to be disclosed. Under certain circumstances, the privilege may be waived if the request is from the patient, a party claiming through or on behalf of the patient, and if there is litigation in which the plaintiff has claimed damages for the injury or death of the patient.

Psychotherapist-Patient Privilege

Whether an APRN who renders psychotherapy is covered by the psychotherapist-patient privilege is a state by state consideration. Each state has the right to legislate a psychotherapist-patient privilege; many do not include nurses, whether or not they provide psychotherapy. The local statute should be closely scrutinized to see when, if ever, the privilege includes a nurse and in what capacity.

There is no privilege preventing disclosure when the therapist has reasonable cause to believe that the patient is in such a mental or emotional condition as to be dangerous to himself or herself or to another, and the communication is necessary to prevent the danger. One of the most difficult decisions facing a therapist is whether to warn a third person of threats of harm that the patient has made against the third person. In Tarasoff, et al v. Regents of the University of California (1976), the court found that a therapist has a special relationship with a patient, which may extend to a victim of that patient. This is the first element of a negligence action. The second element is satisfied when the therapist fails to exercise "that reasonable degree of skill, knowledge, and care ordinarily possessed and exercised by members of [that professional specialty] under similar circumstances." This requires a therapist to use reasonable care in predicting violence to a third person and informing that person or someone who can inform the individual of the threat. This warning does not have severe consequences to the therapist's patient because it does not deprive the patient of his or her liberty. However, it should be done discreetly, in a fashion that would preserve the privacy of the patient while preventing the danger. If no warning is given and harm results, the elements of an action in negligence results.

■ ADMINISTRATIVE LAW

Administrative law is as significant as the civil or criminal branches of law. It arises from statutes enacted by the state or federal legislature that creates administrative agencies. Administrative laws are rules created by administrative agencies. For APRNs, the most important of these agencies are the state boards that regulate the registration of nurses. Their authority has been delegated to them by legislature, and their rules have the force and effect of statutes passed by the legislature.

Board of Registration in Nursing

The primary purpose of the State Boards of Registration in Nursing is to protect the public. They have two functions:

1. To define the responsibilities of the nurse and grant licenses to applicants that meet those standards.
2. To investigate and, if appropriate, take disciplinary action when a nurse is charged with violating those standards.

The disciplinary proceedings can work separately or in parallel with civil legal complaints of malpractice levied against nurses. The Board proceedings are independent of any civil action and can result in the suspension or revocation of licenses to practice as well as other disciplinary actions, such as limitations on the areas in which the licensee may practice, required remedial education, and special reporting requirements. Although the results of these proceedings are subject to judicial review, boards have broad discretionary powers, and a basis for challenging their discretion must be established to overcome adverse decisions.

Rather than initiating a case by a complaint filed with a court, as in a civil case, a case may begin by a disgruntled individual writing or calling and lodging a complaint with the Board. The first time that a nurse may be aware of such a complaint is when the board writes, informally requesting an explanation for the complaint. This is the most critical stage of the entire proceeding. The response to the complaint may resolve the entire matter, with no complaint registered on the nurses' record. An inappropriate response to the complaint, or none at all, will lead to a formal "order to show cause," which lodges the complaint on the nurse's record and should be reported to the National Practitioners Data Bank. Therefore it is vital that the nurse seek legal representation before answering any informal complaint from the Board.

Once an order to show cause is filed, the Board expects a formal response. After the investigation period is complete, a hearing will be convened. Usually the Board or some subset of the Board serves as a hearing panel. They will hear evidence, receive exhibits, and admit almost all evidence on the record, whether testimony or demonstrative. The rules of evidence are considerably relaxed compared with those used in a court of law. Hearsay, which is testimony by an individual who relates what someone else told them, is usually allowed, unlike in a court of law.

In many states, if the complaint against the nurse is the abuse, misuse, or diversion of controlled substances, the Board will not proceed with the full administrative hearing as long as the nurse admits to having a drug problem, enters into a rehabilitation program, and complies with drug testing and other requirements imposed by the Board. This may prevent the action from being reported to the National Practitioners Data Bank if action is taken before an order to show cause is initiated.

The other common cases seen by the Board are negligence and patient neglect, incompetence, abusive behavior, physical or mental impairment, and fraud. A single incident of negligence usually will not lead to disciplinary action unless the negligence was egregious. Unlike negligence (when the nurse is able to render reasonable care but fails to do so), *incompetence* is applied to a nurse who is not qualified to provide the care. This charge can be levied against new and experienced nurses. For instance, if a nurse without experience is floated to a specialty unit, that nurse jeopardizes the patients and her license to practice. Just because the nurse is required to float to the unit does not serve as a defense.

Abusive behavior may be physical or verbal. What is verbal abuse may be subject to interpretation. In one case, a patient, while being assisted to the bed, became disoriented and tried to sit down. The nurse used profanity when telling him to move. This was overheard by an aide who reported it to the supervisor. It was eventually reported to the Board of Registration in Nursing who found that it rose to the level of abuse.

When a nurse has a loss of motor skill or mobility, this may or may not make the nurse unable to provide safe care. The Board may intervene in these situations if there is a risk of harm to the public. This may also include mental illness such as schizophrenia, panic disorders, depression, substance abuse, and others. The Americans with Disabilities Act (ADA) requires an employer to make reasonable accommodations to assist a nurse to provide safe care. The issue, however, is determining what is "reasonable" to accommodate a particular nurse's disability.

Delegation

With the advent of unlicensed assistive personnel (UAP), delegation of nursing duties has come to the forefront, with many cases before the state Boards of Registration in Nursing. Some state legislatures have enacted laws on the exact requirements for delegation, some have added the requirements to the rules and regulations that govern nursing practice, and others have not addressed the issue. Regardless, nurse practice acts identify the scope of the practice of a registered nurse and what care can be provided only by nurses. Delegation issues are likely to arise in both

a malpractice case or a case before the Board of Nursing.

The ANA (1995) defines delegation as "transferring responsibility for the performance of an activity . . . while retaining accountability for the outcome." The National Council of State Boards of Nursing has defined it as "transferring to a competent individual authority to perform a selected nursing task in a selected situation" (Anon, 1995). Regardless of the definition used, a specific framework for making delegation decisions is of utmost importance, as well as a thorough knowledge of the policies and procedures of the facility.

The framework for delegation must include five factors:

1. The decision must be within the scope of the nurse's professional judgment.
2. The nurse must assess the patient's care needs before delegating the activity.
3. A reasonable and prudent nurse should determine that the activity may be delegated.
4. The person to whom the activity is delegated must be capable of performing it.
5. The nurse must be able to supervise the performance of the activity.

Applying the framework for delegation will insulate the APRN from liability for the UAP's actions. Courts generally rule that supervisors are not vicariously liable for the actions of employees under them, provided the supervisor was not negligent in supervision. The institution rather than the APRN is liable.

In one case, a nurse was able to successfully defend herself against disciplinary action by showing that she had complied with appropriate delegation. The facility had a policy and procedure manual that defined the unlicensed assistive personnel's job and training. The nurse showed that the delegated act was allowed to be delegated by the nurse practice act and the facility policy. Based on the training of the UAP and the history of the UAP performing the act, the delegation of the act to the UAP was appropriate. The nurse pointed to her notes in the chart and the documentation of the UAP to show that she had appropriately supervised the act. Further, she proved that a reasonable and prudent nurse would delegate that task to that UAP by showing past assignment sheets in which other nurses had delegated the same duty to that individual. The Board dismissed the allegation of inappropriate delegation.

Prescriptive Authority

APRNs who have prescriptive authority should be aware of the rules of their state that affect their ability to prescribe. A review of the prescriptive problems of physicians dealt with by the Board of Registration in Medicine reveals that the major issues are either the inappropriate prescription practices of the physicians ordering narcotics for their patients or the physician's diversion and abuse of drugs.

The Drug Enforcement Agency (DEA) is a federal administrative agency that investigates the uses of controlled substances. Their interaction with nurses may be the result of an investigation of potentially criminal activities of nurses or patients. If the Board of Registration in Nursing is investigating an APRN for possible drug diversion, the DEA may conduct an investigation of its own. The Board may then use those findings as evidence against the APRN.

Nurses with prescriptive authority must be familiar with the rules and regulations of at least three boards that interact: the Board of Registration in Nursing, the Board of Registration in Medicine, and the Board of Pharmacy. These three boards govern the right to prescribe medications within a given state. The authority is usually limited to designated nurse practitioners who practice within established protocols. The APRN interested in obtaining prescriptive authority should review the state's laws to identify whether the state recognizes the prescriptive authority of APRNs, and if it is regulated within the context of professional nursing practice. The statute should be explicit on the limits, if any, the requirements for obtaining prescriptive authority, the relationship required with a physician, and what drugs the APRN may prescribe. The ANA has suggested legislation on prescriptive authority that urges caution in the dispensing of medication by the APRN. Chapter 13 describes prescriptive practice of APRNs in more detail.

EMPLOYMENT AND ENTREPRENEUR ISSUES

When the APRN's relationship with the employer is as an independent contractor, the employer is not vicariously liable for the negligence or malpractice of the APRN. The status of the APRN is established by the employment contract (which may identify the status explicitly) as well as the practice of the APRN's activities. When the written contract is unclear, a court may look at the activities of the APRN to see how much control is exercised over the practice of nursing.

At-will employees may be terminated at any time with no notice requirements, but they are protected from liability by the principles of respondeat superior. Conversely, an at-will employee may leave a job without notice. The law of the individual state may provide certain remedies or rights for the at-will employee, such as requiring that the employer not fire an employee for "whistle blowing" or for other public policy reasons. Chapter 19 discusses whistle blowing as an ethical act and its implication.

A contract of employment is generally inferred when there is a collective bargaining agreement and is possibly found in the employer's policy and procedure manual. A contract provides that an employee may only be terminated in a certain manner for certain specified reasons. The employee has more rights and may grieve the dismissal or discipline to the collective bargaining group.

APRNs are becoming employers and developing their own businesses as well as developing specialty practices within existing employment areas. No matter what service is being developed, whether it is the APRN's own business or he or she is employed in a supervisory or developmental capacity, certain employment issues must be addressed.

Employee Protections

Several federal statutes protect the employee and provide the employee with causes of action against their employers. Title VII 42 U.S.C. Subsec. E-1 et seq. (Civil Rights Act of 1964) protects employees from discrimination based on race, color, religion, sex, or national origin and requires that pregnant women receive the same protection as any other employee. Sexual harassment claims and other violations of the Civil Rights Act are handled by the Equal Employment Opportunity Commission (EEOC). *Sexual harassment* includes the following:

1. Submission to sexual advances is explicitly or implicitly a condition of employment.
2. Submission to sexual advances is used as a basis for employment decisions.
3. Sexual harassment interferes with job performance even if it only creates an intimidating, offensive, or hostile environment.

The Age Discrimination and Employment Act (ADEA), 29 U.S.C. Subsec. 621 (1967), is also enforced by the EEOC. This law prohibits discrimination against anyone 40 years of age or older in hiring and promotions.

The 1990 Americans with Disabilities Act (ADA) affected nearly every aspect of employment policy from placing job ads to training supervisors. The ADA provides a framework for managing all employees, whether they have a disability or are in a protected class that may not be discriminated against.

A four-part formula was developed by the ADA to define a disability:

1. A physical or mental impairment that substantially limits one or more of major life activities of an individual
2. A record of such an impairment

3. Being regarded as having such an impairment
4. Individuals who have a work, social, or family relationship with a disabled person

The first part of the definition includes someone who is hard of hearing, blind, or in a wheelchair. Part two of the definition protects groups like recovering alcoholics or individuals with a history of mental illness. Individuals protected against discrimination are those who have completed a drug or alcohol rehabilitation program or are in the process of completing one. If an employer has clear evidence of an individual's drug use, the employer does not have to hire the person, and may fire a person based on the clear evidence. However, the employer cannot refuse to hire or fire anyone simply because he or she is an alcoholic. Employers can fire an alcoholic only if the drinking is affecting the job performance. Part two also covers those who have been erroneously classified as having such an impairment.

Part three protects individuals whose employers think might have a disability even though they do not. It also covers those whose perceived disability does not limit their activities. This may include someone who has a vision impairment being perceived as having a disability. It may also include homosexuals, although they are not a protected class under federal law, since they could be seen as carrying the HIV virus, and individuals who are infected with the HIV virus are protected under the law.

Part four offers protection to those who assist those with a disability to more easily support those individuals. Box 8-4 describes the common forms of discrimination that the law clearly bars.

Employment Practices

Job descriptions must be written before an ad is placed. They are the first line of defense to an allegation of discrimination. Writing a description after the employer has been charged with discrimination has no weight with the court.

A good job description separates essential job functions from nonessential job functions. *Essen-*

box

8-4

COMMON FORMS OF DISCRIMINATION THAT THE LAW BARS

1. Limiting the duties of an individual with a disability based on an assumption of what is best for the person or about the person's ability to perform the task.
2. Adopting separate tracks of progression for individuals with disabilities based on an assumption that no one with a disability would be interested in moving into a particular job.
3. Denying employment to someone based on a generalized fear about the safety of the individual or higher rates of absenteeism.
4. Denying a job, promotion, or benefits to a qualified, able-bodied individual because he or she has a relationship or association with a person who has a disability.
5. Denying employment opportunities to a qualified applicant based on the need to make reasonable accommodations.
6. Administering tests in a manner that fails to accurately reflect the skills, aptitude, or other factors intended to be measured.
7. Participating in contractual or other relationships that would subject a qualified individual with a disability to discrimination.
8. Using standards, criteria, or methods of administration that discriminate because of a disability.
9. Failing to make reasonable accommodations for a known physical or mental limitation of a qualified applicant or employee with a disability without clear demonstration that the accommodation imposes undue hardship for the business.

tial functions are those that must be completed to do the job thoroughly. In one recent case, a trial court held that being required to work other shifts than solely the day shift was an essential function. The facility proved that the nonsenior day shift nurses were all required to work the other shifts and that requirement had always been enforced. The court found that it was an essential function and the nurse was not entitled to work solely the day shift. The facility had explored with her other options, which she had not accepted. The ADA says that a person's inability to perform nonessential functions cannot be held against him or her.

The job description should identify and list both essential and nonessential functions. This clearly indicates to employees without disabilities that they are expected to do everything. Employees with disabilities will know what duties they are required to perform and which ones they do not have to do if they are unable.

The job application forms must also avoid discrimination. Questions that could force the applicant to reveal a disability must be avoided. Inappropriate questions could allow that job applicant to charge discrimination if the employer does not hire him or her. The application should focus on the job description itself, including the essential functions and the qualifications for that job.

The application should focus on the job description itself, including the essential functions and the qualifications for that job. Rather than ask if someone can drive a van, the question should ask whether the applicant has a valid driver's license. If rotating shifts are required, the employer cannot ask the person if he or she has a disability that would prevent him or her from working rotating shifts. Instead, the employer should state that the job requires rotating shifts and decide if that applicant can meet that requirement.

The interview site must be accessible. The law requires that barriers preventing access to the interview site be removed on a case by case basis. The interview questions must be nondiscriminatory. Interviewers must not ask applicants about age, marital status, or dependent children; they cannot ask minorities about their national origin, and they cannot inquire about possible disabilities. The interviewer should tell the applicants what the essential functions or duties are, then ask them if they can do those duties without accommodations. If they are unable to perform the job even with accommodations, employers do not have to consider that individual any further. If the applicants can do the job with accommodations, then the employer must ask how they can perform the tasks and what accommodations will be necessary.

When employers are ready to make a job offer, they must make it to the most qualified candidate. If an individual with a disability is the most qualified after accommodations have been made, then that candidate should be offered the job. If there is a tie between a candidate with a disability and one without a disability, and the employer makes a decision against the person on the basis of his or her disability, that is discrimination. The decision must always be based on factors other than the disability. Most hiring decisions are based on how that person will fit into the organization.

Preemployment physical exams are illegal. Only two types of employment physicals are permitted under the ADA: an examination that takes place after a job offer is made, or an examination before a candidate is placed in a specific job. Under no circumstances can the employer single out only certain employees in a job classification to have a physical examination. All employees in that same job classification must complete the physical examination.

The key to the ADA is reasonable accommodations. *Reasonable accommodations* are required for an individual who has a disability to perform the essential functions of the job. The employer has the right to choose the accommodation that fits the employer's purposes best and is the most efficient. If the person with a disability refuses the possible accommodations, then the employer is no longer obligated to employ or keep the individual employed.

Accommodations are not reasonable when it is an undue hardship to the employer. This means that the accommodations would impose a significant difficulty or expense. However, more than just the initial cost should be reviewed. Consideration should be given to the possible tax credits available and outside funding sources. The effects that the accommodations would have on the operation of the facility are a significant factor. For example, if there is a fast work flow and accommodations cause a bottle-neck that disrupts this flow, they may not be reasonable.

Current employees have significantly more rights than prospective employees. If an employee has already demonstrated that he or she can do the essential functions of the job and then develops a disability, the employer must do everything that would be done for a new employee, plus consideration must be given to moving him or her into a vacant position. This should be a lateral move with the same level of pay and authority as the position he or she can no longer hold. If there are no accommodations possible and there is no lateral position to offer the employee, a lesser position can be offered. If the employee refuses the lower position with less pay or benefits, then the employer is no longer obligated to retain that employee.

Once performance standards for employees with disabilities are set, employers are allowed to enforce them just as they would for any other employee. For instance, if an accommodation was made because someone had difficulty getting to work precisely at 8 AM because of transportation problems related to a disability, but then the employee began to arrive after the accommodated time of 9:00 AM, and this was all the accommodation possible, the employee can then be disciplined for poor attendance. Employers are allowed to uphold and enforce current policies if done so consistently.

Performance reviews must be based on the job and not the disability. An objective evaluation process focuses on the employee's ability to do the essential functions. The evaluation should be no different than that of someone without a disability. The evaluator must refrain from asking questions relating to the disability and commenting on how the person's treatment is progressing. The focus must remain on the work performance during the appraisal interview.

IMPLICATIONS FOR ■ THE FUTURE

APRNs are gaining prescriptive authority throughout the country. More APRNs are becoming the owners and operators of their own clinics and businesses. APRNs taking on these roles may look to other professions that have functioned in these roles to identify possible new areas of liability. The APRNs must also be prepared to face the unknown challenges presented by the rapidly changing health care system. The concepts presented in this chapter will prepare APRNs to understand some of the legal implications of future advanced nursing practice.

RESOURCES AND CONNECTIONS

PUBLICATIONS

Aiken, T.D., & Catalano, J. T. (1994). *Legal, ethical and political issues in nursing*. Philadelphia: F.A. Davis.

Guido, G.W. (1988). *Legal issues in nursing: a source book for practice*. Norwalk, CT: Appleton & Lange.

Kjervik, D. (Ed.). *Journal of Nursing Law*. KRM Information Sources.

Laben, J.K., & Powell, C.P. (1989). *Legal issues and guidelines for nurses who care for the mentally ill*. Owings Mills, MD: National Health Publishing.

Sullivan, G.H., & Mattera, M.D. (1997). RN's legally speaking. *Medical Economics* (regular feature).

ASSOCIATIONS

American Association of Nurse Attorneys
7784 Grow Drive
Pensacola, FL 32514
850-484-9987
Email: TAANA@Puetzamc.com

References

Adams v. Murakami, No. C410409 (Los Angeles County Superior Court) [personal communication].

American Nurses Association. (1995). Position statement on registered nurse utilization of assistive personnel. *American Nurse*, 25(2), 7–8.

Anon. (1995). Working with UAPs. *NSO Risk Advisor*, 1–6.

Bost v Riley, 262 S.E. 2d 391 (N.C. App. 1980).

Cook v Highland Hospital, 84 S.E. 352 (N.C. 1915).

Hamburger v Henry Ford Hospital, 91 Mich App 580, 284 NW 2d 155, 1979.

Hammons v Aetna Casualty, 244 F. Supp. 793 (N.D. Ohio, 1965).

Pisel v Stanford Hospital, 430 A 2d 1, 1980.

Tarasoff, et al v. Regents of the University of California, 17 Cal 3d. 425: 551 P.2d 34 (1976).

ADVANCED CLINICAL PRACTICE

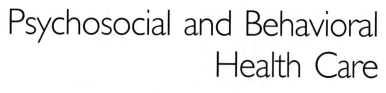

chapter 9

Psychosocial and Behavioral Health Care

ANNE FISHEL

■ INTRODUCTION

This chapter describes scientific advances in the psychosocial knowledge base that are relevant for advanced practice registered nurses (APRNs) in psychiatric and mental health nursing. Current theory, research, and clinical examples focus on cognitive behavioral, interpersonal, supportive, motivational, and brief solution-focused therapies. Changes in the health care delivery system offer more opportunities for brief therapies (Montgomery & Webster, 1994) and a new emphasis

185

on primary mental health care (Haber & Billings, 1995).

Consider the following example. A graduate nursing student approaches her preceptor to discuss her patient, diagnosed with bipolar disorder, who has missed her appointment. The student is concerned that the patient's condition is getting worse, and the student plans to phone her. If unable to reach her patient, the student plans to make a home visit. The preceptor explains that the policy in that agency is not to phone for "no-shows" because the patient's behavior is a sign of resistance. The therapeutic approach is to wait for the patient to call and reschedule. If the patient does not call, then after three missed appointments, the agency will send a form letter explaining that the file will be closed if the patient does not call within a week. A week after the missed appointment, the patient is admitted to the hospital in an acute manic state.

Why did these two therapists differ in their approach to this patient? The rationale for the preceptor's decision was based on psychoanalytic and motivational theories and system policy. The rationale for the student's decision was based on biologic knowledge about bipolar disorder, interpersonal and supportive therapy theories, and an acknowledgment of the need for case management and assertive outreach with persons having a severe and persistent mental illness (SPMI).

To fully understand and treat psychiatric patients, an integration of biologic, psychologic, and sociocultural factors is necessary. Nurse psychotherapists use a variety of theoretical frameworks to both understand mental illness and guide interventions. Because APRNs in psychiatric and mental health care are holistic, they believe in assessing the whole person, including biology, psychology, social systems, culture, and spirituality, before deciding on a course of action. Although pharmacotherapies are used with many psychosocial therapies, this chapter focuses on psychotherapies alone. Nurse psychotherapists have the option of choosing certain models for certain patients or a variety of models with the same patient based

upon the best scientific evidence. Which framework will work best in each situation is not always known, but the APRN tries an intervention based on the current theoretical and scientific evidence and then evaluates the outcome. In the previous example, perhaps the intervention was not successful because the patient was hospitalized. Some would argue that the intervention was successful because hospitalization would enable the patient to receive treatment that would increase the patient's level of functioning in the community. Although there was no research to guide the intervention in this situation, there was nursing knowledge that suggested a therapeutic intervention. Worley (1997) writes that a telephone call reminder the day before a scheduled appointment should be common practice with persons experiencing SPMI, and that every effort should be made to contact a patient who has missed a scheduled appointment. Such nursing knowledge, however, needs to be validated by research.

No longer can decisions be made based on intuition or invalidated approaches. These are the challenges and complexities that are the practice realities of APRNs in psychiatric and mental health care. The field of psychiatric nursing, as in all of health care, is being held accountable to standards of evidence-based practice and measurable outcomes. As Barlow (1996) states, "If we do not promote and disseminate existing evidence for the efficacy of our psychologic interventions, then we will put psychotherapy at a severe disadvantage and risk a substantial deemphasis if not elimination of psychologic interventions in our health care delivery system" (Box 9-1). Therein lies the challenge for nurse psychotherapists.

■ THERAPEUTIC ALLIANCE

The *therapeutic alliance,* defined broadly as the collaborative bond between therapist and patient, is widely considered to be an essential ingredient in the effectiveness of psychotherapy. Several studies have examined the effects of the therapeutic alliance on clinical outcomes. Using data from

box 9-1

DEFINITION OF EFFICACY

Psychologists have proposed a scheme to determine when a psychologic treatment is efficacious or possibly efficacious. Only when a treatment has been found efficacious in at least two studies by independent research teams do they consider its efficacy to have been established. If there is only one study supporting a treatment's efficacy, or if all of the research has been conducted by one team, then they consider the findings promising but would label such treatments as "possibly efficacious, pending replication." In addition, the research teams determined that a sample size of 25 to 30 patients would suffice even though 50 patients are needed per treatment condition to reach the conventional 80% power level for significance testing. In actuality, reports in the literature indicate that the median sample size per treatment condition is 12 patients. The greatest weight was given to efficacy trials, but those trials should be followed by research on effectiveness in clinical settings and with various populations and by cost-effectiveness research.

From Chambless & Hollon, 1998.

the National Institute of Mental Health Treatment of Depression Collaborative Research Program (TDCRP), the relationship between therapeutic alliance and treatment outcome was examined for depressed outpatients who received psychotherapy (Krupnick et al., 1996). Clinical raters scored videotapes of 619 sessions. Outcome was assessed from patients' and clinical evaluators' perspectives and from depressive symptomatology. Therapeutic alliance was found to have a significant effect on clinical outcome with both interpersonal and cognitive behavioral psychotherapy. The ratings of the patient's contribution to the alliance were significantly related to treatment outcome. There was no association between the therapist's contribution and outcome—probably because all of the

therapists were highly skilled and there was little variability.

In an examination of the outcomes of psychotherapy, Miller and colleagues (Miller, Hubble, & Duncan, 1995) reported that extra therapeutic factors explained 40% of the change, relationship factors explained 30%, hope of the patient explained 15%, and technique of the therapists explained 15%. The extra therapeutic factors are the patient's innate abilities (the therapist can emphasize the patient's strengths) and chance or fortuitous events (the therapist can listen for chance events and assist patients in recognizing that they took advantage of them). This research also points out that the therapeutic alliance and the installation of hope are much more influential in bringing about change than are specific techniques. By maintaining belief in their patients' recovery, therapists communicate the confidence necessary for preventing an irreversible sense of hopelessness. Further study supports the finding that the most important aspect of therapist effectiveness is the ability to form a therapeutic alliance (Elliott, Adams, & Hodge, 1992).

Effective treatment involves therapists responding appropriately to their patients' predominant, interpersonal styles. Therapists who were not told about their patient's interpersonal style nevertheless responded with systematically different interventions depending on patients' interpersonal style (Hardy, Stiles, Barkham, & Startup, 1998). Therapists tended to use more affective and relationship-oriented interventions with overinvolved patients and more cognitive treatment methods with underinvolved patients. Outcomes of the interpersonal style groups were approximately equivalent, consistent with the view that the differences in treatment reflected appropriate responsiveness to patients' styles. In another study, high-impact sessions were characterized by higher alliance scores than those for low-impact sessions, and alliance was positively related to therapists' ratings of session depth and smoothness and to patients' ratings of mood (Raue, Goldfried, & Barkham, 1997).

Connectedness

Research indicates that the therapeutic alliance has a significant influence on outcome. APRNs are keenly aware of the importance of the alliance in the psychotherapy relationship. As early as 1952, Peplau was writing about the nurse-patient relationship as an opportunity to transform nursing situations into learning experiences. Drawing upon Sullivan's (1953) theory of interpersonal relations, Peplau developed the theoretical foundation upon which many APRNs are building the science and art of nursing psychotherapy. Thus far, nursing has been more involved in operationally defining the therapeutic alliance (what it is) than in conducting outcome research (whether it works). For example, during structured interviews, participants were encouraged to describe their perceptions of "connectedness" in the nurse-patient relationship (Heifner, 1993). From these data, Heifner identified essential elements that are related to the development of psychiatric nurse-patient relationship (Box 9-2). Perhaps this formulation could be used as the basis for looking at the large number of patients who do not keep their second appointments. By analyzing the first interviews, the APRN researcher could detect where "connectedness" was missing and give direction for building the therapeutic alliance.

Forchuk (1995a) analyzed data from 124 newly formed nurse-patient dyads with patients who had a chronic mental illness. She identified the following factors, which influenced progress in the therapeutic relationship:

1. Longer nurse-patient meetings (one 30 minute session was better than three 10 minute sessions)
2. More total time in meetings
3. Shorter previous patient hospitalizations
4. More experienced psychiatric nurses

Each nurse-patient dyad is unique, and a very different outcome may occur if the patient is transferred to a different nurse (Forchuk, 1995b). Another study found that persons with nonchronic schizophrenia who were able to form a therapeutic alliance within 6 months had better treatment outcomes, including a lower dropout rate, less prescribed medication, greater compliance with medication, and fewer rehospitalizations during the next 2 years (Frank & Gunderson, 1990). These data seem to suggest that APRNs who are working with the severe and persistent mentally ill need to be willing to transfer them to another nurse therapist if significant progress is not made in relationship development within 3 to 4 months.

Empathy

Although the concept of empathy was thought to be borrowed from other disciplines, the phenomenon has been prevalent in nursing since the U.S. Civil War (Sutherland, 1993). In a group of 185 patients treated with cognitive behavior therapy, therapeutic empathy was found to have the major effect on recovery from depression (Burns & Nolen-Hoeksema, 1992). The Empathy Scale, which asks patients to rate how warm, caring, and empathic their therapists are, was used to measure empathy. Depression was measured using the

---

box **9-2**

ESSENTIAL ELEMENTS IN FORMING AN ALLIANCE

Nurse makes initial contact with the patient →
Nurse experiences some tension →
Patient shows vulnerability →
Nurse feels a lessening of tension →
Nurse encourages more disclosure in the vulnerable area →
Nurse recognizes commonalities that the patient may or may not disclose →
Nurse experiences a feeling of reciprocity with the patient →
Nurse feels valued by the patient →
Patient and nurse invest more in the relationship, each taking risks →
Connectedness results.

From Heifner, 1993.

Beck Depression Inventory. The patients of novice therapists improved significantly less than did the patients of more experienced therapists when controlling for therapeutic empathy and homework compliance.

Caring

Caring has been proposed as a paradigm unique to nursing, as the "core," or essence, of the therapeutic alliance (Morse et al., 1990). Some have argued that the affectual nature of caring may be jeopardized or devalued in today's market driven economy. Interactions with professionals and external supports (including relationships) were found to be two of only four factors that influenced hospitalized suicidal patients' ambivalence about suicide (Cardell & Horton-Deutsch, 1994). Often patients who commit suicide are seen in retrospect to have not established a therapeutic alliance with therapists.

In a caring relationship the APRN maintains therapeutic perspective rather than therapeutic objectivity. When distance is needed, the therapist distances from the pathology rather than from the human being (Montgomery, 1993). Another quality that is important in a caring relationship is that caregivers transcend their own ego to find some greater existential or spiritual significance to their involvement (Montgomery & Webster, 1994). Authenticity requires that therapists drop their professional persona and show their human self in a way that can engage with the patient's human self; therefore nurse therapists use more self-disclosure than traditional theory would suggest. For example, while working with a young African-American woman who was referred because she had experienced loss of her baby born at 16 weeks' gestation (resulting from incompetent cervix), the therapist disclosed that she too had lost a premature baby for the same reason. The therapist offered hope by also sharing that with treatment, she carried two additional pregnancies to term, and her children are now adults (Fischel & Lowdermilk, in press).

Empowerment

Empowerment is a technique useful in maintaining the therapeutic alliance. Listening to patients and helping them sort through their fears and expectations encourages them to take charge of their lives. For example, Ms. S, an 86-year-old woman, was living in a retirement center with her 90-year-old husband. She had a long history of severe depression that was stabilized with medications and cognitive and supportive psychotherapy. Her husband was diagnosed with Alzheimer's disease. As his memory became more of a problem, their adult children and the health care staff at the center bombarded Ms. S. with advice about putting him in the special Alzheimer's unit. She had a long history of caring for family members who were sick and maintained much of her self-esteem by doing a good job with nurturing. Only when she was severely depressed was she unable to be a caregiver. As she discussed the dilemma about her husband's illness, it was obvious that she wanted to care for him for as long as possible. Furthermore, placing him in the Alzheimer's unit would be a financial burden. The nurse therapist facilitated her working out her feelings about this and empowered her to make the decision about moving her husband. "You will know when the time is right to move him to the special unit. When you think it is the right time, you can discuss how to pay for it with the staff and your adult children." The patient was noticeably relieved with this empowering suggestion and reported telling the staff and her adult children that she would make the decision and that she would know when it was necessary. In addition, she was able to articulate what would make her caregiving easier and what resources she could request from her church and friends at the retirement center.

The therapist's expertise lies not in fixing the problem but in knowing how to mobilize the patient's own strengths and resources for healing (Montgomery, 1993). Power and expertise do not reside within the therapist but within the patient. Obtaining the best data from interviews requires that a trusting relationship be established. Both outcome and process research as well as randomized clinical trials, single case study designs, and community case-finding research are important to the further development of advanced practice psychiatric-mental health nursing. Concepts basic to the therapeutic alliance, including connectedness, empathy, caring, and empowerment, provide fertile theory to be tested.

COGNITIVE AND BEHAVIORAL ■ THERAPIES

Cognitive and behavioral therapies put patients back in charge of their own lives. The therapist collaborates with the patient in defining the problem, identifying goals, formulating treatment strategies, and evaluating progress. Because the focus is on the patient's self-control, cognitive behavioral therapy is seen as educational and skill building rather than curative, with the therapist taking a facilitative role (Stuart, 1998). From this brief description, it is evident that cognitive behavioral therapy fits well with advanced practice nursing.

The evolution of cognitive behavior therapy (CBT) took place in three stages. Initially, behavior therapy emerged in independent but parallel developments in the United Kingdom and the United States between 1950 and 1970. The second stage, the growth of cognitive therapy, took place in the United States in the mid 1960s. The third stage, the merging of behavior and cognitive therapy into CBT, gathered momentum in the late 1980s and is now well advanced in Europe and North America. CBT is widely accepted and is practiced by growing numbers of clinicians; in all likelihood, it is today the most broadly and confidently endorsed form of psychologic therapy (Rachman, 1997). The British form of behavior therapy concentrated on anxiety disorders (notably agoraphobia) in outpatient adults and was derived mainly from the ideas of Pavlov, Watson, and Hull. The American psychologists were applying Skinnerian ideas and techniques to institutionalized patients with severe problems. Both groups concentrated on behavioral problems, and both groups believed that it was necessary and usually sufficient to change the affected person's behavior. Both groups regarded psychologic problems as problems of faulty learning, but the British group was not dedicated to an unqualified environmentalism, (i.e., the British recognized the importance of cognitive forces). Both espoused the use of strict scientific standards (Rachman, 1997).

Behavioral Therapy

Behavioral techniques are invaluable in child-rearing practices. Techniques have included reinforcement, such as giving stickers or other rewards to children for desirable behaviors, and systematic desensitization in reducing phobias. These techniques are also effective in the treatment of elders. An example of a contemporary behavioral treatment condition was used in a study on geriatric insomnia. The treatment consisted of instructions designed to curtail sleep-incompatible behaviors. Subjects were instructed to do the following (Morin & Azrin, 1988):

1. Go to bed only when sleepy at night.
2. Use the bed and bedroom only for sleep and sex (i.e., no reading, watching television, eating).
3. Get out of bed and go to another room whenever you are unable to fall asleep or return to sleep within 15 to 20 minutes, and return to bed only when you feel sleepy again.
4. Repeat this last procedure as often as necessary throughout the night.
5. Arise in the morning at the same time regardless of the amount of sleep obtained.
6. Do not nap during the day.

The treatment was successful in improving sleep, and the benefits were maintained or enhanced at a 12-month follow-up appointment.

Consider the following examples of behavioral techniques. The APRN used guided imagery with one patient who was very worried about skin breakdown during radiation therapy for breast cancer. She imagined tiny black umbrellas shielding her breast from harmful rays and allowing the good radiation to enter and attack any remaining cancer cells; she had no skin changes during or after the treatment. With children, the APRN may be able to get them through painful procedures by asking them to remember an action hero like Superman and to behave the way Superman would if he were there. Prayer and meditation also are potent ways to decrease anxiety by controlling thoughts. The patient may silently repeat a short prayer, scripture, or word, such as "peace" (Fishel, 1998). Behavioral techniques used frequently by nurse therapists are described in Table 9-1.

Cognitive Therapy

Although there was considerable success in treating anxiety disorders with behavioral techniques,

table 9-1

BEHAVIORAL INTERVENTIONS

THERAPIES	INTERVENTION EXAMPLES
Breathing exercises	Begin in a quiet place with deep or abdominal breathing as the first intervention. Demonstrate how to do abdominal breathing. (Many people are shallow breathers and use only their upper chest, which means that only their shoulders move up and down.) Instruct the patient to breathe in through the nose and fill the lungs so that the diaphragm pushes down and the abdomen pushes out. Instruct the patient to exhale through the mouth, moving the diaphragm up and the abdomen in; count the breaths going in and out at a rate of five counts in, seven counts out, and rest. Encourage the patient to breathe in and breathe out saying to himself or herself, "Breath in calmness, breathe out anxiety."
Progressive muscle relaxation	Begin with the toes and work up, or start the greatest distance from the uncomfortable area. Instruct the patient at every phase (e.g., "Tighten your toes, very tight, hold it, now relax your toes, don't forget to breathe, take a deep breath in, and blow it out"). Make a tape of the guided progressive relaxation exercise. Encourage the patient to play the tape whenever he or she needs to relax. (Offer reasurance with the sound of the APRN's familiar voice on the tape.)
Guided imagery	Before you create an imagery exercise, find out in what kind of place the patient feels most relaxed. Also, instruct the patient to think about whatever event is worrisome and make that go away in the exercise. Let your imagination and your knowledge of the patient guide your visualization. After 5 to 10 minutes of deep breathing, ask the patient to close his or her eyes and imagine a pleasant scene. Ask the patient to engage all of his or her senses (e.g., hear the ocean, smell the flowers, taste the honey, feel the warm sun, see the mountain view).
Exposure	Teach patients with phobias to identify their anxiety-evoking stimuli and to develop a hierarchy or "stimuli map." Help the patient choose an initial item from the hierarchy and design an exposure task to confront this stimulus. After a hierarchy is made of the specific symptoms that cause the patient to have increased anxiety, ask

continued

table 9-1

BEHAVIORAL INTERVENTIONS—cont'd	
THERAPIES	**INTERVENTION EXAMPLES**
	the patient to do the things that cause the symptoms in a gradually increasing, repetitive manner. Use exposure to desensitize patients to catastrophic interpretations of their internal bodily cues, such as tachycardia. (Patients may be asked to jump in place or run up a flight of stairs.) Use flooding, another form of exposure therapy, whereby the patient is immediately exposed to the most anxiety-provoking stimulus instead of being exposed gradually to the feared stimuli. If this technique uses an imaginary as opposed to real life event, it is called *implosion*.
Response prevention	Encourage the patient to face a particular fear without engaging in the accompanying behavior. Repeated exposure to the anxiety-producing stimulus without the presence of the anxiety-reducing response will lead to a reduction in the anxiety behavior.
Eye movement desensitization	Ask the patient to think about past traumatic events while you move your hand back and forth in front of the patient's face; the patient's eyes will follow. The neural tracks become reprogrammed to be less sensitized to anxiety-provoking stimuli. This technique requires special training. Treatment is based on the theory that during early traumatic experiences, the brain lays down biologic memory tracks that are provoked later during seemingly unrelated events, causing anxiety and perhaps depression.

From Fishel, 1998; Schweitzer et al., 1995; Stuart, 1998.

the early attempts to treat depression by rearranging the reinforcement contingencies were not successful. It is not surprising that the emergence of cognitive therapy was in the area of depression. Beck and Ellis shared the view that disturbances arise from faulty cognitions and/or faulty cognitive processing (Rachman, 1997). According to Beck (1976), depressed persons tend to perceive their experiences in an idiosyncratic way, which he called the *cognitive triad*. They saw themselves, the world, and the future as negative. Beck's daughter Judith (1995) has continued to expound on cognitive theory. With this theory, the patient must learn to distance himself or herself emotionally from thoughts with the critical perspective that will enable the patient to judge whether the thoughts are realistic or justified. For example, a young mother was feeling very inadequate because

of one instance when her 2-year-old daughter fell and cut her lip. This is an example of reacting to a single, isolated failure by overgeneralization. She was encouraged to look at other ways in which her parenting was excellent.

Rickelman and Houfek (1995) developed a model to predict suicidal behavior using cognitive theory, such as cognitive rigidity and attributional style, and hopelessness. They recommend "guided discovery" as one form of cognitive retraining that is especially useful with depressed patients who have a particular negative bias in their thinking and who are likely to view suicide as their only option. In the first step, the therapist attempts to teach the patient how to identify his or her automatic negative thinking. In the second step, the patient is asked to identify his or her attributions for success and failure. the repeated patterns of thinking. Then the patient can be encouraged to own his or her successes and therefore increase satisfaction and feelings of competence (Rickelman & Houfek, 1995). Specific examples of cognitive therapy techniques are listed in Box 9-3.

An example of a contemporary cognitive treatment condition comes from the study on geriatric insomnia mentioned previously (Morin & Azrin, 1988). The researchers also used an attention-focusing technique whereby individuals were instructed to imagine a sequence of six common objects—a candle, a light bulb, an hour glass, a kite, a stairway, and a palm tree on a beach. With their eyes closed, subjects concentrated on the image of the designated objects and focused their attention on the purely descriptive properties (e.g., shape, color, movement, and texture) of the stimuli. Color drawings of these objects were initially used as a prompt and then were gradually faded as subjects reported proficiency. Each object was imagined for 2 minutes, and the sequence of the six objects was repeated twice per session. The subjects were instructed to practice the visual-imagery exercises once during the day and whenever they were unable to fall asleep or to return to sleep at night. These subjects also evidenced statistically significant improvement in sleep but not as much as the behavioral group.

Reeder (1991) developed cognitive strategies for helping patients manage anger. Navaco hypothesizes a model for anger arousal that incorporates elements of cognitive theory. He proposes that events are perceived as aversive on the basis of the expectations people have of an event, as well as the appraisal of the event's meaning. When people appraise an event as frustrating, insulting, threatening, and so on, or when they expect a certain outcome and receive a different one, the result is anger (Reeder, 1991).

Cognitive Behavioral Therapy

Cognitive theory and behavior theory merged, and most of today's psychotherapists use the merged theoretical framework. CBT incorporates both behavioral interventions (direct attempts to reduce

box 9-3

COGNITIVE THERAPY TECHNIQUES

- *Questioning the evidence.* Teaching patients to question evidence used to maintain an idea.
- *Examining options and alternatives.* Angry patients have trouble seeing other ways.
- *Decatastrophizing ("what-if" technique).* "What's the worst that can happen?"
- *Examining advantages and disadvantages.* Patients list pros and cons of a belief or behavior to gain perspective and move away from all-or-nothing thinking.
- *Rehearsing.* Visualizing an event in the mind's eye.
- *Labeling of distortions.* Patients can monitor dysfunctional thinking.
- *Exaggerating.* Taking an idea to an extreme.
- *Reasoning through the "downward arrow."* Patients are encouraged to think about "then what" as they go though successive steps in reasoning.
- *Positive self-talk training.* Patients can 1) identify the negative self statements ("I'll never be able to manage my job"), 2) recognize the role that negative self-statements play in influencing increased anxiety and hopelessness, and 3) replace negative self statements with positive self-statements that help the patient cope ("Anxiety won't kill me. I can do this one step at a time. Right now I need to breathe and stretch. I don't have to be perfect").
- *Reframing and redefining.* Patients can adjust themselves psychologically in such a way that events formerly perceived as threatening are now seen in a more positive light. For example, instead of disparaging himself for having high levels of anxiety, the APRN helped the patient reframe that thought to how lucky he was that he had such a sensitive system for protection. Instead of identifying herself as a victim, the patient was helped to think of herself as a survivor. Instead of being concerned about bouts of weeping, the patient was encouraged to think about the weeping as helpful for her "dry eye" condition.

From Fishel, 1998; Reeder, 1991.

dysfunctional emotions and behavior by altering behavior) and cognitive interventions (attempts to reduce dysfunctional emotions and behavior by altering individual appraisals and thinking patterns). The assumption is that prior learning is currently having maladaptive consequences, and the purpose of therapy is to reduce distress or unwanted behavior by undoing this learning, or by providing more adaptive learning experiences (Brewin, 1996). The most solid advances have been achieved in understanding and treating panic disorder, and newer research is looking at obsessive-compulsive disorder (OCD) and hypochondriasis (Rachman, 1997).

Clinical example of CBT with insomnia. An APRN is working with Ms. A., a single parent who had been abused by her male partner for years before she was finally able to move out safely. In her new apartment, she continues to have trouble sleeping and only sleeps about 2 hours a night, catching naps during the day. During therapy Ms. A. realizes that she is still being alert to the possibility of her former partner returning and beating her. The therapist records a tape for her, which begins with acknowledging her fear and her courage in moving out. Then the therapist softly mentions that Ms. A. is safe in this new apartment with several strong locks, that he does not know where she is, that he is in prison, and that she can sleep now. She has been resourceful in finding a safe place for herself and her children. Then the therapist includes a series of relaxation exercises for her to follow. The first night she plays the tape, she sleeps for 6 hours. After a month, she does not need the tape. However, she does repeat the phrases to herself that she heard on the tape.

Coping template. CBT is one of the most widely researched approaches for treating youth (Southam-Gerow et al., 1997). A central treatment goal is to help the child build a "coping template," developing a new cognitive structure or modifying an existing one for processing information about the world. Techniques may include affective education, relaxation training, social problem solving, cognitive restructuring and attribution retraining,

contingent reinforcement, modeling, and role-playing. Clinical trials with both generalized anxiety and OCD have produced very favorable results. When working with depressed youth, in addition to cognitive restructuring and self-control skills, more traditional behavioral techniques are implemented. These include techniques in anxiety reduction (imagery, deep-muscle relaxation, and breathing exercises); increasing pleasant activities (planning realistic goals and rewards after successful completion); social-skills training (conversation skills, planning social activities, strategies in initiating and maintaining friendships, and dealing with conflict); and communication, negotiation, and problem-solving skills (instructing the child how to effect change in his or her environment using assertive behavior and future planning).

The current trend in CBT for children is to encourage parental participation in a parallel course of therapy (Southam-Gerow et al., 1997). Clinical trials report significant results as well as superior outcome over traditional counseling modalities. However, treating aggressive behavior and attention-deficit hyperactivity disorder (ADHD) with CBT has not been as successful. A multisystemic treatment approach is needed, combining child-focused CBT with academic tutoring, parent management training, family therapy, and medication (Nathan, 1992).

Homework assignments. CBT techniques, such as homework assignments, extend the work of therapy beyond the set time with the nurse therapist and have been found in research to have a significant effect on recovery (Burns & Nolen-Hoeksema, 1992). Examples include a daily record of dysfunctional thoughts, social skills training, assertiveness training, relaxation techniques, shame-attacking exercises (Reeder, 1991), taping psychotherapy sessions for patients to listen to between sessions, asking patients to maintain a continuous record of "things learned from therapy," keeping a list of accomplishments, and having the patient take the perspective of "giving advice to a friend" (Jones & Pulos, 1993).

EFFECTIVENESS OF CBT WITH
■ SPECIFIC ILLNESSES

Anxiety Disorders

Until recently, only behavioral techniques such as desensitization, flooding, or response prevention were widely accepted as effective in treating anxiety disorders. Now the effectiveness of cognitive interventions or the combination of cognitive and behavioral interventions is clear (Brewin, 1996).

Generalized anxiety disorder. Adequate evidence exists for concluding that CBT and applied relaxation (AR) are efficacious treatments for generalized anxiety disorder (GAD) (DeRubeis & Crits-Christoph, 1998). However, the clinical significance of change produced by this treatment is somewhat limited, leaving room for further treatment development and testing within this population. Of the two studies that directly compared CBT and relaxation, one (Barlow, Rapee, & Brown, 1992) reported no differences but had low statistical power. The second study (Borkovec & Costello, 1993) demonstrated no difference at posttreatment, but at follow-up the highest gains were maintained in the CBT group (58% of the CBT had clinically significant change on six to eight outcome measures, whereas only 38% of the AR patients showed such change.)

In the Borkovec and Costello (1993) study, a nondirective (ND) treatment modality also was included along with AR and CBT. For the ND therapy, the patients were told that therapy would involve exploration of life experiences with a goal of deepening knowledge about self and anxiety; direct suggestion, advice, or coping methods were prohibited. AR therapy involved learning new coping techniques for reducing anxiety and worry. They were taught to self-monitor, intervene early with a variety of relaxation responses, and focus attention on present experience rather than on mentally created past events. They were trained in diaphragmatic breathing and meditation, and were given homework assignments to practice relaxation techniques and thought focusing. CBT followed the traditional model. Results indicated that both AR and CBT were superior to ND at postassessment.

In another study by nurses, Waddell and Demi (1993) evaluated the effectiveness of a partial hospitalization program for the treatment of anxiety disorders. The 5-week program was based on an integration of biologic, cognitive, and behavioral theories. Significantly lowered at posttest were the patients' "fear of fear," severity of impairment, and general emotional distress. (See Table 9-2 for specific interventions.)

Social phobia. Exposure therapy for social phobia appears to be a potent treatment, and there are indications that its effects persist to at least a moderate degree after cessation of treatment (DeRubeis & Crits-Christoph, 1998). Exposure plus cognitive restructuring treatment exceeded control conditions in benefits to social phobic patients. About 65% of the cognitive behavioral patients experienced a "stringent" level of improvement that was maintained at 6 months (Heimberg et al., 1990).

Obsessive-compulsive disorder. In patients with OCD, CBT involves compensatory skills training in teaching patients not to avoid their negative thoughts, verbal belief modification of the identified automatic thoughts and underlying assumptions, and the overwriting of specific learned associations with behavioral techniques such as response prevention (Brewin, 1996). Patients with OCD received CBT consisting of a detailed explanation of the occurrence and maintenance of obsessive thoughts, exposure to obsessive thoughts, response prevention of all neutralizing strategies, cognitive restructuring, and relapse prevention in a research study. They were significantly improved, and gains were maintained at 6 months (Freeston et al., 1997).

In a particularly rigorous test of the potency of exposure and response prevention therapy (ERP), 32 OCD patients were assigned to ERP, exposure alone, or response prevention alone (Foa et al., 1984). ERP patients improved significantly more than did the patients in either of the control treatments. After 1 month, 80% of the ERP pa-

table 9-2

INTERVENTIONS FOR ANXIETY DISORDERS

THERAPIES AND TRAINING	INTERVENTION EXAMPLES
Behavioral therapy	Exposure, paradoxic intention, and operant procedures
Cognitive therapy	Cognitive restructuring, myth clarification, and recognition of catastrophic thinking
Pharmacotherapy	Assessing need for and monitoring effectiveness
Anxiety management skills	Diaphragmatic breathing, biofeedback, relaxation training; using anger, distraction, and refocusing to inhibit anxiety
Social skills	Assertiveness training, communication skills, problem-solving techniques, time management skills
Psychoeducation	Teaching about biologic, psychologic, and social aspects; treatment modalities and expected results
Group therapy	Identification and confrontation of interpersonal and relationship conflicts through self-disclosure and feedback; learning to deal with factors contributing to high levels of stress, opportunity for growth through group support, realistic self-appraisal, and peer pressure

continued

table 9-2

INTERVENTIONS FOR ANXIETY DISORDERS—cont'd

THERAPIES AND TRAINING	INTERVENTION EXAMPLES
Family therapy	Education about nature of disease process, participation of family as cotherapists to decrease their sense of isolation
Discharge planning	Ensuring adequate support systems, gradual transition from program

From Waddell & Demi, 1993.

tients remained improved, whereas only 27% of those in the single-component groups remained improved.

Panic disorder and agoraphobia. Accumulated studies suggest substantial efficacy for CBT therapy in panic disorders (Barlow, 1997). After reviewing 11 research papers on treatments for panic disorder, DeRubeis and Crits-Christoph (1998) reported that 7 revealed that cognitive therapy surpassed an active comparison condition at posttreatment; the other 4 reported no significant differences between CT and other empirically supported treatments. In addition, cognitive therapy was found to be superior to supportive psychotherapy, pharmacotherapy, AR therapy, and waiting-list. However, in one study by Ost and Westling (1995), they did not find CT to be superior to AR. By the 1-year follow-up, rates of high end-state functioning were neatly identical: 79% in CT and 82% in applied relaxation. Williams and Falbo (1996) reported the superiority of an individual exposure-based treatment for panic disorder with agoraphobia. About 58% of the exposure patients were judged panic free at posttreatment as opposed to 11% of the control patients; 80% were panic free at 1 to 2 years posttreatment. Although AR therapy meets the criteria for an efficacious treatment, considerable variability has been reported with applied relaxation as compared with other treatments, such as cognitive therapy (DeRubeis & Crits-Christoph, 1998).

In the first controlled trial of exposure treatment for agoraphobia, 12 patients were assigned to each of three conditions: exposure (flooding) therapy, systematic desensitization therapy, and a control condition termed *associative psychotherapy* (Gelder et al., 1973). The systematic desensitization condition and the flooding condition yielded effects approximately twice as large as those in the control condition.

For patients experiencing panic and agoraphobia, exposure therapy reduces avoidance but not panic; cognitive therapy reduces panic but not avoidance. An integrated approach using both CBT and pharmacologic approaches is successful for most patients experiencing panic disorder with agoraphobia (Craske, 1996; Rosenbaum et al., 1995). A brief nurse-facilitated group training in CBT significantly reduced symptoms of panic disorder and agoraphobia (Schweitzer et al., 1995). Patients were taught to identify their anxiety-evoking stimuli and to develop a hierarchy or "stimuli map." Each member then chose an initial item from the hierarchy and designed an exposure task to confront this stimulus.

Post-traumatic stress disorder. Three research teams have provided evidence that systematic exposure to traumatic stimuli (such as imaginal flooding or implosive flooding therapy) either alone, or when added to treatment as usual, is superior to waiting-list or other control conditions in the treatment of post-traumatic stress disorder (PTSD) (Boudewyns et al., 1990; Foa et al., 1991; Keane et al., 1989). Eye movement desensitization and reprocessing (EMDR), administered in three 90-minute individual sessions, resulted in greater change than the waiting-list condition (Wilson, Becker, & Tinker, 1995). However, there is as yet no published evidence that EMDR is as effective as standard exposure treatments for PTSD.

CBT research has also focused on the treatment of nightmares. Those in the treatment group were instructed in imagery rehearsal, in which they learned in a waking state to change a nightmare and visualize a new set of images (Krakow et al., 1995). Treated patients showed significant and clinically important decreases in nightmares in terms of both nights per week and actual number of nightmares. They also had a significant improvement in self-rated quality of sleep.

Childhood anxiety. A family-based treatment for childhood anxiety was evaluated (Barrett, Dadds, & Rapee, 1996). Children 7 to 14 years of age who fulfilled diagnostic criteria for separation anxiety, overanxious disorder, or social phobia were randomly allocated to three treatment conditions: CBT, CBT plus family management, and waiting-list. At posttreatment, the results indicated that across treatments, 70% no longer met diagnostic criteria for anxiety disorder, compared with 26% of waiting-list children. At the 12-month follow-up, 70% of the children in the CBT group and 95% of the children in the CBT plus family management group did not meet criteria. Younger children and female participants responded better to the CBT plus family intervention.

Depression

Of the psychologic interventions for serious mental disorders, perhaps the treatment most widely studied and most widely regarded by proponents of clinical trial methodologies is cognitive therapy for depression (DeRubeis & Crits-Christoph, 1998). The primary explanation for effectiveness of CBT with depression is the development of compensatory skills and the repeated application of these skills, which leads to a change in schemata (Brewin, 1996). The function of therapy is to disrupt the repeated synthesis of high-level schematic models containing generalized meanings prototypical of previous depressing situations. Therapists mainly work with consciously available cognitions, even though the aim is to change underlying cognitions. Examining the outcomes of men and women who had experienced CBT, the authors concluded that there are gender-specific differences in the symptoms and treatment utilization of depressed patients. CBT was equally useful for both sexes, but alternative treatment methods may be needed for patients with more severe syndromes (Thase et al., 1994).

In a meta-analysis of 62 studies of CBT for depression using the Beck Depression Inventory as outcome measure, CBT was found to be superior to other forms of psychotherapy and pharmacotherapy (Gaffan, Tsaousis, & Kemp-Wheeler, 1995). However, the findings from the TDCRP (Elkin et al., 1989) have led to skepticism about cognitive therapy (CT) for depression for several reasons. The TDCRP was a large, well-conducted comparative outcome study, it included a stringent control condition, and it found CT especially ineffective among the more severely depressed patients. It performed worse than medications and not demonstrably better than pill placebo with clinical management (DeRubeis & Crits-Christoph, 1998). With the exception of the TDCRP study, the effects of CT are equivalent to those of antidepressant medications. Moreover, follow-up studies suggest that CT yields a relapse prevention effect. Cognitive therapy has an advantage over antidepressant medications when both are withdrawn shortly after remission (De-Rubeis & Crits-Christoph, 1998).

In a large comparative study of behavior therapy (n = 156), McLean and Hakstian (1979) observed significantly greater symptom change in the behavior therapy condition than in each of the other three conditions (psychotherapy, relaxation therapy, and amitriptyline pharmacotherapy). Results were strongest in the comparisons of behavior therapy with psychotherapy; a significant advantage of behavior therapy over amitriptyline was observed on several measures.

In a rigorous experimental study to compare the relative effectiveness of components of CBT, researchers reported that all treatment conditions were equally effective for treating depression (Jacobson et al., 1996). The comparison involved randomly assigning 150 outpatients with major depression to a treatment focused exclusively on the behavioral activation (BA) component of CBT, a treatment that included BA and the teaching of skills to modify automatic thoughts (AT), and a full CBT treatment that included BA and AT and also addressed core schema. The intervention techniques for the BA condition included the following:

- Monitoring daily activities
- Assessing pleasure that is achieved by various activities
- Assigning increasingly more difficult activities that have potential of enhancing pleasure
- Using cognitive rehearsal of anticipated activities to anticipate obstacles
- Discussing specific problems such as insomnia and prescribing behavior therapy techniques to deal with them
- Performing interventions such as assertiveness training to ameliorate deficits in social skills

The intervention techniques for the AT condition included the following:

- Noticing mood shifts in the session and asking for thoughts preceding the shift
- Using a daily record of dysfunctional thoughts as a form of personal diary to record distressing events and thoughts preceding them
- Reexamining thoughts in specific situations to determine if the event warranted the conclusion drawn by the patient
- Helping patients to respond in a more functional manner to negative thinking
- Examining the possibility of attributional biases in which patients view successes and failures in their lives
- Using homework assignments to assess validity of negative interpretations

The intervention techniques for the full CBT condition included the following:

- Asking patients for explanations about why certain problems have emerged
- Identifying explicit underlying assumptions and core beliefs
- Identifying alternative assumptions
- Discussing the advantages and disadvantages of holding various assumptions

- Discussing short-term versus long-term advantages of various assumptions or beliefs
- Giving homework assignments

Based on a meta-analysis of psychotherapy trials, the overall efficacy of cognitive therapy alone was found to be 46.6% (USDHHS, 1993). For adult outpatients, efficacy was 46.9%; for geriatric outpatients, it was 51.3%. The overall efficacy for behavioral therapy alone was 55.3%. Compared with waiting-list, behavioral therapy was 17.1% more effective; compared with all other forms of psychotherapy, behavioral therapy was 9.1% more effective (USDHHS, 1993) (Table 9-3).

Fishel and Jefferson (1983), using the Alberti and Emmons (1974) model of assertiveness training, implemented a group intervention with hospitalized emotionally disturbed women. They reported that the assertively trained patients had significantly higher change scores than did the comparison subjects. Those diagnosed with depression had more success than did patients with other diagnoses.

Gordan's theoretical model about the etiology of depression in women incorporates group interventions that are based on CBT (Gordan & Ledray, 1985). In a series of 12 to 16 sessions, the women use a workbook and progress through structured learning experiences using 1 hour for lecture, education, and discussion about depression and women; and a second hour devoted to specific activities related to issues addressed by that particular session. Weekly topics include goal setting, feelings and depression, cognitions and feelings, self-worth, relationships, communication skills, assertiveness, conflict management, decision making, stress, relaxation, exercise, nutrition, menstruation/menopause, and strength building (Gordan & Ledray, 1986). In a 3-year follow-up study of the Gordan model, the treatment group was found to have significantly lower levels of depression and hopelessness and significantly higher levels of self-esteem than the no-treatment control group (Gordan et al., 1988). In a replication study to examine the differences between groups receiving and not receiving antidepressant

table 9-3

META-ANALYSES OF PSYCHOTHERAPY TRIALS IN OUTPATIENTS WITH MAJOR DEPRESSIVE DISORDER

THERAPY	OVERALL EFFICACY	THERAPY VS. WAITING-LIST	THERAPY VS. PLACEBO	THERAPY VS. OTHER THERAPY	THERAPY VS. DRUG ALONE
Behavior therapy alone	55.3% (9.3) [10]	17.1% (34.0) [5]	N/A	9.1% (19.9) [6]	23.9% (11.6) [2]
Brief psychotherapy alone	34.8% (17.8) [6]	N/A	N/A	−7.6% (14.6) [8]	8.4% (21.3) [2]
Cognitive psychotherapy alone	46.6% (6.9) [12]	30.1% (22.0) [2]	9.4% (8.3) [1]	−4.4% (16.9) [6]	15.3% (26.1) [3]
Interpersonal therapy alone	52.3% (6.1) [1]	N/A	22.6% (8.4) [1]	13.3% (8.6) [1]	12.3% (8.6) [1]
Totals	50.0% (5.3) [29]	26.0% (23.5) [7]	15.7% (13.0) [2]	4.7% (8.5) [21]	14.0% (11.2) [8]

From USDHHS, 1993.
Numbers in parentheses ( ) are the standard deviations of the estimated percentage of responders.
Bracketed numbers [ ] are the numbers of cells on which these estimates are calculated.

medications while participating in Gordan's model program, Sargent-Trolinger (1995) reports that both groups showed similar success.

Studying nursing home patients, Zerhusen, Boyle and Wilson (1991) compared cognitive therapy and music therapy with a control group; depression scores were significantly lower in the cognitive therapy group. In another study involving nursing home residents with slight to moderate cognitive impairment, significant and lasting improvements in overall cognitive status were found with both CBT and focused visual imagery group therapy, but not with the educational discussion groups (Abraham & Reel, 1992). The imagery group interventions consisted of breathing and progressive relaxation exercises along with exercises in imagery content to protect the patients from anxiety and increase self-esteem, energy, and feelings of control. Specific cognitive improvements were in abstraction and conceptual thinking, concentration and linguistic manipulation, and execution of auditorily presented language skills (Abraham & Reel, 1992).

Borderline Personality Disorder

Individuals with borderline personality disorder (BPD) are prevalent in mental health centers and practitioners' offices. They present with severe problems and intense misery, and treatment modalities have been inadequate (Linehan, 1993). The primary dysfunction is one of inadequate affect regulation. Consequently, there is also disregulation in behavior, interpersonal relationships, cognition, and self-concept. Patients frequently engage in "parasuicidal" behaviors. Linehan developed dialectical behavioral therapy (DBT) to address the ineffective coping of individuals with BPD that may result in repetitive suicidal behaviors (Linehan, 1993). Although primarily a CBT framework, several aspects of DBT differentiate it from the usual CBT: 1) the focus on acceptance and validation of behavior as it is in the moment, 2) the emphasis on treating therapy-interfering behaviors, 3) the perspective on the therapeutic

relationship as essential to the treatment, and 4) the use of dialectical processes. DBT assumes that the patients have within themselves all the potential that is necessary for change. Assumptions include that patients are as follows:

1. Doing the best they can
2. Want to improve
3. Need to do better, try harder, and be more motivated to change
4. May not have caused all of their own problems, but they have to solve them anyway
5. Have lives that are unbearable as they are currently being lived
6. Learn new behaviors in all relevant contexts
7. Cannot fail

Another assumption is that therapists treating borderline patients need support (Linehan, 1993). The central dialectical tension is between change and acceptance.

DBT is conceptualized in three stages (Boyd, 1997). Before treatment, there must be agreement on goals for therapy. The first stage targets decreasing suicidal behaviors, decreasing therapy interfering behaviors, and increasing behavioral skills (mindfulness, interpersonal effectiveness, emotion regulation, distress tolerance, and self-management). In the second stage, the target is to decrease posttraumatic stress. The third stage is designed to increase self-respect and meet individual goals. Basic treatment strategies in DBT (Linehan, 1993) are listed in Box 9-4.

A randomized clinical trial was conducted to evaluate the effectiveness of DBT for the treatment of chronically parasuicidal women who met criteria for BPD (Linehan et al., 1991). At most assessment points and during the entire year, the subjects who received DBT had fewer incidences of parasuicide and less medically severe parasuicides, were more likely to stay in individual therapy, and had fewer inpatient psychiatric days.

Miller, Eisner, and Aliport (1994) developed a "creative coping group" to be used in short-term inpatient settings by psychiatric nurses for BPD patients. Based on Linehan's DBT framework, the ten group sessions sought to help patients to iden-

box 9-4

TREATMENT STRATEGIES IN DIALECTICAL BEHAVIOR THERAPY

- Dialectical strategies such as entering the paradox, using a metaphor, and "making lemonade out of lemons"
- Core strategies such as validating, problem solving, and change procedures (including managing contingencies and observing limits); skills training; exposure; and cognitive modification
- Stylistic strategies that deal with the therapist's communication and include self-disclosure, warm engagement, confrontational tone, and "plunging in where angels fear to tread"
- Case management strategies such as entering the patient's environment to give assistance and consultation about handling family and friends

From Linehan, 1993.

tify the emotions they were experiencing and learn skills to reduce intense emotional responses, improve interpersonal effectiveness, and learn to self-soothe to tolerate distress. DBT is an appropriate intervention for APRNs to use in their treatment of persons with BPD (Boyd, 1997; Hampton, 1997).

Smoking

Interventions have been designed to decrease health risk behaviors, such as alcohol and substance abuse and smoking, and increase health promoting behaviors, such as exercise and following a healthy diet. Interventions are available to manage specific symptoms or problems such as chronic pain, including headache, back pain, and chronic abdominal pain. Interventions have been designed to facilitate effective coping with chronic or life-threatening diseases and conditions, including cancer, HIV and AIDS, diabetes, asthma,

Alzheimer's disease, stroke, and brain and spinal cord injuries (Compas et al., 1998).

Smoking cessation is used as an example of this group of health risk behaviors. Depression is overrepresented among smokers. Depressed smokers appear to experience more withdrawal symptoms upon quitting, are less likely to be successful at quitting, and are more likely to relapse (Hall et al., 1993). In addition to antidepressant medications and nicotine replacement, CBT is recommended. Interventions should address overt coping behaviors (which eventually result in increases in reinforcement) and the mental events that are involved in perception and self-administration of reinforcement. Research suggests that affect regulation may be specifically efficacious for smokers with a history of major depressive disorder relapse (Hall et al., 1993).

Hill, Rigdon, and Johnson (1993) randomly assigned 82 chronic older cigarette smokers to receive behavior therapy, behavior therapy plus nicotine gum, behavior therapy plus physical exercise, or physical exercise alone. The group behavior therapy program included educational information on health consequences of smoking, environmental management (e.g., removing ashtrays), setting a specific quit date, and relapse prevention training (e.g., identifying high-risk situations and role-playing coping responses applicable to them). Groups met for 12 sessions over 3 months. The behavioral groups did not differ significantly from one another (averaging 32% abstinence) but were significantly superior to the exercise-only control condition (10% abstinence).

Stevens and Hollis (1989) studied 744 adult smokers who were enrolled in a 4-day (2 hr/day) intensive smoking cessation intervention conducted in groups and teaching numerous CBT techniques, such as relaxation, cognitive restructuring, and behavioral methods of coping with withdrawal symptoms. Participants who achieved smoking cessation (79%) were then randomly assigned to relapse prevention skills training, group discussion, or no further treatment. Group discussion and no-further treatment conditions were equivalent in effectiveness, whereas the skills-training group was significantly superior (41% at 1-year follow-up compared with 33% to 34% in the other groups).

■ INTERPERSONAL THERAPY

Interpersonal therapy (IPT) of depression has evolved over the past 30 years originating from the experiences of the New Haven—Boston Collaborative Depression Research Project. Psychologists such as DiMascio, Prusoff, and most recently Klerman have been the major developers. IPT facilitates recovery from the acute depression by 1) relieving the depressive symptoms and 2) helping the patient develop more effective strategies for dealing with current interpersonal problems associated with the onset of symptoms (Klerman et al., 1984). The first goal is achieved by helping patients understand that their experiences are part of a depressive syndrome. Often the patient is instructed to read educational literature written in lay language. The second goal is to help the patient develop more successful patterns for dealing with current social and interpersonal problems that were associated with the onset of the current depression.

IPT is focused (one to two problem areas in the patient's current interpersonal functioning), time-limited (less than 9 to 12 months), and emphasizes the current interpersonal relations of the depressed patient (Klerman et al., 1984). IPT tries to change the way the patient thinks, feels, and acts in problematic interpersonal relationships. The IPT therapist is nonjudgmental, communicating warmth and unconditional positive regard—a "benign and helpful ally." Confrontation is gentle and timely, and the therapist is careful to foster the patient's positive expectations of the therapeutic relationship. The therapist is optimistic and supportive as well as active in helping the patient focus on bringing about improvement in current interpersonal problems and in guiding the patient to cover the material that is relevant to the treatment goals (Klerman et al., 1984). IPT is intense

and uses the relationship between the patient and therapist as a variable. There is no analysis of transference, and no attention is paid to early life factors that might have been precursors to the current depressed state of the patient, even though theoretically those events are accepted as part of the etiology of depression. The focus is on current relationships and on facilitating the patient to develop more effective ways of relating (Cornes, 1990).

Many of the techniques used in IPT are common to dynamic psychotherapy. They include exploratory techniques (such as supportive acknowledgment), encouragement of affect, clarification, communication analysis (examining and identifying communication failures to help the patient learn to communicate more effectively), use of the therapeutic relationship, and behavior change techniques (such as education, advice, and suggestion) (Klerman et al., 1984). IPT is designed specifically for depressed patients. Common problem areas are unresolved grief, difficult role transitions, interpersonal role disputes, and social skill deficits. Nurse therapists will recognize this approach as very similar to nurse-patient relationship therapy as formulated by Peplau (1952) and expounded on by Beeber (1989) and others.

IPT has been studied in two acute phase randomized trials in outpatients with nonpsychotic major depressive disorder (Elkin et al., 1989; Weissman et al., 1979). In the one study for which meta-analysis was feasible (Elkin et al., 1989), the efficacy of IPT exceeded that of cognitive therapy by 13.2%, that of placebo plus clinical management by 22.6%, and that of imipramine by 12.3%, based on the Beck Depression Inventory as the outcome measure. The overall efficacy was 52.3% (USDHHS, 1993) (see Table 9-1). However, only 26% of the IPT patients recovered and stayed well throughout follow-up; this figure was very similar to the rates obtained in CT (30%), pharmacotherapy (19%), and placebo (10%) (Elkin et al., 1989).

Beeber (1989, 1996; Beeber & Caldwell, 1996) has constructed an intervention model that advances the theories of Sullivan (1953) and Peplau

(1952, 1963). She hypothesizes that the depressed patient, in an attempt to protect the self from anxiety, enacts particular interpersonal patterns designed to create distance and control intimacy. These patterns become evident in both the patient's relationships with others and with the nurse therapist. Through the nurse-patient relationship, a corrective educational experience can occur. Beeber (1989) operationalizes how the nurse-patient relationship evolves when the interpersonal experience is a corrective one (Box 9-5).

To test this theory, research data derived from clinical interventions conducted over a 4-month period with six women revealed four pattern integrations (Beeber & Caldwell, 1996):

- *Complementary pattern.* Helpless patient and helper nurse (most frequent).
- *Mutual pattern.* Both nurse and patient were manifesting the same behavior (e.g., both being helpers for each other).
- *Alternating pattern.* One person was the pursuer while the other was the distancer, and vice versa.
- *Antagonistic pattern.* Patient maintained the relationship with the nurse while complaining that it was not helping.

The patterns usually involved sequences that were hierarchical. If the first relief behavior was not successful, another followed until the patient's repertoire was exhausted. Beeber and Caldwell (1996) advise that the APRN must be vigilant and engage in supervision so that he or she will not be pulled into nonfacilitative patterns. It is these patterns that support depressive symptoms. This work represents a scholarly approach to theory development and testing for the advanced practice of psychiatric nursing, but it must be expanded to include larger groups of patients and controlled clinical trials.

SUPPORTIVE ■ PSYCHOTHERAPY

Although many clinicians have a low regard for supportive psychotherapy, Rockland (1993) asserts that this approach should be taken more seriously. Supportive psychotherapy is eclectic, empirically based (i.e., techniques that have been observed to work), and patient-driven (rather than theory-guided) (Novalis, Rojcewicz, & Peele, 1993). Concepts such as *transference* and *defense mechanisms* are frequently involved, but theories about the supposed cause of the patient's disorder are not required.

Supportive psychotherapy has a long and varied history dating back to the ancient Greeks. In this century, the major developers have been psychiatrists such as Jones, Schilder, Levine,

box 9-5

NURSE-PATIENT RELATIONSHIP CORRECTIVE INTERPERSONAL EXPERIENCE

Nurse presents as a consistent, caring person; empathic linkage between nurse and patient is established →

Patient experiences the tension of need that elicits anxiety; simultaneously, the nurse experiences the tension through empathy →

Patient's anticipation of rebuff or failure activates the self-dynamism designed to protect self-esteem →

Nurse does not respond reciprocally with anger; by remaining in the interpersonal field, the nurse will both raise the patient's anxiety and bring the need for tenderness closer to the syntaxic mode →

To facilitate consensual validation, the nurse continually attempts to elicit verbal descriptions from the patient about what is happening interpersonally; the nurse encourages validation of the anxiety and often encourages the patient to verbalize the need eliciting the anxiety →

Nurse acknowledges the appropriateness of the need →

Patient gathers insight and gives up self-defeating behaviors

From Beeber, 1989.

Bibring, Schlesinger, and Dewald (Novalis et al., 1993). The first two books devoted exclusively to supportive psychotherapy were written by Werman (1984) and Rockland (1989); the most extensive work on supportive psychotherapy is being done at the Mount Sinai School of Medicine in New York City by Pinsker's (1991) team.

The goals of supportive psychotherapy are to reduce behavioral dysfunctions, reduce subjective mental distress, support and enhance the patient's strengths and coping skills and his or her capacity to use environmental supports, maximize treatment autonomy, and achieve maximum possible independence from psychiatric illness (Novalis et al., 1993). Techniques include the following (Rockland, 1993):

- Strengthening of the therapeutic alliance
- Environmental interventions
- Education
- Advice and suggestion
- Encouragement and praise
- Social skills training
- Homework
- Limit setting and prohibitions
- Undermining maladaptive defenses while strengthening adaptive defenses
- Emphasis on strengths and talents.

The therapist is active and involved, willing to develop a real relationship (as compared with the distant and detached relationship in psychoanalysis), able to show empathy and concern for the patient, supportive of the patient's healthy adaptive efforts, and genuinely interested in the patient's life activities and well-being (Novalis et al., 1993).

Traditionally, supportive psychotherapy has been considered the treatment of choice (often in conjunction with psychopharmacology) for patients in crisis or for those with very chronic medical or psychiatric illnesses. In addition, supportive psychopharmacology is now recommended for the elderly and for persons with anxiety disorders, dual diagnosis, and personality disorders.

Relatively little research has been reported on supportive psychotherapy. The research that is available does not consistently demonstrate effectiveness of the therapy across various conditions. In the Boston Psychotherapy Study of persons with schizophrenia (Gunderson, Frank, & Katz, 1984), a sample of 95 persons was treated with either supportive psychotherapy or exploratory, insight-oriented therapy. Two-year outcomes showed minimal differences in only three out of ten areas of assessment, with supportive treatment slightly superior in reducing hospitalizations and improving occupational function. Given the cost of hospitalization, the supportive treatment was clearly more cost-effective. In a study by Hogarty, Anderson, and Reiss (1986), patients with schizophrenia who were given social skills training exhibited only a 20% relapse rate. This was compared with a rate of 41% in patients randomly assigned to a control group in which pharmacotherapy was given along with a yoga, exercise, and stress management group. In addition, the social skills training group experienced fewer rehospitalizations.

In a comparison study of cognitive therapy with brief supportive psychotherapy for patients with varying levels of agoraphobic avoidance, after 8 weeks, 71% of the patients in the CT condition were panic free, compared with only 25% in the supportive psychotherapy condition (Beck et al., 1992). At the end of the comparison period, 94% of the patients in the supportive psychotherapy condition elected to cross over to a 12-week course of CT.

Its usefulness in depression was established in the TDCRP (Elkin et al., 1989). For a less depressed subgroup, no other treatment was more effective than in the placebo-supportive therapy group. This study suggests the therapeutic efficacy of medication combined with supportive psychotherapy and also the effectiveness of supportive therapy alone for less severely depressed patients.

A major clinical trail using supportive group therapy was conducted with metastatic breast cancer patients (Spiegel, Bloom, & Yalom, 1981). The results indicated that, compared with no-treatment control participants, patients who participated in the intervention experienced improved mood and fewer phobic symptoms and reported reduced pain sensation and suffering.

Although many nurse therapists use supportive psychotherapy, research on its effectiveness is sparse. Some mental health systems discourage supportive psychotherapy by separating the case management and therapist roles. When using a supportive psychotherapy framework, the nurse therapist works with the patient on issues that might ordinarily be considered within the realm of case management. For example, a therapist was working with a poor mother of three who was arrested for shop lifting at the local supermarket. The mother had never been to court before and was very frightened. While she was in the office, the therapist telephoned the clerk of court to get information about the process and what was likely to happen when the patient went to court. The therapist discussed these details with the patient, and they rehearsed what she could say when she appeared before the judge. The therapist also went with the patient to court and encouraged her to watch what others were doing as they approached the judge so that she would know what to do when it was her turn. The nurse therapist was criticized by the system for choosing a supportive role. Using this example, a research study could be developed on the comparative effectiveness of supportive psychotherapy versus the traditional psychodynamic role. Nurses need to be more actively involved in turning clinical observations into systematic investigations of effectiveness of practice.

STAGES OF CHANGE AND MOTIVATIONAL ∎ INTERVIEWING

The "stages of change" model (Prochaska & DiClemente, 1992) and motivational interviewing (Miller & Rollnick, 1991) have encouraged clinicians and scientists to examine new interventions where behavior change is the goal. The stages of change model was developed as Prochaska and DiClemente were exploring how change process activities could be measured in smoking cessation.

Currently, they are using stage models in research and intervention projects related to cancer prevention, alcoholism treatment, health promotion, and psychotherapy interventions. The basic processes of change that they have operationalized come from systems of psychotherapy and behavior change. Five stages have been isolated (Prochaska & DiClemente, 1992):

1. *Precontemplation* is the earliest stage, and individuals in this stage are unaware, unwilling, or discouraged about changing problematic behavior. Precontemplators are not convinced that the negative aspects of the problem behavior outweigh the positive. They are not considering changing and would be least responsive to interventions focused on change activities. To move ahead they need to acknowledge or take ownership of the problem.

2. *Contemplation* involves an active consideration of the prospects of change. Contemplators engage in information seeking and begin to re-evaluate themselves in light of the particular target behavior. However, they are not prepared to take action yet.

3. *Preparation* indicates a readiness to change. Individuals are intending to change in the near future and have learned valuable lessons from past change attempts and failures. They are on the verge of taking action and need to make commitments to follow through.

4. *Action* involves the overt modification of the problem behavior. Action individuals must have the skills to use key processes, such as counter-conditioning, stimulus control, and contingency management to interrupt habitual patterns of behavior. They must be aware of pitfalls.

5. *Maintenance* is the final stage in the process of change. Sustaining behavior change is significant and difficult, especially if the environment is filled with cues that can trigger the problem behavior.

A questionnaire to measure the stages of change called the *University of Rhode Island Change Assessment Scale* has been developed (McConnaughy,

Prochaska, & Velicer, 1983). Cluster analysis has revealed five profiles: precontemplation, contemplation, preparation, ambivalent, and discouraged. Over 80% of inpatient alcoholics could be classified into one of the five profiles with a likelihood ratio above 0.70. The scale has solid psychometric properties and has been used with several different populations (Prochaska & DiClemente, 1992).

This stages of change model is referred to as *transtheoretical* because it combines several theoretical concepts. For instance, self-efficacy is an important mediator between knowledge and action. To measure self-efficacy, patients are asked to rate how confident they are (5-point Likert scale) that they can change the problem behavior. Higher efficacy scores among precontemplation and contemplation stage subjects were correlated with greater change process activity. However, in action and particularly in maintenance stages, subjects' higher self-efficacy correlated with decreased change process activity (Prochaska & DiClemente, 1992). This suggests that although confidence is helpful in the early stages of change, confidence may interfere with the vigilance needed to maintain change. This change model is also discussed in terms of utilization and dissemination of research in Chapter 22.

Motivation is considered critical to changing problem behaviors and to engaging in health-protection behaviors. Motivational interviewing is a directive, patient-centered counseling style for helping the patient explore and resolve ambivalence about behavior change (Miller & Rollnick, 1991). The goal of motivational interviewing is not to persuade patients that they should be concerned about a behavior or for the clinician to provide practical solutions to problems identified by professionals, but rather to help patients recognize their problems and to help them move toward making desired changes. Miller and Rollnick (1991) identified five basic principles of motivational interviewing:

1. Express empathy.
2. Develop a discrepancy between individuals' perceptions of where they are and where they want to be.
3. Avoid argumentation.
4. Roll with resistance.
5. Support the patient's sense of self-efficacy.

Motivational interviewing uses many of the principles of empathic communication in a systematic effort to facilitate change. The key to intervention is to identify some goal that is meaningful to the patient and, through the course of working toward the goal, help the patient see how the problem behavior creates barriers to achieving that goal (Smyth, 1996). Resistance is a signal not to blame or label the patient, but for the counselor to back off and change the approach. An example of the motivational interviewing intervention with a smoker is shown in Table 9-4.

After patients are correctly classified by stage of readiness for change, then specific motivational strategies can be tailored for the individuals. Three studies have found that most smokers are in the precontemplation stage (Prochaska & DiClementi, 1992). Is it possible to recruit precontemplators to intervention programs? When a self-help program for smokers who do not want to quit smoking was advertised, 200 people showed up. In one study (Prochaska & DiClementi, 1992), the stages of change scores were the second best predictors of outcome; they were better predictors than age, socioeconomic status, problem severity and duration, goals and expectations, self-efficacy, and social support.

The only variable that outperformed the stages of change as outcome predictors were the processes of change the patients used early in therapy (Prochaska, DiClemente, & Norcross, 1992). Ten processes have been identified as receiving the most theoretical and empirical support: consciousness raising, self-reevaluation, self-liberation, counterconditioning, stimulus control, reinforcement management, helping relationships, dramatic relief, environmental reevaluation, and social liberation (Prochaska, DiClemente, & Norcross, 1992). The stages and processes of change were able to predict with 93% accuracy which patients would drop out prematurely from psychotherapy. Change processes traditionally as-

table 9-4

MOTIVATIONAL INTERVIEWING WITH A SMOKER

PHASE	INTERVENTION EXAMPLES
PHASE I: QUICK ASSESSMENT	
Rapport	"What sort of smoker are you?" "You may be a little fed up with people lecturing you about smoking. I'm not going to do that, but it would help me if I understood how you really feel about your smoking."
Motivation to quit	"If on a scale of 1 to 10, 1 is not at all motivated to give up smoking and 10 is 100% motivated, what number would you give yourself?"
Confidence in ability to quit	"If on a scale of 1 to 10, 1 means that you are not at all confident and 10 means that you are 100% confident, what number would you give yourself now?"
PHASE II: PATIENT IDENTIFIES PROBLEMS AND SOLUTIONS	
Motivation	"Why are you at (chosen number) and not at 1?" "What would need to happen for you to get from (chosen number) to (higher number)?"
Pros and cons	"What do you like about smoking?" When patient responds, ask, "What do you dislike about smoking?" Summarize both sides and ask, "Where does that leave you now?"
Nonjudgmental information about personal risk	"Would up-to-date information about the risks involved help you in your decision making about smoking?"
Confidence	"Why are you at (chosen number) and not at 1?"
	"What would need to happen for you to get from (chosen number) to (higher number)?" If no ideas come from patient, offer range of possibilities.
PHASE III: TARGET AND FOLLOW-UP	
Target	Reinforce value of small gains and openness. Can patient set manageable goal? Relate to numbers of cigarettes smoked (not to increase, but to cut down or quit). Relate to factors that influence smoking, such as relationships, weight, and exercise.
Follow-up	Find out how the patient thinks you can help him attain his target. Ideas could include follow-up visits, telephone calls, or advice on nicotine replacement.

From Rollnick, Butler, & Stott, 1997.

sociated with the experiential, cognitive, and psychoanalytic persuasions are most useful during the precontemplation and contemplation stages. Change processes traditionally associated with the existential and behavioral traditions are most use-

ful during action and maintenance (Prochaska, DiClemente, & Norcross, 1992).

Investigators have been examining the stage model/motivational interviewing with a variety of health behaviors such as mammography screening and exercise programs (Prochaska & DiClemente, 1992), medication self-management (Hayward et al., 1995), smoking (Dijkstra et al., 1998; Rollnick, Butler, & Stott, 1997), alcoholism (Bien, Miller & Tonigan, 1993), diabetes care (Stott et al., 1996), eating disorders (Ward et al., 1996), and dual diagnosis (Smyth, 1996). Thus far, most of the research has been on classifying patients according to the stage of change. With the exception of studies on alcohol, effectiveness of motivational interviewing is not readily available.

In a literature review, 30 controlled studies of brief interventions targeting drinking behavior were found, enrolling over 6000 problem drinkers across 14 nations (Bien et al., 1993). Overall, these studies indicate that brief interventions are more effective than no counseling and often as effective as more extensive treatment.

In a pilot study (n = 21) designed to improve medication compliance, using an intervention adapted from principles of motivational interviewing, patients receiving the intervention showed changes in attitudes towards medication and insight into illness in the desired direction, but the changes failed to reach statistical significance. The authors suggest that replication with larger numbers is needed (Hayward et al., 1995).

OTHER CONTEMPORARY ■ THERAPY MODELS

Theory precedes therapy models, and models precede specific interventions that can then be tested for effectiveness. There are some theory/therapy models that lack evidence-based research. They represent opportunities for future studies by nurse therapist and researchers.

Brief Solution-Focused Therapy

The brief solution-focused therapy model, appropriate for individual, family, and group therapy, builds on the strategic therapy approach that de-emphasizes history and underlying pathology and commits to brevity. Solution-focused therapy moves away from the strategic approach, which focuses on problems. Growing out of Haley's (1963) strategic therapy model, O'Hanlon and Weiner-Davis (1989) and deShazer (1985) have been major developers of this model. Solution-focused therapists help patients focus exclusively on solutions that have worked or might work. Much of the work lies in the negotiation of a goal that is achievable (O'Hanlon & Weiner-Davis, 1989). Clarifying the goal may be accomplished by questions such as, "What will you be doing instead? How will you be doing this? As you leave here today, and you are on track, what will you be doing differently or saying differently to yourself?" (Walter & Peller, 1992).

Solution-focused therapists trust and use the resources of patients to help them reach their goals (Mason, Breen, & Whipple, 1994). They believe that people already have the skills to solve their problems but often have lost sight of these abilities because the problems loom so large. Solution-focused therapy is an extension of *constructivism*, the idea that people create their own realities. If all realities are merely personal constructions, then why not help people construct the reality that their problems are solvable and not so bad (Nichols & Schwartz, 1998)? The interventions in Table 9-5 represent some of the approaches in this therapy (Billings, 1996; deShazer, 1985, 1988; Hillyer, 1996; O'Hanlon & Weiner-Davis, 1989; O'Hanlon & Beadle, 1994).

These three examples help illustrate how to use this therapy technique with patients.

1. One young woman with mild postpartum depression suggested that if she did not cry all the time, her husband would be more attentive. She perceived that her crying upsets him. The therapist discussed what "more attentive" meant—a hug in the morning and at night when he returns home from work and a weekend trip to the beach. When asked how she can make those things happen, she answered that she could ask him. In the next session,

table 9-5

SOLUTION-FOCUSED INTERVENTIONS

NAME OF TECHNIQUE	INTERVENTIONS
Formula tasks	In the first session, ask patients to observe what happens in their life or relationships that they want to continue.
Miracle question	"Suppose one night, while you were asleep, that there was a miracle and this problem was solved. How would you know? What would be different?" This question gives people a clear vision of their goal.
Exception question	Ignore the problem that patients bring up and instead direct their attention to the opposite of that problem—times in the past when they did not have the problem when, ordinarily, they would have. By exploring these times and what was different, patients find clues to what they can do to expand these exceptions. Also, when patients realize that they were able to control the problem, their outlook toward it changes.
Reorienting in the direction of strengths	Sometimes when adolescents come in, they paint a picture that portrays themselves as all bad—argue with parents, do not study, refuse to get a part-time job, etc. When asked what they are doing well, they reluctantly reveal that they are an A-B student, do not use substances, and always obey curfew. Ask about what is going well and encourage patients to do more of it. Ask for the exception when an argument could have developed but did not.
Open possibilities	Put the problem in the past and the solution in the future. Get a detailed description of what life will be like and what the family will be doing when they are no longer experiencing this problem. For example, when the husband reports, "We're fighting all the time," the therapist replies, "So you used to fight a lot; we'll know we're successful when you are getting along a lot better most of the time."
Reframing	Help patients adjust themselves psychologically in such a way that events formerly perceived as threatening are now seen in a more positive light. Instead of the patient disparaging himself or herself for high levels of anxiety, reframe that thought to "how lucky I am that I have such a sensitive system for self-protection."
Empowering	Remind patients of their solutions, resources, and contexts of competence. Recall times in the past when they were successful.

From Billings, 1996; Deshazer, 1985; Hillyer, 1996; O'Hanlon & Beadle, 1994.

her crying had decreased from "just about all day every day" to "several times a day." When the therapist exclaimed, "Wow! How did you do that?" she reported that she talked with her husband. He admitted that her crying upset him because he thought he should fix it and did not know how. He was very responsive to her requests for hugs, and they have planned a trip to the beach for the next weekend.

2. A postpartum woman recalled one time in the previous week when she felt like crying and did not. When encouraged to focus on that occasion, she was able to recall (after first saying she did not know) that she parked her car

and felt like she was going to cry. Instead, she took several deep breaths while staring at a lovely tree in front of her car. The urge to cry passed and she was able to buy her groceries. From that example, the therapist could develop a plan with the patient to give her more control over her crying, which included that she find a safe place to cry at least several times a day.

3. The therapist was working with a young woman who is a rape survivor. She is from an Appalachian mountain culture where rape is considered to be God's punishment for sins of the victim; therefore much blame is placed and guilt is experienced by the rape survivor. One of the patient's goals for therapy was to be able to tell her parents about the rape that she kept a secret for about 3 years. She was very frightened about their reactions. First, the therapist externalized the problem to be the mountain culture. Then the patient was encouraged to bring into therapy a sister who she thought would be supportive. She shared the rape experience with this sister, and the two of them planned how to tell the parents. The patient was encouraged to take her time, do it when she was ready, etc. The patient completed eight therapy sessions with the agreement that she will write to the therapist when she accomplished her goal. About 2 months later, the therapist received the letter stating that the family had dealt with this revealing of the secret in a very supportive manner. The therapist wrote her a letter commenting on the patient's strength to complete this important task and on the courage of her parents to be supportive and not just reenact the mountain culture's solution to this critical life event. This therapy was effective because the patient met her goals.

Abstinence is no longer considered necessary for recovery in all individuals, especially those with mild to moderate alcohol problems (Rosenberg & Davis, 1994). Instead of an illness model, a "learned habit" paradigm is used to guide interventions. The first level of intervention consists of brief intervention strategies such as educational materials and feedback to the patient about the specific ways in which alcohol affects physical and emotional health and social functioning (Minicucci, 1994). Guidelines are discussed for safer levels of consumption, and the patient is encouraged to keep ongoing records of alcohol intake. The second level of intervention consists of brief therapy, a form of behavioral treatment. It involves engaging the patient to set goals, self-monitor, and identify high-risk situations and gives instruction of procedures for avoiding drinking or overdrinking (Minicucci, 1994).

Berg (1995) has developed an effective approach for substance abusers using such techniques as the miracle question, the relationship question (How do others see your drinking behavior?), the hidden miracle question (Are some of these things already happening?), scaling questions (On a scale from 1 to 10, how badly do you want to stop using drugs? How badly do other family members want you to stop? How do you get from 1 to 4?), and coping questions (What about using drugs is helpful for you? Therapist accepts the patient's answer, and then asks, "How come what are you doing isn't worse?"). It is most important that the therapist pay attention to successes, and when relapse occurs, ask patients how they get themselves back on the right track (Berg, 1995).

The following is an example of Berg's approach. These interventions were used with a young single woman who shared that she thought she had an alcohol problem. Several nights a week, she went out to local bars with friends and drank about six beers. While driving after one such drinking incident, she almost missed her driveway. Her goal was to drink only two to three beers a night. Her strategy was to alternate sparkling water or nonalcoholic beer between beers. She kept a record of drinking behavior and noted what enabled her to meet her goal. She also shared her concern and plan with her friends and asked for their help. After a month she has been successful every night except for one. That night she had a friend drive her home.

(Re)defining the Self

In a grounded theory study, Schreiber (1996) reported that the basic psychosocial process of women's recovery from depression could be described as "(re)defining the self." This model considers the woman a holistic organism existing within a complex network of social interactions and consists of six phases. "My Self Before" is the woman as she was before she encountered depression. When the woman confronts her depression, she is "Seeing the Abyss." The woman then engages in two phases: "Telling My Story" and "Seeking Understanding." The woman may spend a long time in the fourth phase and never progress further. To come to a true understanding of herself, the woman must "Clue In." Clueing In combines insight, readiness, and motivation so that she is making changes in her world. The last phase is "Seeing With Clarity," looking back and accepting where she has been (Schreiber, 1996). Essential psychotherapeutic strategies include the following:

- Establishing a trusting relationship
- Accepting the woman as she presents herself
- Gently inquiring about what is troubling her
- Normalizing
- Asking directly if she has been in an abusive relationship
- Caring without controlling
- Giving factual information about depression

In addition, the woman needs to hear that the therapist understands and appreciates that she is feeling "pretty rough" right now but that things will likely improve. Loaning self-help books and making referrals to self-help groups can be very helpful in the seeking understanding phase (Schreiber, 1996).

Mourning-Liberation Process

A contemporary developmental framework developed by Pollock (1986) based on his work with mid- and late-life adults is the *mourning-liberation process*. Pollock views late life as a time of mourning for what one has or has not achieved. He argues that unless this work of mourning is achieved, an older person is at risk of turning his or her rage and despair onto himself or herself and becoming depressed.

A first step in formulating research questions may be to test a theory in clinical practice and see if it fits and if it works. For example, a therapist was working with a 65-year-old, recently retired professor from a New England university. Much of his depression seemed to center around a book that he had not completed. Even with much encouragement, he was unable to return to the book. Grieving about that loss then became the goal. The grieving was especially difficult because the current situation resurrected feelings of abandonment and loss when his mother left and moved to a distant state, leaving him to be raised by relatives. Another goal of therapy then became to help him gain insight into why his mother left—an understanding that was different from his feeling that somehow it was his fault. The theme of an overwhelming sense of guilt and unfinished business was evident in his recurring nightmares. He was able to feel good about what he had accomplished during his career as well as grieve for the unfinished book, which he was finally able to chuckle about. Through recalling observations of his parental interactions, he was able to see that they had a very unhappy relationship. Recalling visits to see his mom, he was reassured that she loved him very deeply. Nurse psychotherapists have the potential to make important contributions to the growing elderly population in the areas of clinical practice, research, and theory-building (Turner, 1992). One of the prime questions for investigation is whether APRNs are assessing the elderly and identifying those who could benefit from psychotherapy.

■ INTEGRATIVE CASE STUDY

Even though theory/therapy models are discussed separately in this chapter and psychopharmacology is discussed in other chapters, in actual practice, most nurse therapists use a variety of theoretical frameworks and therapeutic treatment strategies. APRNs must stay abreast of scientific advances, determine which theory fits with the philosophical bases of nursing, and continue to evaluate outcomes of treatment. Case studies, such as the one to follow, enable APRNs to capture the essence of psychiatric-mental health nursing. This particular example illustrates a short-term therapeutic relationship using an eclectic approach.

Joy is a 32-year-old married mother of two sons, a 6 year old and a 7-week-old infant. Current difficulty began when she was seen for routine follow-up by the obstetrician who performed her cesarean section. She was crying all the time, and he prescribed sertraline, 25 mg. Twelve hours after taking the first pill, she broke out in hives, and the medication was discontinued promptly. She was referred to a nurse therapist by the women's health nurse practitioner after her postpartum visit. During the interview with the therapist, Joy cried the entire time. She appeared tired and reported sleeping only about 3 hours a day. The baby had colic and cried frequently. She reported feeling depressed with uncontrollable crying, which began several days after delivery. She had no appetite, with a 20 lb weight loss since coming home from the hospital. Several times during the session, she had a flushing of the face and neck and fanned herself saying, "I get these hot flashes, especially when I'm around a crowd." She also reported feeling overwhelmed—finding it difficult to care for the baby and her son and getting housework done. "I have a lot on me." She was critical of her husband who she said does not understand. "My crying turns him away." She also reported that he would not agree to watch the children so that she could get out of the house for a walk. "He says he doesn't know what to do when the baby cries." She reported feeling irritable and sometimes argued with him, but most of the time she "just gets quiet and says nothing." She knows several "mothers" who live close by and are very supportive.

History

There is no family history of mental illness. She was raised by her grandparents after being in a foster home. She described herself as always being a "nervous type" person. She felt very uneasy when her first child was born and wondered about her ability to care for him, but she reported no depression after that birth. She planned to have a tubal ligation at the time of her second delivery, but when she went (at 36 weeks' gestation) to have the baby turned (breech presentation), she went into labor and required a cesarean section. Since the papers had not been signed, she could not get the tubal ligation. She admitted to some anger about that. Joy is self-employed as a day care provider for children in her home. At present she is unemployed but plans to resume paid child care in her home as soon as she feels able emotionally.

Mental Status Examination

This young woman appeared in acute psychologic distress, crying throughout the session. She was neatly dressed in shorts and a T-shirt. She had no unusual psychomotor behavior, and her handshake was firm. She had a sad affect and was critical of her husband's lack of support. She seemed particularly upset about her older son's crying when she dropped him off at school and expressed helplessness about what to do about that. She completed stage 5 on attention and concentration with five numbers forward and four backwards. When asked the proverb about crying over spilled milk, she responded, "don't get upset." Her short-term memory was intact. She answered questions but did not talk voluntarily. She seemed dependent on the therapist to direct the use of the time. Her speech was at a usual rate. Crying did not prevent her from talking about her concerns. There was no evidence of thought disorder. She denied suicidal thoughts or thoughts of harming the children or other family members.

Physical Examination and Laboratory Test

Joy's postpartum physical examination, which was completed by the nurse practitioner, was normal except for her emotional status. Her menstruation had resumed. A blood sample for thyroid-stimulating hormone (TSH) levels was drawn.

Clinical Formulation

Pertinent factors included the missed opportunity to have tubal ligation, oldest son starting kindergarten, perceived lack of support by husband, and hormonal fluctuations caused by pregnancy and postpartum leading to postpartum depression. The patient is a work-at-home mom and may be enmeshed with her oldest son. Her own foster home placement and being raised by grandparents also may have left her more vulnerable to deal with stresses of pregnancy and childbirth. See Table 9-6 for *DSM-IV* and Nursing Diagnosis, and Table 9-7 for the treatment plan and associated therapy model.

Outcome

By the third visit, Joy only cried when talking about her son going to school. She reported feeling better and was sleeping about 5 hours a night. She washed and styled her hair. She talked with her husband about her specific needs. Her husband told her that he knew she needed help and was going to help more. She felt heard and hopeful about their relationship. She plans to take her oldest son to the fair; and her husband has plans to take him fishing. The family has made plans to go to the beach for a weekend (one of Joy's specific requests). Her mother-in-law takes care of the baby so that she and her husband and older son can go out to eat. For the first time, her older son did not cry (and neither did Joy) when she dropped him off at school. She was encouraged to discuss how she did that, and the therapist acknowledged that she was taking important steps to make things better for herself (empowerment).

table 9-6

DSM-IV AND NURSING DIAGNOSES IN CASE STUDY

DIAGNOSIS CATEGORY	PATIENT'S DIAGNOSES
DSM-IV diagnosis	*Axis I.* Major depressive disorder with postpartum onset 296.22
	Axis II. Deferred, 799.9
	Axis III. 7 weeks postpartum
	Axis IV. Role change with new baby and son starting school; perceived lack of support from husband.
	Axis V. 55
Nursing diagnoses	Anxiety related to postpartum hormonal fluctuation and role changes as evidenced by hot flashes, and more intense crying when talking about son starting school.
	Self-esteem disturbance related to stresses associated with role changes as evidenced by feeling unable to care for baby, son, and housework.
	Potential for violence towards self or children related to postpartum depression.

table 9-7

TREATMENT PLAN AND THERAPY MODELS

TREATMENT PLAN	THERAPY MODEL
Fluoxetine, 10 mg; monitor closely for hives	Biologic
Teach about medications and side effects, and reinforce need to take every day and to continue even when starting to feel better	Psychoeducation
Contract for eight sessions and evaluate at that time	Brief solution focused
Normalize experience of depression postpartum and assure her that it is treatable	Supportive psychotherapy
Assist her in figuring out how to negotiate with husband for more support (i.e., need for hugs, need to get out of house and go for a walk)	Behavior therapy
Help her reexamine her conclusion that husband is not supportive; offer alternative explanations about husband's behavior (i.e., concerned about her and feeling overwhelmed and helpless)	Cognitive therapy
Allow for expression of feelings of anger	Supportive psychotherapy
Discuss ways to help her and older son with school drop-off; ask about times when he did not cry when she left him and what she did to facilitate that happening	Brief solution focused
Encourage her to spend regular time with mother-in-law with whom she feels close and supported	Supportive psychotherapy
Plan ways to spend time alone with older son	Developmental
Encourage her to use support system for respite	Supportive psychotherapy
Monitor sleep pattern and intervene as necessary	Biologic

She continues to have a few hot flashes and has days when she cries "a little."

She decided on the sixth visit that she did not need to come to therapy anymore. She was feeling fine and resumed full family responsibilities, including her job providing day care for other children. Follow-up phone calls revealed sustained progress at 1 month and 6 months. At the 6-month follow-up, she had stopped taking her medication and was doing well.

IMPLICATIONS FOR THE ■ FUTURE

Under ideal conditions, theory guides research and research guides practice. The practice of the nurse therapist, however, is not always evidence-based because of the complexity of mental health phenomena and the relative immaturity of the science. Borrowing research from other mental health disciplines is necessary for now as psychiatric-mental health nursing continues to develop its own knowledge base. Theory evolves from observation. Beeber and Gordan are two nurse therapists who used their observations to generate theory, design therapy interventions, and then implement research projects to test effectiveness in a systematic manner.

Research on effectiveness has been published primarily by psychologists (cognitive behavioral interventions) and by psychiatrists (double-blind clinical trials involving psychotherapies and psychotropic medications). In contrast, nursing research on effectiveness and outcomes is sparse, and pilot studies that occur during graduate study often do not get published because of small sample sizes and less rigorous designs. Furthermore, nursing research studies are not often referenced in the literature by other disciplines. Research on cognitive behavioral therapies has been extensive and much of it supports the efficacy of these therapies. Of the psychologic interventions for serious mental disorders, perhaps the treatment most widely studied and best regarded by proponents of clinical trial methods is cognitive therapy for depression (DeRubeis & Crits-Christoph, 1998). The caution with cognitive behavioral research is that most of the studies were conducted by carefully selected and trained therapists, and most of the patients were carefully screened to include those with only the disorder of interest, often excluding those with comorbid diagnoses. This leaves an uncertainty about the ability to generalize the findings to treatments, therapists, patients, and settings outside the control of the university-based researcher (DeRubeis & Crits-Christoph, 1998). Many of the studies reported lack of sustained progress at follow-up. The percentage of persons who were effectively treated never approach 100%. So how does one account for those who do not get better? Although there is some information about what works best with whom, the knowledge base at this time is comparable with the tip of the iceberg. Nurse researchers have a unique opportunity to contribute to the state of the science because of their eclectic understanding of human behavior.

Clinicians disagree about how useful the results of randomized controlled trials (RCTs) are to psychotherapists (Persons & Silberschatz, 1998). Persons argues that information from RCTs is vital to clinicians, and Silberschatz argues that information from RCTs is irrelevant to clinicians. Persons argues that clinicians cannot provide top quality care to their patients without attending to findings of RCTs. Further, history states that clinicians have an ethical responsibility to inform patients about, recommend, and provide treatments supported by RCTs before informing patients about, recommending, and providing treatments shown to be inferior in RCTs or not evaluated in RCTs. Silbershatz argues that RCTs do not and cannot answer questions that concern practicing clinicians. He advocates alternative research approaches (e.g., effectiveness studies, quasi-experimental methods, case specific research) for studying psychotherapy. Although this debate is useful, APRNs need not be concerned about the primacy of one methodology; all kinds of research are applicable to nursing.

Goldfried and Wolfe (1998) give direction for the future:

Despite the advances in psychotherapy outcome research, findings are limited because they do not fully generalize to the way therapy is conducted in the real world. Research's clinical validity has been compromised by the medicalization of outcome research, use of random assignment of clients without regard to appropriateness of treatment, fixed number of therapy sessions, nature of the therapy manuals, and use of theoretically pure therapy. The field needs to foster a more productive collaboration between clinician and researcher; study theoretically integrated interventions, use process research findings to improve therapy manuals, make greater use of replicated clinical case studies; focus on less heterogeneous, dimensionalized clinical problems; and find a better way of disseminating research findings to the practicing clinician.

APRNs must participate in clinical research so that psychiatric nursing will continue to be respected as one of the key mental health professions in the future.

RESOURCES AND CONNECTIONS

American Psychiatric Nurses Association (APNA) homepage www.apna.org
American Psychological Association Psych-NET www.apa.org
Behavior Online www.behavior.net
ERIC Clearinghouse on Assessment and Evaluation ericae2.educ.cua.edu/main.hum
Evidence-Based Mental Health Care www.psychiatry.ox.ac.uk/cebmh/frames.html
Health Guide Online—Clinical Tools Inc www.healthguide.com
Internet Mental Health—Improving understanding, diagnosis, and treatment of mental illness throughout the world www.mentalhealth.com/main.html

Mental Health Net—Review guide to mental health, psychology, and psychiatry online
www.emhc.com

National Association of Cognitive Behavioral Therapists (NACBT) www.nacbt.org

National Institute of Mental Health: Publications List, Room 7C-02, 5600 Fishers Lane, Rockville, MD 20857, 800–421-4211
www.nimh.nih.gov

The Substance Abuse and Mental Health Services Administration of the U.S. Department of Health and Human Services
www.samhsa.gov/index.htm

References

Abraham, I., & Reel, S. (1992). Cognitive nursing interventions with long-term care residents: effects on neurocognitive dimensions. *Archives of Psychiatric Nursing, 6*(6), 356–365.

Alberti, R., & Emmons, M. (1974). *Your perfect right*. San Luis Obispo, CA: Prometheus.

Barlow, D. (1996). The effectiveness of psychotherapy: science and policy. *Clinical Psychology: Science and Practice, 3*, 236–240.

Barlow, D. (1997). Cognitive behavioral therapy for panic disorder: current status. *Journal of Clinical Psychiatry, 58*(supplement 2), 32–37.

Barlow, D., Rapee, R., & Brown, T. (1992). Behavioral treatment of generalized anxiety disorder. *Behavior Therapy, 23*, 551–570.

Barrett, P., Dadds, M., & Rapee, R. (1996). Family treatment of childhood anxiety: a controlled trial. *Journal of Consulting and Clinical Psychology, 64*(2), 333–342.

Beck, A. (1976). *Cognitive therapy and the emotional disorders*. New York: International Universities Press.

Beck, A., et al. (1992). A crossover study of focused cognitive therapy for panic disorder. *American Journal of Psychiatry, 149*, 778–783.

Beck, J. (1995). *Cognitive therapy*. New York: Guilford Press.

Beeber, L. (1989). Enacting corrective interpersonal experiences with the depressed client: an intervention model. *Archives of Psychiatric Nursing, 3*(4), 211–217.

Beeber, L. (1996). Pattern integrations in young depressed women. Part I. *Archives of Psychiatric Nursing, 10*(3), 151–156.

Beeber, L., & Caldwell, C. (1996). Pattern integrations in young depressed women. Part II. *Archives of Psychiatric Nursing, 10*(3), 157–164.

Berg, I.K. (1995). *Brief solution work with substance abuse*. Paper presented at the Family Therapy Networker Symposium, Washington, DC.

Bien, T., Miller, W., & Tonigan, J. (1993). Brief interventions for alcohol problems: a review. *Addiction, 88*, 315–336.

Billings, C. (1996). Brief solution-focused therapy. In Lego, S. (Ed.). *Psychiatric nursing: a comprehensive reference*. Philadelphia: J.B. Lippincott.

Borkovec, T.D., & Costello, E. (1993). Efficacy of applied relaxation and cognitive behavioral therapy in the treatment of generalized anxiety disorder. *Journal of Consulting and Clinical Psychology, 61*, 611–619.

Boudewyns, P.A., et al. (1990). PTSD among Vietnam veterans: an early look at treatment outcome using direct therapeutic exposure. *Journal of Traumatic Stress, 3*, 359–368.

Boyd, M.A. (1997). *Dialectical behavior therapy in a long term care facility: implications for nursing practice*. Paper presented at the annual meeting of SERPN, Washington, DC.

Brewin, C. (1996). Theoretical foundations of cognitive behavior therapy for anxiety and depression. *Annual Review of Psychology, 47*, 33–57.

Burns, D., & Nolen-Hoeksema, S. (1992). Therapeutic empathy and recovery from depression in cognitive behavioral therapy: a structural equation model. *Journal of Consulting and Clinical Psychology, 60*(3), 441–449.

Cardell, R., & Horton-Deutsch, S. (1994). A model for assessment of inpatient suicide potential. *Archives of Psychiatric Nursing, 8*(6), 366–372.

Chambless, D., & Hollon, S. (1998). Defining empirically supported therapies. *Journal of Consulting and Clinical Psychology, 66*(1), 7–18.

Cornes, C. (1990). Interpersonal therapy of depression. In Wells, R., & Giannetti, V. (Eds.). *Handbook of the brief psychotherapies*. New York: Plenum Press.

Compas, B., et al. (1998). Sampling of empirically supported psychological treatments from health psychology: smoking, chronic pain, cancer, and bulimia nervosa. *Journal of Consulting and Clinical Psychology, 66*(1), 89–112.

Craske, M. (1996). An integrated treatment approach to panic disorder. *Bulletin of the Menninger Clinic, 60*(2, supplement A), A87-A104.

DeRubeis, R., & Crits-Christoph, P. (1998). Empirically supported individual and group psychological treatments for adult mental disorders. *Journal of Consulting and Clinical Psychology, 66*(1), 37–52.

deShazer, S. (1985). *Keys to solution in brief therapy*. New York: Norton.

deShazer, S. (1988). *Clues: investigation solutions in brief therapy*. New York: Norton.

Dijkstra, A., et al. (1998). Tailored interventions to communicate stage-matched information to smokers in different motivational stages. *Journal of Consulting and Clinical Psychology, 66*(3), 549–557.

Elkin, I., et al. (1989). National Institute of Mental Health Treatment of Depression Collaborative Research Program: general effectiveness of treatments. *Archives of General Psychiatry, 46*, 971–982.

Elliott, C., Adams, R., & Hodge, G. (1992). Cognitive therapy: possible strategies for optimizing outcome. *Psychiatric Annals 22*(9), 459–463.

Fishel, A. (1998). Management of anxiety and panic. *Nursing Clinics of North America, 33*(1), 135–151.

Fishel, A., & Jefferson, C. (1983). Impact of assertiveness training on hospitalized emotionally disturbed women. *Journal of Psychosocial Nursing, 21*(1), 22–27.

Fishel, A., & Lowdermilk, D. (in press). Complications of pregnancy. In Lowdermilk, D., Perry, S., & Bobak, I. (Eds.). *Maternity nursing* (ed. 5). St. Louis: Mosby.

Foa, E., et al. (1991). Treatment of post-traumatic stress disorder in rape victims: a comparison between cognitive behavioral procedures and counseling. *Journal of Consulting and Clinical Psychology, 59, 715 723.*

Foa, E., et al. (1984). Deliberate exposure and blocking of obsessive-compulsive rituals: immediate and long-term effects. *Behavior Therapy, 15*, 450–472.

Forchuk, C, (1995a). Development of nurse-client relationships: what helps? *Journal of the American Psychiatric Nurses Association, 1*(5), 146–151.

Forchuk, C. (1995b). Uniqueness within the nurse-client relationship. *Archives of Psychiatric Nursing, 9*(1), 34–39.

Frank, A., & Gunderson, J. (1990). The role of the therapeutic alliance in the treatment of schizophrenia: relationship to course and outcome. *Archives of General Psychiatry, 47*, 228–236.

Freeston, M., et al. (1997). Cognitive behavioral treatment of obsessive thoughts: a controlled study. *Journal of Consulting and Clinical Psychology, 65*(3), 405–413.

Gaffan, E., Tsaousis, I., & Kemp-Wheeler, S. (1995). Researcher allegiance and meta-analysis: the case of cognitive therapy for depression. *Journal of Consulting and Clinical Psychology, 63*(6), 966–980.

Gelder, M.G., et al. (1973). Specific and non-specific factors in behaviour therapy. *British Journal of Psychiatry, 123*, 445–462

Goldfried, M., & Wolfe, B. (1998). Toward a more clinically valid approach to therapy research. *Journal of Consulting and Clinical Psychology, 61*(1), 143–150.

Gordan, V., & Ledray, L. (1985). Depression in women: the challenge of treatment and prevention. *Journal of Psychosocial Nursing, 23*(1), 26–33.

Gordan, V., & Ledray, L. (1986). Growth-support intervention for the treatment of depression in women of middle years. *Western Journal of Nursing Research, 8*(3), 263–268.

Gordan, V., et al. (1988). A 3-year follow-up of a cognitive behavioral therapy intervention. *Archives of Psychiatric Nursing, 2*(4), 218–226.

Gunderson, J., Frank, A., & Katz, H. (1984). Effects of psychotherapy in schizophrenia. Part II. Comparative outcome of two forms of treatment. *Schizophrenia Bulletin, 10*, 564–598.

Haber, J., & Billings, C. (1995). Primary mental health care: a model for psychiatric-mental health nursing. *Journal of the American Psychiatric Nurses Association, 1*(5), 154–162.

Haley, J. (1963). *Strategies of psychotherapy.* New York: Grune & Stratton.

Hall, S., et al. (1993). Nicotine, negative affect, and depression. *Journal of Consulting and Clinical Psychology, 61*(5), 761–767.

Hampton, M. (1997). Dialectical behavior therapy in the treatment of persons with borderline personality disorder. *Archives of Psychiatric Nursing, 11*(2), 96 101.

Hardy, G., Stiles, W., Barkham, M., & Startup, M. (1998). Therapist responsiveness to client interpersonal styles during time-limited treatments for depression. *Journal of Consulting and Clinical Psychology, 66*(2), 304–312.

Hayward, P., et al. (1995). Medication self-management: a preliminary report on an intervention to improve medication compliance. *Journal of Mental Health, 4*, 511–517.

Heifner, C. (1993). Positive connectedness in the psychiatric nurse-patient relationship. *Archives of Psychiatric Nursing, 7*(1), 11–15.

Heimberg, R., et al. (1990). Cognitive behavioral group treatment for social phobia: comparison with a credible placebo control. *Cognitive Therapy and Research, 14*, 1–23.

Hill, R., Rigdon, M., & Johnson, S. (1993). Behavioral smoking and cessation treatment for older chronic smokers. *Behavior Therapy, 24*, 321–329.

Hillyer, D. (1996). Solution oriented questions: an analysis of a key intervention in solution-focused therapy. *Journal of the American Psychiatric Nurses Association, 2*(2), 3–10.

Hogarty, G., Anderson, C., & Reiss, D. (1986). Family psychoeducation, social skills training and maintenance chemotherapy in the aftercare treatment of schizophrenia. *Archives of General Psychiatry, 43*, 633–642.

Jacobson, N., et al. (1996). A component analysis of cognitive behavioral treatment for depression. *Journal of Consulting and Clinical Psychology, 64*(2), 295–304.

Jones, E., & Pulos, S. (1993). Comparing the process in psychodynamic and cognitive behavioral therapies. *Journal of Consulting and Clinical Psychology, 61*(2), 306–316.

Keane, T., et al. (1989). Implosive (flooding) therapy reduces symptoms of PTSD in Vietnam combat veterans. *Behavior Therapy, 20*, 245–260.

Klerman, G., et al. (1984). *Interpersonal psychotherapy of depression*. New York: Basic Books.

Krakow, B., et al. (1995). Imagery rehearsal treatment for chronic nightmares. *Behaviour Research and Therapy, 33*, 837–843.

Krupnick, J., et al. (1996). The role of the therapeutic alliance in psychotherapy and pharmacotherapy outcome: findings in the National Institute of Mental Health Treatment of Depression Collaborative Research Program. *Journal of Consulting and Clinical Psychology, 64*(3), 532–539.

Linehan, M. (1993). *Cognitive behavioral treatment of borderline personality disorder*. New York: Guilford Press.

Linehan, M., et al. (December, 1991). Cognitive behavioral treatment of chronically parasuicidal borderline patients. *Archives of General Psychiatry, 48*, 1060–1064.

Mason, W., Breen, R., & Whippie, W. (1994). Solution-focused therapy and inpatient psychiatric nursing. *Journal of Psychosocial Nursing, 32*(10), 46–49.

McLean, P., & Hakstian, A. (1979). Clinical depression: comparative efficacy of outpatient treatments. *Journal of Consulting and Clinical Psychology, 47*, 818–836.

McConnaughy, E., Prochaska, J., & Velicer, W. (1983). Stages of change in psychotherapy: measurement and sample profiles. *Psychotherapy: Theory, Research and Practice, 20*, 368–375.

Miller, C., Eisner, W., & Allport, C. (1994). Creative coping: a cognitive-behavioral group for borderline personality disorder. *Archives of Psychiatric Nursing, 8*(4), 280–285.

Miller, S., Hubble, M., & Duncan, B. (Mar-Apr, 1995). No more bells and whistles. *Family Therapy Networker,* 53–58, 62–63.

Miller, W., & Rollnick, S. (1991). *Motivational interviewing: preparing people to change addictive behaviour*. New York: Guilford Press.

Minicucci, D. (1994). The challenge of change: rethinking alcohol abuse. *Archives of Psychiatric Nursing, 8*(6), 373–380.

Montgomery, C.L. (1993). *Healing through communication: the practice of caring*. Newbury Park, CA: Sage.

Montgomery, C.L., & Webster, D. (1994). Caring, curing, and brief therapy: a model for nurse psychotherapy. *Archives of Psychiatric Nursing, 8*(5), 291–297.

Morin, C., & Azrin, N. (1988). Behavioral and cognitive treatments of geriatric insomnia. *Journal of Consulting and Clinical Psychology, 56*(5), 748–753.

Morse, J., et al. (1990). Concepts of caring and caring as a concept. *Advances in Nursing Science, 13*(1), 1–14.

Nathan, W. (1992). Integrated multimodal therapy of children with attention-deficit hyperactivity disorder. *Bulletin of the Menninger Clinic, 56*(3), 283–312.

Nichols, M., & Schwartz, R. (1998). *Family therapy*. Boston: Allyn & Bacon.

Novalis, P., Rojcewicz, S., & Peele, R. (1993). *Clinical manual of supportive psychotherapy*. Washington, DC: American Psychiatric Press.

O'Hanlon, W.H., & Beadle, S. (1994). *A field guide to possibility land: possibility therapy methods*. Omaha, NE: Possibility Press.

O'Hanlon, W.H., & Weiner-Davis, M. (1989). *In search of solutions: a new direction in psychotherapy*. New York: Norton.

Ost, L., & Westling, B. (1995). Applied relaxation vs cognitive behavior therapy in the treatment of panic disorder. *Behaviour Research and Therapy, 33*, 145–158.

Peplau, H. (1952). *Interpersonal relations in nursing*. New York: G.P Putnam's Sons.

Peplau, H. (1963). A working definition of anxiety. In Burd, S.F., & Marshall, M.A.(Eds.). *Some clinical approaches to psychiatric nursing*. London: Macmillan

Persons, J., & Silberschatz, G. (1998). Are results of randomized controlled trials useful to psychotherapists? *Journal of Consulting and Clinical Psychology, 61*(1), 126–135.

Pinsker, H., Rosenthal, R., McCullough, L. (1991). Dynamic supportive psychotherapy. In Crits-Christoph, P., & Barbee, J. (Eds.). *Handbook of short-term psychotherapy*. New York: Basic Books.

Pollock, G.H. (1986). The psychoanalytic treatment of older adults with special reference to the mourning-liberation process. In Masserman, J.H. (Ed.). *Current Psychiatric Therapies*, vol. 23. Orlando: Grune & Stratton.

Prochaska, J., & DiClemente, C. (1992). Stages of change in the modification of problem behaviors. In Hersen, M., Eisler, R., & Miller, P. (Eds.). *Progress in behavior modification*, vol. 28. Sycamore IL: Sycamore Publishing Company.

Prochasaka, J., DiClemente, C., & Norcross, J. (1992). In search of how people change. *American Psychologist, 47*(9), 1102–1114.

Rachman, S. (1997). The evolution of cognitive behaviour therapy. In Clark D., & Fairburn C. (Eds.). *Science and practice of cognitive behaviour therapy*. Oxford: Oxford University Press.

Raue, P., Goldfried, M., & Barkham, M. (1997). The therapeutic alliance in psychodynamic-interpersonal and cognitive behavioral therapy. *Journal of Consulting and Clinical Psychology, 65*(4), 582–587.

Reeder, D. (1991). Cognitive therapy of anger management: theoretical and practical considerations. *Archives of Psychiatric Nursing, 5*(3), 147–150.

Rickelman, B., & Houfek, J. (1995). Toward an interactional model of suicidal behaviors: cognitive rigidity, attributional style, stress, hopelessness, and depression. *Archives of Psychiatric Nursing, 9*(3), 158–168.

Rockland, L. (1989). *Supportive therapy: a psychodynamic approach.* New York: Basic books.

Rockland, L. (1993). A review of supportive psychotherapy, 1986–1992. *Hospital and Community Psychiatry, 44*(11), 1053–1060.

Rollnick, S., Butler, C., Stott, N. (1997). Helping smokers make decisions: the enhancement of brief intervention for general medical practice. *Patient Education and Counseling, 31,* 191–203.

Rosenbaum, J., et al. (1995). Integrated treatment of panic disorder. *Bulletin of the Menninger Clinic, 59*(2, supplement A), A4-A26.

Rosenberg, H, & Davis, L. (1994). Acceptance of moderate drinking by alcohol treatment services in the United States. *Journal of Studies on Alcohol, 55,* 167–172.

Sargent-Trolinger, J. (1995). *The effects of cognitive therapy combined with antidepressant therapy in the treatment of depression for women.* Unpublished masters thesis, University of North Carolina, Chapel Hill.

Schreiber, R. (1996). Understanding and helping depressed women. *Archives of Psychiatric Nursing, 10*(3), 165–175.

Schweitzer, P., et al. (1995). Outcomes of group cognitive behavioral training in the treatment of panic disorder and agoraphobia. *Journal of the American Psychiatric Nurses Association, 1*(3), 83–90.

Southam-Gerow, M., et al. (1997). Cognitive behavioral therapy with children and adolescents. *Child and Adolescent Psychiatric Clinics of North America, 6*(1), 111–136.

Smyth, N. (December, 1996). Motivating persons with dual disorders: a stage approach. *Families in Society: The Journal of Contemporary Human Services,* 605–614.

Spiegel, D., Bloom, J., & Yalom, I. (1981). Group support for patients with metastatic cancer. *Archives of General Psychiatry, 38,* 527–533.

Stott, N., et al. (1996). Professional responses to innovation in clinical method: diabetes care and negotiating skills. *Patient Education and Counseling, 29,* 67–73.

Stevens, V., & Hollis J. (1989). Preventing smoking relapse, using an individually tailored skills-training technique. *Journal of Consulting and Clincial Psychology, 57,* 420–424.

Stuart, G. (1998). Cognitive behavioral therapy. In Stuart, G.,& Laraia, M. (Eds.). *Stuart & Sundeen's principles and practice of psychiatric nursing* (ed. 6). St. Louis: Mosby.

Sullivan, H.S. (1953). *The interpersonal theory of psychiatry.* New York: Norton.

Sutherland, J. (1993). The nature and evolution of phenomenological empathy in nursing: an historical treatment. *Archives of Psychiatric Nursing, 7*(6), 369–376.

Thase, M., et al. (1994). Do depressed men and women respond similarly to cognitive behavior therapy? *American Journal of Psychiatry, 151,* 500–505.

Turner, M. (1992). Individual psychodynamic psychotherapy with older adults: perspectives from a nurse psychotherapist. *Archives of Psychiatric Nursing, 6*(5), 266–274.

U.S. Department of Health and Human Services. (1993). *Depression in primary care,* vol. 2, Rockville, MD: Public Health Service.

Waddell, K., & Demi, A. (1993). Effectiveness of an intensive partial hospitalization program for treatment of anxiety disorders. *Archives of Psychiatric Nursing, 7*(1), 2–10.

Walter, J., & Peller, J. (1992). *Becoming solution-focused in brief therapy.* New York: Brunner/Mazel.

Ward, A., et al. (1996). To change or not to change—'How' is the question. *British Journal of Medical Psychology, 69,* 139–146.

Weissman, M., et al. (1979). The efficacy of drugs and psychotherapy in the treatment of acute depressive episodes. *American Journal of Psychiatry, 136*(4B), 555–558.

Werman, D. (1984). *The practice of supportive psychotherapy.* New York: Brunner/Mazel.

Williams, S.L., & Falbo, J. (1996). Cognitive and performance-based treatments for panic attack in people with varying degrees of agoraphobic disability. *Behaviour Research and Therapy, 34,* 253–264.

Wilson, S., Becker, L., & Tinker, R. (1995). Eye movement desensitization and reprocessing (EMDR) treatment for psychologically traumatized individuals. *Journal of Consulting and Clinical Psychology, 63,* 928–937.

Worley, N. (1997). *Mental health nursing in the community.* St. Louis: Mosby.

Zerhusen, J., Boyle, K., & Wilson, W. (1991). Out of the darkness: group cognitive therapy for depressed elderly. *Journal of Psychosocial Nursing, 29*(9), 16–21.

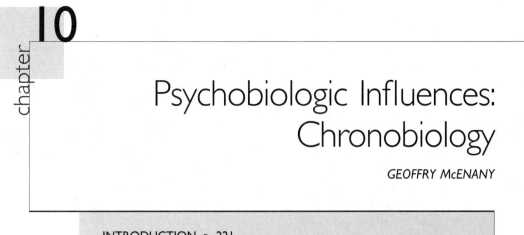

chapter 10

Psychobiologic Influences: Chronobiology

GEOFFRY McENANY

■ INTRODUCTION

The end of the 1990s stands witness to a variety of significant and noteworthy events, the least of which is the beginning of a new century. As with most things, beginnings and endings provide a contiguous experience, as seen in the culmination of *The Decade of the Brain* adjoining the old millennium with the new.

Psychiatric nursing pledged at the beginning of the 1990s to examine and evaluate its approaches to both the scientific and artistic dimensions of the work of the specialty. This process of change mainly involved the infusion of biologically based concepts into the established norms of thinking in both the art and science of psychiatric nursing. In articles published in the beginning of

The Decade of the Brain (McBride, 1991; McEnany, 1991), discussion focused on the challenges facing the specialty in the philosophy of science. The discussion is briefly reviewed to give contextual understanding of the issues currently facing psychiatric-mental health nursing and how those issues have guided the application and synthesis of new areas of science, such as chronobiology, for psychiatric-mental health nursing.

PHILOSOPHY OF SCIENCE IN PSYCHIATRIC-MENTAL ■ HEALTH NURSING

At the beginning of the 1990s, psychiatric-mental health nursing was faced with the arduous task of reconsidering the foundations of a philosophy

221

long believed to provide structure to what psychiatric-mental health nurses do in practice. This philosophy could be called *holism,* referring to the epistomologic understanding of the inseparable nature of mind and body. Discussion of holism was commonplace in the psychiatric-mental health nursing literature of the time (Agan, 1987; Benoliel, 1987; Kobert & Folan, 1990). There seemed to be agreement among psychiatric-mental health nurses that the phenomena of concern to the specialty required an integrated perspective, which was provided with a philosophical foundation such as holism. However, support for holism shifted when the conceptual equation included an infusion of psychobiologic knowledge in a way that challenged the accepted definition of holism of the time. Operationalizing holism in practice began to mean having to acquire and maintain a grasp of the biology of emotional experience in the same way in which nurses had traditionally used psychosocial or psychodynamic viewpoints to understand the experience of those receiving psychiatric-mental health nursing care. However, by the end of the 1990s, psychiatric-mental health nursing had embraced the challenge of shifting its philosophy, creating the conceptual connections that allowed for a broadened definition of holism. One pragmatic example of this shift is the change in prescribing privileges for advanced practice nurses across the United States within this decade. The public has acknowledged the integrated knowledge of advanced practice psychiatric-mental health nursing and through legislated changes has imbued the practice arena with new responsibilities.

This philosophical shift in practice has influenced some other consequential and fundamental changes within psychiatric-mental health nursing, namely how the enriched definition of holism has been taught to nursing students. The warnings set forth by Pothier and colleagues (1990) about the potential consequences of omitting content germane to the biologic sciences in psychiatric-mental health nursing were well heeded. Despite the integration of psychiatric content throughout the curriculum in the early 1990s, academicians worked collaboratively within the specialty to re-shape teaching-learning approaches to help students meet the demands of a shifting paradigm in science, particularly neuroscience.

Professional organizations also made efforts to ensure that guidelines were available to shape a psychobiologically based curriculum for students. An excellent example of such an effort was seen in the Psychopharmacology Task Force project sponsored by the American Nurses Association (ANA). This project involved an impressive effort by psychiatric-mental health nurse experts in the area of psychopharmacology from across the country. The product of these efforts was a monograph (ANA, 1994) that included essential information about the various dimensions of psychopharmacology applications in psychiatric-mental health nursing practice. Of greatest interest to both clinicians and academicians was a data-based compilation of content areas recommended for inclusion in the teaching of any nurse who was involved in either the prescription or dispensing of medications. This seminal work continues to be widely used across the United States to guide curriculum development. It is often used with documents prepared by the professional organizations within psychiatric-mental health nursing, focused on assuring sound approaches to teaching this specialized content to students of the discipline.

The last area to be addressed by the shift in the conceptual face of holism is evident in nursing research. At the beginning of the 1990s, there was significant tension within the specialty of psychiatric-mental health nursing in the area of research, and a great deal of this consternation focused on differences in qualitative and quantitative methods. The idealization of one approach led to the devaluation of the other, further polarizing the members of the discipline at a time when strength through diversity could have been used to the benefit of the advancement of nursing science. This split between quantitative and qualitative methods provided an uncanny parallel to the dualistic notions challenging the holistic philosophy that was occurring in science. What became clear was that nursing science needed both quantitative and qualitative approaches, given the sorts of questions to be addressed in research by nursing scientists.

Psychiatric-mental health nursing has rallied to the challenges of the 1990s, yet it faces a new series of challenges in the years ahead. Given the advances in the development, communication, and testing of philosophy, one of the pressing challenges facing the specialty of psychiatric-mental health nursing is that of synthesis. Psychiatric-mental health nursing must now take this new knowledge and weave it securely into the fabric of the work of the specialty in a way that advances the art and science of nursing's work, ensuring viability of the discipline into the twenty-first century. This chapter provides a template for appreciating the synthesis of new knowledge in one area of emerging science, chronobiology, and its salient applications to psychiatric-mental health nursing practice.

CHRONOBIOLOGY:
■ FUNDAMENTAL CONCEPTS

Chronobiology refers to the sequencing of human rhythms occurring within an environment that also has rhythmic properties. It is the study of human clocks or timing systems, which regulate the sequencing of biologic processes in a synchronous fashion within environmental timing. Such synchrony is critical to well-being and to the absence of symptoms common to illness. For example, everything within the human body occurs in a rhythm. Every subsystem of the human body (e.g., neurologic, endocrine, cardiac, respiratory, reproductive, gastrointestinal) has a rhythmic base. The neurochemicals of the central nervous system (CNS) function rhythmically, allowing for periods of wakefulness and sleep. The endocrine system demonstrates rhythms that peak at certain points in the clock and are at their nadirs at other points. This is the case with all hormones but well demonstrated with growth hormone and cortisol.

What is crucial to the quality of human experience is the notion that these rhythms function in synchrony to provide a sense of so-called "wellness." Examples of desynchronized rhythms are common in everyday experience and in illness and can be appreciated by anyone who has had jet lag, has had to work discontiguous rotating shiftwork, or who has felt fatigued in the day or two after the time change associated with daylight savings time. In all of these examples, the body's biologic rhythms provide a dissonant contrast with the established environmental rhythms of day and night. The consequence is one of not feeling well. Examples of rhythm desychrony abound in the practice of psychiatric-mental health nurses. Examples include difficulties with either getting to sleep, staying asleep, or early morning awakening. Daytime fatigue and anergia are often early symptoms of rhythm desynchronization and are common to any illness, yet they are not well understood in the absence of a chronobiologic framework with which to appreciate the symptom experience. Other examples of rhythm desynchronization are seen in behaviors common to illness such as appetite disturbance, loss of interest in usual activities, difficulty with concentration, and loss of libido. All of these experiences reflect biologic dimensions that clinicians do not generally understand. The lack of understanding often results in the application of a model of thinking that does not give consideration to the interconnectedness of the body's clocks, referred to as the *human circadian timing system*.

Chronobiology in human systems implies a complexity that is often ignored when the clinician confronts the patient's symptom presentations. For example, if a person presents at the office of an advanced practice registered nurse (APRN) with a complaint of "stomach pain," the usual workup will include a series of tests and examinations aimed at yielding a set of differential diagnoses, which are geared toward understanding the multifaceted nature of the complaint. With correct diagnosis, an intervention strategy is planned that addresses the essence of the complaint. In this example, the intervention may be stress modulation, change in diet, and the prescription of a medication such as an H_2 blocking agent. This example provides an excellent template for current approaches to contained and predictable symptom management.

Clinicians tend to fare less successfully in symptom management when chronobiologic indices are clearly prominent. Examples of such phenomena include fatigue, anergia, sleep-pattern disturbance, and lethargy. These bothersome symptoms are difficult for clinicians to address in part because they may lack a clear understanding of them from a physiologic perspective. All an APRN needs to do to appreciate this fact is to spend time with persons who suffer conditions such as chronic fatigue syndrome or fibromyalgia. These individuals often report symptom constellations that do not meet the usual criteria of a well circumscribed presentation as in the previous example of stomach pain. Part of the complexity in figuring out the symptom presentation has to do with the limitations of the clinician's clinical lenses. For example, how is the diurnal pattern of fatigue assessed? How is sleep assessed? What are the strategies used to intervene in phenomena such as fatigue and sleep-pattern disturbance?

Traditional medical approaches have proven less than effective with such complex symptoms as anergia, fatigue, and sleep-pattern disturbance. Probably the most common intervention with sleep-pattern disturbance is pharmacological, which in most cases will yield symptomatic relief. However, such an intervention does not take into consideration some of the chronobiologic dimensions of the symptom (addressed later in this chapter). Other clinical examples are easily given, such as symptom constellations seen in the experiences of women going through the perimenopausal period. Some women report incredible fatigue, lack of energy, sleep-pattern disturbance, and often mood instability. However, these experiences are often difficult to target effectively. Inquiries into the reasoning behind such difficulty leads the cli-

nician back to the issue of chronobiology. These symptom constellations are complex consequences of dysregulated rhythms in contrast to the example of the individual with simple gastritis.

What is acutely compelling for APRNs is that many of the phenomena of concern in the psychiatric-mental health nursing specialty are chronobologic indices that parallel the early patterns of self-care discussed by Orem (1980) and applied to the work of psychiatric-mental health nursing by Underwood (1980): patterns of rest and activity; patterns of appetite and satiety; patterns of elimination; and patterns of solitude and socialization. Understanding the rudiments of chronobiology, dimensions of the human circadian timing system, and the application of these constructs to clinical practice will advance a more complete appreciation of the symptom presentations of those receiving care from psychiatric-mental health nurses. These applications have consequences for both the generalist RN and the APRN engaged in psychiatric-mental health nursing practice. Chronobiologic concepts can enhance the clinical understanding of symptom constellations. In turn, this understanding may potentially affect symptom appraisal and symptom-related intervention strategies and assist persons receiving care to understand their symptoms in a more comprehensive fashion, thereby avoiding the dualistic approaches of the past.

This leads to the consideration of several important questions:

1. What is the nature of biologic rhythms within the body, and how do these rhythms become so tightly aligned with environmental rhythms?
2. What is the normative range of rhythms?
3. What occurs in rhythms in illness states and in circumstances where illness is absent but clear examples of rhythm dysregulation exist, as in jet lag, or in normative circumstances such as menopause?
4. What are the implications of such questions for current and future advanced practice in psychiatric-mental health nursing?

CHARACTERISTICS OF ■ BIOLOGIC RHYTHMS

If all biologic functions occur rhythmically, then it stands to reason that there are some unifying characteristics that allow concordance of rhythm functioning. Fig. 10-1 demonstrates the fundamental characteristics of biologic rhythms. The main features of a biologic rhythm are defined by the shape of the rhythm and the time necessary for its enactment. Terms used to describe these characteristics are *acrophase, nadir, mesor, amplitude,* and *periodicity. Acrophase* and *nadir* refer to the highest and lowest points in the rhythm respectively. *Mesor* is the chronobiologic parallel to the arithmetic mean. The *amplitude* of a given rhythm refers to the distance between the mesor and the acrophase, and the *periodicity* refers to the length of time it take for the rhythm to occur normatively. Each of these terms is applied to every rhythm, regardless of their periodicity.

These terms are important to understand because they have direct parallels with the lived experience of an individual. Applying these concepts to the biologic rhythm of brain stem-

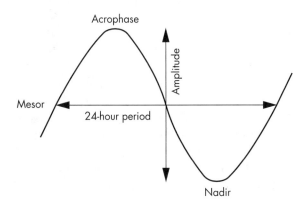

Figure 10-1 Depiction of a normal biologic rhythm. (Adapted from Lee, K.A. [1991]. Nursing care of patients with disturbances in arousal and sleep patterns. In Woods, M.P., et al. [Eds.]. *Medical surgical nursing: pathophysiological concepts.* Philadelphia, J.B. Lippincott).

regulated core body temperature provides an illustration of how these work. Normally, persons are warmer during the day and cooler at night. The warm daytime temperatures correspond with alertness, activity, and cognitive capacity. Conversely, the cooler nighttime temperatures correspond with physiologic conditions required for sound sleep. Given the periodicity of 24 hours for a temperature rhythm, the timing of the peak and nadir in relation to the environmental day is critical. For most people, the peak or acrophase occurs around noon, and the temperature nadir occurs around 2:00 AM. Imagine the consequences of inverting the acrophase and nadir! The affected person would not be able to sleep at night and would have incredible difficulty staying awake during the day. Consider the effect of a significant decrease or increase of the temperature mesor on day-to-day functioning. Having the core body temperature mesor change as little as 0.5° C will potentially alter both day and night experience significantly. Women who ovulate can attest to such an experience as the core body temperature mesor increases about a half degree at ovulation. The mesor remains elevated until the woman begins her menstrual period, at which time the temperature drops back to preovulation levels (Lee, 1988). The symptoms of sleep-pattern disturbance, daytime fatigue, and possibly mood changes are related to such a slight shift in the chronobiologic rhythm of core body temperature, providing a good example of the effects of chronobiologic variables on performance and experience.

In addition to having individual rhythm characteristics as discussed previously, rhythms may also be clustered according to their periodicity. Probably the most commonly discussed rhythms are *circadian rhythms,* referring to those rhythms based on a 24-hour cycle. Examples of circadian rhythms include core body temperature, endocrine functions, sensory processing, and cognitive performance (Mistlberger & Rusak, 1994). *Ultradian rhythms* refer to rhythms of less than 24 hours' duration. Many examples of rhythms of this type abound and can be seen in respiratory functions, gastrointestinal transit times, and certain neurochemical rhythms regulating sleep and wakefulness. *Infradian rhythms* occur in periods greater than 24 hours; the menstrual cycle is an excellent example.

Circadian Rhythms

The research focus on circadian rhythms carries with it a rich history of study, beginning with early scientific attempts to understand the nature of rhythmicity and its application to human experience. Challenging the early beliefs that daily variations in activity cycles of both plants and animals were nothing more than passive responses to environmental stimuli, the works of de Mairan (1729) and de Candolle (1832) demonstrate that certain rhythms in plants persist without routinized environmental cues. De Candolle (1832) illustrated that organisms will either gain or lose time according to the environment and are considered to be free running from the 24-hour clock. Some of the early investigations of free running rhythms in humans involved the use of time-free environments (i.e., environments that are in isolation from all cues of time). As with other mammals tested in time-free environments, humans demonstrated a persistent rhythmicity in cycles related to rest and activity and temperature (Aschoff, 1965), often referred to as *free running rhythms*. These rhythms stand in direct contrast to *entrained rhythms*, which are reliant on some form of environmental cue to keep their enactment in synchrony with the natural environment. Studies indicated that the free running period in humans is approximately 25 hours. Providing that there is no resetting of the circadian clock via environmental means, referred to as *environmental entrainment*, the rhythm would delay about 1 hour each day in relation to the actual clock time (Weaver, 1979). This is referred to as a *phase delay* and is evident in the sleep patterns of many people with psychiatric illness. For example, phase delay

can be seen in the person who goes to bed at 11:00 PM but is unable to get to sleep until 1:00 AM. When the usual wake-up time of 6:00 AM arrives, the person has great difficulty getting out of bed. The propensity would be to sleep the additional 2 hours that he or she lost in the beginning of the night.

The opposite pattern is also seen, although less commonly. An example is referred to as a *phase advance* and is seen in persons who want to go to bed well before their usual sleep time. If they follow their inclination and go to bed at this early time, they find that they are awake in the early morning hours, perhaps 3:00 AM or 4:00 AM, with an inability to get back to sleep. This pattern of phase advance is often normative among elders but is pathologic in many other circumstances, as is the case in psychiatric illness. The underlying physiology of either phase advance or phase delay, commonly referred to as *phase shifts,* has to do with dysregulation of rhythms, particularly that of core body (brain stem regulation) temperature as previously described.

In the natural light-dark environment provided by the earth's diurnal rotation, rhythm delays are not always apparent, pointing to an environmentally based influence on the synchronization of rhythms. This potent influence is natural light as discovered by Richter (1965). Given that an environmental influence is evident in the regulation of rhythms, subsequent research focused on isolation of an anatomic transducer of light, which demonstrated a capacity to regulate rhythms. Richter (1965) conducted a variety of experiments on blind rats and sequentially destroyed neurologic and endocrine tissues that might confound the tracking of a free running rhythm. His results demonstrated that the hypothalamus was the only place where lesions affect free running rhythms. With the collaborative work of other researchers (Moore & Lenn, 1972; Rusak & Zucker, 1979), a retinohypothalamic projection was identified, which terminated in the suprachiasmatic nuclei of the anterior hypothalamus. Fig. 10-2 shows the location of the nuclei in the hypothalamus of the

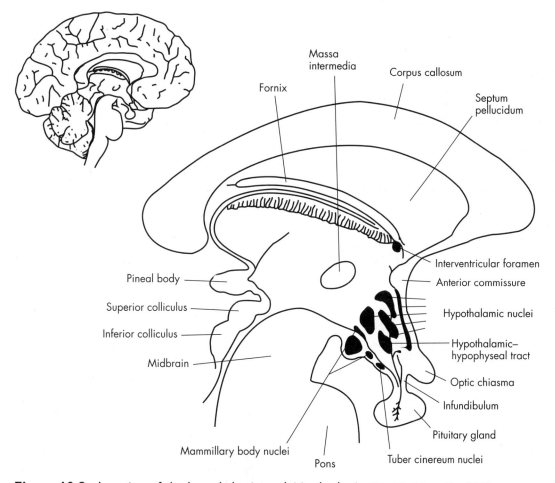

Figure 10-2 Location of the hypothalamic nuclei in the brain. (Modified from Kandel ER: *Principles of Neural Science*, ed 2, 1985, Simon & Schuster International.)

brain. Destruction of these nuclei yields loss of rhythm capacity (Moore & Eichler, 1972).

Given that there is a 24-hour rhythm propensity in humans, the presence of light is critical in maintaining synchrony with a light-dark environment, and such a mechanism is the result of a functioning retinohypothalamic projection and suprachiasmatic nuclei in the hypothalamus. Provided physiologic substrates for the circadian system are intact, rhythm entrainment is possible with the influence of environmental timekeepers referred to as *zeitgebers*. Light, although the most powerful, is not the only zeitgeber. Researchers have demonstrated the nonphotic sources of

rhythm entrainment such as food (Boulos & Terman, 1980), states of arousal (Richter, 1965) and social cues (Miles, Raynal, & Wilson, 1977). However, the most powerful source of entrainment is light, and this has become the source of several applications of light across a variety of conditions and illness states (Lin et al., 1990; Avery et al., 1991; Mackert et al., 1991; Parry et al., 1993; Lam et al., 1994; McEnany, 1997).

The variance around a 24-hour periodicity for different individuals raises some important questions about the understanding of disorders that arise from circadian rhythm dysregulation. The normal range for entrainment for a single human being is 23.5 to 26.5 hours. If a person's internal "clock" is forced to advance approximately $\frac{1}{2}$ hour or delay more than $2\frac{1}{2}$ hours, it is generally not tolerated in one whose internal "clock" is 24 hours long (Moore-Ede, Sulzman, & Fuller, 1982). These rhythms can be modified by influences such as light intensity and hormones (Sack & Lewy, 1997) and have significant implication for changes in circadian rhythmicity in psychiatric illnesses.

Given the evidence of free-running and entrained rhythms, the question of whether more than one "clock" exists within the human timing system gives rise to the development of several chronobiologic models. Of those models, a commonly accepted one is the two oscillator model developed by Weaver (1979). This model postulates that one of the two oscillators is stronger than the other, and they are responsible for different functions. This model has received support over time as repeated studies have demonstrated the persistence of weaker circadian rhythms subsequent to the destruction of the suprachiasmatic nuclei (Mistlberger & Rusak, 1994). Normally in light-dark environments, the two oscillators are coupled or linked. However, the two oscillators become free running in conditions of constant light (Kupferman, 1991). The weaker oscillator is believed to be the one more easily influenced by the presence of other zeitgebers and is alleged to regulate slow wave sleep, calcium excretion, and growth hormone. The stronger oscillator controls rapid eye movement (REM) sleep, core body temperature, corticosteroid secretion, and potassium excretion (von Zerssen, 1987). According to classic research conducted by Schulz and Lavie (1985), the notion for whether the "master clock" for the body's rhythmicity is in the suprachiasmatic nucleus is supported when those nuclei are surgically isolated and the neural rhythms outside the suprachiasmatic nucleus island cease.

Normative Range of Rhythmicity

The question often arises about what variance is considered normal in rhythms, which raises the issue of rhythm propensity. Specifically, *rhythm propensity* refers to rhythm strength. Examples of normal variation are seen in persons whose basic rhythm structure characterize them as either morning types (larks), evening types (owls), or as neither. What distinguishes an owl from a lark is the placement of the rhythm acrophase and nadir in relation to the rhythm periodicity (Fig. 10-3). For example, the lark is more likely to have an earlier acrophase and an earlier nadir, and their rhythms tend to be less than 24 hours. Conversely, the owl has a later onset of acrophase and a later nadir with a periodicity of probably more than 24 hours. This categorization is seen behaviorally in those who need to be to work at 7:00 AM. The larks are energetic, but by the end of the work day are beginning to slow down and report feeling fatigue. The antithesis is seen in those who are characterized as owls. They may have difficulty functioning in the morning, sharply contrasting with the larks, whereas they become more activated as the day progresses. While the lark's energy is waning, the owl's is cresting, and the behavioral differences provide an ongoing source of discussion between these two groups. Despite the obvious incongruity between the rhythm propensities of owls and larks, most people do not have strong inclinations toward either.

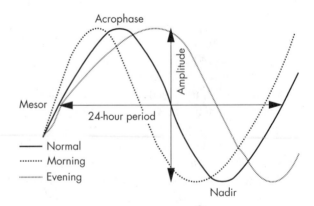

Figure 10-3 Chronotyping of biologic rhythms. (From McEnany GW: Rhythm and blues revisited: biological rhythm in depression, *J Am Psych Nurses Assoc* 2(1):15, 1996.)

Some of the earliest investigations into circadian phenomena related to psychiatric illness date to the latter part of the nineteenth century with the works of Kraft-Ebing (1874). This area of knowledge is particularly interesting because of its applicability to understanding dimensions of depression that span from cellular mechanisms to behavioral manifestations of illness. Clusters of data exist that examine prominent and interrelated biologic markers in depression, including temperature, sleep, and various neuroregulators and their metabolites (Nemeroff, 1998). Part of the challenge embedded in this body of literature is the need to determine the main chronobiologic abnormalities that occur as a dimension of psychiatric illness. The issue of which circadian variables are involved in the etiology of the illness has yet to be fully understood.

It is clear that core body temperature is an entrained circadian rhythm, but the mechanism for that entrainment is unclear (Mistlberger & Rusak, 1994). Temperature regulation is a cumulative response to input from a variety of the body's systems including the CNS, the endocrine system, and muscle responses to ambient temperature. The seat of the body's temperature regulation is the hypothalamus, which is also involved in the endocrine indices of temperature (e.g., thyroid-related regulation of heat production) (Kupferman, 1991).

Temperature plays an important role in sleep-wake periods. It has been long documented that humans have a daily variance in temperature that spans 1.5° F with a peak in the late morning or early afternoon and a nadir at some point in the night. The fact that there is a low point in the temperature rhythm during sleep is critically important for the smooth transitioning from one sleep stage to another (referred to as *sleep architecture*) and a restful experience.

Changes in temperature in sleep are influenced in three ways:

1. The circadian rhythm for core body temperature is as described previously. Influences on the circadian rhythm include the propensity for morningness or eveningness in rhythm strength. Additionally, there is a gender effect on temperature rhythm in women who are ovulating or perimenopausal. The works of Lee (1988) have shown that there is an increase in core body temperature mesor along with a dampening of the temperature amplitude post-ovulation.

2. Temperature varies within the sleep period. Part of this variability is related to the circadian influence on temperature rhythm in sleep, but the other component is an artifact of sleep stage changes. For example, thermoregulation is inhibited in REM sleep, and conversely, the mechanisms for thermoregulation remain intact in non-REM sleep (Goltzbach & Heller, 1989).

3. There is an influence from the environment in which the individual sleeps, namely ambient or room temperature. With warm ambient temperatures, studies note reductions in both REM and non-REM sleep, whereas cold ambient temperatures yield more awake time after sleep onset, more movement time during sleep, and more difficulty getting to sleep (Carskadon & Dement, 1994).

In some forms of psychiatric illness, several circadian-based events occur that may include either a phase advance (Czeisler et al., 1987) or phase delay for the body's rhythm for temperature, or a blunting of the body's circadian rhythm for temperature (Rosenthal et al., 1990). Behaviorally, these influences include difficulties initiating and maintaining sleep and varying levels of daytime fatigue.

Given the fact that temperature is a reliable indicator of circadian rhythm strength and phase, it provides a benchmark of the circadian timing system, which potentially could be more widely applied to understanding symptom constellations in psychiatric illness. The monitoring of circadian rhythm related to temperature requires frequent data points over a 24- to 48-hour period to be able to fully examine the dimensions of the rhythm (e.g., the highest [acrophase] and lowest [nadir] point in the temperature rhythm as indices of rhythm phase). Equally important is the rhythm strength. The mean (mesor) temperature is a critical index in understanding both daytime fatigue and nighttime sleep-pattern disturbances (Glotzbach & Heller, 1994).

Many factors potentially change sleep patterns, such as age, history of sleep-pattern disturbance, disruption of circadian rhythms, core body temperature, menstrual cycle patterns, drug ingestion, and disease (Reite, Ruddym, & Nagel, 1997). Table 10-1 delineates the sleep variables of concern in psychiatric illnesses.

The actual process of sleeping and remaining awake is expressed in a circadian pattern and varies according to a multitude of individual factors. This pattern generally reflects the adaptation of the individual to the environment. Sleep has both homeostatic and biorhythmic properties. The homeostatic features of sleep are juxtaposed on some very powerful biorhythmic fluctuations that are not only circadian but also ultradian and infradian throughout the sleep period (Broughton et al, 1990).

Two types of sleep alternate rhythmically throughout the entire sleep period: rapid eye movement (REM) and non-rapid eye movement (non-REM, or NREM). REM is considered to be active sleep. In REM, the sleeping person is generally immobile with paralysis of the large muscle groups. Characteristically, the person's eyes dart back and forth. Most dreaming occurs in REM sleep.

REM is further delineated into phasic REM and tonic REM. In phasic REM, the person who sleeps is generally immobile, but minute twitches of the face, body, and fingers are common. Snoring ceases and respirations become irregular. Cerebral blood flow increases and the metabolic activity of the brain increases. Concurrently, the brain's temperature also increases. Tonic REM seems to be far less complex in its presentation. Tonic REM

table 10-1

DEFINITIONS OF SLEEP VARIABLES

VARIABLES	DEFINITIONS
Total sleep time (TST)	Total minutes of sleep actually occurring during a period when sleep is attempted
Sleep period time (SPT)	Total time spent in bed attempting to sleep
Sleep latency (SL)	The amount of time passed between going to bed and actual sleep onset
Sleep efficiency index (SEI)	The percentage of the sleep period actually spent in a sleep stage.
REM sleep	Rapid eye movement sleep; commonly referred to as *dream sleep* and occupies approximately 20% of the total sleep time in adults
Non–REM sleep (NREM)	Non–rapid eye movement sleep; divided into four stages: stages 1 and 2 are light sleep, and stages 3 and 4 are deep, restorative sleep; NREM occupies approximately 80% of the night in adults, with the majority of this time spent in stage 2
REM latency (REML)	Period of time between sleep onset and the appearance of the first REM period; normally in adults it occurs between 90 and 120 minutes, but many factors influence this timing; this is considered to be a biologic marker for some types of psychiatric illnesses, particularly depression

is a state within REM sleep that is characterized by similar brain activity as noted in phasic REM. However, there is an absence of the twitching of small muscles. The electroencephalographic (EEG) recordings of brain activity in REM sleep parallel those of a person who is awake, except for the rapid eye movements.

NREM is often described as an idling brain in an active body. NREM consists of four stages with stages 1 and 2 being lighter sleep and stages 3 and 4 being deep sleep. Dreaming is by far less common in this type of sleep. Throughout the night, REM and NREM cycles alternate to create *sleep architecture,* a mapping of the brain's activity in sleep. Normally, NREM-REM cycles vary in duration from 70 to 110 minutes, but the average is 90 minutes, and the first appearance of REM sleep, referred to as *REM latency,* is approximately 90 minutes after sleep onset. Again, these parameters will change normatively with age, gender, and the aforementioned variables. Early night sleep is characteristically NREM, particularly stages 3 and 4. However, as the night progresses, REM periods can last 60 minutes or longer, and the interspersed NREM is nearly all light sleep.

Several changes in sleep patterns of those with psychiatric illnesses distinguish them from those classified without illness. As clinicians, APRNs know this fact from a phenomenologic perspective because it is both observable in sleep quality and quantity, as well as reflected in the person's self reports of sleep. However, using findings from other data sources to be discussed here offers not only a different perspective on the phenomenon of concern (sleep-pattern disturbance) but also sheds light on the chronobiologic indices of the illness. For example, approximately 90% of persons diagnosed with major depressive disorder show some form of EEG-verified alteration in sleep (Nathan et al., 1995). More specifically, the changes noted in the sleep of persons with major depression include shortened REM latency and sleep discontinuity disturbances, prolonged sleep latency (difficulty getting to sleep), awakenings in the middle of the night, and early morning awakening. Other EEG-verifiable changes include diminished NREM stages 3 and 4, an altered temporal distribution of REM sleep within the night, and an overall increase in the amount of REM sleep in a given night (Benca et al., 1992). These factors combined yield sleep that is more fragmented and less efficient, often leaving the person feeling unrested and fatigued upon awakening.

In a landmark meta-analytic study of sleep architecture changes across psychiatric illnesses, Benca and colleagues (1992) examined the EEG data from 177 studies, which included 7151 study participants and controls. Across diagnostic categories, the findings of this study revealed significantly reduced sleep efficiency. *Sleep efficiency* refers to the amount of time actually slept during a period when sleep was attempted. For example, if a person was in bed from 12:00 AM to 6:00 AM but was only able to get to sleep and stay asleep between 3 AM and 6 AM, his or her sleep efficiency index ranges around 50%. The longer one is in bed and is able to sleep during that time span without interruption, the greater the sleep efficiency. Additionally, the meta-analysis revealed other noteworthy findings, including a general reduction in total sleep time in the diagnosed groups. REM sleep was relatively preserved across diagnostic groups, but the percentage of REM sleep was increased in affective disorders. Reduction in REM latency was very common to affective disorders but occurred in other groups as well. Although no single sleep variable appeared to have absolute specificity for any particular psychiatric disorder, patterns of sleep-pattern disturbance could be clustered according to diagnostic category. Overall, the findings from the affective disorders groups differed most frequently and significantly from those classified as controls. Table 10-2 reviews the findings of the Benca and colleagues (1992) study according to diagnostic category as compared with data from controls.

It is important to ask some very cogent and compelling questions when evaluating findings of a study such as the one conducted by Benca and colleagues (1992). The majority of the questions to be asked need to address concerns over specificity of these findings. One of the major benefits of meta-analysis is that it permits an evaluation of a large data set originating from the compiled results of various studies. Because of the statistical maneuvers involved in meta-analysis, the unit of analysis no longer is a test result wrought in scores from a research instrument but an evaluative appraisal of the size of effect from a given intervention. This is referred to as *effect size* (Cohen, 1988). In the evaluation of effect size of various sleep parameters in groups of persons within a given diagnostic category, it is important to question whether the effect seen is an inherent trait of the persons under study or a reflection of the state of the illness. For example, shortened REM latencies have been consistently documented in

persons with affective disorders as previously discussed. When these individuals return to states of wellness, do the shortened REM latencies self correct or do they persist? Although the answer to such questions remains uncertain, sound reasoning drives the line of questioning concerning specificity measures before applying these data directly to clinical circumstances.

Neurochemical Regulation and Dysregulation of Sleep

It stands to reason that if sleep-wake cycles are chronobiologic phenomena with patterns of rhythmicity and an entrained basis for enactment, then there must be traceable biochemical foundations to these patterns within very specific re-

table 10-2

SLEEP IN PSYCHIATRIC DISORDERS: SLEEP ARCHITECTURE PARAMETERS

DIAGNOSIS	TST	SE	SL	SWS%	REM LATENCY	REM%
Mood disorders	↓	↓	↑	↓	↓	↑
Alcoholism	↓	N/A	↑	↓	Same	↑
Anxiety disorders	↓	↓	↑	Same	Same	Same
Borderline personality	↓	↓	↑	Same	Same	Same
Dementia	↓	↓	↑	Same	Same	Same
Eating disorders	↓	Same	Same	Same	Same	Same
Schizophrenia	↓	↓	↓	Same	↓	Same
Insomnia	↓	↓	↑	↓	Same	Same
Narcolepsy	Same	↓	↓	↓	↓	Same

Modified from Benca et al., 1992.
TST, Total sleep time; *SE,* sleep efficiency; *SL,* sleep latency or time from going to bed to when stage 1 sleep occurs; *SWS%,* % deep restorative sleep across the night; *REM latency,* time from sleep onset to 1st REM period; *REM%,* % REM sleep across the night.

gions of the CNS. A brief review of those regions of the brain provides a neuroanatomic and neurophysiologic understanding of the chronobiologic phenomena of sleep and wakefulness. The implications of these structures and functions may be extrapolated onto neurochemical processes at play in psychiatric disease states.

Intact patterns of sleep and wakefulness rely on unimpaired communication of the neurons within the brainstem reticular formation. These specific neurons form the ascending reticular activating system, project into the thalamus, and excite cells that project to widespread areas of the cerebral cortex (Fig. 10-4). Such activity produces the cortical activation that occurs during wakefulness.

Additionally, brainstem reticular neurons project into the hypothalamus and basal forebrain where neurons are located that also project to the cerebral cortex and participate in the maintenance of an alert state of awareness (Sleep Research Society, 1993).

Very specific neurochemicals are involved in the enactment of wakefulness and are found in cell clusters within the reticular formation. The six main neurochemicals involved in wakefulness are noradrenaline, dopamine, acetylcholine, histamine, glutamate, and aspartate. Table 10-3 delineates the locations and functions of these chemicals in their roles in wakefulness. Additionally, there are peptides such as corticotropin-

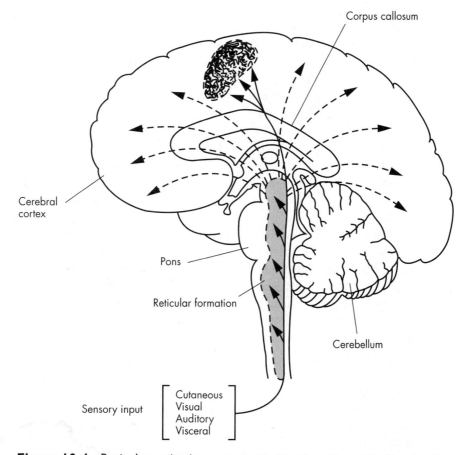

Figure 10-4 Reticular activating system. (Modified from Kandel ER: *Principles of Neural Science*, ed 2, 1985, Simon & Schuster International.)

table 10-3

NEUROCHEMICALS IMPLICATED IN SLEEP AND WAKE STATES

SLEEP	WAKE
Serotonin (sleep induction)	Catecholamines, particularly dopamine and norepinephrine
Adenosine (deep sleep)	Acetylcholine
Gamma-aminobutyric acid (deep sleep)	Histamine
Peptides (sleep promotion)	Glutamate
Opiate peptides (sensory modulation)	Cerebrospinal fluid peptides
Insulin (deep sleep induction)	Blood-borne epinephrine
Cholecystokinin	

releasing factor, thyrotropin-releasing factor, and others that are believed to be involved in the cortical activation through central mechanisms. Blood-borne hormones can enhance arousal or wakefulness as is the case with epinephrine, thyroid-stimulating hormone (TSH), or adrenocorticotropin hormone (ACTH).

In many ways, sleep is a more complex phenomenon as compared with wakefulness because the brain has different anatomic areas for the different types of sleep (i.e., REM and NREM sleep). Sleep is an active process, not one whereby certain cells *turn off* while others *turn on*. In NREM sleep, the basal forebrain is the most prominent area of control for this type of sleep (Sleep Research Society, 1993). Lesions in this part of the brain create significant disturbances in the enactment of NREM sleep. It is currently believed that a variety of widely separated brain regions are involved in NREM sleep (e.g., the midbrain raphe), but that the basal forebrain is the most crucial of these areas. Serotonin and gamma-aminobutyric acid (GABA) are involved in NREM sleep as are various peptides, the endogenous opiates, alpha melanocyte-stimulating hormone, and somatostatin (Reite, Ruddy, & Nagel, 1997).

REM sleep mechanisms have been localized in the brain and are distinctly different from those areas involved in NREM sleep patterns. For example, of great interest are the areas of the lateral pontine and medial medullary reticular areas.

These areas contain cells that are very actively discharging during REM sleep but not in NREM sleep. There is very little discharge activity from these cells during wakefulness. Cholinergic mechanisms are essential to the enactment of REM sleep, and monoaminergic mechanisms are important to its interruption (Reite, Ruddy, & Nagel, 1997). These systems may also control many of the other manifestations of REM sleep such as rapid eye movements, skeletal muscle paralysis, and the characteristic EEG arousal that accompanies both REM sleep and dreaming.

In psychiatric illness, the prevailing belief is that there is a dysregulation of the neurochemical systems that deal with cognitive and emotional experiences, yielding symptoms common to psychiatric illness. The notion that one neurochemical is responsible for the totality of a given emotional state is both naive and incomplete, which was the nemesis of both the catecholamine hypothesis of depression and the dopamine hypothesis of psychosis. Both of these hypotheses are reflections, however, of the linear and monocausal thinking that led to their development. Such unidimensional thinking is countered by more holistic approaches to the understanding of behavior and behavioral disturbances characteristic of psychiatric illness states.

Given such a perspective, it is important to recognize that the CNS is simply a system. Given the principles of systems logic, if one part of the system is changed, then the entire system undergoes transformation. Neurochemically, this means that if one neurochemical index undergoes a pathophysiologic change in its metabolic course, then other related chemicals will reflect that disruption. This exact principle applies to chronobiologic phenomena as well. For example, of interest and significance to a chronobiologic perspective is the notion that sleep is probably the most sensitive indicator of the onset of psychiatric illness. Additionally, sleep patterns can be viewed as indicators of the underlying course of the illness. To be able to address sleep as a true symptom of the illness and not a byproduct thereof provides an opportunity to use a common chronobiologic marker (sleep pattern) as a gauge of the course of the illness rather than an isolated symptom to be ameliorated symptomatically. Details of such applications of chronobiology are addressed in the section that follows.

APPLICATION OF CHRONOBIOLOGIC ■ PRINCIPLES

The disciplines involved in the care and treatment of those who live with mental illnesses have been forced to reconsider the ways in which they view the phenomena of concern in their work. In the arena of mental health and illness, this reconceptualization has taken the shape of a revolution in scientific ideology, especially in the normative understanding of the psychobiologic dimensions of behavior in general and of psychiatric illnesses in particular. The psychobiologic revolution of the last several years has forced a reconceptualization of mind as a process of the brain in interaction with the environment. Such a new perspective suggests a paradigm shift in psychiatry that negates biologic or structural reductionism, and in turn triggers a rethinking of the psychologic paradigm. This psychobiologic revolution offers APRNs in psychiatric and mental health care an opportunity to operationalize a new form of

holism that includes the enrichment offered by chronobiology to mental health sciences. This perspective allows for the integration of the biologic, psychologic, spiritual, and social realms to yield what humans have come to know as *experience*.

Nursing science has begun to explore the dimensions of biologic rhythms and their applications to practice. These explorations are likely to broaden the perspective of APRNs on behaviors encountered in practice. For example, do mental health professionals fully understand the phenomenon of sleep in relation to psychiatric disease? Although these professionals recognize the importance of balance between rest and activity, they often do not use a chronobiologic lens on the phenomenon. Consequently, they may not be fully aware of the interplay between, for example, models of temperature regulation and sleep-wake patterns. Without such understanding, difficulty falling asleep, staying asleep, or early morning awakening may be viewed at worst as something under the volitional control of the individual. Cognitive influences play an important role in some dimensions of sleep and alertness. However, *not* including an understanding of biologic rhythm in the APRN's perception of sleep behavior is inadequate, if not precarious, for clinical assessment and intervention. Lack of this type of knowledge may lead to a more extensive use of biomedical interventions rather than chronobiologic nursing strategies.

Continuing with the sleep example, if APRNs were to understand sleep-wake patterns as seen through a chronobiologic lens, they might be more amenable to enhancing competence in intervention strategies such as phototherapy or sleep manipulations (McEnany, 1996; McEnany & Lee, 1997). Given nursing's domain of "person in interaction with environment," new and potentially more effective strategies for clinical care would include some means of shaping rhythm-based disturbances in health and illness across the life span. In dealing with clinical trials of chronobiologic intervention strategies for women with major depression (McEnany, 1994; McEnany & Lee,

1998), the potential application of such strategies in nursing practice seems very promising.

CHRONOBIOLOGIC
■ ASSESSMENT OF SLEEP

Sleep is a very sensitive index of both chronobiologic functioning and onset as well as course of psychiatric illness. It therefore provides a good example upon which to discuss a prototypical approach to assessment of psychiatric symptom presentations.

Routinized Assessment of Sleep-Wake Patterns

Recognizing that sleep-wake patterns are simply different dimensions of the same continuous phenomenon, it is important to consider both when appreciating disturbances in one realm or the other. The first place to begin with assessment of sleep is with a thorough sleep history. Assessment in this arena must include an evaluation of daily sleep-wake patterns and some of the potential confounders of these patterns. Morin (1996) points out that there are several risk factors that potentially yield sleep difficulties: cognitive and physical hyperarousal; obsessive thinking; propensity toward emotional repression; medical or psychiatric illnesses; increasing age; family history of insomnia; and female gender, given some of the normative changes that women experience in relation to women's health variables. Clinical questioning needs to follow the lines of the risk factors as outlined here. Of the factors noted in the above list, three stand out as requiring particularly close attention: medical or psychiatric illnesses, age, and gender.

Influence of Medical or Psychiatric Illnesses

Under this category, it is critical to use complete data from the standard history and physical examination, recognizing the potential effects of symptom constellations from various illnesses on sleep-wake pattern. The APRN needs to be apprised of the rudiments of formal sleep disorders to recognize symptom clusters that are related to sleep disorder and not necessarily related to psychiatric illness. This is an area of particular challenge to the psychiatric clinician of any discipline because of the nature of the frameworks provided to understand behavioral disturbance. More often than not, the frameworks taught to students of a given discipline are spare in their teaching of formal sleep disorders. However, the consequences are significant. An undiagnosed sleep disorder being inappropriately treated as a psychiatric illness will not respond to the prescribed intervention (e.g., obstructive sleep apnea syndrome [OSAS]). On the surface, the symptoms of OSAS appear like those of depression (e.g., symptoms of daytime fatigue, nonrestorative sleep, difficulty concentrating, anergia, mood disturbances). However, these patients are often the ones who have had two or three trials of thymoleptics, none of which have adequately dealt with

box 10-1

COMMON DRUGS CAUSING SLEEP-PATTERN DISTURBANCE

Beta blockers
Corticosteroids
Adrenocorticotropic hormone
Monoamine oxidase inhibitors
Diphenylhydantoin
Calcium channel blockers
Bronchodilators
Stimulating tricyclic antidepressants
Caffeine
Thyroid hormones
Oral contraceptives
Stimulating selective serotonin reuptake inhibitors
Antimetabolites
Select decongestants
Thiazides
Stimulants

the symptoms. On closer evaluation, the symptom constellation relates to OSAS rather than major depression. More often than not, once the OSAS evaluation is completed and appropriate treatment is begun, the symptom constellation clears quickly.

Of equal importance, and often the most obvious culprit in sleep-wake pattern disturbance, is the role of medications. Box 10-1 summarizes some of the most commonly cited medications that create problems with patterns of efficient sleep and alert wakefulness. As the APRN notes, the complexity of illness and iatrogenesis related to an intervention strategy can themselves be responsible for the symptom constellation under assessment. It is important to realize that the dis-

box **10-2**

SLEEP HYGIENE INSTRUCTIONS

A. The Body's Drive for Sleep
   1. Avoid naps, except for a brief 10- to 15-minute nap 8 hours after arising.
   2. Restrict sleep period to average number of hours you have actually slept per night in the preceding week. Quality of sleep is important. Too much time in bed can decrease quality on subsequent night.
   3. Get regular exercise each day, preferably 40 minutes per day of an activity that causes sweating. It is best to exercise about 6 hours before bedtime.
   4. A warm bath should be reserved for more than 2 hours before bedtime. A hot drink may relax you, but it may warm you as well.
B. Circadian Factors
   1. Keep a regular bedtime seven times per week.
   2. Do not expose yourself to light if you have to get up at night.
   3. Get at least one half hour of sunlight within 30 minutes of your out-of-bed time.
C. Drug Effects
   1. Do not smoke to get yourself back to sleep.
   2. Reduce or avoid smoking after 7 PM.
   3. Limit caffeine use to no more than three cups of caffeinated coffee or tea no later than late morning. Avoid caffeine entirely if possible.
D. Arousal in Sleep Setting
   1. Keep clock face turned away, and do not find out what time it is when you wake up at night.
   2. Avoid highly strenuous exercise for which you are not conditioned.
   3. Do not eat or drink heavily for 3 hours before bedtime. A light bedtime snack may be okay.
   4. Do not retire too hungry or too full. Raise the head of the bed if you have regurgitation.
   5. Keep your sleep room dark, quiet, well ventilated, and at a comfortable temperature. Ear plugs and eye shades are okay.
   6. Use the bedroom only for sleep; do not work or do other activities that lead to prolonged arousal.
   7. Use a bedtime ritual. Reading before lights out may be okay if it is not related to occupation.
   8. Learn simple self-hypnosis to use if you wake up at night. Do not try too hard to sleep; instead, concentrate on the pleasant feeling of relaxation.
   9. Use stress management in the daytime.
   10. An occasional sleeping pill is probably alright.

From Kryger MH, Roth T, Dement WC, editors: Principles and practice of sleep medicine, ed 2, Philadelphia, 1994, WB Saunders.

ruption in sleep-wake patterns, whether a dimension of morbidity of illness or a result of iatrogenic causes, reflect dysregulation of chronobiologic indices, yielding sleep-pattern disturbance. Of major importance in this area of assessment is that of substance use. This category of assessment includes obvious substances such as alcohol, tobacco, illicit drugs, caffeine, over-the-counter preparations, and excesses in dietary consumption of foods.

As a dimension of assessment in this area, the APRN needs to assess basic sleep hygiene. Box 10-2 offers guidelines to the assessment of sleep hygiene. This is a critical dimension of the assessment and should include whenever possible the use of a sleep-wake diary as presented in Fig. 10-5.

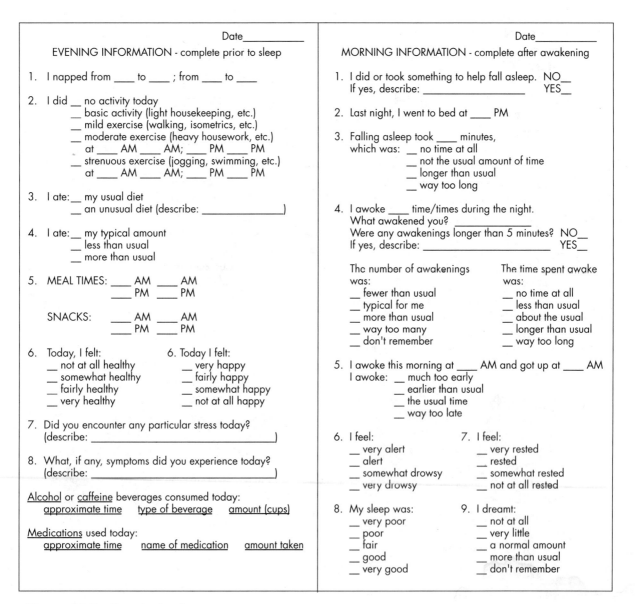

Figure 10-5 Sleep/wake diary.

To assess patterns, the patient should complete several days of the sleep-wake diary. The clinician can compare the data with the guidelines for sleep hygiene and make recommendations for appropriate adjustments in sleep-wake patterns. Additionally, the use of sleep-wake diaries will permit identification of chronobiologic phenomena such as phase advance and phase delay (formally called *circadian rhythm sleep disorder* in the *DSM IV*) (APA, 1994). Intervention strategies in dealing with advanced or delayed sleep phases are described in Box 10-3.

Influence of Age and Gender

It is important to assess the influence of age and gender on chronobiologic functioning. Fig. 10-6 depicts the normative changes in sleep across the lifespan. As is clear from the figure, as a person ages there is a lessening of all types of sleep stages and an increase in awake time. To expect that sleep will remain unchanged in adulthood is based on erroneous assumptions that in turn can have a deleterious effect on sleep. The best predictor of a poor night's sleep is the expectation of a poor night's sleep. This information needs to become part of any APRN's teaching related to sleep and sleep hygiene.

In relation to gender, women and men sleep differently because of hormonal differences and biologic processes, such as the menstrual cycle and menopause. Both of these phenomena are chronobiologic in nature and should be viewed from this perspective. Sleep in women experiencing menopause is directly related to temperature rhythm dysregulation, for which adequate chronobiologically based interventions have yet to be developed. However, using the available data on sleep, fatigue, and mood related to chronobiologic phenomena in women may yield two beneficial outcomes. First, these data enhance the APRN's perspective on the phenomena under evaluation, which improves assessment, teaching, and understanding of the lived experience. Second, these data may enhance and augment women's under-

---

box 10-3

INTERVENTION STRATEGIES WITH ADVANCED OR DELAYED SLEEP PHASE SYNDROMES

DELAYED SLEEP PHASE SYNDROME

Difficulty falling asleep, difficulty awakening, daytime sleepiness and fatigue

- *Strict adherence to sleep hygiene principles seven days/week.* Avoid variability in this schedule at all costs because the goal is to re-entrain disturbed sleep-wake rhythms.
- Exposure to bright light (approximately 10,000 lux) for 30 to 60 minutes in the morning. Monitor for potential side effects of agitation, headache, eye strain, or hypomania.
- *Selective use of 0.5 to 1 mg melatonin at bedtime.* This should be avoided in persons with a history of seasonal depression.
- If there is no response with ensured adherence to this regimen within 2 to 3 weeks, refer to a sleep disorders center for more thorough evaluation.

ADVANCED SLEEP PHASE SYNDROME

Early evening sleepiness with a bedtime much earlier than is desirable, early morning awakening

- *Exposure to bright light (approximately 10,000 lux) between 6 pm and 8 pm for 30 to 60 minutes.* Monitor for potential side effects of agitation, headache, eye strain, or hypomania.
- *Selective use of 0.5 to 1 mg melatonin at bedtime.* This should be avoided in persons with a history of seasonal depression.
- Consider delaying the bedtime by 15 minutes every 3 days.
- *Use of chronotherapy.* This involves having the person go to bed earlier by 3 hours each night until the sleep phase has advanced back to a normal bedtime.

Adapted from Reite, Ruddy, & Nagel, 1997.

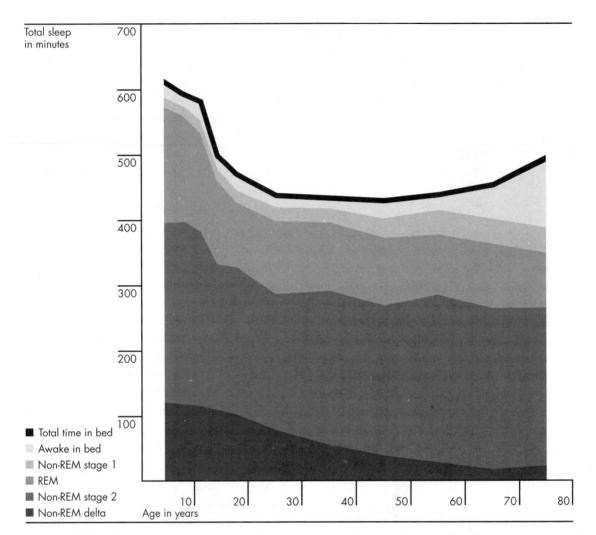

Figure 10-6   Sleep architecture across the life span. (Adapted with permission from Williams, R.L., Karacan, I., & Hursch, C.J. (1974). *Electroencephalography (EEG) of human sleep: clinical applications.* New York: John Wiley & Sons).

standing of their own sleep-wake experiences. This allows for an opportunity to understand the sleep-wake pattern as a normative dimension of a chronobiologic event, although one that may carry with it significant discomfort. Such a framework can potentially shift perspectives, enhancing the affected individual's appreciation of her own experience.

IMPLICATIONS FOR ■ THE FUTURE

Although the emerging facet of science encompassing chronobiology has been reviewed here in some detail, it is important to realize that there is much more to be learned. Some of the directions for chronobiologic research within mental health that will affect nursing practice include advancements in chronopharmacology, phototherapy, and other forms of intervention aimed at resetting the human circadian timing system. For example, chronopharmacology is the emerging branch of pharmacologic science that aims to recommend the administration of medications at optimal points in the circadian clock. This is now fairly common in chemotherapy related to oncology but is not yet practiced in psychiatry. Given variables such as diurnal variation, common to some forms of psychiatric illness, it stands to reason that such strategies would be of potential benefit. However, the research needed to substantiate these approaches has yet to be conducted in humans.

In the meantime, advanced practice in psychiatric-mental health nursing has its own set of challenges regarding the integration of chronobiologic principles into nursing science in ways that benefit the recipients of nursing care. Although some of those potential applications have been discussed here, the challenge lies in gaining a fuller understanding of chronobiologic phenomena aided by advances in nursing research. With this work underway, new strategies for nursing intervention based on chronobiologic principles can be developed, tested, and implemented. In turn, such advancements in nursing science will contribute to the larger body of emerging branches of science applied to the challenges of clinical work.

RESOURCES AND CONNECTIONS

Sleep Research Society
American Sleep Disorders Association
1610 14th Street NW, Suite 300
Rochester, MN 55901

Society for Light Treatment and Biological Rhythms
10200 West 44th Avenue, Suite 304
Wheat Ridge, Colorado 80033–2840
303-424-3697
Fax: 303-422-8894
Email: sltbr@resourcenter.com
www.websciences.org/sltbr/

Bio-Brite, Incorporated (Phototherapy)
7315 Wisconsin Avenue, Suite 1500W
Bethesda, Maryland 20814
800-621-5483
Fax: 301-961-0414
Email: biobrite@aol.com

Lighting Specialties, Incorporated (Phototherapy)
78 NW Couch Street
Portland, OR 97209
503-226-3461
Fax: 503-222-9975

Goroll, A.H., May, L.A., & Mulley, A.G. (1995). *Primary care medicine* (ed. 3). Philadelphia: J.B. Lippincott.

Kryger, M.H., Roth, T., & Dement, W.C. (1994). *Principles and practice of sleep medicine* (ed. 2). Philadelphia: W.B. Saunders.

References

Agan, R.D. (1987). Intuitive knowing as a dimension of nursing. *Advances in Nursing Science, 10*(1), 63–70.

American Nurses Association. (1994). *Psychiatric-mental health nursing psychopharmacology project*. Washington, DC: Author.

Aschoff, J. (1965). Circadian rhythms in man: a self sustained oscillator with an inherent frequency underlies human 24 hour periodicity. *Science, 148*, 1427–1432.

Avery, D., et al. (1991). Morning or evening bright light treatment of winter depression? the significance of hypersomnia. *Biological Psychiatry, 29*, 117–126.

Benca, R.M., et al. (1992). Sleep and psychiatric disorders: a meta analysis. *Archives of General Psychiatry, 49*, 651–668.

Benoliel, J.Q. (1987). Response to "Toward holistic inquiry in nursing: a proposal for synthesis of patterns and methods." *Scholarly Inquiry for Nursing Practice: An International Journal, 1*(2), 147–152.

Boulos, Z., & Terman, M. (1980). Food availability and daily biological rhythms. *Neuroscience and Biobehavioral Review, 4*, 119–131.

Broughton, R., et al. (1990). Sleep-wake biorhythms and extended sleep in man. In Montplasir, J., & Godbout, R. (Eds.). *Sleep and biological rhythms*. New York: Oxford University Press.

Carskadon, M.A., & Dement, W.C. (1994). Normal human sleep: an overview. In Kryger, M.H., Roth, T., & Dement, W.C. (Eds.). *Principles and practice of sleep medicine* (ed. 2). Philadelphia: W.B. Saunders.

Cohen, J. (1988). *Statistical power analysis for the behavioral sciences*. Hillsdale, NJ: Lawrence Erlbaum Associates.

Czeisler, C., et al. (1987). Biologic rhythm disorders, depression and phototherapy: a new hypothesis. *Sleep Disorders, 11*, 687–709.

de Candolle, A. (1832). *Vegetable physiology*. Paris: Bechet Jeune.

de Mairan, J. (1729). *Plant observations*. Paris: Histoire de L'Acadamie Royale des Sciences.

Goltzbach, S., & Heller, H. (1989). Thermoregulation. In Kryger, M.H., Roth, T., & Dement, W.C. (Eds.). *Principles and practice of sleep medicine*. Philadelphia: W.B. Saunders.

Kobert, L., & Folan, M. (1990). Coming of age in rethinking the phiosophies behind holism and nursing process. *Nursing and Health Care, 11*(16), 308–312.

Kraft-Ebing, R. (1874). *The depression*. Enke, Germany: Erlangen.

Kupferman, I. (1991). Hypothalamus and limbic system: motivation. In Kandel, E., Schwartz, J., & Jessell, T. (Eds.). *Principles of neural science*. New York: Elsevier.

Lam, R.W. (1994). Morning light therapy for winter depression: predictors of response. *Acta Psychiatrica Scandanavica, 89*(2), 97–101.

Lee, K.A. (1988). Circadian temperature rhythm in relation to menstrual cycle phase. *Journal of Biological Rhythms, 3*, 255–263.

Lin, M., et al. (1990). Night light alters menstrual cycles. *Psychiatry Research, 33*, 135–138.

Mackert, A., et al. (1991). Phototherapy in nonseasonal depression. *Biological Psychiatry, 30*, 257–268.

McBride, A.B. (1990). Psychiatric nursing in the 1990s. *Archives of Psychiatric Nursing, 4*(1), 21–28.

McEnany, G.W. (1991). Psychobiology and psychiatric nursing: a philosophical matrix. *Archives of Psychiatric Nursing, 5*(5), 255–261.

McEnany, G.W. (1994). *Effects of late partial sleep deprivation on major depression in women*. Dissertation. University of California, San Francisco.

McEnany, G.W. (1996). Rhythm and blues revisited: biological rhythm disturbance in depression. *Journal of the American Psychiatric Nurses Association, 2*(1), 15–22.

McEnany, G.W, & Lee, K.A (1997). Effects of phototherapy on nonseasonal depression in women. In review.

McEnany, G.W., & Lee, K.A (1998). A meta analysis on the effectiveness of phototherapy in nonseasonal depression. In review.

Mistlberger, R., & Rusak, B. (1994). Mechanisms and models of the human circadian timekeeping system. In Kryger, M.H., Roth, T., & Dement, W.C. (Eds.). *Principles and practice of sleep medicine* (ed. 2). Philadelphia: W.B. Saunders.

Miles, L., Raynal, D, & Wilson, M. (1977). Blind man living in normal society has circadian rhythms of 24.9 hours. *Science, 198*, 421–423.

Moore-Ede, M.C., Sulzman, F.M, & Fuller, C.A (1982). *The clocks that time us*. Cambridge, MA: Harvard University Press.

Moore, R., & Eichler, V. (1972). Loss of a circadian corticosterone rhythm following suprachiasmatic lesions in the rat. *Brain Research, 42*, 201–206.

Moore, R., & Lenn, N. (1972). A retinohypothalamic projection in the rat. *Journal of Comprehensive Neurology, 146*, 1–14.

Morin, C.M. (1996). *Relief from insomnia*. New York: Doubleday.

Nathan, K.I., et al. (1995). Biology of mood disorders. In Schatzberg, A.F., & Nemeroff, C.B. (Eds.). *Textbook of psychopharmacology*. Washington, DC: APA Press.

Nemeroff, C.B. (June, 1998). The neurobiology of depression. *Scientific American, 278*(6), 42–48.

Orem, D.E. (1980). *Nursing: concepts of practice* (ed. 2). New York: McGraw-Hill.

Parry, B, et al. (1993). Light therapy of late luteal phase dysphoric disorder. *American Journal of Psychiatry, 150*, 1417–1419.

Pothier, P.C., et al. (1990). Dilemmas and directions for psychiatric nursing in the 1990s. *Archives of Psychiatric Nursing, 4*(5), 284–291.

Reite, M., Ruddy J., & Nagel, K. (1997). *Evaluation and management of sleep disorders* (ed. 2). Washington, DC: APA Press.

Richter, C. (1965). *Biological clocks in medicine and psychiatry*. Springfield, Illinois: Charles C. Thomas.

Rosenthal, N., et al. (1990). Effects of light treatment on core body temperature in seasonal affective disorder. *Biological Psychiatry, 27*, 39–50.

Rusak, B., & Zucker, I. (1979). Neural regulation of circadian rhythms. *Physiology Review, 59*, 499–526.

Sack, R.L., & Lewy, A.J. (1997). Melatonin as a chronobiotic: treatment of circadian desynchrony in night workers and the blind. *Journal of Biological Rhythms, 12*(6), 595–603.

Schulz, H., & Lavie, P. (1985). *Ultradian rhythms in physiology and behavior*. New York: Springer-Verlag.

Sleep Research Society. (1993). *Basics of sleep behavior*. Los Angeles: University of California at Los Angeles.

Underwood, P.R (1980). Facilitating self care. In Pothier, P. (Ed.). *Psychiatric nursing*. Boston: Little-Brown.

Von Zerssen, D. (1987). What is wrong with circadian clocks in depression? In Halaris, A. (Ed.). *Chronobiology and psychiatric disorders*. New York: Elsevier.

Weaver, R. (1979). *The circadian system of man: results of experiments in time isolation*. New York: Springer-Verlag.

Complementary Therapies and Practices

CAROLYN CHAMBERS CLARK and WAILUA BRANDMAN

■ INTRODUCTION

This chapter introduces the field of complementary practice and related research. The groundbreaking study by Eisenberg and colleagues (1993) revealed that in 1990, Americans made an estimated 425 million visits to providers of complementary practices. This exceeds the 388 million visits to all U.S. primary care physicians. The money spent, $10.3 billion, was paid out of pocket and is comparable with the $12.8 billion spent annually for all U.S. hospitalizations. One in three respondents (34%) reported using at least one complementary therapy in the year, and a third of these saw providers for therapy. The average charge per visit was $27.60. About 83% also sought treatment for the same condition from a physician, and 72% did not inform their medical practitioner that they were doing so (Eisenberg et al., 1993).

Although there are hundreds of complementary approaches, the ones presented in this chapter are those for which there is a readily available research base. Because 1 in 3 individuals seeing traditional practitioners may also be using complementary approaches, it behooves advanced practice registered nurses (APRNs) in psychiatric-mental health nursing to have a basic understanding of complementary procedures and their effects. APRNs may also wish to query their patients about their use of such practices to see if they work in concert or are at odds with their traditional treatment program. Some APRNs may wish to take education offerings, become proficient in the practices, and add them to their repertoire of procedures. Combining traditional and complementary practices can provide a powerful new way for APRNs to influence patient behavior and enhance health status.

COMPLEMENTARY AND ALTERNATIVE MEDICINE AT THE NATIONAL INSTITUTES ■ OF HEALTH

The Office of Alternative Medicine (OAM) was created in early 1992 to facilitate the fair evaluation of various alternative treatment modalities by the National Institutes of Health (NIH). Initiated by Senator Tom Harkin and former House Representative Berkley Bedell, Congress appropriated $2 million to launch the OAM. Its official mandates are to facilitate the evaluation of alternative modalities that might offer promise for addressing serious health problems, establish an information clearinghouse to exchange information with the public, and support research training in alternative-complementary areas (Rubik, 1995). The OAM is also involved in developing a database for disseminating information on alternative-complementary research to researchers and the public, organizing conferences, grant writing and clinical research workshops, and networking with NIH institutes and other government agencies (OAM Mission Statement, 1998).

In 1994, the Office developed ten administrative centers for alternative-complementary research. Each center focuses on a particular disease or health problem, such as cancer, acquired immunodeficiency syndrome (AIDS), mental conditions, or pain. Their charge is to identify alternative-complementary practitioners and researchers who would like to conduct research on complementary therapies, network with them, assist them in preparing experimental protocols, evaluate their research proposals, and award small seed grants to conduct either retrospective studies or new research (Rubik, 1995).

By 1998, the budget had grown ten times and the number of complementary-alternative study citations in the literature in MEDLINE had grown 12% per year from 1966 to 1995. The number of studies more than doubled from under 4000 to almost 9000 (Office of Alternative Medicine, 1996).

■ COMPLEMENTARY PRACTICES

Acupuncture

Acupuncture is an ancient Chinese therapy based on the belief that channels (meridians) exist in the human body to transport the life energy (*qi*, or sometimes called *chi*) throughout the body. In illness, this energy gets blocked or otherwise out of balance. To reestablish harmony throughout the meridian system of twelve major pathways, special needles are inserted through the skin into certain channels at specific points. It is thought that these points act as amplifiers, boosting minute electrical signals that normally travel throughout the body.

The World Health Organization (WHO) has cited 104 conditions that acupuncture can treat, including pain, infections, inflammations, high blood pressure, addictions and detoxification, near-sightedness, hormonal imbalances, mental disorders, gastrointestinal disorders, paralysis from stroke, nervous disorders, speech aphasia, osteoarthritis, rheumatoid conditions, and environmental poisoning (Jayasuraiya, 1987). Acupuncture is believed to stimulate and direct mood-altering substances, including endorphins and enkephalins, to supply the needs of specific receptor sites. For this reason, acupuncture may be of value in addictions therapy for patients addicted to nicotine, alcohol, cocaine, or heroin (Holder, 1991).

A consensus panel convened by the NIH (Kessler, 1998) supported widespread use of acupuncture in pain and symptom management. The 12-member panel concluded that acupuncture is effective for postoperative and chemotherapy nausea and vomiting, nausea of pregnancy, and postoperative dental pain. The procedure may also be effective as adjunctive therapy for addiction, stroke, rehabilitation, headache, menstrual cramps, tennis elbow, fibromyalgia, low back pain, and asthma. The panel also recommended more research into the modality's physiologic effects and clinical potential, improved training and accreditation, and expanded insurance coverage.

State regulations for the practice of acupuncture vary. Twenty-two states license, certify, or register acupuncturists. Twelve states limit acupuncture to MDs, DOs, and DCs. Others allow acupuncture under the supervision of a licensed physician. Certification examinations are conducted by the National Commission for Certification of Acupuncturists (NCCA) (Collinge, 1996). See the Resources and Connections section for more information.

Animal-Assisted Therapy

Pets have long been known to hasten healing and reduce stress, perhaps because they give unconditional love. There is no single accepted theory that explains the therapeutic advantages of human-animal interactions. Some positive human outcomes associated with human-animal interaction include nurturance, security, touch, and social lubrication (Gammonley, 1999).

Animal-assisted therapy (AAT) is a goal-directed procedure that makes an animal an integral part of the human treatment process. AAT is directed by health professionals with special expertise and within the scope of their practice. There is no certification process for the procedure (Gammonley, 1999).

The following are some ways that animal-assisted therapy can be used (Gammonley, 1999):

- A nurse can ask a nursing home resident to care for a caged parakeet to increase communication and coordination.
- A depressed patient can be assigned to watch an exotic bird show with another depressed patient to increase stimulation and social interaction.
- A group of adolescents with behavioral problems can be given a therapeutic assignment to visit a city aquarium and then instructed about how to set up their own aquarium together.
- Speech therapists often ask patients to practice talking to an animal, possibly because there will be no negative criticism elicited.
- In rehabilitation hospitals, brushing, petting, and teaching animals to fetch provides needed movement.

Any or all of these approaches could prove useful to APRNs. See the Resources and Connections section for more information.

Aromatherapy

Aromatherapy is the practice of using the distilled essence (essential oils) of plants to promote well-being and health. Aromatherapy has been used since ancient times in Egypt, Italy, India, and China for embalming, anointing, and purifying the spirit. The term *aromatherapy* was coined by a French chemist, Ren-Maurice Gattefoss, in 1937. In aromatherapy, the essential oils of any part of plants are used to affect the human body in several ways: diffusion of microparticles of the oil into the air; external application via baths, hot and cold compresses, massages, or simply topical application; sprays of floral waters onto the body or into the air; or oral, nasal, or rectal applications via enemas.

Essential oils are believed to have antibacterial, antiviral, antispasmodic, diuretic, and vasoactive properties. They interact effectively with the immune system, nervous system, digestive system, and circulatory system, and they also modulate moods and emotions. Torri's 1988 study shows that inhalation of various essential oils leads to a change in brain wave activity. Oils were measured for an increase or decrease in brain wave activity. The most stimulating oils were jasmine, clove, basil, patchouli, peppermint, rose, and ylang ylang. The most relaxing were lavender, chamomile, bergamot, lemon, sandalwood, and marjoram.

More research is needed before the practice of aromatherapy can be integrated into mainstream health care. As with many complementary therapies, politics and health care economics also play a major role in that integration. APRNs in the future may use aromatherapy to modulate disturbed behavior in patients (Brooker et al., 1997); to alter cognition, mood, and social behavior (Martin, 1996); and to manage pain (Urba, 1996).

There is no national certification process, but the National Association for Holistic Aromatherapy is working to establish educational standards in the field. See Table 11-1 for some possible psy-

---

table 11-1

ESSENTIAL OIL USES AND CAUTIONS

ESSENTIAL OIL	USES	CAUTIONS
Chamomile	Antidepressant action, antifatigue, calms crying hyperactive children	Avoid if allergic to flowers.
Coriander	Stimulates appetite and nervous system, arouses sexual desire	
Rosewood	Dimishes depression, stimulates sexual feelings, stimulates brain, clears thinking	
Sandalwood	Releases negative emotions, promotes understanding, increases sociability, strengthens resolve, clears thought processes	
Tea tree	Restores energy, calms during emotional stress	May be irritating to sensitive skin.
Vetiver	Calms nervousness, may help with anorexia nervosa, induces restful sleep, may help overcome sexual dysfunction caused by stress	
Ylang Ylang	Calms heart palpitations, relaxes tense muscles, calms menopausal women, lifts depression, arouses sensuality	

From Wilson, 1995.
Essential oils are strong and should never be used near the eyes or taken internally. If the odor of the oil is not pleasant to a patient, do not use it. Almost all oils are used in a carrier oil such as apricot, olive, canola, or peanut. Before using essential oils with patients, consult an aromatherapy text or aromatherapist for further instructions.

chiatric-mental health uses of essential oils. See the Resources and Connections section for more information.

Biofeedback

The theory behind biofeedback is a holistic one: body and mind are interrelated. The approach originated from research in the fields of psychophysiology, learning theory, and behavioral theory (Good, 1998). Learning to self-regulate autonomic functions such as heart rate, temperature, and blood pressure occurs through biofeedback. Signals from monitoring equipment (sensors or electrodes) are converted to immediate electronic visual or audio cues that appear on a screen visible to the patient. Changes in the body produced by the patient's will are immediately fed back to the patient. Skin temperature measured by the galvanic skin response, brainwaves measured by electroencephalgrams (EEGs), and muscle tensions measured by electromyograms are some of the parameters that can be controlled by will. A beep or an illumination signals learners that they have altered bodily functions. Becoming aware of these subtle body changes by seeing them on the monitor assists patients to further alter their physiologic responses by altering the displayed signals. Additional practice improves self-regulation (Strohecker, 1994).

Biofeedback has applications for many conditions, including tension headaches, migraine headaches, chronic pain, attention-deficit hyperactive disorder (ADHD), addictions, anxiety, phobias, panic attacks, irritable bowel syndrome, hypertension, incontinence, hyperhidrosis, and Raynaud's disease (Foster, 1999). See the Resources and Connections section for more information.

Breathing Therapy

Breathing is the only body function that can be under either voluntary or automatic control. Therefore it can be a bridge between the conscious and unconscious. Observing the breath provides information about inner feeling states.

The breath is a physical, biochemical, energy, and expressive system. All of these overlap, but the different segments interact with one another, creating feeling and mirroring feeling and physical states. Spiritual teachers emphasize diaphragmatic breathing as a major vehicle for opening the heart. Negative experiences from injuries, poor posture, stress, and repressed feelings can inhibit healthful breathing. One theory holds that people who feel a lack of connectedness with themselves frequently suffer from restricted breathing patterns that may not respond to verbal therapy and other conventional treatments.

The breath is a natural biofeedback apparatus. By observing the breath, patients can learn about and alter habits, including chronic tension and anxiety (Leeds, 1985).

Dance

Dance is an "inner experience of one's being, as well as a universal means of communicating one culture to another" (Heber, 1999). The therapist and patient have an inner awareness and open interaction with the environment. This interaction provides a therapeutic self-process that can help release tension and anxiety and rechannel anger and frustration through self-expressive movements.

Dance/movement therapists work with individuals and groups at all ages and levels of physical and psychologic functioning. Children and adults often respond positively to treatment. It has been used for addictions (alcohol, drugs, eating disorders), for anxiety and affective disorders, to enhance self-esteem, to increase sensory awareness, to increase reality orientation, to enhance assertiveness, to promote interactional skills, to establish improved communication, to decrease maladaptive behaviors, and to broaden the range of emotional response (Terry, 1999). See the Resources and Connections section for more information.

Exercise

Exercise is movement of the body that promotes health and fitness. It can include dance, gardening, and various other daily activities. Exercise has been associated with a sense of accomplishment, improved mood, decreased tension, and enhanced self-image. Movement also strengthens the body, making it easier to effectively deal with mental and physical stressors (Sibille, 1999).

Herbs

Herbal therapies have been in existence from the earliest civilizations. Today, many cultures have traditional medical practices that include herbology or phytology. Many modern medicines were originally prepared from plants, and some of them are prepared synthetically today to mass market them and control quality. Herbal medicine is a licensed profession in Germany, and physicians there must study phytology before they take their certification boards. The use of herbs is practiced widely in Great Britain as well.

An *herb* is any part of a plant, including its flower petals, roots, and bark. These plant parts contain naturally occurring chemicals that interact biologically with the human physiology when taken internally or applied topically. Herbs have many actions, including anthelmintic, antiinflammatory, antimicrobial, antispasmodic, astringent, carminative, demulcent, diuretic, emmenagogue, expectorant, hepatic, hypotensive, laxative, and tonic. Herbal medicines are available in the form of teas, whole herbs, capsules, tablets, powders, extracts, tinctures, salves, balms, essential oils, and ointments. Today, grocery stores, health food stores, and drug stores sell many forms of herbal medicines. Ingestion of herbs should always be undertaken with the guidance of an expert practitioner to ensure high-quality, safe products.

Herbs work slowly and so are believed to be most effective on chronic and degenerative diseases. They are an excellent complementary therapy for APRNs to consider in their treatment plans; however, more research and articles on the effects of these substances is needed. There is no national certification process in this country, but the School of Phytotherapy in East Sussex, England provides a course that meets the requirements for medical herbalist in the United Kingdom. See Table 11-2 for herbs that may be useful for psychiatric-mental health complaints. See the Resources and Connections section for more information.

Homeopathy

Homeopathy was founded by Samuel Hahnemann, an eighteenth century German physician. Today it is an accepted practice in the United States, Europe, South America, Central America, and India. French pharmacies are required to carry homeopathic remedies, and England has homeopathic hospitals and outpatient clinics. There are several colleges of homeopathy in the United States, and the Food and Drug Administration (FDA) regulates homeopathic remedies, recognizing them officially as drugs.

The main principles of homeopathy are the law of similars (like cures like), the law of the infinitesimal dose (the more a remedy is diluted, the greater its potency), and the principle that illnesses are specific to the individual. Homeopathic therapy treats presenting symptoms, which often mask underlying emotional or physical states. Patients may get worse before they get better, because the masking conditions are removed, revealing deeper, more chronic conditions that can then be recognized and treated. This is known as the *healing crisis*, during which symptoms can increase. Once the crisis passes, healing occurs (Strohecher, 1994). Certification information is available from the Council for Homeopathic Certification. See the Resources and Connections section for more information.

table 11-2

HERBS AND THEIR USE

HERBS	CONDITIONS	CONTRAINDICATIONS
1. 2 to 3 capsules/day of valerian root, passion flower, wood betony, black cohosh root, skullcap, hops, ginger root combination	Anxiety, fear, being overworked, hysteria, insomnia, hyperactivity, restlessness	Do not use while driving (pp. 213–221)
2. 2 to 6 capsules/day of cayenne, siberian ginseng, gotu kola, kelp, peppermint leaves, ginger root combination	Depression, emotional exhaustion, fatigue	None (pp. 101–106)
3. 4 to 8 capsules/day of licorice root, gotu kola, siberian ginseng, ginger combination	Fatigue, exhaustion	Ensure adequate serum potassium levels (pp. 25–30)
4. 4 capsules, three times/day of garlic, valerian, black cohosh root, cayenne, and kelp combination	Anxiety attacks	None (pp. 9–16)
5. Gingko	Depression	See Schubert & Halama, 1993
6. St. John's wort	Mild-moderate depression	See Linde et al., 1996; Nordfors & Hartvig, 1997

All page numbers refer to information in Mowry, 1986.

Humor Therapy

Humor therapy uses laughter to decrease stress and pain. Humor has been in use since biblical times. The modern use of humor therapy began in the 1930s when clowns were brought into hospitals to cheer up children hospitalized with polio (Bennett, 1999).

Psychoneuroimmunology (PNI) theory explains how humor affects health status. According to PNI theory, interventions that lead to changes in hormones, neurotransmitters, and immune functioning can influence health status (Solomon, 1987). Although humor could be misinterpreted by those with poor reality testing, for others humor may be a useful intervention.

Imagery

Imagery is a means of communication among body, mind, and spirit, making information available through imagination to the five senses (Dossey, 1995). Humans are constantly using imagery, although not everyone is aware of it. Imagery affects physiology (Taylor, Lee, & Young, 1997) through neuropeptides, hormones, and endorphins offering pain relief, relaxation, stress reduction, and mood modulation. Through association and synthesis, imagery can provide insight and perspective into health (Rossman, 1989). Emotions, and therefore health, are intimately connected to mental images (Strohecker, 1994).

There are two types of images: active and receptive. *Active imagery* includes forming an image consciously and can be used to direct physiologic or emotional processes. *Receptive imagery* occurs when external images are presented and can be used to discover or assess physical illness. Relaxation and imagery have a complementary relationship, each enhancing the other. Relaxation, through breathing exercise and suggestion, precedes imagery sessions; imagery can be used to enhance relaxation. Images can be guided by a therapist during a session, learned from a therapist for later self-administration (using videotapes or audiotapes), or patient-developed once the process has been learned (Clark, 1996).

Imagery is already practiced by many nurses. In the future, advanced practice will rely more on this unobtrusive, noninvasive therapy for prevention and treatment of chronic illnesses (e.g., hypertension, pain, and depression) and acute problems (e.g., panic disorder and phobias). It has also been used to treat chemical dependence. The Academy for Guided Imagery provides professional training and a certification program in interactive guided imagery. See the Resources and Connections section for more information.

Light and Color Therapy

Upon entering the human eye, light activates the color- and light-sensitive receptor cells (photoreceptors) to send neurotransmitters, via the optic nerve, to the hypothalamus. The endocrine system is stimulated there to regulate the immune system, the autonomic nervous system, the digestive system, the limbic system, circadian rhythm, sexual functioning, and the aging process. Cerebral and motor cortex activities are now believed to be affected by visually perceived light as well. Full-spectrum light, which contains all the light wavelengths, is necessary to maintain health. A 1990 study by the U.S. Navy (Garland et al., 1990) demonstrates that the incidence of melanoma is higher in those with restricted exposure to sunlight and lower in those who work both indoors and outdoors in the sunlight. This suggests that vitamin D production (from exposure to sunlight) inhibits melanoma growth, and brief, regular exposure to sunlight maintains appropriate levels of this important vitamin.

Melatonin, a sedative, is produced only during darkness. It is important for people who work night shifts or keep irregular work shift schedules to get enough regular exposure to sunlight to reduce their melatonin production to normal levels or face the risk of developing seasonal affective disorder (SAD), heart disease, back pain, respiratory problems, sleep disorders, and ulcers (Strohecker, 1994).

Several forms of light therapy, including bright light, cold laser, colored light, full-spectrum light, syntonic optometry, ultraviolet light, and whole-brain light therapy are currently available. A wide range of conditions respond to light therapy, including hyperactivity in children, SAD, bulimia, altered menstrual cycles, jaundice, delayed sleep phase syndrome, jet lag, vitiligo, psoriasis, symptoms of AIDS, infections, cancer, asthma, rheumatoid arthritis, traumatic brain injury, headache, and photocurrent deficiency. Whole-brain therapy is said to improve mood, physical coordination, poor self-esteem, SAD, depression, anxiety, fear, night blindness, and other conditions.

Color therapy is the application of colored light to the body for the purpose of correcting disharmony (Strawn, 1999). The power of color therapy is decribed in the biblical book of Genesis (the rainbow as a sign of God's protection) and used in the Hindu tradition (each of the seven chakras, or energy centers, is associated with a color of the rainbow).

Colors represent light waves in motion, vibrating at measurable and distinct rates (Strawn, 1999). One system of color healing theorizes that disease is either acute (hot) or chronic (cold) and that cold or warm colors can treat the disorder. Hot colors are scarlet, red, orange, yellow, and lemon. Cold colors are purple, violet, indigo, and turquoise (Strawn, 1999). There is no certification program in light or color therapy.

Massage

Massage is the oldest known healing art. Massage was used in Asia at least since 3000 BC. In China, it was one of the four classical forms of medical treatment, along with acupuncture, moxabustion (heat energy), and herbalism. In the East, massage remains an integral part of family life and is taught to children in much the same way youngsters are taught to brush their teeth in the United States.

The effects of massage are physiologic, mechanical, psychologic, and reflexive. Massage is a unique form of communication and caring. It is also a science; a systematic manipulation of body tissue produces nervous, muscular, circulatory, visceral, and metabolic effects (Knaster, 1996). The American Massage Therapy Association provides information about certification. See the Resources and Connections section for more information.

Meditation

Several thousand years old, meditation is a complementary therapy that is easy to use, can be done in any setting, and is available to everyone. The two major categories of meditation—mindfulness and concentrative—include almost all the many different types of meditation.

Mindfulness meditation is a process that is like perceiving the world through the wide-angle lens of a camera. In a relaxed state, one maintains awareness of all the perceptions that enter the mind without becoming attached or involved in them but simply noting them and letting them pass by. Walking meditation is an example of this type. It is done with eyes open, paying attention to the experience of each foot making contact with the ground. The focus is on the experience of the sensations of the whole body as it is involved in breathing and walking.

Concentrative meditation is the simplest form of meditation. It aims to quiet the mind by focusing on a sound, image, or the breath while becom-

ing more relaxed, ultimately allowing an increased clarity and awareness to emerge into consciousness (Strohecker, 1994). Both of these states of meditation increase the production of alpha waves by the brain. In a meditative state, the cortisol level, heart rate, and blood pressure drop to normal levels. The general metabolic rate declines, and the meditator enters a hypometabolic state that is more conducive to healing and creativity (Taylor, 1997). Meditation benefits the body, mind, and spirit: anxiety, pain, blood pressure, and chronic illnesses are regulated; mood improves, psychologic response to stress is reduced, one is more alert and creative; and long-term meditators report an interest in spirituality. APRNs are learning to recommend and teach meditation to their patients. There is no certification process for meditation. See the Resources and Connections section for more information.

Music

Music can promote change and enhance living. It is a healing art based on tonal sound intervals and harmonies that give meaning through rhythm, volume, and lyrics. Music can be used to improve physical coordination, concentration skills, fine motor movement, socialization skills, and self-esteem; to develop basic life skills; and to expand the quality of life.

Music is often used to decrease anxiety and stress and prevent depression by using hypnotic suggestion. Music is also used as a backdrop for relaxation tapes (Music Therapy Program, 1997; National Association for Music Therapy, 1997; Oz et al., 1996).

Nutritional Approaches

Nurses learn nutritional information in nursing school, but in today's world of commercial agriculture and special interest politics, it is not enough to know which foods provide which nutrients.

More contaminated and processed foods are being eaten. These foods contribute to poor health and degenerative diseases, indirectly accounting for more than two thirds of deaths in the United States (Strohecker, 1994).

Foods can contain any or all of the following detrimental substances: dyes, stabilizers, preservatives, pesticides, hormones, antibiotics, and industrial pollutants. Ingested over a lifetime, these contaminants may increase the risk of decreased immune function, neurotoxicity, allergic reactions, birth defects, and cancers.

It is recommended that the best diet (whole diet) is from plants that are lower on the food chain. These foods, as natural and as whole as possible, with the least amount of processing and additives, are high in carbohydrates and fiber, low in animal fats and saturated oils, and low in sugar and salt (Steinman, 1990; Clark, 1996).

Prevention is now, and will be even more in the future, of major importance in the role of advanced practice nursing. The use of foods and supplements to maintain health will likely increase in importance as the knowledge base grows. See the Resources and Connections section for more information.

Self-Hypnosis

Hypnosis has been used for at least 200 years, and the art of suggestion has been used by folk healers for millennia. Hypnosis includes focusing awareness or concentration while deeply relaxed (Rossi, 1993). Self-hypnosis begins by relaxing and focusing on slow, deep, regular breaths. Once in a relaxed state, a person can speak or think statements to himself or herself that reflect a desired change.

Autogenics is a form of self-hypnosis that allows the participant to induce the feeling of warmth and heaviness associated with a trance state. Johannes H. Schultz, a Berlin psychiatrist, combined autosuggestion with some yoga techniques and developed the system of autogenics. The exercises have been used to increase resistance to stressors, reduce sleep disorders and anxiety, and enhance the workings of many body systems (Murphy, 1999).

The exercises can be completed in a comfortable sitting or lying position, in an attitude of passive concentration. The therapy is not recommended for children under 5 years of age or for adults who lack motivation or have severe emotional disorders. Early exercises are focused on heaviness ("My left [nondominant] arm is heavy. Both my arms are heavy. My right leg is heavy. My left leg is heavy. Both my legs are heavy"). Later exercises focus on warmth with an objective of attaining relaxation in blood vessels ("My right [dominant] arm is warm. My left [nondominant] arm is warm. Both my legs are warm. My right leg is warm. Both my legs are warm. My arms and legs are warm"). In later sessions, the patient focuses on the heartbeat being calm and regular and breathing being calm and relaxed. Other exercises are used to treat ulcers, diabetes, or any condition involving bleeding, dizziness, pain, and tightness. Additional statements are interspersed with standard themes including, "I feel quiet. I withdraw my thoughts from the surroundings, and I feel serene and still. I am at peace. I feel inward quietness, and deep within my mind I can visualize and experience myself as relaxed and comfortable and still" (Davis, Eshelman, & McKay, 1995).

The statements can also be on an audiotape. Relaxing music or sounds of nature can be used to heighten the state of relaxation. According to the WHO, 90% of the general population can be induced into a superficial hypnotic state, and 20% to 30% are highly receptive to hypnotherapy, which enables them to enter a deeper trance state called the *somnambulistic state* (Bannerman et al., 1983). These individuals benefit most from the hypnosis.

Once in a hypnotic state, a person's physiology begins to change, as it has been shown to do in states of relaxation. Activation switches from the sympathetic nervous system to the parasympathetic system. Cortisol levels drop, extremity temperatures rise, blood pressure drops, and the heart rate slows. In this state, physical and emotional healing can take place. Hypnotism is a skill and an art that APRNs can learn in order to teach self-hypnosis to their patients (Clark, 1998). The American Society for Clinical Hypnosis certifies hypnotherapists.

Therapeutic Touch

Many nurses are familiar with the complementary practice called *therapeutic touch* (TT). TT was developed in 1972 by Dolores Krieger and her colleague Dora Kunz, a healer. Krieger has taught this practice to more than 48,000 health care professionals, and TT is now practiced in 75 countries throughout the world (Horrigan, 1998). TT is founded on the precept that human beings are energy fields.

The practice begins with the practitioner "centering" or attuning with his or her higher self. Centering and the intent to heal are essential components of the process. During the diagnostic phase, the practitioner passes the hands slowly parallel to the subject's body, sensing disturbance in the subject's energy field with sensors in the palms of the hands while keeping centered. The field is then unruffled with the hands, pushing the pressure out away from the body, dissipating the energy and releasing it into the ethers. Another assessment is completed after unruffling to see if the field is balanced (Horrigan, 1998).

TT is used with neonates, children, adults, and elders for pain relief, reduction of blood pressure, activation of enzymes, and production of hemoglobin (Strohecker, 1994). It has also been used for mood disorders and anxiety (Fig. 11-1).

As with so many complementary practices, the research that has been conducted is often with small samples, with questionable protocols and statistical measures, and/or without control groups. As a result, findings have been inconsistent. As more research is completed and APRNs learn about and become certified in TT, the practice will be integrated into advanced practice nursing. There is no certification process for TT, but

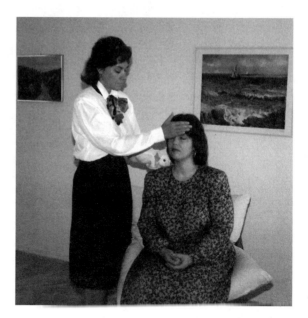

Figure 11-1 Therapeutic touch.

it may be practiced by any practitioner who has successfully completed a beginning workshop addressing the cognitive and experiential aspects of TT (Nurse Healers-Professional Associates). See the Resources and Connections section for more information.

Yoga

Yoga was one of the first alternative-complementary practices to influence the emergence of mind/body medicine through research studies conducted at the Menninger Clinic on yogis decades ago. Yoga's purpose is to integrate the body, mind, and spirit and is based on the yoga Sutra teaching that, "if the mind is chronically restless and agitated, the health of the body will be compromised, and if the body is in poor health, mental strength and clarity will be adversely affected" (Strohecker, 1994).

The practice of yoga consists of yogic postures, breath control, purification and detoxification of the body, and meditation. Yoga initiates the relaxation response, which is known to aid healing through regulation of the autonomic nervous system. It also appears to control blood flow through its various positions and breathing, as well as stimulating the flow of prana (life energy) and strengthening the immune system. Yoga is beneficial for children, adults, and the elderly. It is also an integral part of Ayurvedic medicine. There are many schools of yoga, including Hatha, Siddha, Tantra, Iyengar, Kriya, Sivananda, Kundalini, Integral, and Ashtanga.

In the future, many APRNs may find themselves practicing yoga as a way of taking care of the care giver. They may also recommend it to many of their patients for health maintenance and prevention. The Rocky Mountain Institute of Yoga and Ayurveda offers certificate programs in yoga teaching and Ayurveda and yoga therapy. See the Resources and Connections section for more information.

RESEARCH FINDINGS AND ■ CLINICAL USES

Research in most complementary practices is in its infancy. Findings are often mixed, and complementary practitioners are not always sophisticated researchers. Many Asian and old world procedures have been used for hundreds and sometimes thousands of years and proved their efficacy and lack of side effects over the years. Although the gold standard in the United States is the experimental study, it must be remembered that most medical and nursing procedures have not been validated by scientific study either (Collinge, 1996) and that adverse medication reactions account for up to 140,000 deaths annually in the United States and cost over $136 billion (Classen, 1997).

There is a need for more research on almost every complementary practice; however, the general public is flocking to complementary practitioners, some because they appreciate the listening skills of many complementary practitioners, dislike the side effects of medications and surgery, and/or have been told that there is nothing further that traditional health care can provide (Clark, 1999). Evidence for the use of complementary practices with ADHD, aging, Alzheimer's disease, anger, anxiety, and depression follows.

Attention-Deficit Hyperactivity Disorder

Research findings are available for complementary practices in the treatment of ADHD. Acupuncture, aromatherapy, exercise, food and supplements, and other lifestyle factors have been studied.

Acupuncture. Sonenklar (1997) investigated the efficacy of using single-point acupuncture (ear) treatment for a small number of children with ADHD. Seven children completed the study. Three of them showed improvement during the treatment phase, one showed improvement during the placebo phase, and two showed worsening throughout. The researcher suggested that acupuncture, a simple procedure with minimal risk, might be effective for children.

Foods and supplements. In a double-blind, placebo-controlled food challenge with 16 children, Boris and Mandel (1994) demonstrated a significant improvement on placebo days compared with open-challenge days when children reacted to many foods, dyes, and/or preservatives. The study demonstrated the beneficial effect of eliminating reactive foods and artificial colors in children with ADHD. The researchers concluded that dietary factors may play a significant causal role in ADHD.

Carter and colleagues (1993) studied 78 children referred to a diet clinic because of hyperactive behavior. All of the children were placed on a few-food elimination diet. Fifty-nine improved their behavior during this open trial. For 19 of the participants, it was possible to disguise foods or additives by mixing them with other tolerated foods and testing their effect. The provoking foods significantly worsened behavior ratings and impaired psychologic test performance.

Rowe and Rowe (1994) used a 21-day double-blind, placebo-controlled, repeated-measures study of 200 children to show that behavioral changes in irritability, restlessness, and sleep disturbance were associated with intake of tartrazine, a synthetic food coloring, in 24 children. The use of a food diary to identify potential behavioral irritants followed by nutritional counseling may be of benefit to advanced nurse practitioners who wish to understand and influence irritability, hyperactivity, restlessness, and sleep disturbance.

Lifestyle factors: smoking. Milberger and colleagues (1996) investigated the role of maternal smoking during pregnancy in the etiology of ADHD in 140 boys between 6 and 17 years of age and a normal comparison group (n = 120). About 22% of the ADHD children had a maternal history of smoking during pregnancy compared with 8% of the non-ADHD children. This positive association remained significant after adjustment for parental intelligence quotient (IQ) and ADHD and socioeconomic status. Significant differences in IQ were found between those children whose mothers smoked during pregnancy and those whose mothers did not smoke. Counseling pregnant women regarding ways to cease smoking is a preventive measure with the potential to affect the development of ADHD in offspring.

Symmetric tonic neck reflex exercises. Bender and colleagues' research (Bender, 1971; Cook, 1973) and clinical writings (O'Dell & Cook, 1997) indicate that many children experience behavioral and academic difficulties, including ADD/ADHD, as a result of an immature symmetric tonic neck reflex (STNR).

During normal growth and development, the STNR governs head position until 2 years of age. Retention of this reflex past that age is abnormal and can lead to muscular tension in the child's arms and legs in relation to head movements, and involuntary movements that can interfere with the child gaining bodily control. When a child is unable or not allowed to crawl sufficiently, the reflex remains in control (O'Dell & Cook, 1997).

Children with immature STNR are often diagnosed with ADHD when any of the following difficulties may actually be due to immature STNR: sitting "inappropriately," squirming, daydreaming, writing poorly, writing laboriously, moving awkwardly or clumsily, reversing letters or numbers, and avoiding athletics or poor development of needed athletic skills.

Bender and her students developed exercises that can be used with anyone over 5 years of age (O'Dell & Cook, 1997) that may be useful to APRNs. Practitioners can counsel mothers to allow their children to crawl and not walk too soon, refer mothers and their children to Bender practitioners, or try Bender's exercises with ADHD patients who are not responding to other treatments. Like so many complementary practices, the Bender exercises are noninvasive and have no known side effects when used correctly.

Aging and Psycho-Geriatric Concerns

Several complementary procedures may positively influence the aging process in older adults and other patients. Evidence is accumulating that specific behaviors can enhance performance despite age. For example, although brain cells may shrink by 10% between 20 and 70 years of age, response time may be reduced, but not significantly. The power to think is the same even though it may take a little longer to remember things or solve complex problems. Challenging the brain at any age helps sprout dendrites that enhance communication between cells. Although it is believed that sensory perception diminishes with age, after 6 years of volunteers smelling lemons and some 40 other scents, including natural gas and bubble gum, Dr. Marc Heft (Daughtry, 1997) determined that aging has little effect on smell, taste, or touch. Using the Pennsylvania Smell Identification Test, in which participants scratched and sniffed cards with different scents on them ranging from licorice to paint thinner, the researchers found that women were better able to identify different scents than men. There were no differences between gender for the other senses. Clinical practices recommended by Heft for enhancing sensory and thought processes in older adults include engaging in regular exercise and activities that stretch the mind (such as reading) and staying out of the sun, which speeds the aging process and indirectly affects the skin's senses.

Animal-assisted therapy. Fick (1993) conducted a study to determine the effect of the presence and absence of a dog on the frequency and types of social interactions among nursing home residents during a socialization group. Point sampling was used to evaluate the behavior of 36 male residents at a VA Medical Center. A significant difference in verbal interactions occurred among residents with the dog present, providing additional support for the value of animal-assisted therapy for increasing socialization among residents in long-term care facilities.

Thomas (1994) reported on using birds, dogs, cats, rabbits, and plants in a nursing home environment. Results indicate a significant reduction in the use of psychotropic drugs as well as a 15% reduction in resident deaths compared with a control group who did not use animals, birds, and plants. Zisselman and colleagues (1996) also reported positive results from using pet therapy with geriatric psychiatry patients. Based on these results, animal-assisted therapy should be considered by APRNs as a vehicle for enhancing communication, reducing medication intake in older adults, and enhancing health status.

Exercise. Moderate-intensity exercise programs can improve self-reported sleep in healthy older adults between 50 and 76 years of age according to a study by King and colleagues (1997). Forty-three adults participated in the research. Exercise group participants had four sessions of exercise per week, two sessions at the local YMCA lasting 1 hour, and two sessions at home lasting 40 minutes, for 16 weeks. Controls continued their usual activities. Exercise participants had significant improvement on the self-report Pittsburgh Sleep Quality Index for sleep duration, quality, and onset. Sleep disturbances are a major symptom for many psychiatric and mental health conditions. Exercise could be recommended by APRNs as a method of improving sleep quality in patients.

Foods and supplements. Perrig, Perrig, and Stahelin (1997) examined the relationship between antioxidants and memory performance in the old and very old. Noting that aging processes, and specifically brain aging, are believed to be associated with free radical action, they hypothesized that plasma antioxidant vitamin levels would correlate with cognitive performance in healthy older adults. In a total of 442 participants, the researchers found that free recall, recognition, and vocabulary were correlated significantly with vitamin C and beta-carotene. The two antioxidants remained significant predictors, especially of semantic memory, after controlling for possible confounding variables including age, education, and gender. Memory is certainly a factor in the ability to work through psychiatric-mental health issues and one that should be of interest to APRNs. Nutritional skills may increasingly complement counseling skills.

Lindenbaum and colleagues (1994) found that vitamin B_{12} deficiency was extremely common in older people. None showed signs of pernicious anemia, the classic cause of B_{12} deficiency. A more likely cause identified by the lead researcher was that a sizable group of the elderly population did not secrete enough acid and pepsin to liberate B_{12} from food. Part of the problem could be corrected by taking crystalline B_{12} in supplements, which can be absorbed by older adults who secrete too little stomach acid. Because B_{12} deficiency is dangerous and can lead to irreversible damage to the nervous system, Lindenbaum advised that anyone with an unexplained neuropsychiatric problem should be tested for B_{12} deficiency. If the result is less than 258 pmol/L, not the usual 149 pmol/L cutoff, there is a definite suspicion of B_{12} deficiency.

Dance. Twenty-six individuals were selected at random from the psychogeriatric population at the Psychiatric Hospital in Havana, Cuba. During a year of participation in psychoballet, there was an improvement in interpersonal relationships and a decrease in the need for psychopharmaceuticals (Acanda Roque, Gonzales Valente, & Fialio Sanza, 1990).

Herbs. Drabaek and colleagues (1996) tested the effects of *Ginkgo biloba* extract versus a placebo in a randomized, double-blind cross-over study. Questionnaires based on visual analog scales were used to quantify the severity of leg pain, impairment of concentration, and inability to remember. The researchers did not find any significant changes in either peripheral blood pressures, walking distances, or the severity of leg pain. Systemic blood pressure was reduced both by placebo and by the Ginkgo. The impairment of concentration and the inability to remember were both reduced when comparing results during active treatment (Ginkgo) with the those during placebo treatment. The researchers concluded that treatment with the *Ginkgo biloba* extract did improve some cognitive functions in older individuals with moderate arterial insufficiency.

Alzheimer's Disease

Crawford (1997) reviewed the literature and found a link between reduced cerebral blood flow and Alzheimer's disease. Neurofibrillary tangles, senile plaques, cell loss, and impaired synaptic function characterize the problem. Cholinergic, noradrenergic, and dopaminergic neurons are lost. Oxidative stress and the accumulation of free radicals lead to neuronal degeneration and excessive lipid peroxidation in the brain. Several complementary approaches have been found helpful for enhancing cerebral blood flow and cognitive ability. A discussion of researched complementary practices for symptoms of Alzheimer's disease follows.

Foods and supplements. Sugar has been identified as a risk factor in Alzheimer's disease because it is linked to reduced cerebral blood flow (Crawford, 1997). Some other foods and supplements have proved helpful, including vitamins A, C, and E; beta-carotene; and L-carnitine.

A double-blind, placebo-controlled, randomized, multicenter trial was conducted with 341 individuals with Alzheimer's disease of moderate severity. All participants received either 10 mg of the monoamine oxidase (MAO) inhibitor, selegine, 2000 IU of vitamin E, or a placebo. Both selegiline and vitamin E slowed the progression of Alzheimer's disease (Sano et al., 1997).

A 20-year study at the University of Basel by geriatric professor Hannes Staehelin (1997) of Switzerland on Swiss men and women between 65 and 94 years of age found that those who had high levels of vitamin C and beta-carotene in their blood performed better in memory tests. Vitamin C and beta-carotene were significant predictors of ability in tests of vocabulary and beta-carotene in tests of recognition. The research showed that memory functions could be linked to increased oxidative stress with aging. Neurons in brain cells are challenged by free radicals and antioxidants that protect the neurons from damage. Shaehelin suggested that antioxidants are ideally obtained from natural sources such as fruits and vegetables, but supplements might be necessary.

Pettegrew and colleagues (l995) used a double-blind placebo study to test the effect of acetyl-L-carnitine (an amino acid–like substance) with seven probable Alzheimer's disease individuals who were then compared over the course of a year by clinical and 31P magnetic resonance spectroscopic measures with five placebo-treated probable Alzheimer's disease individuals and 21 age-matched healthy controls. Compared with Alzheimer's disease individuals on placebo, acetyl-L-carnitine–treated participants showed significantly less deterioration in their mini-mental status and Alzheimer's Disease Assessment Scale test scores. Also, the decrease in phosphomonoester levels observed in both the acetyl-L-carnitine and placebo Alzheimer's disease groups at entry was normalized, as were high-energy phosphate levels, but only in the treatment group.

Thal and colleagues (1996) also studied the effect of acetyl-L-carnitine, using an acetyl-L-carnitine hydrochloride (ALCAR) formulation. Their 1-year, double-blind, placebo-controlled, randomized, parallel-group study compared the efficacy and safety of ALCAR with placebo in individuals with mild to moderate probable Alzheimer's disease 50 years of age or older. The participants were given 3 g/day of ALCAR or placebo (l g tid) for 12 months. Of the 4311 individuals who entered the study, 83% completed 1 year of treatment. Early onset Alzheimer's disease individuals (65 years of age or younger at study entry) on ALCAR declined more slowly than those on placebo and tolerated the supplement well.

Herbs. Itil (1995) reported findings from a pilot bioequivalency study. Findings indicate significant quantitative CNS effects in *Ginkgo* similar to other psychoactive compounds classified as cognitive activators. Kanowski and colleagues (1996) used a prospective, randomized, double-blind, placebo-controlled, multicenter study using *Ginkgo biloba* special extract EGb 761 (240 mg) or placebo with 216 individuals diagnosed with presenile or senile primary degenerative dementia of the Alzheimer type (DAT). Those taking Ginkgo showed a significant positive difference from the placebo group on the Clinical Global Impressions Test, the Syndrom-Kurz test for attention, and memory, and the Nurnberger Alters-Beobachtungsskala test for behavioral assessment of activities of daily life. Haase, Halama, and Horr (1996) had similar results with short-term intervenous infusion therapy for those with moderate dementia. Results include an improvement in cognitive performance and increased ability to cope with the demands of daily living.

LeBars and colleagues (1997) at the New York Institute for Medical Research reported that an extract of *Ginkgo biloba* (EGb 761) may be as effective as any drug, hormone (primarily estrogen), or vitamin (E) currently used to treat Alzheimer's disease. About 27% of participants (n = 309 with a 1/3 dropout rate) who took 120 mg/day of the herb for 6 months or longer showed improvement in mental functioning (reasoning, memory, and ability to learn) compared with those who took a placebo (14%).

Mirror use. Tabak, Bergman, and Alpert (1996) reported the use of the mirror as a therapeutic tool for patients with dementia. One hundred people suffering from dementia (67 women and 33 men between 67 and 95 years of age) comprised the sample. Most responses to looking in the mirror were positive and raised awareness regarding self-care. In a few participants, looking into the mirror aroused feelings of anger or despair, but this was followed by relief and calmness. The use of mirrors allowed caregivers to communicate more clearly with participants. Staff reported that the use of mirrors was an inexpensive and efficient therapeutic tool for improving care.

Music. Dinner music can help nursing home residents eat more calmly; feed themselves more than usual; decrease restlessness (Ragneskog et al., 1996a); appear less depressed, irritable, and fearful (Ragneskog et al., 1996b); and significantly reduce the cumulative incidence of total agitated behaviors, physically nonaggressive behaviors, and verbally agitated behaviors (Goddaer & Abraham, 1994).

Anger

Although release of anger can be adaptive, alerting humans that something is wrong, it often causes problems by creating additional frustration and anger. Holding anger in can also lower self-esteem, lead to depression (Tavris, 1984; Thomas, 1993), and affect work performance (Brooks, Thomas, & Droppleman, 1996). Several complementary therapies have shown promise for patients who wish to manage their anger expression constructively.

Breathing therapy. Appels and colleagues (1997) reported the use of breathing therapy to reduce anger in 30 postangioplasty participants and the 65 controls who comprised the sample that was followed for an average period of 16 and 18 months, respectively. The results indicated that breathing therapy can reduce exhaustion and hostility, thereby reducing the risk of a new cardiac event. Teaching patients breathing techniques may assist in reducing anger and hostility and could become a standard advanced practice nursing procedure.

Exercise. Petajan and colleagues (1996) randomly assigned 54 people diagnosed with multiple sclerosis to exercise or nonexercise groups. As a result of participating in an exercise group, anger scores were significantly reduced.

Jette and colleagues (1996) reported a videotaped, home-based strength-training program (Strong-for-Life) with older adults between 66 and 87 years of age. Participants were identified from the Medicare beneficiary list and randomized to exercise or no exercise. Older males who exercised achieved significant differences in perceived anger, tension, and overall social functioning. Exercise should be considered as a regular treatment for patients with anger.

Humor and laughter. Keltner and Bonanno (1997) investigated the use of laughter to reduce distress and anger. To test their hypothesis that laughter facilitates an adaptive response by increasing the psychologic distance from stress and enhancing social relations, they created measures of bereaved adults' laughter and smiling. Duchenne laughter, which involves orbicularis oculi muscle action, related to self reports of reduced anger and increased enjoyment, dissociation of distress, better social relations, and positive responses from strangers.

Anxiety

Complementary therapies are effective treatments for moderate and intense anxiety. Some approaches for which there is clinical, but not significant, research support include avoiding drinking more than four cups of coffee, tea, or cola drinks a day; pressing acupressure calming points; using Bach flower remedies; breathing from the abdominal area; keeping a panic diary of each attack, what triggers it, and individual coping responses to the attack; using homeopathic remedies such as *Aurum metallicum* and *Ignatia*; and taking antistress vitamins (B-complex or B-complex and C).

Autogenic training. Sakai (1996) reported the use of the second autogenic training exercise for panic disorder with 34 individuals treated by the researcher. Fifteen participants had no further

symptoms, nine were much improved, five improved, and five remained unchanged.

Combined treatments to reduce anxiety. Field and colleagues (1997) reported a study testing the immediate effects of brief massage therapy, muscle relaxation with visual imagery, muscle relaxation, and a social support group session for job stress among health care workers. All groups reported decreases in anxiety, depression, fatigue, and confusion as well as increased vigor, which suggests that all therapies were equally effective.

Gagne and Toye (1994) found that both relaxation (treatment) and therapeutic touch (placebo, control group) produced significant reductions in reported anxiety in 30 individuals in a psychiatric facility. Rest, music therapy, and music-video therapy were equally helpful in producing a relaxation response in a study of individuals undergoing heart surgery (Barnason, Zimmerman, & Nieveen, 1995).

Dance. Leste and Rust (1984) studied the effects of modern dance on anxiety. State anxiety was assessed before and after a 3-month education program using the Spielberger State-Trait Anxiety Inventory. The class in modern dance was compared with a physical education group, a music group, and a mathematics control group. Dance training significantly reduced anxiety, but no control activities did. Noreau and colleagues (1995) investigated the use of aerobic dance-based exercise for 19 people with rheumatoid arthritis who participated in a 12-week biweekly program. Ten people served as controls. Besides improvement in movement and decrease in pain, the treatment group also showed positive changes in anxiety and other negative feelings.

Exercise. Positive changes in anxiety and tension were observed after a 12-week exercise program for individuals with arthritis (Noreau et al, 1995). Exercise was also found useful in significantly decreasing anxiety in women during radiation therapy treatment for breast cancer (Mock et al., 1997). Kugler, Seelbach, and Kruskemper (1994) completed a meta-analysis of 15 studies on the psychologic effects of exercise programs on people diagnosed with coronary heart conditions. They found a positive effect for anxiety and depression.

Pierce and Pate (1994) examined the effects of a single bout of physical activity among older participants. Sixteen trained women completed an abbreviated Profile of Mood States before and immediately after a 75-minute session of aerobic line dancing. A series of one-way analysis of variance with repeated measures from pretest to posttest scores showed significant decreases in scores of tension.

O'Connor and colleagues (1993) reported the effect of resistance exercise in females on state anxiety and ambulatory blood pressure. Young women undergoing high-intensity exercise reported significantly less stress than participants in the less intense exercise groups. The relationship between stress and anxiety, depression, and hostility weakened at the end of the training period but strengthened in the less intense exercise groups. The study provided evidence that for an adolescent population, aerobic exercise has positive effects on well-being.

Raglin, Turner, and Eksten (1993) also provide evidence for the use of exercise as an anxiety-reducer. Eleven female and 25 male collegiate varsity athletes completed 30-minute sessions of leg cycle ergometry or weight training in a randomized order on separate days. State anxiety, systolic blood pressure (SBP), and diastolic blood pressure (DBP) were measured at baseline before exercise and 20 and 60 minutes after exercise. State anxiety increased significantly after weight training, but decreased significantly below baseline 50 minutes after ergometry. The SBP (but not the DBP) was reduced by 6.5 mm Hg below baseline at 60 minutes after ergometry.

Rejeski and colleagues (1992) evaluated the experimental hypothesis that aerobic exercise (AE) buffers psychosocial stress responses in low to moderately physically fit women. Forty-eight (24 Caucasian, 24 African-American) 25- to 40-year old women participated in either an attention control group or a 40-minute bout of AE at 70%

heart rate reserve. Both groups were followed by 30 minutes of quiet rest, exposure to mental and interpersonal threat, and 5 minutes of recovery. AE reduced both the frequency and intensity of anxiety-related thoughts after the interpersonal threat as compared with the placebo group.

Homeopathy. Individually selected homeopathic remedies were used on an outpatient basis to treat 12 adults who had social phobia, panic disorder, or major depression. Overall response rates were 58% according to the clinical global improvement scale and 50% on the SCL-90 and the Brief Social Phobia Scale (Davidson et al., 1997).

Meditation. Miller, Fletcher, and Kabat-Zinn (1995) found that an intensive, time-limited group-stress reduction based on mindfulness meditation significantly reduced anxiety and panic for 22 individuals with DSM-III-R-defined anxiety disorders.

Music. A convenience sample of 97 adults receiving chemotherapy for the first time was assigned to either experimental taped music and a message from their physician (n = 47), or "no intervention" control group (n = 50). After the fourth chemotherapy treatment, Sabo and Michael (1996) found significant results on the Spielberger State Anxiety Inventory (as compared with initial evaluation) for the taped music group but not for the control group. These preliminary findings indicate that this simple and cost-effective intervention can decrease anxiety.

Relaxation, breathing, imagery, and guided imagery. Using a conceptual framework of holism, Weber (1996) investigated the effects of relaxation exercises on anxiety levels in an inpatient general psychiatric unit. The researcher used a convenience sample of 39 participants. Anxiety levels were measured before and after the relaxation exercises using the state portion of the State-Trait Anxiety Inventory. Treatment included progressive muscle relaxation, meditative breathing, guided imagery, and soft music. There was a significant reduction in anxiety level on the posttest.

Self-hypnosis. Ashton and colleagues (1997) hypothesized that self-hypnosis relaxation techniques would have a positive effect on individuals' mental and physical condition after coronary artery bypass surgery. They used a prospective, randomized trial (n = 32) and followed participants from one day before surgery until the time of discharge. The treatment group was taught self-hypnosis relaxation techniques preoperatively, while the control group received the usual care. Individuals who were taught self-hypnosis were significantly more relaxed postoperatively compared with the control group. Pain medication requirements were also significantly less for the treatment group.

Therapeutic touch. Simington and Laing (1993) studied the effects of TT versus a back rub on anxiety level in 105 institutionalized elderly. A double-blind, three-group, experimental design was used. State anxiety was measured using the Speilberger State-Trait Anxiety Inventory. The anxiety level of subjects who received TT was significantly lower than those who received a back rub without TT. The researchers suggest that TT has a potential for enhancing quality of life for this population.

Depression

Acupuncture. Allen and Schnyer (1994) reported the use of acupuncture for unipolar depression for 33 women between 18 and 45 years of age. The treatment group received acupuncture designed to treat depressive symptoms. The nonspecific group first received acupuncture for symptoms not related to depression and later for depressive symptoms. The wait list group received no treatment for 8 weeks, followed by specific acupuncture treatment. About 64% of the women who received treatment specifically designed for depression experienced full remission, indicating sufficient promise to warrant a larger clinical trial. Yang and colleagues (1994) compared the use of acupuncture (n = 20) with the use of amitriptyline (n = 21) for depression. Measured with Hamil-

ton's scale, the factor of anxiety somatization decreased significantly in the acupuncture group (as compared with the antidepressant group). After 6 weeks, slow-wave delta decreased in the treatment group, while fast-wave alpha increased significantly more than in the antidepressant group.

Biofeedback. Rosenfeld and colleagues (1995) reported the use of biofeedback to teach depressed undergraduates to control left-right frontal (brain) alpha power differences. Two studies of five 1-hour sessions on each of 5 days were used. In the first study, 6 of 8 students met learning criteria by showing a significant difference between baseline and training scores. In the second study, 3 of 5 students met learning criteria.

Dance. Noreau and colleagues (1995) examined the use of a dance-based exercise program in a group of 19 persons with arthritis (mean age 49.3 years) in a 12-week, twice-weekly format. Health status, use of medication, joint pain and swelling, physical fitness, activities of daily living, and psychologic state were assessed at baseline after the 12-week training program and 6 months after the end of the program. Positive changes occurred in depression, anxiety, fatigue, and tension in participants.

Exercise. Singh, Clements, and Fiatarone (1997) tested the use of a progressive resistance training (PRT) program, hypothesizing that it would reduce depression while improving physiologic capacity, quality of life, morale, function, and self-efficacy without adverse events in an older, significantly depressed population. Volunteers 60 years of age and above were randomly assigned to a 10-week exercise program or an attention-control group. PRT significantly reduced all depression measures (Beck Depression Inventory and Hamilton Rating Scale of Depression) and improved quality of life, social functioning, role emotion (morale), and strength.

Testing a group (n = 58) of ethnically diverse pregnant adolescents, Koniak-Griffin (1994) found that aerobic exercise significantly decreased depressive symptoms and increased total self-esteem. Thayer, Newman, and McClain (1994) completed four studies evaluating the success of behaviors and strategies used to self-regulate depressed mood, raise energy, and reduce tension. The four studies (open-ended questionnaire, fixed-response surveys, therapist- and self-rating measures) confirmed previous findings that exercise is the most effective mood-regulating behavior, and the best general strategy to elevate mood is a combination of relaxation, stress management, exercise, and cognitive techniques.

Guided imagery and music therapy. McKinney and colleagues (1997) found that healthy adults who participated in 13 weeks of the Bonny Method of Guided Imagery and Music (a depth approach to music psychotherapy) sessions reported significant decreases between pre- and post-session depression, fatigue, and total mood disturbance (on the Profile of Mood States) as opposed to a wait-list control group. According to blood tests, they also exhibited a reduced level of cortisol, which may have health implications for chronically stressed people.

Herbs. The ability of *Ginkgo biloba* extract (GBE) to improve the general mood in people suffering from cerebral vascular insufficiency led researchers to investigate the antidepressive effects of the herb. Forty depressed participants (ranging 51 to 78 years of age) who did not benefit fully from standard antidepressant drugs were given either 80 mg of GBE three times daily or a placebo. By the end of the fourth week of treatment, the total score on the Hamilton Depression Scale was reduced from an average of 14 to an average of 7. After 8 weeks of treatment, the total score in the GBE group dropped to 4.5. In comparison, the placebo group dropped from 14 to 13. The researchers concluded that GBE offers significant benefits as an antidepressant on its own or in combination with standard drug therapy (Schubert & Halama, 1993).

Two meta-analyses of 23 (Linde, 1996), and 25 (Nordfors & Hartvig, 1997) randomized trials showed that extracts of *Hypericum perforatum* (St. John's wort) were more effective than placebo in the treatment of depression and as effective as standard antidepressive treatment. St. John's wort also had fewer side effects than the standard antidepressant drugs.

Lifestyle behaviors. Koenig and others (1997) examined models of relationships between religious activities, physical health, social support, and depressive symptoms for a sample of 4000 people 65 years of age and over. Frequency of church attendance was positively related to physical health and negatively related to depression but unrelated to social support. Frequent churchgoers were about half as likely to be depressed. Private prayer and Bible reading was negatively associated with physical health and positively associated with social support but unrelated to depression. Religious television watching and radio listening was unrelated to social support, negatively associated with good physical health, and positively associated with depression.

Light therapy. Seasonal affective disorder (SAD) represents a subgroup of depression that includes hypersomnia, anergia, increased appetite, weight gain, and carbohydrate craving. The symptoms occur in autumn and winter in northern climates and are in full remission in spring and summer.

Light therapy, or phototherapy, continues to be under study as a treatment for the depressive symptoms. To treat SAD, individuals are exposed to a full light screen 2 hours early in the morning, between 6:00 AM and 9:00 AM. The most common side effects are headache, eyestrain, and muscle pain. It is not used with tricyclic antidepressants, neuroleptics, and other medication containing a tricyclic, heterocyclic, or porphyrin ring system because of the potential negative reaction (Sartori & Poirrier, 1996). Beauchemin and Hays (1997) randomly assigned depressed inpatients to high and low levels of artifical light. Both unipolar and bipolar depression responded when phototherapy was used as an adjunct to pharmacotherapy. Mood improvement was significantly related to intensity of illumination.

Massage and relaxation therapy. Field and colleagues (1996) examined the effects of relaxation and massage therapy on depression and anxiety in teen mothers who recently gave birth and were recruited from an inner-city hospital maternity ward. All mothers showed elevated scores on the Beck Depression Inventory but were not being treated for depression or taking medications. They were randomly assigned to either a relaxation therapy (RT) group or a massage therapy (MT) group for 30 minutes a day for 2 successive days for 5 successive weeks. The MT group reported less anxiety, anxiety behaviors, depression, and stress than the RT group. Participants perceived the RT as "too much work," so results may have been biased, suggesting that further research is needed to avoid this bias.

Meditation. Smith, Compton, and West (1995) reported the use of meditation to enhance Fordyce's Personal Happiness Enhancement Program (PHEP) to reduce depression and anxiety. A control group received no instruction. The Happiness Measure, Psychap Inventory, Beck Depression Inventory, and State-Trait Anxiety Scale were dependent measures. The meditation plus PHEP group significantly improved on all dependent measures, including depression, over both the PHEP only group and the control group.

Yoga. Berger and Owen (1992) found that both yoga and swimming participants reported greater decreases in scores on anger, confusion, tension, and depression than did the control group. Among

table 11-3

SUMMARY OF COMPLEMENTARY THERAPIES FOR SPECIFIC CONDITIONS

THERAPIES	ADHD	AGING	ALZHEIMER'S	ANGER	ANXIETY	DEPRESSION
Acupuncture	X					X
Animal-assisted therapy		X				
Aromatherapy	X					
Biofeedback		X	X			X
Breathing				X		
Dance		X			X	X
Exercise	X	X		X	X	X
Herbs		X	X			X
Homeopathy					X	
Humor therapy				X		
Imagery					X	X
Light/color therapy						X
Massage						X
Meditation					X	X
Mirror feedback			X			
Music			X		X	X
Nutrition	X	X	X			
Other lifestyle factors	X					X
Self-hypnosis					X	
Therapeutic touch					X	
Yoga						X

the men, marked decreases in tension, fatigue, and anger after yoga were significantly greater than those after swimming. The researchers concluded that aerobic exercise was not necessary to reduce depression and other negative feelings. See Table 11-3 for a summary of complementary therapies for specific conditions.

CASE STUDY WITH COMPLEMENTARY AND ■ TRADITIONAL PRACTICES

Mr. Hopkins is a 47-year-old computer programmer who suffers from bouts of extreme anxiety, accompanied by rapid heartbeat, dryness of mouth, restlessness, and insomnia. He has been receiving disability benefits for 3 months and is taking an antidepressant. His anxiety is so severe, meeting all the criteria for panic disorder, that he has to be driven to his appointment by a friend. After three sessions with an APRN skilled in psychotherapy, he is able to drive to sessions himself but still is unable to return to work. When the patient discussed an article on therapeutic touch

and guided imagery with his nurse therapist, they agree to try a combined program of guided imagery, meditation, and breathing. The nurse psychotherapist refers the patient to a nurse practitioner with therapeutic touch skills. The nurse psychotherapist develops a guided imagery and meditation audiotape for the patient during the next session and helps him practice some breathing exercises. Two weeks later the patient returns to work and continues to see the nurse psychotherapist biweekly for another month. The nurse is so impressed with the combination of complementary practices with her counseling skills that she takes a continuing education course in therapeutic touch and advanced guided imagery and begins to incorporate them into her practice.

■ CERTIFICATION

Before adding any complementary approaches to practice, it is wise to achieve the minimum education for certification or at least safe practice. Many universities now incorporate complementary practices and holistic mind-body-spirit theoretical

table 11-4

COVERAGE FOR COMPLEMENTARY TREATMENTS

COMPANY	COMPLEMENTARY PRACTICES COVERED
Oxford Health Plans (800) 444-6222	In all states: yoga, massage therapy, acupuncture, chiropractic, nutrition, naturopathy
Blue Shield of California (800) 535-8000	Chiropractic and biofeedback with an MD
Alternative Health Insurance Services (800) 966-8467	In all states except California: acupuncture, massage therapy, bodywork, biofeedback, herbal medicine, meditation, chiropractic, Ayurveda, chelation therapy, naturopathy, traditional Chinese medicine, midwifery
Group Health Insurance Services (800) 358-8815	Western Washington state only and only with doctor approval: naturopathy, acupuncture, massage therapy, up to 10 visits; chiropractic, more visits
Bienestar Gold (888) 692-4363	In New York, New Jersey, Connecticut, Florida, and rapidly expanding to other areas: acupuncture, nutritional counseling, massage therapy, homeopathy, smoking cessation, stress management, and over 90 modalities

frameworks into master's programs and offer continuing education courses in complementary practices. Skilled APRNs in private practice often offer workshops, seminars, and training in therapeutic touch, guided imagery, nutrition, and hypnosis, among other topics.

IMPLICATIONS FOR
■ THE FUTURE

The future for complementary practices is bright. Third-party payers are beginning to provide reimbursement for a number of complementary procedures (Table 11-4). Nursing programs are incorporating complementary procedures into their curricula. As more practitioners learn about and become expert in these procedures, they will find novel ways to combine traditional psychotherapeutic procedures with complementary ones and test the effect through systematic study. This will provide a bridge to interdisciplinary collaboration with other health care professionals.

RESOURCES AND CONNECTIONS

ACADEMIC CENTERS

Academy for Guided Imagery, Inc.
P.O. Box 2070
Mill Valley, CA 94942
1-800-726-2070
Fax: 415-389-9342

American Institute for Mental Imagery
351 E. 84th Street, Suite 10D
New York, NY 10028
212-988-7750 or 534-4373

The Ayurvedic Institute
11311 Menaul NE
Albuquerque, NM 87112
505-291-9698

Bastyr University
144 NE 54th Street
Seattle, WA 98105
206-523-9585

Center for Human Caring at the University of Colorado Health Sciences Center
4200 E 9th Avenue, Box C288-8
Denver, CO 80262
303-270-6157
Fax: 303-270-5666

College of New Rochelle, Graduate School of (Holistic) Nursing
29 Castle Place
New Rochelle, NY 10805
914-654-5437
Fax: 914-654-5994

Southeastern Institute for Music-Centered Psychotherapy (SIMCP)
2801 Buford Highway, Suite 225
Atlanta, GA 30329
404-633-8224

Turtle Island Project
602-345-6112

CERTIFYING BODIES

American Dance Therapy Association
2000 Century Plaza
Columbia, MD 21044

American Massage Therapy Association
820 Davis Street, Suite 100
Evanston, IL 60201-444
708-864-0123

American Society of Clinical Hypnosis (ASCH)
2200 East Devon Avenue, Suite 291
Des Plaines, IL 60018
708-297-3317
Fax: 708-297-7309

Biofeedback Certification Institute of America
10200 W 44th Avenue, Suite 304
Wheatridge, CO 80033
303-420-2902

Council for Homeopathic Certification
P.O. Box 157
Corte Madera, CA 94976

National Association for Holistic Aromatherapy (NAHA)
P.O. Box 17622
Boulder, CO 80308

National Association for Music Therapy
www.namt.com/NAMT.html

National Commission for Certification of Acupuncturists
1424 16th Street NW, Suite 501
Washington, DC 20036
202-232-1404
Fax: 202-462-6157

North American Society of Homeopaths
10700 Old County Road 15, #350
Minneapolis, MN 55441
612-593-9458

Rocky Mountain Institute of Yoga and Ayurveda
P.O. Box 1091
Boulder, CO 80306.
303-443-6923

Vedic Sciences Institute (offers a hundred-hour supervised internship leading to the designation Certified Ayurvedist [C.Av.])
P.O. Box 2537
Jupiter, FL 33468-2537
407-745-2164

CONTINUING EDUCATION COMPLEMENTARY COURSES

American Holistic Nurses' Association
P.O. Box 2130
Flagstaff, AZ 96003-2130
800-278-AHNA
Fax: 520-526-2752
Email: nightingale@ahna.org
Website: ahna.org/nightingale.htm

Artemis Institute of Natural Therapies/ Herbal Medicine
P.O. Box 1824
Boulder, CO 80206
303-443-9289
Fax: 303-443-6361

Biofeedback Training Associates
255 West 98th Street
New York, NY 10025
212-222-5665

Nurse Healers—Professional Associates, Inc. Cooperative
P.O. Box 444
Allison Park, PA 15101-0444
412-355-8476

University of South Florida, Division of Lifelong Learning, Educational Outreach
13301 Bruce B. Downs Blvd
Tampa, FL 33612-3899
813-974-5146
Fax: 813-974-5732

Wellness Resources
3451 Central Avenue
St. Petersburg, FL 33713
727-321-0841
Email: sfe4hy@scfn.thpl.lib.fl.us

GOVERNMENT

Office of Alternative Medicine Clearinghouse
P.O. Box 8218
Silver Spring, MD 20907-8218
Phone and TTY: 888-644-6226
Fax: 301-495-4957
Website: altmed.od.nih.gov.

OTHER RESOURCES

Alternative health practitioner: the journal of complementary and natural care. New York: Springer.

Encyclopedia of complementary practices. (1999). New York: Springer.

Delta Society (Animal-Assisted Therapy)
289 Perimeter Road East
Renton, WA 98055-1329
800-869-6898.

Herb Network
P.O. Box 12937
Albuquerque, NM 87195

Holistic Discussion Group. To subscribe write to listserv@siucvmb.siu.edu with the following text: SUBscribe HOLISTIC

Paracelsus Mailing List. To subscribe write to majordomo@SUBSCRIBE PARACELSUS.
Send a biographical note indicating training, practice, and interests to paracelsus@teleport.com

REFERENCES

Acanda Roque, M.C., Gonzales Valente, A., & Fialio Sanza, A. (1990). Psychogeriatrics and psychoballet. *Rev Cubana Enferm, 6*(2), 198–204.

Allen, J.J. & Schnyer, R.N. (1994). *An acupuncture treatment study for unipolar depression.* altmed.od.nih.gov/oam/cgi-bin/research/search_imple.cgi.

Appels, A., et al. (1997). The effect of a psychological intervention program on the risk of a new coronary event after angioplasty: a feasibility study. *Journal Psychosomatic Research, 43*(2), 209–217.

Ashton, C., Jr., et al. (1997). Self-hypnosis reduces anxiety following coronary artery bypass surgery: a prospective, randomized trial. *Journal of Cardiovascular Surgery, 38*(1), 69–75.

Bannerman, R.H., Burton, J., & Wen Chieh, C. (Eds.). (1983). *Hypnosis: traditional medicine and health care coverage.* Geneva: World Health Organization.

Barnason, S., Zimmerman, L., & Nieveen, J. (1995) The effects of music interventions on anxiety in the patient after coronary artery bypass grafting. *Heart and Lung, 24*(2), 124–132.

Beauchemin, K.M. & Hays, P. (1997). Phototherapy is a useful adjunct in the treatment of depressed in-patients. *Acta Psychiatrica Scandinavica, 95*(5), 424–427.

Bender, M.L. (1971). *A study of the relationships between persistent immaturity of the symmetric tonic neck reflex and learning disabilities in children.* Ph.D dissertation, Purdue University.

Bennett, M.P. (1999). *Humor as a complementary therapy: the encyclopedia of complementary health practices.* New York: Springer.

Berger, B.G., & Owen, D.R. (1992). Mood alteration with yoga and swimming: aerobic exercise may not be necessary. *Perceptual and Motor Skills, 75*(3 part 2), 1331–1343.

Boris, M., & Mandel, F.S. (1994). Foods and additives are common cause of the attention deficit hyperactive disorder in children. *Annals of Allergy, 72*(5), 462–468.

Brooker, D.J., et al. (1997). Single case evaluation of the effects of aromatherapy and massage on disturbed behaviour in severe dementia. *British Journal of Clinical Psychology, 36*(2), 287–296.

Brooks, A., Thomas, S., & Droppleman, P. (1996). From frustration to red fury: a description of work-related anger in male registered nurses. *Nursing Forum, 31*(3), 4–15.

Carter, C.M., et al. (1993). Effects of a few food diet in attention deficit disorder. *Archives of Disease in Childhood, 69*(5), 564–568.

Clark, C.C. (1996). *Wellness practitioner: concepts, research, and strategies.* New York: Springer.

Clark, C.C. (1998). *The power of suggestion: how self-hypnosis can assist your patients.* In press.

Clark, C.C. (1999). Why clients try complementary therapies. *Alternative Health Practice: Journal of Complementary Natural Care, 5*(1), 3–4.

Classen, D.C. (1997). Adverse drug reactions. *Journal of the American Medical Association, 277*(4), 301–306.

Collinge, W. (1996). *The American Holistic Health Association complete guide to alternative medicine.* New York: Warner Books.

Cook, P. (1973). *The relationship of Bender facilitating exercises to ocular control and to achievement test scores.* Ph.D. dissertation, Purdue University.

Crawford, J.G. (1997). Alzheimer's disease risk factors as related to cerebral blood flow. *Medical Hypotheses, 46*(4), 367–377.

Daughtry, C. (September 12, 1997). *UF study reveals loss in sensory perception may not be linked to aging.* Press Release, University of Florida, Health Science Center Communications.

Davidson, J.R., et al. (1997). Homeopathic treatment of depression and anxiety. *Alternative Therapies in Health and Medicine, 3*(1), 46–49.

Davis, M., Eshelman, E.R., & McKay, M. (1995). *The relaxation and stress reduction workbook.* Oakland, CA: New Harbinger.

Dossey, B.M. (1995). Using imagery to help your patient heal. *American Journal of Nursing, 95*(6), 40–46.

Drabaek, H., et al. (1996). The effect of *Ginkgo biloba* extract in patients with intermittent claudication. *Ugeskrift for Laeger, 158*(27), 3928, 3931.

Eisenberg, D.M., et al. (1993). Unconventional medicine in the United States. *New England Journal of Medicine, 328,* 246–252.

Fick, K.M. (1993). The influence of an animal on social interactions of nursing home residents in a group setting. *American Journal of Occupational Therapy, 47*(6), 529–534.

Field, T., et al. (1997). Job stress reduction therapies. *Alternative Therapies in Health and Medicine, 3*(4), 54–56.

Field, T.M., et al. (1996). Massage and relaxation therapies' effect on depressed adolescent mothers. *Adolescence, 31*(124), 903–911.

Foster, S. (1999). Biofeedback. In *The encyclopedia of complementary health practices.* New York: Springer.

Gagne, D., & Toye, R.C. (1994). The effects of therapeutic touch and relaxation therapy in reducing anxiety. *Archives of Psychiatric Nursing, 8*(3), 184–189.

Gammonley, J. (1999). Animal-assisted therapy. In *The encyclopedia of complementary health practices.* New York: Springer.

Garland, F.C., et al. (1990). Occupational sunlight exposure and melanoma in the U.S. Navy. *Archives of Environmental Health, 45,* 261–267.

Good, M. (1998). In Snyder, M., & Lindquist, R. *Complementary/alternative therapies in nursing* (ed. 3). New York: Springer.

Goddaer, J., & Abraham, I.L. (1994). Effects of relaxing music on agitation during meals among nursing home residents with severe cognitive impairment. *Archives of Psychiatric Nursing, 8*(3), 150–158.

Haase, J., Halama, P., & Horr, R. (1996). Effectiveness of brief infusions with *Ginkgo biloba* special extract Egb 761 in dementia of the vascular and Alzheimer type. *Zeitschrift fur Gerontologie und Geriatrie, 29*(4), 301–309.

Heber, L. (1999). Dance and movement. In *The encyclopedia of complementary health practices.* New York: Springer.

Holder, J. (1991). *New auricular therapy formula to increase retention of the chemically dependent in residential treatment.* Research study funded by the State of Florida, Department of Health and Rehabilitative Services.

Horrigan, B. (1998). Dolores Kreiger, RN, PhD: healing with therapeutic touch. *Alternative Therapies in Health and Medicine, 4*(1), 87–92.

Itil, T., & Martorano, D. (1995). Natural substances in psychiatry: *Ginkgo biloba* in dementia. *Psychopharmacology Bulletin, 31*(1), 147–158.

Jayasuraiya, A. (1987). *Open International University's textbook on acupuncture.* Columbo, Sri Lanka: Open University.

Jette, A.M., et al. (1996). A home-based exercise program for nondisabled older adults. *Journal of the American Geriatric Society, 44*(6), 644–649.

Kanowski, S., et al. (1996). Proof of efficacy of the *Ginkgo biloba* special extract Egb 761 in outpatients suffering from mild to moderate primary degenerative dementia of the Alzheimer type or multi-infarct dementia. *Pharmacopsychiatry, 29*(2), 47–56.

Keltner, D., & Bonanno, G.A. (1997). A study of laughter and dissociation: distinct correlates of laughter and smiling during bereavement. *Journal Personal and Social Psycology, 73*(4), 687–702.

King, A.C., et al. (1997). Moderate-intensity exercise and self-rated quality of sleep in older adults: a randomized controlled trial. *Journal of the American Medical Association, 277*(1), 32–37.

Kessler, R. (in press). Alternative medicine update. *Alternative Health Practitioner: Journal of Complementary and Natural Health.*

Knaster, M. (1996). *Discovering the body's wisdom.* New York: Bantam.

Koenig, H.G., et al. (1997). Modeling the cross-sectional relationships between religion, physical health, social support, and depressive symptoms. *American Journal of Geriatric Psychiatry, 5*(2), 131–144.

Koniak-Griffin, D. (1994). Aerobic exercise, psychological well being, and physical discomforts during adolescent pregnancy. *Research in Nursing and Health, 17*(4), 253–263.

Kugler, J., Seelbach, H., & Kruskemper, G.M. (1994). Effects of rehabilitation exercise programmes on anxiety and depression in coronary patients: a meta-analysis. *British Journal of Clinical Psychology, 33*(3), 401–410.

LeBars, P.L., et al. (1997). A placebo-controlled, double-blind, randomized trial of an extract of *Ginkgo biloba* for dementia. *Journal of the American Medical Association, 278*(16), 712–718.

Leeds, A. (1985). The anatomy of breath. In Bauman, E., et al. (Eds.). *The new holistic health handbook.* Lexington, MA: Penguin.

Leste, A., & Rust, J. (1984). Effects of dance on anxiety. *Perceptual and Motor Skills, 58*(3), 767–772.

Linde, K., et al. (1996). St. John's wort for depression: an overview and metanalysis of randomized clinical trials. *British Medical Journal, 313*(7052), 253–258.

Lindenbaum, J., et al. (1994). Prevalence of cobalamin deficiency in the Framingham elderly population. *American Journal of Clinical Nutrition, 60*(1), 12–14.

Martin, G.N. (1996). Olfactory remediation: current evidence and possible applications. *Social Science and Medicine, 43*(1), 63–70.

McKinney, C.H., et al. (1997). Effects of guided imagery and music (GIM) therapy on mood and cortisol in healthy adults. *Health Psychology, 6*(4), 390–400.

Milberger, S. et al. (1996). Is maternal smoking during pregnancy a risk factor for attention deficit hyperactivity disorder in children? *American Journal of Psychiatry, 153*(9), 1138–1142.

Miller, J.J., Fletcher, K., & Kabat-Zinn, J. (1995). Three-year follow-up and clinical implications of a mindfulness meditation-based stress reduction intervention in the treatment of anxiety disorders. *General Hospital Psychiatry, 17*(3), 192–200.

Mock, V., et al. (1997). Effects of exercise on fatigue, physical functioning, and emotional distress during radiation therapy for breast cancer. *Oncology Nursing Forum, 24*(6), 991–1000.

Mowry, DB. (1986). *The scientific validation of herbal medicine.* New Canaan, CT: Keats.

Murphy, M.C. (1999). Autogenic training. In *The encyclopedia of complementary health practices.* New York: Springer.

Music therapy program. (1997). California State University. www.csun.edu/-hcmus006/Music Therapy.html1#2.

National Association for Music Therapy. (1997). www.namt.com/NAMT.html.

Noreau, L., et al. (1995). Effects of a modified dance-based exercise on cardiorespiratory fitness, psychological state and health status of persons with rheumatoid arthritis. *American Journal of Physical Medicine and Rehabilitation, 74*(1), 7019–7027.

Nordfors, M., & Hartvig, P. (1997). St. John's wort against depression in favour again. *Lakartidningen, 94*(25), 2365–2367.

Nurse Healers-Professional Associates. *Therapeutic touch policy and procedures for health professionals.* New York.

OAM Mission statement. (1998). *Complementary and alternative medicine at the NIH, 5*(1), 8.

Office of Alternative Medicine. (1996). *Growth of CAM studies.* altmed.od.nih.gov/oam/resources/present/oam-core/27.html.

O'Connor, P.J., et al. (1993). State anxiety and ambulatory blood pressure following resistance exercise in females. *Medicine and Science in Sports and Exercise, 25*(4), 516–521.

O'Dell, N.E., & Cook, P.A. (1997). *Stopping hyperactivity: a new solution.* Garden City Park, NY: Avery.

Oz, M.C., et al. (1996). Treating CAD with cardiac surgery combined with complementary therapy. *Medscapes Women's Health 1*(10), 2–17.

Petajan, J.H., et al. (1996). Impact of aerobic training on fitness and quality of life in multiple sclerosis. *Annals of Neurology, 39*(4), 432–441.

Perrig, W.J., Perrig, P., & Stahelin, H.B. (1997). The relation between antioxidants and memory performance in the old and very old. *Journal of the American Geriatric Society, 45*(6), 718–724.

Pettegrew, J.W., et al. (1995). Clinical and neurochemical effects of acetyl-L-carnitine in Alzheimer's disease. *Neurobiology of Aging, 16*(1), 1–4.

Pierce, E.F., & Pate, D.W. (1994). Mood alterations in older adults following acute exercise. *Perceptual and Motor Skills, 79*(1 part 1), 191–194.

Ragneskog, H., et al. (1996a). Dinner music for demented patients: analysis of video-recorded observations. *Clinical Nursing Research, 5*(3), 262–277.

Ragneskog, H., et al. (1996b). Influence of dinner music on food intake and symptoms common in dementia. *Scandinavian Journal of Caring Sciences, 10*(1), 11–17.

Raglin, J.S., Turner, P.E., & Eksten, F. (1993). State anxiety and blood pressure following 30 minutes of leg ergometry or weight training. *Medicine and Science in Sports and Exercise, 25*(9), 1044–1048.

Rejeski, W.J., et al. (1992). Acute exercise: buffering psychosocial stress responses in women. *Health Psychology, 11*(6), 355–362.

Rosenfeld, J.P., et al. (1995). Operant (biofeedback) control of left-right frontal alpha power differences: potential therapy for affective disorders. *Biofeedback and Self Regulation, 20*(3), 241–258.

Rossi, E.L. (1993). *The psychobiology of mind-body healing: new concepts of therapeutic hypnosis.* New York: W.W. Norton & Co.

Rossman, N. (1989). *Healing yourself: a step-by-step program for better health through imagery.* New York: Pocket Books.

Rowe, K.S., & Rowe, K.J. (1994). Synthetic food coloring and behavior: a dose response effect in a double-blind, placebo controlled, repeated-measures study. *Journal of Pediatrics, 125*(5), 691–698.

Rubik, B. (1995). The NIH Office of Alternative Medicine: what has it accomplished in its 3 years? *Alternative Health Practitioner: Journal of Complementary and Natural Care, 1*(1), 7–12.

Sabo, C.E., & Michael, S.R. (1996). The influence of a personal message with music on anxiety and side effects associated with chemotherapy. *Cancer Nursing, 19*(4), 283–289.

Sakai, M. (1996). A clinical study of autogenic training-based behavioral treatment for panic disorder. *Fukuoka Igaku Zasshi, 87*(3), 77–84.

Sano, M., et al. (1997). A controlled trial of selegiline, alpha-tocopherol, or both as treatment for Alzheimer's disease. *New England Journal of Medicine, 336*, 1216–1222.

Sartori, S., & Poirrier, R. (1996). Seasonal affective syndrome and phototherapy: theoretical concepts and clinical applications. *Encephale, 22*(1), 7–16.

Schubert, H., & Halama, P. (1993). Depressive episode primarily unresponsive to therapy in elderly patients: efficacy of *Ginkgo biloba* (EGb 761) in combination with antidepressants. *Geriatric Forsch 3*, 45–53.

Sibille, K. (1999). Physical exercise. In *The encyclopedia of complementary health practices.* New York: Springer.

Simington, J.A., & Laing, G.P. (1993). Effects of therapeutic touch on anxiety in the institutionalized elderly. *Clinical Nursing Research, 2*(4), 438–450.

Singh, N.A., Clements, K.M., & Fiatarone, M.A. (1997). A randomized controlled trial of progressive resistance training in depressed elders. *Journals of Gerontology. Series A, Biological Sciences and Medical Sciences, 52*(1), M27–35.

Smith, W.P., Compton, W.C., & West, W.B. (1995). Meditation as an adjunct to a happiness enhancement program. *Journal of Clinical Psychology, 52*(2), 269–273.

Solomon, G. (1987). Psychoneuroimmunologic approaches to research on AIDS. *Annals of the New York Academy of Science, 494*, 628–636.

Sonenklar, N.A. (1997). *Acupuncture point treatment for attention deficit hyperactivity disorder.* altmed.od.nih.gov/oam/cgi.

Staehelin, H. (August 18–22, 1997). *Dietary therapy for Alzheimer's disease.* Research paper presented at the World Congress of Gerontology in Adelaide, Australia.

Steinman, D. (1990). *Diet for a poisoned planet.* New York: Ballantine.

Strawn, J. (1999). Color therapy. In *The encyclopedia of complementary health practices.* New York: Springer.

Strohecker, J. (Ed.). (1994). *Alternative medicine: the definitive guide.* Fife, WA: Future Medicine.

Tabak, N., Bergman, R., & Alpert, R. (1996). The mirror as a therapeutic tool for patients with dementia. *International Journal of Nursing Practice, 2*(3), 155–159.

Tavris, C. (1984). On the wisdom of counting from one to ten. *Review of Personality and Social Psychology, 5,* 270–291.

Taylor, E., Lee, C., & Young, J. (1997). Bringing mind-body medicine into the mainstream. *Hospital Practice, 32*(5), 183–196.

Terry, N. (1999). Dance therapy. In *The encyclopedia of complementary health practice.* New York: Springer.

Thal, L.J., et al. (1996). A 1-year multicenter placebo-controlled study of acetyl-L-carnitine in patients with Alzheimer's disease. *Neurology, 47*(3), 705–711.

Thayer, R.E., Newman, J.R., & McClain, T.M. (1994). Self-regulation of mood: strategies for changing a bad mood, raising energy, and reducing tension. *Journal of Personal and Social Psychology, 67*(5), 910–925.

Thomas, S.P. (1993). *Women and anger.* New York: Springer.

Thomas, W. (1994). *The Eden alternative: nature, hope, and nursing home.* Cherburne, NY: The Eden Alternative.

Torri, S., Fukuda, H., & Kanemoto, H. (1988). Contingent negative variation (CNV) and the psychological effects of odour. In Van Toller, S., & Dodd G.H., (Eds.). *Perfumery: the psychology and biology of fragrance.* London: Chapman and Hall.

Urba, S.G. (1996). Nonpharmacologic pain management in terminal care. *Clinical Geriatric Medicine, 12*(2), 301–11

Weber, S. (1996). The effects of relaxation exercises on anxiety levels in psychiatric inpatients. *Journal of Holistic Nursing, 14*(3), 196–205.

Wilson, R. (1995). *Aromatherapy for vibrant health and beauty.* Garden City Park, NY: Avery.

Yang, X., et al. (1994). Clinical observation on needling extrachannel points in treating mental depression. *Journal of Traditional Chinese Medicine, 14*(1), 14–18.

Zisselman, M.H., et al. (1996). A pet therapy intervention with geriatric psychiatry patients. *American Journal of Occupational Therapy, 50*(1), 47–51.

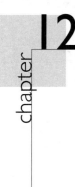

12

Practice Guidelines and Outcome Evaluation

GEORGE B. SMITH

■ INTRODUCTION

Practice guidelines and outcome evaluation are currently among the hottest topics in mental health service delivery. Payers, managed care companies, government regulators, and consumers are demanding consistent, effective quality treatment while producing quantitative data that demonstrate efficiency and valid outcomes. Changes in how mental health care services are organized and delivered have created a demand for meaningful tools to help guide practitioners in treatment selection and evaluation of relevant clinical outcomes. Practice guidelines that integrate outcome evaluation provide advanced practice registered nurses (APRNs) in psychiatric-mental health care with useful tools for delivering consistent and high-quality care.

Historically, practice patterns and treatment outcomes in mental health care have been difficult to evaluate because of inconsistencies among numerous types of treatments and the lack of clear, valid outcomes research. Practice guidelines provide the needed consistency in treatment approaches and delineate meaningful clinical outcomes. Practice guidelines summarize and present available treatment options and expected outcomes in a practical and orderly manner (Zarate, 1997). However, the practice guidelines that have been developed in recent years have been based primarily on global subjective judgments and opinions by experts rather than rigorous criteria for analysis of evidence (Geyman, 1998). For practice guidelines to be used by APRNs to improve quality of care, dictate effective practice patterns, and provide meaningful outcomes, they must be grounded in evidence from literature and research. Evidence-based practice guidelines are clearly written, contain specific current recommendations, and explicitly identify the primary source or research of the evidence (McIntyre, Zarin, & Pincus, 1996).

Evidence-based practice is the conscientious, explicit, and judicious use of the best data currently available in making clinical decisions about the care of individual patients (Sackett et al., 1996). Evidence-based practice requires the integration of the APRN's clinical expertise and judgment with the best available relevant external evidence. Practice guidelines based on evidence provide the APRN and patient with applicable research information in selecting treatment options and in measuring outcomes.

By using well-developed, current practice guidelines that are evidence based and comprehensive, APRNs can continually improve their practice patterns and incorporate feedback from an outcome evaluation system into clinical decisions. Outcome data can be used for the following:

1. To supplement the APRN's professional judgment about treatment decisions and choices
2. To modify the course and duration of treatment in terms of goal, modality, and intervention strategies by focusing on changes in health status, symptoms, and functioning
3. To develop practice guidelines that have a significant effect on the quality and efficacy of treatment choices and expected outcomes.

■ PRACTICE GUIDELINES

Definition (What)

Practice guidelines are official statements or polices of major organizations, professional associations, and/or agencies on the proper indications for performing a procedure or treatment or the appropriate management for specific clinical problems (Woolf, 1990). The Institute of Medicine (IOM) defines clinical practice guidelines as systematically developed statements that assist practitioner and patient in decisions about appropriate health care for specific clinical circumstances (Field & Lohr, 1990).

In mental health, these guidelines are written strategies or protocols for mental health care delivery that are developed to facilitate clinical decision making and to provide patients with critical information concerning the different treatment options available to them (McIntyre, Zarin, & Pincus, 1996; Stuart, 1998). The American Psychiatric Association (APA) defines clinical practice guidelines as a "set of patient care strategies developed to assist physicians in clinical decision making" (Zarin, McIntyre, & Pincus, 1996). Practice guidelines provide a wide range of possibilities and are usually broad. Some provide comprehensive recommendations for the diagnosis and management of a specific clinical condition, such as depression, anxiety, or substance abuse. Others provide recommendations for a less comprehensive set of issues, such as selection of medications or types of psychotherapeutic interventions.

Practice guidelines are known by many different names including practice parameters, protocols, evidence-based practice guides, consensus statements, practice standards, and others. Practice guidelines are often mistaken for standards but they are not standards. Guidelines are intended to be flexible, whereas standards are rigid (Berger & Rosner, 1996). They are strategies that should be followed in the majority of cases; exceptions are more common and require minimal justification for alternative treatment approaches. Standards, on the other hand, are recommendations that should be followed in virtually all cases, exceptions are rare and require extensive justification (McIntyre, Zarin, & Pincus, 1996). However, practice guidelines have become de facto standards through enforcement by health care agencies and in litigation of malpractice suits (Berger & Rosner, 1996).

Guidelines are developed from the consensus of a group of research and clinical experts in the field and an exhaustive review of the literature. For example, in developing its practice guidelines, the APA adopted a method of rating the scientific literature based on the strength of evidence of treatment efficacy (APA, 1993). The group of experts systematically develops the guidelines as statements about health care for specific clinical conditions. They usually specify steps based on clear clinical and research evidence resulting from multiple randomized, controlled trials. However, the APA guidelines do not indicate the next step in treatment for a patient who continues to fail to respond, but it instead offers alternative treatments at the same step or level.

Purpose (Why)

Practice guidelines provide practitioners with a tool to manage quality of care, improve efficiency of treatment provision, decrease costs, reduce liability risk, provide for medical training, and assist in the utilization of services. According to Stuart (1998), the primary goals of practice guidelines are as follows:
- Document preferred practice patterns
- Increase consistency in care and treatment
- Facilitate outcome evaluation and research
- Enhance the quality of care
- Improve staff productivity
- Reduce the cost of care

APRNs use guidelines to obtain the advice of recognized clinical experts, stay abreast of the latest clinical research, and assess the clinical significance of often conflicting research findings (Rieve, 1998). Practice guidelines provide APRNs with the following (Kelly, 1994):
- An authoritative source of information on important clinical issues
- A comprehensive evaluation of relevant scientific literature
- A source of reliable expert opinions
- Clarification of significant clinical controversies
- A specific, practical recommendation for patient management
- An evaluation of economic consequences of alternative patient management strategies
- An identification of specific patients who will benefit from the use of specific clinical recommendations
- A useful basis for effective case management or disease management activities

Studies have consistently demonstrated the benefits of practice guidelines in improving quality, utilization, and outcomes of clinical care (Kelly, 1994). Practice guidelines provide for consistency in practice patterns between practitioners and across geographic boundaries. With the rapid advances in mental health care, it is increasingly difficult for APRNs to remain abreast of current useful and practical information and research findings for use in clinical practice. Practice guidelines summarize research findings and present the resulting data in a practical and useful manner. In addition, practice guidelines that incorporate outcome evaluation provide a vehicle to continually improve quality by validating or calling into question the current treatments and interventions with their resulting outcomes.

Practice guidelines may have an effect on utilization of resources by reducing inappropriate treatment, controlling geographic variations in practice patterns, and making more effective use of health care resources (Woolf, 1990). Practice guidelines are intended to direct treatment toward clinically appropriate and cost-effective interventions and outcomes based on the best available scientific evidence. Practice guidelines provide two key benefits in managing resources: 1) identification of key clinical decision points along the management continuum for a specific patient problem and 2) valuable information regarding the suggested sequence and timing of specific interventions and processes (Kelly, 1994).

Based on relevant evidence, practice guidelines provide the compilation and analysis of the latest scientific research and literature. The analysis of the literature details the strengths and weaknesses of the evidence and identifies gaps in the current knowledge of treatments and outcomes. From these gaps, research studies can be conducted to further support the recommendations in practice guidelines or identify new research areas. According to Kelly and Bernard (1996), since practice guidelines provide access to the recommendations of recognized experts, they allow for the identification of areas of consensus and controversy, facilitate determination of clinical areas in which particular interventions might be effective, and provide useful information to guide clinical practice and research.

APRNs may be concerned that practice guidelines will increase their exposure to professional liability or malpractice claims. Many health care professionals share concern that they will be automatically liable if, for legitimate medical reasons, they choose to digress from relevant practice guideline recommendations and subsequently an undesirable outcome occurs. However, comprehensive analysis of the legal implications of practice guidelines indicates that these concerns are unfounded (Johnson, Hirshfield, & Ile, 1990). To avoid having practice guidelines used against practitioners in a malpractice case, they should remember that guidelines are recommendations only (Murphy, 1997). Guidelines are based on current available knowledge and research and may not fit all patients in all circumstances. According to Murphy (1997), practice guidelines cannot anticipate every condition and complication that an APRN might encounter with a given patient and therefore should be viewed as recommendations with implementation being tailored to the patient

and his or her needs. APRNs can protect themselves by clearly documenting why the variation from the guideline was appropriate and in the patient's best interest. Practice guidelines do not create new liabilities for practitioners; instead, they may serve to assist practitioners to manage their liability risks (Kelly, 1994).

OUTCOME RESEARCH OF ■ PRACTICE GUIDELINES

There is no question that practice guidelines and outcome research are closely coupled. The consistent and wide-spread use of practice guidelines in clinical practice will expedite the collection of valid outcome data, as well as link the data from outcome studies to the development of more explicit, definitive, and evidence-based practice guidelines (McIntyre, Zarin, & Pincus, 1996).

Practice guidelines can be evaluated by using the structure, process, and outcome framework outlined by Donabedian (1966). To improve clinical practice from the outcome data obtained, APRNs must understand the context within which the interventions and services are provided. In other words, the effect of the setting or provider specific variables (structure) upon provider actions, as well as treatment efficiency (process) and patient participation, influence changes in the recipient of care (outcomes). The structures of care within this framework include the characteristics of the community, organization, provider, and the population served. The processes include the technical excellence, interpersonal excellence, and the efficiencies within a practice setting.

The use of practice guidelines provides practitioners and researchers with consistent structures and processes that assist them in isolating key interventions and treatments that can be tested for effectiveness. Practitioners are able to isolate specific medications, treatment modalities, and outcomes that affect specific mental illnesses and populations. Without an examination of the causal relations among the structure, process, and outcomes, outcome evaluation would be a meaningless exercise (Mark, 1995). For practice guidelines to be used in research, they must be developed with recommendations that are as specific as possible without excessively stretching the conclusions that are based on existing scientific evidence. Practice guidelines with vague or general recommendations can result in considerable variation in the interventions or outcomes that actually occur. Outcomes evaluation may result in erroneous conclusions if incorrect or incomplete assumptions are made about the treatment actually delivered (McIntyre, Zarin, & Pincus, 1996).

Currently there is a lack of standardization in guideline process development, use of scientific data, purpose, mechanisms for updating, methods for measuring guideline validity, and other features of practice guidelines (Berger & Rosner, 1996). Few research studies exist on the outcomes of the use of practice guidelines in psychiatric-mental health clinical practice. Schulberg and colleagues (1996) demonstrated that the treatment principles recommended by the Depression Guideline Panel of the Agency for Health Care Policy and Research (AHCPR) were supported. The recommendations for pharmacotherapy and psychotherapy treatments were effective in treating major depression in primary care patients.

The IOM (Field & Lohr, 1990) has outlined attributes of recommendations within a well written practice guideline. These attributes should be evaluated by the APRN in selecting a useful and valid practice guideline. The attributes include ensuring that practice guidelines recommendations are as follows:

• Valid and accurate
• Reliable and reproducible
• Clinically applicable
• Clinically flexible
• Clearly written
• Subjected to scheduled reviews
• Well documented

Hayward and colleagues (1995) identified three critical questions that a clinician must ask in evaluating the validity, importance, and applicability of practice guidelines:

1. Are the recommendations valid?
2. What are the recommendations?
3. Will the recommendations help the clinician in caring for the patient?

When confronted with the first question, the APRN should analyze the practice guideline to ensure that all important options and outcomes are clearly specified. The APRN must ensure that an explicit and sensible process was used to identify, select, and combine supportive evidence, as well as consider the relative value of different outcomes. The practice guideline must be current, reevaluated often, and account for important recent developments in treatments and outcomes. In evaluating the practice guideline for validity, the practitioner must ensure that the guideline has been subjected to rigorous peer review and testing.

In addressing the second question, Hayward and colleagues (1995) suggested that the practitioner ensure that the recommendations are practical and clearly important to the identified problems and expected outcomes. The APRN must ensure that the recommendations are concise, have strong supportive evidence, and that the guideline addresses the effects of uncertainty associated with the evidence and values used.

For the last question, the APRN should evaluate the primary objective of the guideline and ensure that it is consistent with his or her own objectives and goals. In addition, the practice guideline must have recommendations that are applicable to the practitioner's patients' identified needs and problems.

There are primarily three acceptable methods of practice guideline development: informal and formal consensus development, evidence-based guideline development, and explicit guideline development (Woolf, 1992). Current practice guidelines have been developed primarily based on a consensus process. Consensus processes use uniformity of opinion among a specific group of expert clinicians and researchers and are influenced by biases and/or in explicit integration of scientific data. Especially in the specialty of psychiatric-mental health, significant disagreement exists among practitioners about indications for many diagnostic and therapeutic interventions, which makes reliance on opinion consensus questionable. The quality of evidence upon which practice guidelines are based range from simply expert opinion to well-designed, blinded, randomized controlled trials. Expert opinion may differ from standard practice, and the interpretations of data may vary, as may the weight and generalizability of the evidence (Berger & Rosner, 1996). New advances in practice guideline development call for more rigorous use of evidence in developing and evaluating practice guidelines.

DEVELOPMENT OF
■ PRACTICE GUIDELINES

Government Agencies

The National Institutes of Health (NIH) Consensus Development Program was established in 1977. Under this program, the Office of Medical Application of Research at the NIH organizes major conferences that produce consensus statements and technology assessment statements. NIH Consensus Development Conferences convene a panel of experts and researchers to develop consensus statements on controversial issues in health care that are important to health care providers, patients, and the general public. The most recent consensus statements in mental health include *Effective Medical Treatment of Opiate Addiction* (November 17–19, 1997) and *Interventions to Prevent HIV Risk Behaviors* (February 11–13, 1997). Other consensus statements developed by the NIH include *Diagnosis and Treatment of Depression in Late Life*—1991; *Treatment of Panic Disorder*—1991; *Treatment of Destructive Behaviors in Persons With Developmental Disorders*—1989; *Differential Diagnosis of Dementing Diseases*—1987; and *Electroconvulsive Therapy*—1985.

The AHCPR was established in 1989 and replaced the National Center for Health Services Research and Health Care Technology Assessment (NCHSR). For more than 20 years, NCHSR supported research on quality, cost, and access of health care and funded the development of many of the first health care acuity computer-based systems such as COSTAR and APACHE. In becoming an agency, two additional responsibilities were added to AHCPR's mission—supporting research on outcomes, effectiveness, and efficiencies in health care and developing clinical practice guidelines. The AHCPR's primary mission is to generate and disseminate information that improves the delivery and quality of health care. The agency is charged with helping consumers, providers, purchasers, health plan managers, and policymakers meet the challenge of improving the quality of health care services while reducing cost. The AHCPR has been recognized as funding the development of "gold standard" clinical practice guidelines and is the source of unbiased, science-based information on what works and does not work in health care (McCormick, Cummings, & Kovner, 1997).

The AHCPR developed two specific practice guidelines related to psychiatric conditions: depression and Alzheimer's disease. However, in 1996 the AHCPR ended its sponsorship of these two and 18 other developed clinical practice guidelines. The Agency initiated a new program called the Clinical Improvement Program. The program will fund the work in laying scientific foundations (including literature searches, meta-analyses, and information syntheses) through professional societies, health plans, purchasing groups, states, and others developing their own clinical practice guidelines. The Clinical Improvement Program has three new initiatives: the creation of evidence-based practice centers, a National Guideline Clearinghouse, and a Research and Evaluation Plan on the development and use of practice guidelines (McCormick, Cummings, & Kovner, 1997).

The AHCPR, in partnership with the American Association of Health Plans (AAHP) and the American Medical Association (AMA), sponsored the development of the National Guideline Clearinghouse to promote widespread access to practice guidelines. The National Guideline Clearinghouse was designed as a comprehensive database of clinical practice guidelines. For inclusion in the National Guideline Clearinghouse, the clinical practice guideline must meet all of the following criteria (AHCPR, 1998):

- The clinical practice guideline contains systematically developed statements that include recommendations, strategies, or information that assists physicians, APRNs, and other health care practitioners, and patients make decisions about appropriate health care for specific clinical circumstances.
- The clinical practice guideline was produced under the auspices of medical specialty associations; relevant professional societies; public or private organizations; government agencies at the federal, state, or local level; or health care organizations or plans. A clinical practice guideline developed and issued by an individual not officially sponsored or supported by one of the above types of organizations does not meet the inclusion criteria for the National Guideline Clearinghouse.
- Corroborating documentation can be produced and verified that a systematic literature search and review of existing scientific evidence published in peer reviewed journals was performed during the guideline development. A guideline is not excluded from the National Guideline Clearinghouse if corroborating documentation can be produced and verified detailing specific gaps in scientific evidence for some of the guideline's recommendations.
- The guideline is in the English language, current, and the most recent version produced.
- Documented evidence can be produced or verified that the guideline was either developed, reviewed, or revised within the last five years.

State governments have also shown an interest in practice guideline development. Although not directly involved in development and distribution of practice guidelines, some states have implemented committees or legislation for practice guidelines. The state of Maine initiated the Medical Liability Demonstration Project in January 1992. Practice parameters and risk management protocols were developed for specialists in obstetrics and gynecology, emergency medicine, radiology, and anesthesiology. An outcome of the guideline development was that physicians who could demonstrate compliance with the practice criteria might be able to establish an affirmative defense against medical malpractice claims. In 1993, a Florida statute (Chapter 408.02), titled *Practice Parameters*, created the Agency of Health Care Administration under the Office of Health Policy. The Agency was charged with coordinating the development, endorsement, implementation, and evaluation of scientifically sound, clinically relevant practice parameters. The goal of the practice parameters was to decrease unwarranted variation, improve the quality of medical care, and promote appropriate utilization of health care resources (McIntyre, Zarin, & Pincus, 1996). Although the primary focus of these practice parameters was toward physicians, a nurse practitioner was included on the practice parameter development committee.

Professional Association Initiatives

As of June 1998, the American Psychiatric Nurses Association (APNA) has addressed practice guidelines by forming a partnership with two organizations: the Best Practice Network and the Practice Guideline Coalition. The Best Practice Network is a forum for nurses, physicians, and other health care professionals to share ideas, creative solutions, and best practices. The Best Practice Network was formed in 1997 and currently has 28 professional partner organizations of which APNA is a founding member. The primary communication for the Network is its website (www.best 4health.org) and *The Best Practice Directory* (Sherwood, 1998). The Best Practice Network defines a best practice as a program or service in health care, which has been recognized for excellence. To qualify as a Best Practice, the program or service must meet the following criteria:

- Provide significant health care benefits for patients or the community, and

- Be successfully implemented, evaluated, and documented, and
- Represent a substantial improvement in current practices or procedures, or
- Demonstrate an innovative approach to solving a problem.

Best Practice Programs or services are selected through a peer review process. This selection of a Best Practice is a twofold process. Upon receipt, the submission undergoes a screening review to ensure that the basic components of the application, abstract, and report have been submitted in a complete format that meets the criteria. Next, the content evaluation portion of the review process ensures that the content of the submission is meaningful to health care; has been implemented and contributes positively to patient care or community well-being; is consistent with the best practice components; is supported by relevant literature, data, or information; and enhances health care intelligence. The content evaluation is conducted by appointed experts within partnering professional associations or others recognized for their expertise as it relates to the submission. Once a Best Practice has been accepted, it is published on the Best Practice Network website and in the *Best Practice Directory* (Sherwood, 1998).

The Practice Guidelines Coalition is an interdisciplinary, multiorganizational partnership between stakeholders in behavioral health care that intends to improve behavioral health services through the dissemination and implementation of nonpropriety clinical practice guidelines. The Coalition intends to develop two demonstration guidelines. The practice guidelines developed will represent the views of consumers and providers. It is an important initiative for the field as an attempt to develop practice guidelines that are not "guild sponsored" (Stuart, 1998b). Gail Stuart (APNA member and past president) will serve as a Scientific Panel Member for the Panic Disorder Guideline, which is one of the two demonstration guidelines. The Practice Guideline Coalition can be accessed through the APNA website (www.apna.org) or through the Coalition website (www.unr.edu/psych/pgc/).

Clinical practice guidelines have been slow to be accepted by behavioral health care practitioners. However, practice guidelines are effective in managing complex problems of patients with mental illnesses. Practice guidelines based on reliable scientific research and expert clinical judgment will continue to be valuable tools for ensuring quality patient care. APRNs in psychiatric-mental health care must provide leadership in the development, implementation, and evaluation of these practice guidelines in clinical practice.

■ OUTCOME EVALUATION

Changes in the organization; delivery and financing of health care; and the continued pressure on the psychiatric-mental health care system to be more accountable to consumers, policymakers, and the general public have made outcome evaluation a critical issue for APRNs. Employers, consumers, insurers, competing providers, and others are calling on APRNs to document their contributions to health care outcomes and the psychiatric-mental health care system (Girouard, 1996). APRNs in psychiatric-mental health care have become more focused on quality and accountability for treatments and services based on outcome measurements (APNA, 1998; Barrell, Merwin, & Poster, 1997; Sperry, 1997).

Managed behavioral health care and managed competition have greatly affected mental health service delivery. A full discussion of the role of the APRN in managed care is presented in Chapter 2. Managed behavioral health care has been both an organizational strategy for managing care structures and processes and a utilization and cost-control strategy for managing outcomes (Merwin et. al., 1997). These strategies have demanded that APRNs quantify outcomes within their practice and use outcome evaluation data to enhance the value of their clinical care. This emphasis on outcomes and accountability provides APRNs with an opportunity to gather and present convincing evidence on the value of their contributions to psychiatric-mental health care. The ability to understand, define, and explain the outcomes achieved by APRNs is critical to the continued acceptance and growth of the psychiatric nursing profession. Key questions that the APRN must address are as follows:

1. What does outcome evaluation mean to the APRN in psychiatric-mental health care?
2. What are patient outcomes in which the APRN has the greatest influence?
3. How can outcome data and evaluation be used to improve the quality of patient care within an APRN practice?

Outcomes Defined

Simply stated, outcomes are the results of treatments and interventions. Outcomes are the results of changes, both desirable and undesirable, in an individual's or population's health that can be attributed to the care provided (Donabedian, 1990). These changes include the following:

- Health status
- Knowledge acquired
- Behaviors
- Quality of life
- Satisfaction with care
- Satisfaction with the outcome of care.

Marek (1989) defined *outcome* as "a measurable change in a client's [patient's] health status related to the receipt of nursing care." According to Stuart (1998a), outcomes are the extent to which services are cost-effective and have a favorable effect on the patient's symptoms, functioning, and well-being. Outcomes include what happens to the patient and family while they are receiving mental health services. Therefore outcome evaluation can focus on a clinical condition, an intervention, or a caregiver process. Outcome domains examined in psychiatric-mental health services include clinical, functional, satisfaction, and financial indicators (Box 12-1).

The definition of *outcome* should include both positive (well-being) and negative (disease status) dimensions. Patient outcomes have been examined predominantly in terms of mortality or morbidity, selected aspects of functional status, and

---

box 12-1

CATEGORIES OF OUTCOME INDICATORS OR DOMAINS

CLINICAL OUTCOME INDICATORS

High-risk behaviors
Symptomatology
Coping responses
Relapse
Recurrence
Readmission
Number of treatment episodes
Medical complications
Incidence reports
Mortality

FUNCTIONAL OUTCOME INDICATORS

Functional status
Social interaction
Activities of daily living
Occupational abilities
Quality of life
Family relationships
Housing arrangements

SATISFACTION OUTCOME INDICATORS

Patient and family satisfaction with:
Outcomes
Providers
Delivery system
Caregiving process
Organization

FINANCIAL OUTCOME INDICATORS

Cost per treatment episode
Revenue per treatment episode
Length of inpatient stay
Number of mental health care visits
Use of health care resources
Costs related to disability

From Stuart, 1998a.

---

patient satisfaction with services and outcomes of treatment. Only recently have broader outcomes such as physical status, health status, functional abilities, return to work, residential status, social functioning, and quality of life been examined as outcomes of care (Kleinpell, 1997).

Outcome assessment or evaluation has three levels: outcome measurement, outcome monitoring, and outcome management. *Outcome measurement* is the quantification or measurement of clinical and functional outcomes during a specific treatment period. Outcome measures have traditionally been collected at the beginning and end of treatment; however, serial or concurrent assessment is becoming more common. Measures often include change in symptoms, well-being, functioning, and patient satisfaction (Sperry, 1997).

In measuring outcomes, they must be viewed as the result of a particular process. As outlined by McGlynn (1996), the term *outcome* itself implies a longitudinal perspective—an observation of an occurrence between two points in time. In determining the optimal time frame for outcome evaluation, the expected rate of change in outcomes for the intervention being evaluated and the anticipated attribution of outcomes should be considered. Both short-term and long-term outcomes are important. *Short-term outcomes* might refer to the immediate effect of a treatment intervention (e.g., response to a new antipsychotic medication), whereas *long-term outcomes* might refer to an assessment of whether results are maintained after intensive treatment interventions cease (e.g., several months after a behavioral skills training course has been completed). The more time that passes between the assessment and the intervention being studied, the greater the chance that intervening factors will influence the observed outcomes, thus diminishing the ability to attribute results to the intervention. On the other hand, assessments that occur too quickly may prevent an observation of the real benefits of an intervention. For example, many antipsychotic medications may take 6 weeks or more to affect symptoms; assessments done within 2 weeks of starting treatment may give a biased view of the efficacy or effectiveness of treatment (McGlynn, 1996).

Outcome monitoring is the serial or concurrent use of outcome measures during the course of treatment. The goal of outcome monitoring is comparison against a standard of expected results to monitor progress or lack of progress during the course of treatment. Monitoring can be done after each session, after every third session, or on some other scheduled basis. Outcome monitoring data are then used to alter treatment when it is off course or stagnating. It can be used to follow progress in a single case, or it can be summed and adjusted for risk to compare several patients or programs. Outcome monitoring can only be accomplished with repeated or concurrent measures, and the information must be available during the treatment (Sperry, 1997).

Outcome management of data is the most critical level in outcome evaluation. Outcome management is the use of outcome data in a way that allows practitioners and health care systems to learn from experience. Usually, this "learning" results in reshaping or improving the overall administrative and clinical processes of services provided. Patient profiling, provider profiling, and site profiling are three common aspects of an outcome management system (Sperry, 1997). Outcome management is the linkage of outcomes with clinical practice. Therefore outcome management is a necessary step in identifying and measuring relevant outcomes for clinical practice guideline development and evaluation. The clinician can use outcome data and analysis to lend support for decisions about treatment with regard to expected outcomes from a clinical practice guideline.

Quality and Performance Improvement

The evolution of quality in health care has led to an emphasis on performance improvement and measuring outcomes. Although organizational performance improvement remains important, the primary focus continues to shift toward measuring the specific patient outcomes achieved from the treatments and services provided and to benchmark those outcomes both internally as well as externally. Timely and effective feedback is required to improve any practice or system. Outcome data can be used to improve both the practice patterns of individual practitioners and the performance of the organization or health care system. Specific purposes of outcome measurement are as follows (Stuart, 1998a):

- Evaluate the outcomes of services and care
- Suggest changes in treatments
- Evaluate program or treatment course effectiveness
- Profile the practice pattern of practitioners
- Determine the most appropriate level of treatment
- Predict the trajectory of a patient's illness and recovery
- Contribute to quality improvement

Mental health treatment is complex. In mental health care, over 200 models of therapy are practiced across several disciplines (Burlingame et al., 1995) in the treatment of over 200 mental illness diagnoses (APA, 1994). The APRNs in psychiatric-mental health nursing must demonstrate the unique and valuable services that they provide (APNA, 1997). The APNA Work Group on Measuring Outcomes (1997) emphasized the APRN's key role in addressing issues of health behavior and illness prevention, in assisting with identifying social roles and supports for maintaining or changing these over the developmental stages, and in sustaining patients' efforts to overcome the complexities of day-to-day living and the inertia that challenges these efforts. All of these parameters must be examined in the context of the APRN's practice. APRNs should examine the effects of their interventions on symptoms, symptom clusters, functional status, and satisfaction (APNA, 1997).

Historically, outcome evaluation focused on outcome research with rigorous controlled trials. This outcome research studied the effects of discrete treatment interventions under controlled, experimental conditions. However, emphasis is now being placed on the evaluation of patients under the naturalistic conditions in hospitals, clin-

ics, and the community (Sederer, Dickey, & Hermann, 1996). According to Girouard (1996), outcome evaluation emphasizes applied research rather than basic research methods. Basic research methods employ controlled trials within an experimental design, whereas outcome evaluation research uses applied research methods. This involves the application of social-science research methods in collecting, analyzing, and interpreting data to determine the need, implementation, effectiveness, and efficiency of interventions. The data analysis is used to evaluate achievement or lack of achievement of desirable outcomes to improve practice as well as health care systems.

Outcome Measures

As discussed earlier in this chapter, outcome is the third dimension of Donabedian's (1966) quality improvement model of structure, process, and outcome. This model provides a tripartite framework for studying the quality of care and the context from which outcomes are achieved. Using Donabedian's framework, Irvine, Sidani, and Hall (1998) identified the RN's role and influence in affecting outcomes in health care. These same concepts can be modified to apply to the APRN role. Donabedian outlined structure as the characteristics of the delivery system (community, organizational, and provider characteristics) and the patient population served (clinical and demographic characteristics). The structure dimensions for APRNs refer to their experience; advanced knowledge and skills; the organizational structure and resources within which they practice; and the patients' health status, severity, and morbidity. Donabedian's process component is the specification of procedures or treatment modalities provided to the patient. The process dimension for APRNs refers to their independent as well as their interdependent roles. Outcomes of care, according to Donabedian, include clinical and functional status, quality of life, expenditures, patient satisfaction, and life expectancy. Outcomes refer to the specific clinical results of treatments and service efforts (e.g., symptomatic and functional changes), the costs of those efforts, and the degree of satisfaction experienced by the recipients of services (Sederer, Dickey, & Eisen, 1997). For APRNs the outcome dimension must include APRN-sensitive outcomes that are defined as a "general patient state, behavior, or perception resulting from nursing [APRN] interventions" (Johnson & Maas, 1997).

According to the APNA Work Group on Measuring Outcomes (1997; refer to the report in Appendix E), outcome measurement in advanced nursing practice for psychiatric-mental health care should focus primarily on the following:

1. Symptoms, symptom clusters, and their progression over time
2. Functional status related to the ability to participate in day-to-day living
3. Patient satisfaction
4. Family satisfaction

Outcomes are multidimensional. One of the most critical steps in outcome evaluation is the careful selection of the appropriate measurement, which will address the clinical questions being asked. Depending upon the questions asked, different information about the outcome and satisfaction of care may be obtained. Outcome instruments are available that address global well-being, symptoms and functioning, symptoms alone, functioning alone, and satisfaction (Sederer, Dickey, & Eisen, 1997). Instruments are designed to measure patient responses, family or significant others' responses, and/or practitioner responses. No specific instrument can answer every study question or concern. However, when multiple perspectives are obtained, the results can be complementary and enhance the understanding of the patient and health care services (Sederer, Dickey, & Eisen, 1997).

Choosing an outcome measure is a crucial step to successful outcome evaluation. Sederer, Dickey, and Eisen (1997) identified four areas that need to be addressed in selection of the appropriate measurement instrument. The questions to pose when choosing an outcome measure are listed in

box 12-2

QUESTIONS IN SELECTING AN OUTCOME MEASURE

1. Questions about the variables
   a. What do you want to measure?
   b. Which domains or indicators of outcomes do you want to study?
      (1) Global well-being?
      (2) Symptoms?
      (3) Functioning?
      (4) Both symptoms and functioning?
2. Questions about whose perspective
   a. Whom do you want to measure?
   b. Do you want to query the patient, clinician, family, employer, teacher, or payer?
3. Questions about when to measure
   a. When do you want to measure?
   b. Are you seeking to measure an episode of care?
   c. An episode of illness?
   d. Short-term (<30 days) or long-term?
   e. Do you want two, three, or more points of measurement and why?
4. Questions about the users of the data
   a. For what audience?
   b. Who needs the outcome data to make decisions, such as clinicians and administrative staff?

Box 12-2. APRNs may want to measure only one indicator or choose several to measure at the same time. In addition, they may choose to vary the indicators over time, such as by starting with measures of symptoms and functioning and concluding by adding global well-being and quality of life. A second consideration is whose perspective to measure. The more perspectives measured, within practical limits, the more the findings complement one another and something approaching the truth of the matter is obtained. What APRNs measure will also influence when they measure (e.g., changes in symptoms may be measured in short time frames, whereas functioning requires an extended period of time for evaluation). In addition for APRNs in private practice, the cost and convenience of follow-up mail and phone assessment should also be considered relative to face-to-face evaluation of the patient during an episode of care. In addition to clinicians and administrators, payers want to know about access, cost, and value (the relationship between outcome and cost) and often require clinicians to collect this information to meet payer regulatory and accreditation standards (e.g., National Committee for Quality Assurance).

In developing an outcome evaluation program, the APRN should consider using the principles outlined by the Outcome Roundtable. The Outcome Roundtable is a group of mental health consumer, professional, service, and policy-making organizations. Under the auspices of the National Alliance for the Mentally Ill, the Outcome Roundtable articulated in a white paper a set of 12 broadly applicable principles of outcomes assessment (Smith et al., 1997). These principles are listed in Box 12-3. The implementation of outcome evaluation is a complex task over and above the use of these principles. Careful attention to implementation is needed if patient outcomes are to become a routine aspect of mental health services, analogous to the use of the standard laboratory tests in internal medicine practice (Smith et al., 1997).

---

box **12-3**

PRINCIPLES OF CONSUMER OUTCOME ASSESSMENT SYSTEMS

1. Outcome assessments appropriate to the application or question being answered
2. Outcome assessment tools and systems with demonstrated validity and reliability and must be sensitive to clinically important change over time

continued

---

box **12-3**

PRINCIPLES OF CONSUMER OUTCOME ASSESSMENT SYSTEMS— cont'd

3. Outcome assessments that include the consumer perspective as well as outcome assessment obtained from providers and family members or caregivers enhancing what is learned
4. Outcome assessments that have a minimal respondent burden and have the ability to be adapted to different health care systems and practices
5. Outcome assessments that include general health status as well as mental health status
6. Outcome assessments that include measures of consumer evaluation of treatment and outcomes
7. Outcome assessments that quantify the type and extent of treatment that the consumer receives (the process of care) for the target condition to understand the clinical relationship between the outcomes of care and treatment
8. Outcome assessments that include generic and disorder-specific information that is predictive of expected consumer outcomes; this prognostic information may include case mix and severity characteristics and may be associated with choice of and/or success of treatment
9. Outcome assessments that include those areas of personal functioning affected by the condition or conditions of interest
10. Outcome assessments that are initially assessed and reassessed at clinically meaningful points in time given the course of the disorder
11. Outcome assessments that use an appropriate scientific design and representative sample
12. Outcome assessment of consumers who prematurely leave treatment; this is as important as for those who are still in treatment

NURSING-SENSITIVE
■ OUTCOMES

APRNs in mental health care must demonstrate accountability for their practice by identifying and evaluating the outcomes of their performance (Barrell, Merwin, & Poster, 1997). APRN nursing-sensitive outcomes are patient outcomes that can be directly linked to the APRN's nursing interventions. In addition, they are patient outcome measures that can be used to directly evaluate the quality of APRN nursing care. Outcome data and analyses that delineate the unique contributions of APRNs will provide needed documentation for articulating the value of their work.

As outlined by Brush and Capezuti (1997), APRNs should measure their direct effect on care outcomes as well as cost savings. The increasing pressure for APRNs to document their contribution has made access, quality, and cost important outcome measures because they directly influence health outcomes. These outcome measures are crucial for APRNs to articulate to consumers, payers, and policy-makers. As outlined by Girouard (1996), APRN's should ask several questions to evaluate the effect of advanced nursing practice on patient outcomes. Some key questions APRNs in psychiatric-mental health should ask are as follows:

- What is the APRN's effect on patients' access to care providers? Does the presence of an APRN provider or a program developed by an APRN increase the number of people receiving care? How has this influenced health indicators in the community?
- Has the APRN provided cost-effective care and improved the quality of care in particular settings as measured by changes in health status and mental health status of individuals or groups of patients? Has the physical, functional, and/or psychosocial health status of patients improved? Are consumers satisfied with care received from the APRN? Has coordination of care had a positive effect on clinical outcomes?

- What is the cost of providing APRN services? How does this cost compare with other mental health providers? Is the APRN cost-effective in delivering care? Are the outcomes achieved worth the cost? What is the effect of the APRN on rates of service utilization such as unnecessary hospitalization, length of stay, and readmissions?

Nursing-sensitive outcomes can be attributed to nursing care—both basic level and advanced practice nursing. Lang and Marek (1992) identified 15 outcome indicators used in nursing research that are nursing-sensitive (Box 12-4).

box **12-4**

NURSING-SENSITIVE OUTCOMES

1. *Physiological status.* Measures physical parameters such as blood pressure, pulse, temperature, skin integrity, and weight.
2. *Psychosocial status.* Measures intrapersonal and interpersonal aspects of patient functioning, including communication patterns and relationships. Other measures include emotion, attitude, mood, affect, and coping.
3. *Functional status.* Measures activities of daily living, instrumental activities of daily living, mobility, and self-care ability. Patient's family or caregiver is often included in this measure.
4. *Behavioral.* Measures activities, skills, and actions of the patient. Other measures include application of knowledge, problem solving, adherence, motivation, and therapeutic competence.
5. *Knowledge.* Measures the cognitive level of understanding of the patient. Measures of knowledge of diagnosis, problems, diet, medication, and treatment have received the greatest attention.

continued

From an historical perspective, these identified nursing-sensitive indicators are crucial in selecting measures to identify APRN-sensitive patient outcomes. However, more recently within the scientific literature for mental health care, the seven most prevalent domains of outcomes being measured are symptomatology (psychiatric and substance abuse), social/interpersonal functioning, work functioning, satisfaction, treatment utilization, health status/global well-being, and health-related quality of life (Doherty & Streeter, 1997). Using these seven indicators alone may not serve the APRN well because of the difficulty of assigning which discipline or disciplines receive the credit for achievement of outcomes. APRNs must balance outcome selection between the seven most used indicators in mental health with the fifteen indicators that are sensitive to nursing and APRN interventions. The APRN must conduct studies that demonstrate how APRNs make a difference in the outcomes of care. For example, Baradell (1995) studied the clinical outcomes and patient satisfaction with clinical nurse specialists in psychiatric-mental health nursing (CNS-PMH). She

---

box 12-4

NURSING-SENSITIVE OUTCOMES—
cont'd

6. *Symptom control.* Measures the most frequently occurring symptom and is closely tied to physiologic measures. Symptom measures include pain, discomfort, depression, anxiety, and psychotic symptoms.
7. *Quality of life.* Measures the level or degree of the patient's satisfaction with perceived present life circumstances. These measures typically cover a range of dimensions known to contribute to quality of life, such as the physical, psychologic, social, material, and structural areas of life.

continued

---

box 12-4

NURSING-SENSITIVE OUTCOMES—
cont'd

8. *Home functioning.* Measures the functioning of the patient in the home environment.
9. *Family strain.* Measures the functioning of the family caregiver, which may have a significant effect on the patient's recovery.
10. *Goal attainment.* Measures outcomes by obtaining expected outcomes or goals at the beginning of treatment, and attainment of the goals is measured at designated intervals or at discharge from treatment. This type of outcome measure is more sensitive to individual patient differences and outcome achievement.
11. *Utilization of services.* Measures health care resource used and may include variables such as length of stay, number of clinic visits, number of home visits, and number of hospitalizations or rehospitalizations.
12. *Safety.* Measures outcomes from nursing interventions aimed at promoting safety and preventing injury. Measures include fall prevention, suicide prevention, and prevention of injury in using medical devices.
13. *Resolution of nursing diagnoses or nursing problems.* Measures the identification and resolution of relevant nursing diagnoses. Lang and Marek (1992) suggest that because nursing diagnoses are often more temporary than medical diagnoses, the resolution of nursing diagnoses would be more sensitive to changes in patient status.
14. *Patient satisfaction.* Measures the degree of satisfaction with services, providers, and outcomes of care.
15. *Caring.* Measures caring as an outcome versus caring as a process. Outcomes associated with caring are multidimensional; however, the patient's subjective perception related to care provided appears to be a key factor.

From Davis, 1994.

found from a sample of 100 patients of CNS-PMHs, a significant improvement in all clinical symptoms measured: anxiety, depression, anger, confusion, fatigue, and vigor as well as significant improvement in quality of life in terms of family, social life, and job. Satisfaction with care provided was rated very high. This research lends strong support to the value of the APRN's practice to psychiatric-mental health patients.

Another promising framework for evaluating nurse-sensitive outcomes is the Iowa Nursing Intervention Project (McCloskey & Bulechek, 1995). The Iowa Intervention Project developed nursing intervention classification (NIC) codes, nursing outcome classification (NOC) codes, and a taxonomy for arranging nursing interventions and outcomes into groups, sets, or levels. Although this classification system applies to all levels of nursing, the NIC and NOC codes are applicable to the APRN's practice because many of the interventions and outcomes require advanced education, experience, and skill. The University of Iowa College of Nursing established the Center for Nursing Classification (www.nursing.uiowa.edu) to facilitate the continued development of this important work. In August 1991, a research team with the NIC project began conducting a study of nursing-sensitive patient outcomes and the development of the Nursing Outcomes Classification (NOC). The purposes of this ongoing research are as follows (McCloskey & Bulechek, 1995):

1. Identify, label, validate, and classify nursing-sensitive patient outcomes and indicators
2. Evaluate the validity and usefulness of the classification in clinical field testing
3. Define and test measurement procedures for the outcomes and indicators

The contribution of this project is a focus on multiple nursing specialties, a well defined research methodology, a uniform language for nursing interventions and outcomes, and a clear linkage between specific APRN interventions and nursing-sensitive patient outcomes.

CASE STUDY: PUTTING IT ALL TOGETHER

Mr. E. is a 38-year-old married accountant with no history of depression. On his first visit to the mental health clinic, his chief complaints are an inability to work, decreased concentration, difficulty falling asleep with early morning awakening without being able to fall back to sleep, fitful and disturbing dreams when asleep, poor appetite, and feelings of worthlessness and hopelessness. He also reports experiencing a sad or depressed mood every day for the past 2 months with feelings of guilt for not being able to provide for his family. He says that he has been unable to fulfill his family role as a provider and be a source of strength for his wife and two young children. He describes his symptoms and level of impairment as moderate to severe. Mr. E. reports occasionally feeling suicidal with vague plans but without a desire to carry it out. Mr. E. is unable to recall any manic episodes. He has been referred to an APRN in psychiatric-mental health by his employer because of a decrease in occupational functioning over the past 2 months and an inability to get along with co-workers. In the APRN's visit with Mr. E., the diagnosis of major depression is identified and a treatment plan is developed.

The APRN can choose one of the following as an appropriate clinical practice guideline for Mr. E.

- AHCPR's Clinical Practice Guideline on Depression in Primary Care
- APA Practice Guideline on Depressive Disorders
- A behavioral health managed care approved practice guideline for major depression

In this case study, the APRN chose the AHCPR's Clinical Practice Guideline for Depression in Primary Care (1993). The AHCPR guideline is appropriate for this patient because he has never been diagnosed with depression or any other mental disorder in the past. This practice guideline was developed to assist and guide primary care providers (general practitioners, family practitioners, internists, APRNs, registered nurses, mental health nurse specialists, physician assistants, and others) in the detection, diagnosis, and treatment of depression (Depression Guideline Panel, 1993a).

Is this the correct diagnosis? What documentation can the APRN use to support this diagnosis? Using the Clinical Practice Guideline's (Depression Guideline Panel, 1993a) diagnostic decision tree, major depression would be the correct primary diagnosis. The Clinical Practice Guideline uses the same diagnostic criteria as outlined in the *Diagnostic and Statistical Manual of Mental Disorders*, or *DSM-IV*, (APA, 1994) for major depressive disorders. For a major depressive disorder, at least five of the symptoms in Box 12-5 are present during the same time period, and at least one of the first two symptoms must be present. In addition, symptoms must be present most of the day, nearly daily, for a period of at least 2 weeks.

box **12-5**

DIAGNOSTIC CRITERIA FOR MAJOR DEPRESSIVE DISORDERS

- Depressed mood most of the day, nearly every day
- Markedly, diminished interest or pleasure in almost all activities most of the day, nearly every day (as indicated by subjective account or observation by others of apathy most of the time)
- Significant weight loss or gain
- Insomnia or hypersomnia
- Psychomotor agitation or retardation
- Fatigue (loss of energy)
- Feelings of worthlessness (guilt)
- Impaired concentration (indecisiveness)
- Recurrent thoughts of death or suicide

From APA, 1994.

Following the decision tree on differential diagnosis of primary mood disorder in the Clinical Practice Guideline (Depression Guideline Panel, 1993a), the APRN would find that Mr. E. exhibits at least six of the nine symptoms with depressed mood or sadness most of the day as well as reporting no prior manic episodes. The APRN would correctly diagnose Mr. E. with major depressive episode. In addition to detecting and diagnosing the disorder, the Clinical Practice Guideline provides direction on identifying associated conditions that may be causing or exacerbating the depression. Associated conditions include substance abuse; concurrent medication; general medical disorder; causal, nonmood psychiatric disorder, or grief reaction. The Clinical Practice Guideline recommends that an associated condition should be treated before treatment of depression. Once the associated condition is treated, the underlying depression may resolve without further treatment. However, failure to treat the associated cause may prevent the successful treatment of depression. After a complete history and physical examination, the APRN determines that Mr. E. does not have any listed associated conditions.

What forms of treatments are acceptable? Cognitive behavioral therapy? Pharmacotherapy? Would a mono-treatment selection be as effective and cost-saving as combination therapy? Now that the APRN has confirmed the diagnosis for Mr. E. as major depression, the next step is to develop a treatment plan. According to the Clinical Practice Guideline (AHCPR, 1993), the treatment for major depressive disorder may include three phases: acute, continuation, and maintenance. The overall aim of the three phases is the attainment of a stable, fully asymptomatic state and full restoration of psychosocial function. Acute treatment aims at removing all depressive symptoms. Once the patient improves with treatment, a response is declared. A remission may occur either spontaneously or with treatment. If the symptoms return and are severe enough to meet diagnostic criteria within 6 months after remission, a relapse is declared. Continuation treatment aims at preventing this relapse. Once the patient is asymptomatic for at least 6 months after an episode, recovery from the episode is declared. At recovery, continuation treatment may be stopped. For those with recurrent depression, however, a new episode (recurrence) may occur months or years later. Maintenance treatment aims at preventing a recurrence. Recurrence is expected in 50% of cases within 2 years after continuation treatment.

For Mr. E., the APRN will begin the Clinical Practice Guideline (Depression Guideline Panel, 1993a) in the acute phase to eliminate the symptoms and restore psychosocial functioning. According to the Clinical Practice Guideline, all treatments are administered in the context of clinical management. Clinical management refers to education of and discussion with patients and families about the nature of depression, its course, and the relative costs and benefits of treatment options. Clinical management is different from supportive therapy, which itself is a "formal" therapy, or which can be combined with medication. Supportive therapy goes beyond clinical management and focuses on the management and resolution of current difficulties and life decisions through the use of the patient's strengths and available resources.

The APRN weighs the certainty of treatment response against the likelihood and severity of potential adverse treatment effects. Treatment selection is based on an evaluation of the potential benefits and harms of each alternative. Second- and third-line treatments are considered if first-line treatments are contraindicated, ineffective, or inappropriate. The Clinical Practice Guideline provides an overview of treatment for depression (Depression Guideline Panel, 1993b). Formal treatments of major depression include medication, psychotherapy, the combination of medication and psychotherapy, and electroconvulsive therapy (ECT). According to the Clinical Practice Guideline, the routine use of both medication and psychotherapy is not recommended as the initial treatment for most patients. The Depression Guideline Panel (1993b) consensus and research suggest that combined treatment may be useful in the following instances:

- Either treatment alone, optimally given, is only partially effective.
- The clinical circumstances suggest two discrete targets of therapy.
- The prior course of recurrent depression is chronic.

Based on the information from the Clinical Practice Guideline, the APRN decides on treating Mr. E.'s depressive episode by prescribing a selective serotonin reuptake inhibitor (SSRI) and monitoring the effects every week.

What outcome measures should be selected to evaluate the outcomes for this patient? The Clinical Practice Guideline (Depression Guideline Panel, 1993a) includes a section on measuring outcomes. The Guideline suggests that initial evaluation include asking the patient about the nine criteria symptoms of a major depressive episode, as well as the current level of interpersonal and occupational functioning. In addition to the clinical interview, the guideline suggests patient self-report or clinician symptom-rating scales be used to permit rapid assessment of the nature and severity of depressive symptoms. Interviewing a spouse or close friend about the patient's day-to-day functioning and specific symptoms may also provide information in determining the course of the illness, current symptoms, and level of functioning. Follow-up visits during the acute treatment are used to evaluate the level of symptom relief and restoration of function. Symptom evaluation allows both the APRN and the patient to assess response to treatment, determine whether the medication dosage should be adjusted, and clarify whether and when alternative treatments are needed (Depression Guideline Panel, 1993b).

One of the major drawbacks to the AHCPR Clinical Practice Guidelines, as well as most other practice guidelines, is the lack of identified outcome measures that could be used universally by APRNs and other practitioners to measure and compare patient outcomes within populations, within health care systems, and between practitioners and practices. Dorwart (1997) identified outcomes for patients with major depressive disorders as being divided into clinical and functional categories. Clinical outcomes describe the psychiatric and physiologic signs and symptoms of disease or disorders, and functional outcomes describe levels of social role performance. Outcome measures that would be appropriate for use in outcome evaluation for Mr. E. include the following:

- Depression Outcome Module (DOM)
- Beck Depression Inventory (BDI)
- Hamilton Rating Scale for Depression (HRSD)
- Symptom Checklist-90-Report Revised (SCL-90-R)
- Brief Symptom Inventory (BSI)
- Health Status Survey Short Form 36 (SF-36)
- Behavior and Symptom Identification Scale (BASIS-32)
- Global Assessment of Functioning (GAF)
- Clinical Global Impressions (CGI)

See Outcome Measurement Tools in the Resources and Connections section for more information.

IMPLICATIONS FOR
■ THE FUTURE

Clinical Implications

The consistent use of practice guidelines and outcome evaluation in clinical practice provides APRNs with a unique opportunity to demonstrate their contributions to the health care system. Practice guidelines will provide unified treatments and services for similar mental illnesses and populations based on expert consensus, as well as evidence based on research. The APRN's practice and that of other practitioners will be evaluated based on managing patients using these clinical practice guidelines and the achievement of expected patient outcomes. Nurses at all levels of practice have a major role to play in outcome evaluation

and management (APNA, 1997). APRNs must provide leadership in developing practical strategies for incorporating outcome evaluation into their clinical practice. APRNs should be active members of the interdisciplinary team and work with others to select critical outcome indicators of care, the types of instruments that will be used to evaluate patient outcomes, the most effective method for collecting outcome data, and the most meaningful and easily understood way to disseminate outcome data to consumers, payers, practitioners, policy makers, and the public.

Administration should ensure that practice guidelines and outcome evaluation are critical parts of the health care infrastructure. Practice guidelines and outcome evaluation must be integrated as routine parts of care and services. In addition, practitioners require timely feedback on evaluated outcomes to assess the effectiveness of practice guidelines, practice patterns, and outcomes. These data also enhance existing guidelines and inform development of new ones. Administrators can use outcome data for allocating resources, developing new clinical programs, and establishing priorities for quality improvement initiatives. Administrators should actively seek value in the services provided and work to balance competing demands between quality services and limited resources. The selection of particular outcomes and the interpretation of data are powerful tools for setting priorities and allocating resources. Access to outcome data provides more accurate assessment of services and appropriate administrative actions. Administrators must ensure that systems will collect outcome data and feed that data back to practitioners in a timely fashion. It is critical that outcome data be integrated into the performance improvement strategies of the health care system.

Research Implications

Merwin and Mauck (1995) provided a comprehensive literature review of the current status of RN and APRN outcome research in psychiatric-mental health care. The need for research challenges APRNs to articulate their accountability and responsibility for the outcomes of their interventions. Researchers have studied outcomes of APRN practice in psychiatric-mental health in the areas of mood, symptom management, quality of life, functional status, patient and family satisfaction, hospitalization, family relationships, social relationships, and financial cost reduction (Barrell, Merwin, & Poster, 1997; Cornwell & Chiverton, 1997). As discussed earlier in this chapter, the framework of structure-process-outcome evaluation may be used by researchers to identify and articulate the effects of the APRN's practice on patient outcomes. The structure-process-outcome framework allows the researcher to examine how setting- and provider-specific variables (structure variables) affect provider actions or interventions (process variables) and how these, in turn, may relate to changes in the recipient of care (outcome variables) (APNA, 1997; Cornwell & Chiverton, 1997). Researchers, with APRN clinicians, must identify through systematic and deliberate predictive outcome studies which APRN interventions provide the most value (cost-benefit ratio) and which populations are better served with APRNs in the psychiatric-mental health delivery system. Outcome evaluation research will allow researchers to measure the cost effectiveness of APRN practices compared with other practitioners and to measure the effectiveness of clinical practice guidelines used in practice.

Education Implications

Like health care, the system for educating the APRN continues to evolve. To meet the challenges of the future, APRNs must be cognizant of practice guidelines and outcome evaluation. Priorities of nursing educational institutions should be to give APRNs the knowledge, skills, and tools to understand, analyze, and evaluate clinical practice guidelines and to develop and implement an outcome evaluation system. The challenge for educa-

tors is to provide a clear link between clinical practice guidelines used in practice with the outcomes achieved from practice. Educators should require students to analyze practice guidelines for completeness and accuracy, evidence to support recommendations, and the use of outcome evaluation. Educators should participate with students in identifying critical outcomes of APRN practice in psychiatric-mental health. APRN education should include outcome domains and APRN nursing-sensitive outcomes, instrument selection, program development, and research evaluation. Also important is knowledge about the hardware and software technology that supports these processes.

In conclusion, mental health care treatment and service delivery are rapidly evolving and changing. APRNs must remain informed and provide leadership in meeting these evolving challenges. Demands for accountability will continue well into the twenty-first century. Practice guidelines and outcome evaluation will provide the needed tools for APRNs to meet the challenges of accountability with the emerging health care system. Although relatively new, practice guidelines and outcome evaluation will continue to have a profound effect on mental health care delivery over the next few decades. Outcome data will be used to guide development of sound, evidence-based practice, with practice guidelines providing a meaningful structure and process for collecting valid and reliable outcome measures. According to Sederer, Dickey, and Hermann (1996), integrating outcome evaluation into psychiatric-mental health clinical practice will serve three primary functions:

- Promote the development and adoption of treatment guidelines that can be linked to specific outcomes
- Produce data that will legitimize and validate the treatment options of psychiatric illness and substance abuse problems
- Regain public trust with mental health services by offering accountability for outcome management

Outcome evaluation has become an imperative for demonstrating effectiveness in clinical practice. APRNs must demonstrate a balance in cost and treatment effectiveness in the provision of services. With the continued health care movement toward deinstitutionalization; the lack of coordinated, community-based mental health services; and the decreasing resource dollars to provide treatment, it is imperative for APRNs to examine ways to foster continuity of care across the entire continuum of mental illness and health and to focus on a wide range of services that demonstrate cost-effective, quality outcomes.

RESOURCES AND CONNECTIONS

PRACTICE GUIDELINES IN BEHAVIORAL HEALTH

Managed behavioral health programs

Organization	Description
Comprehensive Behavioral Care, Inc. 4200 West Cypress Street, Suite 300 Tampa, Florida 33607	CBC Best Practice Guidelines (1995)
MCC Behavioral Care, Inc. 11095 Viking Drive, Suite 350 Eden Prairie, Minnesota 55344	MCC Clinical Guidelines for Mental Health and Substance Abuse (1996)
Human Affairs International 10150 South Centennial Parkway Sandy, Utah 84070	Best Practices Guidelines (1995)

Professional associations and other sources

Organization	Description
Agency for Health Care Policy and Research www.ahcpr.gov/fund/ngcguidl.htm	Invitation to submit guidelines to the National Guideline Clearinghouse.
American Academy of Child and Adolescent Psychiatry 3515 Wisconsin Avenue, NW Washington, DC 20016 202-966-7300	Various practice parameters: anxiety, ADHD, bipolar disorder, conduct disorder, depressive disorder, schizophrenia, substance use disorder, others
Association for Ambulatory Behavioral Healthcare 301 North Fairfax Street, Suite 109 Alexandria Virginia 22314 703-836-2274	Partial hospitalization • Child/adolescent • Adult • Geriatric • Chemical dependency
American Psychiatric Association 1400 K Street, NW Washington, DC 20005 202-682-6288	Various guidelines: psychiatric evaluation, depression, bipolar disorder, schizophrenia, substance use disorder, eating disorders, Alzheimer's disease, and other dementias of late life
American Psychological Association Practice Directorate 750 First Street, NE Washington, DC 20002 202-336-5865	Template for developing guidelines: interventions for mental disorders and psychological aspects of physical disorders
Institute for Healthcare Quality 8000 West 78th Street Minneapolis, Minnesota 55439 612-829-3500	Behavioral Health Best Practice Guidelines (1995)

Other resources

Milliman & Robertson, Inc.
Healthcare Guidelines
206-624-7940

Mosby-Year Book Case Management Guidelines
800-426-4545

The Zitter Group
Center for Outcomes Information
Guidelines Conferences
415-495-2450

Books

Chan, P.D. (1996). *Practice parameters in medicine, primary care, and family practice.* Laguna Hills, CA: Current Clinical Strategies.

Dambro, M.R. (1998). *Griffith's 5 minute clinical consult.* Baltimore: Williams & Wilkins.

Mozena, J.P., Emerick, C.E., & Black, S.C. (1996). *Clinical guideline development: an algorithm approach.* Baltimore: Aspen Publishers.

Tierney, L.M., McPhee, S.J., & Papadakis, M.A. (1998). *Current medical diagnosis and treatment 1998.* Stamford, CT: Appleton & Lange.

Uphold, C.R., & Graham, M.V. (1994). *Clinical guidelines in family practice* (ed. 2). Gainesville, FL: Barmarrae Books.

OUTCOME EVALUATION IN BEHAVIORAL HEALTH

Organizations

Medical Outcomes Trust
8 Park Plaza, #503
Boston, MA 02116
617-426-4046
Fax: 617-426-4131
Email: info@outcomes-trust.org
Website: www.outcomes-trust.org

Stratis Health (formerly Health Outcomes Institute and the Foundation for Health Care Evaluation)
2901 Metro Drive, Suite 400
Bloomington, MN 55425
612-853-1815
Email: info@stratishealth.org
Website: www.stratishealth.org

Institute for Healthcare Improvement
135 Francis Street
Boston, MA 02215
617-754-4800
Fax: 617-754-4848
Email: ihi@world.std.com
Website: www.ihi.org

Outcome measurement tools in the public domain

INSTRUMENT	AREAS MEASURED	TYPE	INFORMATION
Beck Depression Inventory (BDI)[a]	Depressive disorders	Self report	21 items 4-point scale
Behavior and Symptom Identification Scale (BASIS-32)[b]	Psychiatric symptoms and functioning	Self report	32 items 5-point scale 5 subscales
Brief Psychiatric Rating Scale (BPRS)[c]	Psychiatric symptoms and functioning	Clinician rated	18 symptoms constructs 7-point scale 7 subscales
Brief Symptom Inventory (BSI)[d]	Psychiatric symptoms	Self report	53 items Abbreviated SCL-90-R
Child Behavior Checklist (CBCL)[e]	Psychiatric symptoms Social competence Academic performance	Parent rated Teacher rated	Two versions: • Ages 2 to 4 years • Ages 4 to 18 years

INSTRUMENT	AREAS MEASURED	TYPE	INFORMATION
Clinical Global Impressions (CGI)[f]	Overall improvement	Clinician rated	3 items: severity, improvement
Consumer Satisfaction Questionnaire[g]	Satisfaction survey	Self report	8 Items 4-point scale
Geriatric Depression Scale (GDS)[h]	Depressive disorders in geriatric patients	Interviewer or self report	11 items
Global Assessment of Functioning (GAF)[i]	Psychiatric functioning and ADL skills	Clinician rated	Single rating Scored 0–100
Goal Attainment Scale[j]	Individually defined goals	Clinician rated	Behaviorally defined outcomes 5-point scale
Group Health Association of America (GHAA) Consumer Satisfaction Survey[k]	Satisfaction survey	Self report	63 items 5-point scale
Hamilton Rating Scale for Anxiety (HRSA)[l]	Anxiety disorders	Interviewer	14 items 4-point scale
Hamilton Rating Scale for Depression (HRSD)[m]	Depressive disorders	Interviewer	21 items 4-point scale
Health Status Survey Short Form 36 (SF-36)[n]	Quality of life Well-being	Self report	36 items 8 subscales
Patient Satisfaction Questionnaire (PSQ III)[o]	Satisfaction survey	Self report	50 items 5-point scale
Rapid Disability Rating Scale[p]	Functional status and ADL skills	Clinician rated	18 items 4-point scale
Speilberger State-Trait Anxiety Inventory (STAI)[q]	Anxiety disorders	Self report	20 items 4-point scale
Symptom Checklist-90-Revised[r]	Psychiatric symptoms	Self report	90 items 5-point scale 9 subscales, 3 global scores
UM-Composite International Diagnostic Interview (UM-CIDI)[s]	Overall psychopathology and distress	Interview	Brief Gold standard

continued

INSTRUMENT	AREAS MEASURED	TYPE	INFORMATION
Yale Brown Obsessive-Compulsive Scale[t]	OCD	Self report	10 items 5-point scale

[a]Beck, A., et al. (1961). An inventory for measuring depression. *Archives of General Psychiatry, 42*, 667–675.

[b]Eisen, S.V., Dill, D.L., & Grob, M.C. (1994). Reliability and validity of a brief patient-report instrument for psychiatric outcome evaluation. *Hospital Community Psychiatry, 45*, 242–247.

[c]Overall, J., & Gorham, D. (1962). The brief psychiatric rating scale. *Psychology Report. 10*, 782–812.

[d]Derogatis, L.R., & Lazarus, L. (1994). SCL-90-R, brief symptom inventory, and matching clinical rating scales. In Maruish, M. (Ed.). *Treatment planning and outcome assessment.* New York: Lawrence Earlbaum Associates.

[e]Achenbach, T., & Edelbrock, C. (1983). *Manual for the Child Behavior Checklist and Revised Child Behavior Profile.* Burlington, VT: Department of Psychiatry, University of Vermont.

[f]Guy, W. (1976). *ECDEU assessment manual for psychopharmacology.* Washington, DC: NIMH.

[g]Larsen, D.L., et al. (1979). Assessment of client/patient satisfaction: development of a general scale. *Evaluation and Program Planning, 4*, 443–453.

[h]Yesavage, et al. (1983). Development and validation of a geriatric depression screen scale: a preliminary report. *Journal of Psychiatric Research, 17*, 37–49.

[i]American Psychiatric Association. (1994). *Diagnostic and statistical manual of mental disorders* (ed. 4). Washington, DC: the Association.

[j]Kiresuk, T.J., & Sherman, R.E. (1968). Global attainment scaling. *Community Mental Health Journal, 4*, 197–207.

[k]Davies, A.R., & Ware, J.E. (1991). *GHAA's consumer satisfaction survey.* Washington, DC: Group Health Association of America, Inc.

[l]Hamilton, M. (1959). The assessment of anxiety states by rating. *British Journal of Medical Psychology, 32*, 50–55.

[m]Hamilton, M. (1960). Rating depressed patients. *Journal of Clinical Psychiatry. 41*, 21–24.

[n]Ware, J.E., & Sherbourne, C.D. (1992). The MOS 36-item short-form health status survey (SF-36). *Medical Care, 30*, MS253-MS265.

[o]Hays, R.D., Davies, A.R., & Ware, J.E. (1987). *Scoring the patient satisfaction questionnaires: PSQIII. Mos Memo No. 866, Medical Outcomes Study.* Santa Monica, CA: Rand.

[p]Linn, M.W., & Linn, B.S. (1982). The rapid disability rating scale - 2. *Journal of the American Geriatric Society, 30*, 378–382.

[q] Speilberger, C., Gorsuch, R., & Lushen, R. (1970). *Manual for the state-trait anxiety inventory.* Palo Alto, CA: Consulting Psychologist Press.

[r]Derogatis, L.R., Lazarus, L. (1994). SCL-90-R, brief symptom inventory, and matching clinical rating scales. In Maruish, M. (Ed.). *Treatment planning and outcome assessment.* New York: Lawrence Earlbaum Associates.

[s]Kessler, et al. (1994). Lifetime and 12 month prevalence of DSM-III-R psychiatric disorders in the US: results from the national comorbidity survey. *Archives of General Psychiatry, 51*, 8–19.

[t]Goodman, et al. (1989). The Yale Brown obsessive-compulsive scale. *Archives of General Psychiatry, 46*, 1006–1011.

For additional outcome evaluation tools, see the Report of the American Psychiatric Nurses Association Congress on Advanced Practice in Psychiatric Nursing, Measuring Outcomes in APRN-PMH Practice Work Group; and Barrell, L.M., Merwin, E.I., & Poster, E.C. (1997). Patient outcomes used in advanced practice psychiatric nursing to evaluate effectiveness of practice. *Archives of Psychiatric Nursing, 11*(4), 184–197.

INTERNET

Clinical practice guidelines

The American Psychiatric Nurses Association
  www.apna.org

The Best Practice Network www.best4health.org

National Institutes of Health (NIH) Consensus Development Program
odp.od.nih.gov/consensus/

National Association of Healthcare Quality—Practice Guideline Resources
  www.nahq.org/clinical.htm

Emory WebNet Practice Guideline Connections www.gen.emory.edu/MEDWEB/keyword/clinical_practice/guidelines.html

The Expert Consensus Guideline Series www.psychguides.com/eks_gls.htm

The American Academy of Child and Adolescent Psychiatry—Practice Guidelines www.aacap.org/clinical

Nurse Practitioner Web www.npweb.org

Outcome evaluation

National Committee for Quality Assurance www.ncqa.org

Association of Managed Care Providers www.comed.com/amcp

Institute for Behavioral Health Care www.ibh.com

Behavioral Health Outcomes—Newsletter www.manisses.com/manisses-pubs/out/outcurrent.htm

Open Minds: The Behavioral Health and Social Service Industry Analyst www.openminds.com

LISTSERV

Send request to LISTSERV@MAELSTROM.ST JOHNS.EDU: OUTCMTEN—Topical Evaluation Network Outcome Research List

REFERENCES

Agency for Health Care Policy and Research. (April 13, 1998). Invitation to submit guidelines to the National Guideline Clearinghouse. *Federal Register, 63*(70), 18–27.

American Psychiatric Association. (1993). APA practice guidelines for major depressive disorders in adults. *American Journal of Psychiatry, 150,* 1–26.

American Psychiatric Association. (1994). *Diagnositic and statistical manual of mental disorders* (ed. 4). Washington, DC: Author.

American Psychiatric Nurses Association. (1998). *Psychiatric-mental health nurse roles in outcome evaluation and management.* [Position statement]. Washington, DC: Author.

APNA Work Group on Measuring Outcomes. (1997). *Measuring outcomes in advanced practice registered nurses: psychiatric mental health practice. Report of the APNA Congress on Advanced Practice in Psychiatric Nursing.* Washington, DC: American Psychiatric Nurses Association.

Baradell, J.G. (1995). Clinical outcomes and satisfaction of patients of clinical nurse specialists in psychiatric-mental health nursing. *Archives of Psychiatric Nursing, 9*(5), 240–250.

Barrell, L.M., Merwin, E.I., & Poster, E.C. (1997). Patient outcomes used by advanced practice psychiatric nurses to evaluate effectiveness of practice. *Archives of Psychiatric Nursing, 11*(4), 184–197.

Berger, J.T., & Rosner, F. (1996). The ethics of practice guidelines. *Archives of Internal Medicine, 156,* 2051–2056.

Brush, B.L., & Capezuti, E.A. (1997). Professional autonomy: essential for nurse practitioner survival in the 21st century. *Journal of the American Academy of Nurse Practitioners, 9*(6), 265–269.

Burlingame, G.M., et al. (1995). Pragmatics of tracking mental health outcomes in a managed care setting. *Journal of Mental Health Administration, 22,* 226–236.

Cornwell, C., & Chiverton, P. (1997). The psychiatric advanced practice nurse with prescriptive authority: role development, practice issues and outcome measures. *Archives of Psychiatric Nursing, 11*(2), 57–65.

Davis, T. (1994). Patient outcomes research. Part II. *Canadian Journal of Cardiovascular Nursing, 5*(4), 29–32.

Depression Guideline Panel. (1993a). *Depression in primary care: Volume 1, Detection and diagnosis. Clinical Practice Guideline, number 5.* Rockville, MD: U.S. Department of Health and Human Services, Public Health Service, Agency for Health Care Policy and Research [AHCPR]. AHCPR Publication No. 93–0550.

Depression Guideline Panel. (1993b). *Depression in primary care: Volume 2, Treatment of major depression. Clinical Practice Guideline, number 5.* Rockville, MD: U.S. Department of Health and Human Services, Public Health Service, Agency for Health Care Policy and Research [AHCPR]. AHCPR Publication No. 93–0551.

Doherty, J.P., & Streeter, M.J. (1997). Measuring outcomes. In Sederer, L.I., & Dickey, B. (Eds.). *Outcomes assessment in clinical practice.* Baltimore: Williams & Wiklins.

Donabedian, A. (1966). Evaluating the quality of medical care. *Milbank Quarterly, 44,* 166–203.

Donabedian, A. (1990). *Exploration in quality assessment and monitoring.* Ann Arbor, MI: Health Administration Press.

Dorwart, R.A. (1997) Outcomes management strategies in mental health: application and implications for clinical practice. In Sederer, L.I., & Dickey, B. (Eds.). *Outcomes assessment in clinical practice.* Baltimore: Williams & Wilkins.

Field, M.J., & Lohr, K.N. (Eds.). (1990). Committee to Advise the Public Health Service on Clinical Practice Guidelines, Institute of Medicine. *Clinical practice guidelines: directions for a new program.* Washington, DC: National Academy Press.

Geyman, J.P. (1998). Evidence-based medicine in primary care: an overview. *Journal of the Association of British Family Practice, 11*(1), 46–56.

Girouard, S. A. (1996). Evaluating advanced nursing practice. In Hamric, A.B., Spross, J.A., & Hanson C.M. (Eds.). *Advanced nursing practice: an integrative approach.* Philadelphia: W.B. Saunders.

Hayward, R.S.A., et al. (1995). Users' guides to the medical literature. VII. How to use clinical practice guidelines. A. Are the recommendations valid? *Journal of the American Medical Association, 274*(7), 570–574.

Irvine, D., Sidani, S., & Hall, L.M. (1998). Linking outcomes to nurses' roles in health care. *Nursing Economics, 16*(2), 58–64.

Johnson, K.B., Hirshfield, E.N., & Ile, M.L. (1990). *Legal implications of practice parameters.* Chicago: American Medical Association.

Johnson, M., & Maas, M. (Eds.). (1997). *Nursing outcome classification (NOC).* St. Louis: Mosby.

Kelly, J.T. (1994). The interface of clinical paths and practice parameters. In Spath, P.L. (Ed.). *Clinical paths: tools to outcomes management.* Chicago: American Hospital Publishing.

Kelly, J.T., & Bernard, D.B. (1996). Clinical practice guidelines: foundation for effective disease management. In Todd, W.E., & Nash, D. (Eds.). *Disease management: a systems approach to improving patient outcomes.* Chicago: American Hospital Publishing.

Kleinpell, R.M. (1997). Whose outcomes: patients, providers, or payer? *Nursing Clinics of North America, 32*(3), 513–520.

Lang, N.M., & Marek, K. (1992). Outcomes that reflect clinical practice. In *Proceedings of the State of Science Conference on Patient Outcomes Research sponsored by the National Center for Nursing Research,* NIH Publication No. 93-3411, 27–38.

Marek, K. (1989). Outcome measurement in nursing. *Journal of Nursing Quality Assurance, 4*(1), 1–9.

Mark, B.A. (1995). The black box of patient outcomes research. *Image: Journal of Nursing Scholarship, 27*(1), 42.

McCloskey, J.C., & Bulechek, G.M. (Eds.). (1995). *Nursing intervention classification (NIC).* (ed. 2). St. Louis: Mosby.

McCormick, K.A., Cummings, M.A., & Kovner, C. (1997). The role of the Agency for Health Care Policy and Research in improving outcomes of care. *Nursing Clinics of North America, 32*(3), 521–542.

McGlynn, E.A. (1996). Domains of study and methodological challenges. In Sederer, L.I., & Dickey, B. (Eds.). *Outcomes assessment in clinical practice.* Baltimore: Williams & Wilkins.

McIntyre, J.S., Zarin, D.A., & Pincus, H.A. (1996). Practice guidelines and outcomes research. In Sederer, L.I., & Dickey, B. (Eds.). *Outcomes assessment in clinical practice.* Baltimore: Williams & Wilkins.

Merwin, E.I., & Mauck, A. (1995). Psychiatric nursing outcome research: the state of the science. *Archives of Psychiatric Nursing, 9*(6), 311–331.

Merwin, E.I., et al. (1997). Advanced practice psychiatric nursing: a national profile. *Archives of Psychiatric Nursing, 11*(4), 182–183.

Murphy, R.N. (1997). Legal and practical impact of clinical practice guidelines on nursing and medical practice. *The Nurse Practitioner, 22*(3), 138, 147–148.

Rieve, J.A. (1998). The value of case management guidelines. *The Case Manager, 9*(3), 29–30.

Sackett, D.L., et al. (1996). Evidence-based medicine: what it is and what it isn't. *British Medical Journal, 312,* 71–72.

Schulberg, H.C., et al. (1996). Treating major depression in primary care practice: eight-month clinical outcomes. *Archives of General Psychiatry, 53*(10), 913–919.

Sederer, L.I., Dickey, B., & Eisen, S. V. (1997). Assessing outcomes in clinical practice. *Psychiatric Quarterly, 68*(4), 311–325.

Sederer, L.I., Dickey, B., & Hermann, R.C. (1996). The imperative of outcome assessment in psychiatry. In Sederer, L.I., & Dickey, B. (Eds.). *Outcomes assessment in clinical practice.* Baltimore: Williams & Wilkins.

Sherwood, R. (1998). Best practice network has much to offer. *APNA News, 10*(3), 6–7.

Smith, G.R., et al. (1997). Principles of assessment of patient outcomes in mental health care. *Psychiatric Services, 48,* 1033–1036

Sperry, L. (1997). Treatment outcomes: an overview. *Psychiatric Annals, 27*(2), 95–99.

Stuart, G. (1998a). Environmental context of psychiatric nursing care. In Stuart, G.W., & Laraia, M.T. (Eds.). *Principles and practice of psychiatric nursing* (ed. 6). St. Louis: Mosby.

Stuart, G. (May 18, 1998b). Personal communication. Practice Guideline Coalition.

Woolf, S.H. (1990). Practice guidelines: a new reality in medicine. I. Recent developments. *Archives of Internal Medicine, 150,* 1811–1118.

Woolf, S.H. (1992). Practice guidelines: a new reality in medicine. II. Methods of developing guidelines. *Archives of Internal Medicine, 152,* 946–952.

Zarate, C.A. (1997). Treatment guidelines and algorithms in acute care psychiatry. In Sederer, L.I., & Rothschild, A.J. (Eds.). *Acute care psychiatry: diagnosis and treatment.* Baltimore: Williams & Wilkins.

Zarin, D.A., McIntyre, J.S., & Pincus, H.A. (1996). Introduction. In *Practice guidelines.* Washington, DC: American Psychiatric Association.

chapter 13

Framework for Prescriptive Practice

KATHARINE BAILEY

■ INTRODUCTION

The forces of health care reform during the last decade have resulted in the rapid transformation of most aspects of psychiatric care. A major trend has been the move to a managed care approach in both the private and public sectors. Additionally, a greater emphasis on the biologic aspects of psychiatric disorders and a rapidly expanding pharmacopoeia of efficacious psychotropic agents have resulted in the increased use of psychopharmacotherapy in the treatment of mental illness. Between 1975 and 1985, the proportion of visits to office-based psychiatrists that included medication increased from 27% to 46%, and by 1988, over half of psychiatrists' patients in outpatient settings reportedly received pharmacologic treatment (Olfson, Pincus, & Sabshin, 1994).

These trends have also greatly altered the scope and nature of advanced practice registered nurse (APRN) practice in psychiatric and mental health nursing. They have challenged the psychiatric nursing specialty to integrate a broader repertoire of health-related, neurobiologically based knowledge and intervention. The prescribing of medications is rapidly becoming an integral component of advanced practice in psychiatric nursing. As mental health care delivery systems strive to address goals of cost containment, access to care, quality of care, and patient satisfaction, the expanded use of APRNs is a logical conclusion. Prescriptive authority allows for the independence and latitude of the full scope of advanced nursing practice.

HISTORICAL CONTEXT OF ■ PRESCRIPTIVE AUTHORITY

For APRNs across specialties to attain the legalization of prescriptive authority for their profession, they have had to challenge the widely held assumption that physicians have always had the sole, preeminent authority to prescribe. However, in the United States before 1900, consumers could obtain any available drug through their pharmacists without a prescription. Consulting a physician's advice about drugs, although sometimes done, was neither mandatory nor frequently practiced. The first federal legislation to place controls on the dispensing of drugs was the Pure Food Act of 1906. This law made it illegal to misrepresent drug contents by false and misleading labeling. The law also gave physicians prescriptive authority for drugs containing narcotics, whereas all nonnarcotic drugs were still available to the consumer without a prescription. In 1919, less than one third of all medicines bought were prescribed by physicians (Starr, 1982).

In 1938, after the death of more than 100 people as a result of the release of a toxic preparation by a pharmaceutical company, the Federal Food, Drug, and Cosmetic Act was passed, extending the mandate of the Food and Drug Administration (FDA) to issue a regulation distinguishing over-the-counter drugs from prescription drugs. The authority to designate prescriptive versus nonprescriptive drugs was delegated to the manufacturer. Physicians, by virtue of their dominant position in the health care field, were given the authority to control access to these prescription items (Temin, 1980). After the Humphrey-Durham Amendment in 1951, which provided for an expert review board to decide whether a drug was safe for use, almost all new drugs were placed in the prescription-only class. The Drug Amendment in 1962 gave the FDA authority to regulate which drugs could be used for which illnesses. These regulations took control from the consumer and embedded the prescription of medications more firmly into the existing medical hierarchy, increasing consumer dependence on the physician (Temin, 1980).

The nursing profession did not keep pace with these changes. The original nurse practice acts depended on the support of legislator and physician groups for passage, and the original licensing boards of nursing contained physicians and required letters of support from physicians for licensure, helping to create the perception of nursing as a physician-controlled occupation (Greenlaw, 1985). Although, historically, nurses had been working independently of physicians and making recommendations regarding drug therapy as a matter of course, the FDA legislation of 1938 forced this accepted practice into the domain of informal counseling with no instrumental authority for nurses to prescribe. Additionally, the disclaimer in the 1955 model nurse practice act developed by the American Nurses Association (ANA) explicitly excluded the acts of diagnosis and prescription as nursing functions, and this disclaimer was incorporated into the nurse practice acts in a number of states (Greenlaw, 1985). The ANA finally amended its model definition in 1970 to recognize the responsibility that nurses have for diagnosing and prescribing (Harkless, 1989). Two ANA 1994 publications further defined and expanded these responsibilities (ANA, 1994a, 1994b).

Historically, there has been a gap between actual nursing practice and the statutory parameters of nursing practice. Nurses have assumed a great deal of unofficial critical patient management, including drug-related decisions, without formal or legal recognition. The move toward prescriptive authority for APRNs represents an attempt to make these functions official and to acknowledge the APRN's expanding scope of practice. APRNs now have some form of prescriptive privileges in 48 states (Pearson, 1998), and APRNs are making efforts in many other states to enact legislation allowing prescriptive authority where it does not yet exist (Howard & Greiner, 1997).

In the last few years educational guidelines, credentialing, and the skills and knowledge base needed for APRN psychopharmacotherapy practice have been clearly defined (ANA, 1994b). Models, both for preparing for the practice as well as implementing the role, have also been described comprehensively in the literature (Bailey & Snyder, 1995; Bailey, 1996; Hales et al., 1998; Sovner, Bailey, & Weisblatt, 1990). The purpose of this chapter is to address and discuss the issues related to the role of the APRN as prescriber in psychiatric and mental health care.

PSYCHOPHARMACOTHERAPY KNOWLEDGE BASE FOR ■ ADVANCED PRACTICE

In 1994, the ANA developed and published guidelines designed to describe the knowledge base needed by APRNs to inform and guide their education, practice, and research in the area of psychopharmacotherapy (ANA, 1994). Box 13-1

box 13-1

PSYCHOPHARMACOLOGY GUIDELINES FOR PSYCHIATRIC-MENTAL HEALTH NURSES

NEUROSCIENCES

Commensurate with level of practice, the psychiatric-mental health nurse integrates current knowledge from the neurosciences to understand etiologic models, diagnostic issues, and treatment strategies for psychiatric illness.

continued

box 13-1

PSYCHOPHARMACOLOGY GUIDELINES FOR PSYCHIATRIC-MENTAL HEALTH NURSES— cont'd

PSYCHOPHARMACOLOGY

The psychiatric-mental health nurse involved in the care of patients taking psychopharmacologic agents demonstrates knowledge of psychopharmacologic principles, including pharmacokinetics, pharmacodynamics, drug classification, intended and unintended effects, and related nursing implications.

CLINICAL MANAGEMENT

The psychiatric-mental health nurse applies principles from the neurosciences and psychopharmacology to provide safe and effective management of patients being treated with psychopharmacologic agents. Clinical management includes assessment, diagnosis, and treatment considerations.

Assessment

The psychiatric-mental health nurse has the knowledge, skills, and ability to conduct and interpret patient assessments of psychopharmacologic agents. Assessments include physical, neuropsychiatric, psychosocial, and psychopharmacologic parameters.

Diagnosis

The psychiatric-mental health nurse has the knowledge, skills, and ability to use appropriate nursing, psychiatric, and medical diagnostic classification systems to guide the psychopharmacologic treatment of patients with mental illness.

Treatment

The psychiatric-mental health nurse takes an active role in the treatment of patients with mental illness and integrates prescribed psychopharmacologic interventions in a cohesive, multidimensional plan of care.

summarizes the guidelines that specifically apply to practice. Contemporary APRN practice of pharmacotherapy is based on the integration and application of knowledge from the biologic, behavioral, social, and neurosciences. APRNs must have a basic knowledge of central nervous system structures and functions and current biologic hypotheses implicated in mental illness and the use of psychotropic agents. Other important aspects of knowledge from the neurosciences are normal sleep stages and circadian rhythm disturbances, psychiatric uses of neuroimaging techniques, and the purposes and limitations of current biologic tests used in the diagnosis and monitoring of psychiatric disorders and their treatment.

APRNs must be able to apply this knowledge and knowledge of psychopharmacotherapeutics to provide safe and effective patient care. The components of clinical management are also identified in Box 13-1. Areas to be evaluated in a thorough neuropsychosocial and psychopharmacologic assessment are listed in Box 13-2. In addition, standardized rating scales are ideal for both objective baseline data and for monitoring symptomatic and behavioral changes throughout the course of treatment. Table 13-1 lists behavioral rating scales that can be used to clarify diagnoses and to evaluate change in symptoms after the initiation and titration of pharmacologic interventions.

Part of a comprehensive assessment also includes the identification of the patient's ethnic/cultural background, developmental stage, cognitive ability, educational level, reading level and comprehension, socioeconomic status, capacity to ask questions and seek answers, motivation for treatment, and any other patient-related variables pertinent to the risk/benefit assessment of psychopharmacologic treatment.

APRNs must then be able to use these findings to develop a pharmacologic treatment plan that considers similarities and differences among psychotropic agents of the same and different classes and the mechanisms of action of individual agents. They must be aware of psychiatric symptoms that are unlikely to respond to pharmacologic intervention, the differences between targeted psychiatric symptoms and medication side effects, and the appropriate interventions to minimize each. Drug-related variables important in the risk/benefit assessment of psychotropic agents are listed in Box 13-3.

Knowledge and skills related to the other components of care (stabilization, maintenance, and follow-up) include the ability to use data obtained from therapeutic drug monitoring, laboratory values, standardized rating scales, and patient and family reports to monitor target symptoms, medication effects, and functional status throughout the course of treatment. The integration of health promotion and rehabilitation techniques with pharmacologic treatments is also an important consideration. APRNs must be able to recognize indications for modifying dosing and tapering schedules, choosing alternative medication strategies as needed, managing the discontinuation of medication and potential sequelae (i.e., withdrawal, rebound, or return of symptoms of illness), and differentiating between changes in the

---

box 13-2

AREAS TO BE EVALUATED IN A NEUROPSYCHOSOCIAL AND PSYCHOPHARMACOLOGIC ASSESSMENT

Patient's identifying data
Patient's chief complaint
History of present problem
Symptoms that medications target
History of past treatment
Response and adverse effects to prior medication trials
Family and social history
Personality structure and coping style
Medical history and current treatment
Drug and other kinds of allergies
Past and current substance use or abuse and treatment
Mental status examination

table 4-1

BEHAVIORAL RATING SCALES

CONTENT AREA	SCALE
General Health	MOS Health Survey (SF-36)
General Psychiatric	Acculturation Scale
	Assessing Coping Strategies (COPE)
	Behavior and Symptom Identification Scale (BASIS-32)
	Brief Symptom Inventory (BSI)
	Client Satisfaction Questionnaire (CSQ)
	Clinical Global Impression (CGI)
	Colorado Client Assessment Record (CCAR)
	Family Burden Interview Schedule (FBIS)
	Functional Status Questionnaire (FSQ)
	General Health Questionnaire (GHQ)
	Global Assessment Scale (GAS)
	Global Assessment of Functioning Scale (GAF)
	NIMH Global Consensus Rating Scales
	Nurse Observation Scale for Inpatient Evaluation (NOSIE)
	Quality of Life Interview (QOLI)
	Service Satisfaction Questionnaire (SSQ-30)
	Severity of Psychosocial Stressors Scale
	Symptoms Checklist-90 (SCL-90)

CONTENT AREA	SCALE
Eating Disorders	Body Attitudes Test
	Diagnostic Survey for Eating Disorders (DSED)
	Eating Habits Checklist
	Eating Behaviors Diary
	Eating Disorders Inventory 2 (EDI-2)
Organic Mental Disorders	Alzheimer's Disease Assessment Scale (ADAS)
	Cohen-Mansfield Agitation Inventory
	Blessed Dementia Scale
	Cornell Scale for Depression in Dementia
	Face-Hand Test
	Haycox Dementia Behavioral Scale
	Memory and Behavior Problems Checklist
	Neurobehavioral Rating Scale for Dementia (NRS)
Psychotic Disorders	Andreasen Scale for Assessment of Negative Symptoms (SANS)
	Andreasen Scale for Assessment of Positive Symptoms (SAPS)
	Brief Psychiatric Rating Scale (BPRS)
	Life Skills Profile: Schizophrenia (LSP)
	Schizophrenia Outcomes Module (SOM)
	University of Washington Paranoia Scale

continued

table 4-I

BEHAVIORAL RATING SCALES—cont'd

CONTENT AREA	SCALE	CONTENT AREA	SCALE
Affective Disorders	Assessment of Suicidal Potentiality Back Depression Inventory (BDI) Carroll Self-Rating Scale Center for Epidemiologic Studies Depression Scale (CES-D) Depression Outcome Module (DOM) Family Burden Interview Schedule (FBIS) Geriatric Depression Scale (GDS) Hamilton Depression Scale (Ham-D) Inventory for Depressive Symptomatology (IDS) Manic-State Scale Montgomery-Asberg Depression Rating Scale (MADRS) Raskin Depression Scale Young Mania Scale Zung Self-Rating Depression Scale (ZSRDS)	Substance Use Disorders	Addiction Severity Index (ASI) Alcohol Use Scale (AUS) Brief Drug Abuse Screening Test (B-DAST) CAGE Questionnaire Children of Alcoholics Screening Test (CAST) Clinical Institute Withdrawal Assessment-Alcohol, Revised (CIWA-AR) Drug Use Scale (DUS) Michigan Alcoholism Screening Tool (MAST) Substance Abuse Outcome Module (SAOM) Substance Abuse Treatment Schedule (SATS) Treatment Services Review (TSR)
Anxiety Disorders	Beck Anxiety Inventory (BAI) Covi Anxiety Scale Dissociative Experience Scale Dissociative Disorders Interview Schedule (DDIS) Hamilton Rating Scale for Anxiety (Ham-A) Maudsley Obsessional Compulsive Inventory Panic Disorder Outcomes Module (PDOM) Spielberger Anxiety State-Trait Taylor Anxiety Scale Yale-Brown Obsessive Compulsive Scale (YBOCS) Zung Anxiety Scale	Child/Adolescent	Behavior Problems Checklist Brief Psychiatric Rating Scale for Children Child Behavior Checklist (CBCL) Children's Global Assessment Scale (CGAS) Competency Skills Questionnaire (CSQ) Conners Parent Rating Scale Home and School Questionnaire Self-Control Rating Scale Yale-Brown Obsessive Compulsive Scale (YBOCS) for Children
		Medication Effects	Abnormal Involuntary Movement Scale (AIMS) Simpson-Angus Extrapyramidal Symptoms Scale

From Stuart, G., & Laraia, M. (1998). *Practice of psychiatric nursing* (ed. 6). St. Louis: Mosby.

box 13–3

VARIABLES IMPORTANT IN RISK/ BENEFIT ASSESSMENT

Drug pharmacokinetics and pharmacodynamics
Drug half-life
Steady state
Absorption
Distribution
Metabolism
Patient's age, gender, race, organ system function
Food and drug-drug interactions
Drug safety and efficacy
Therapeutic ranges
Short- and long-term side effects
Contraindications
Cost

patient as a result of illness effects, drug effects, environmental effects, or premorbid personality characteristics.

Patient education is an important element of any modality of nursing practice. However, there are certain special considerations related to the practice of pharmacotherapy regarding patient education. Psychiatric symptoms may constitute an obstacle to the patient's understanding of risks and benefits of treatment or of treatment directives. APRNs must be able to develop an individualized patient education program and plan of care in collaboration with the patient, family, and other care providers that address the patient's cognitive limitations. They must adhere to ethical and legal parameters in informing patients about pharmacologic treatments, risks/benefits, concurrent and alternative treatments, and obtaining informed consent. The application of principles of health education include self-monitoring techniques and teaching tools. Many pharmaceutical companies offer a variety of free written pamphlets, audio tapes, video cassettes, and telephone call-in lines, all of which can be useful in enhancing patient education. These materials can be obtained through local drug company representatives or by calling the company directly.

IMPLEMENTING THE ROLE OF APRN PRESCRIBER

Practice Considerations

Before beginning. APRNs are expanding into the role of prescriber from varying levels of experience with medication management. Both the training and clinical experience of registered nurses and APRNs provide a substantial knowledge base regarding clinical assessment and the monitoring of patients around many aspects of pharmacologic treatment. However, it is unlikely that APRNs will have had experience with the full range of responsibilities and the independent decision making inherent in the role of prescriber.

The APRN prescriber has the authority and the responsibility for the overall care of the patient. In general, nonprescribers rarely make the final treatment decisions regarding, for example, choice of drug for initial treatment, augmentation, or subsequent choice of agents or combinations of agents used in treatment-resistant disorders. Because APRNs usually expand into the role from a solid foundation of clinical experience, they generally learn these skills quickly. Nevertheless, this kind of decision making is an important component of any prescribing clinician's training.

Consequently, although typically the APRN is adequately trained for the role of prescriber, the implementation of the role is often initially based on the traditional supervisor-supervisee relationship with the "APRN-in-training" progressively developing independent practice. The initial phase of implementation may be seen as a kind of internship of a duration that will be tailored to the APRN's level of knowledge and expertise. The ultimate goal of this collaboration is that the APRN will become an independent prescriber (insofar as individual statutory regulations allow) who uses more experienced colleagues as consultants on an as-needed basis. All aspects of the role should be addressed during this initial phase, including issues regarding clinical care, coverage, the supervisory relationship, quality assurance, documentation, and ethical or legal issues.

Initial phase. The best way to begin the practice of pharmacotherapy in terms of patient selection is for the APRN to assume the pharmacologic management of patients he or she is already treating in some other modality and/or patients for whom the supervisor is already prescribing. These patients' histories, target symptoms, dynamic issues, medical statuses, and medication regimens will already be relatively familiar to at least one or both clinicians. Unlike a newly assessed patient, these patients offer an opportunity to review all aspects of care and to discuss in depth target symptoms, rationale for current drug regimens, side effects, dosages, and any other elements of treatment. The APRN can begin writing out and signing prescriptions in the supervisor's presence and address any related questions that might arise.

In addition to building the APRN's clinical skills and familiarity with independent decision making, both clinicians can use this initial phase of practice to become familiar with each other's knowledge level. The goals of this initial phase of practice are as follows:

- Develop a basic level of trust between the APRN and the supervising clinician.
- Build the APRN's confidence in his or her own skills and knowledge of psychopharmacotherapy.
- Ensure both clinicians that the APRN is prepared to assume a more independent role as prescriber.

Final phase. The APRN can move to more independent levels of practice when both clinicians mutually agree that the APRN is ready. This may occur in a natural, spontaneous way or may be planned in steps that are characteristic of a training situation. First, the supervisor does the initial assessment with the APRN observing, initiates treatment, then refers the patient to the APRN for follow-up. Then the APRN can begin doing initial assessments with the supervisor observing, and later on his or her own. The supervisor may want to meet the patient briefly after the APRN's initial assessment and before initiation of treatment or within some specified period of time after initiation of treatment.

Until APRNs are comfortable moving into independent prescriptive practice, clinicians may want to institute a system of periodic review. The supervisor may want to review each patient and each prescription during supervision, but as the practice progresses, a less frequent system of review may be developed. For example, the APRN could keep a confidential loose-leaf notebook that contains a page for each patient with the following information:

- Identifying data (name, birth date, medical record number)
- Names of current providers in all modalities
- Drug names, date of initiation, dosage changes, discontinuation, number of refills
- Disorder for which the drug is being prescribed
- Coexisting medical or psychiatric conditions
- Concurrent medications
- Dates of supervisory review

The supervisor and APRN can review some agreed-upon minimum percentage of all new prescriptions or dosage changes at regular intervals as part of the supervisory sessions. Such a review system should be considered a supervisory tool and not a substitute for adequate documentation in patient records. Eventually, the frequency and nature of reviews will be based on quality assurance standards dictated by the particular practice setting or by statutory regulations. Clinicians can mutually determine the appropriateness of individual patients for the APRN's caseload in the supervisory sessions. Medically complicated or treatment-resistant patients may require more frequent consultation. The APRN may also request that the supervisor see a patient for consultation.

Both clinicians need to feel confident that the APRN is ready to move on to more independent practice at each progressive step. At some point along this continuum the APRN can assume full responsibility for prescribing for patients. The eventual goal of practice is that the APRN will do the initial assessment, make a diagnosis based on the fourth edition of the *Diagnostic and Statistical Manual of Mental Disorders, or DSM-IV* (APA, 1994), make treatment decisions based on these findings, and prescribe and monitor medications independently throughout the course of treatment, using the supervisor or other colleagues for consultation as appropriate.

Guidelines for Clinical Supervision

Experienced APRN prescribers may offer an advantage over psychiatrist supervisors because they are more familiar with APRNs' background knowledge and training. Therefore the APRN may be able to assess the "trainee's" level of knowledge and skills and to address specific training needs more quickly. However, there are many jurisdictions that require psychiatrist supervision by law. Psychiatrist supervision may also be indicated in institutional settings where there are no experienced APRN prescribers or where prescriptive practice supervision would be a natural extension of an already existing, close-working relationship between an APRN and psychiatrist.

The amount of time scheduled for routine supervision will probably be more frequent during the initial phase of practice and decrease as the APRN becomes more independent. Although the caseload will be smaller in the beginning, supervision time is an opportunity for teaching and review of any clinical concerns as well as quality assurance and risk management issues. Clinicians should be guided in case discussions by all of the essential elements of biologic psychiatry:

- Diagnosis
- Familiarity with each class of psychotropic medications
- Familiarity with medications that treat the side effects of psychotropics
- Indications for use and contraindications to use
- Side effects
- Dosages
- Drug-drug interactions
- Pharmacokinetics and pharmacodynamics

Unless routine supervision is required by statutory regulations or by institutional policies, once the APRN progresses to independent practice, supervision or consultation can be used for the purposes of addressing diagnostic or treatment dilemmas, sustaining clinical currency, or developing further professional expertise.

Before beginning the practice, to ensure quality of care, the supervisor and APRN should develop specific guidelines and parameters of practice based on quality assurance considerations. In some jurisdictions mutually agreed-upon written guidelines or protocols are required. In states where this is not the case, it may be desirable to develop written guidelines that can be reviewed and modified periodically as the practice evolves. Guidelines ensure clear role boundaries, respective areas of individual responsibility, and safety and quality of practice. They can address and define practice arrangements but should not be confused with treatment protocols, which are discussed later. Modifications in guidelines usually reflect the increasing skills and experience of the APRN and the mutual trust and respect in the APRN-supervisor relationship. If not required by law, when the APRN becomes an independent prescriber, the guidelines may be obsolete.

Clinicians must develop arrangements to deal with statutory limitations on their practice. For example, if statutory regulations dictate that APRNs cannot prescribe Schedule II drugs and that these prescriptions must be signed by a physician, a system must be developed to accommodate this situation. The clinicians should be absolutely clear about the nature and scope of the APRN's practice—which patients will or will not be seen, which medications will or will not be prescribed. The clinicians should identify as clearly as possible the circumstances under which a referral to another provider is required or when a consultation with a professional other than the supervisor who has a recognized expertise in a particular aspect of care is indicated. The clinicians should also specify how medical conditions and emergencies will be handled. Standards of documentation and coverage during absences of either the supervisor or the APRN should be agreed upon. Clinical supervision should be seen as a fluid situation with a good deal of inherent flexibility. Over time, any of these parameters can be the subject of continuous review and modification.

Credentialing

If the supervisor is a psychiatrist, he or she should hold an unrestricted full license, have completed training in psychiatry approved by the Accreditation Council for Graduate Medical Education (ACGME) or the Royal College of Physicians and Surgeons of Canada or be board-certified in psychiatry; be registered with the U.S. Drug Enforcement Administration (DEA) and, if applicable, with the state agency that regulates controlled substance prescriptive practice; and be covered by professional liability insurance.

APRNs should hold a valid registered nurses license, be certified by the American Nurses Credentialing Center (ANCC), and be covered by professional liability insurance. Both psychiatrists and APRNs who practice in institutional settings may be covered by insurance provided by the institution. If not, they can obtain insurance through their professional organizations. If APRNs can legally prescribe Schedule II drugs, they must also be registered with the DEA and with their state agency regulating controlled substance prescriptive practice. Educational and clinical experience requirements for APRN prescriptive privileges vary among jurisdictions but usually include some designated number of hours of academic and/or continuing educational credits. Additionally, clinicians who work in institutional settings may need to comply with credentialing requirements dictated by the institution.

Risk Management and Liability Issues

One of the controversial risk management and liability issues related to prescriptive practice is the use of drug or treatment protocols (Moniz, 1992). These are sometimes viewed as a means to improve quality of care and thereby decrease liability risk. However, protocols are often rigid, and protocol standards of practice are often too high to be reasonably met by clinicians at all times under all circumstances. For example, some patients require medication dosages that are above amounts recommended by drug company package inserts. If the dosing guideline in a particular protocol does not specify dosages at a higher range than recommended and the patient experiences an adverse effect, this can potentially increase liability risk. When a clinician breaches a specific standard, an attorney representing a patient plaintiff may attempt to use the breach as damaging evidence.

If protocols are to be used, either voluntarily or because they are legally required, they should be based on a minimum safe level rather than the ideal; they should be realistic and be updated on a routine basis (Moniz, 1992). The use of nationally recognized guidelines that can be the basis for establishing clinical pathways and making treatment decisions allows for necessary flexibility. Guidelines that are currently available or in development are mentioned in Chapter 12.

There are two main sources of law pertaining to psychopharmacotherapy practice: statutory law and medical malpractice. There are three specific areas in which professionals engaged in prescriptive practice may experience exposure to liability (Bailey & Snyder, 1995):

1. *Liability related to licensing authorities for practice not in compliance with statutory and regulatory requirements.* Of primary importance is that APRNs must fully understand and comply with the unique statutory and regulatory requirements in the jurisdiction in which they practice. Failure to meet the relevant requirements of state boards of nursing, medicine, pharmacy, or public health or other regulatory requirements may result in disciplinary complaints before professional licensing boards.

Professional boards also typically act when a prescriber has been convicted of a felony or has engaged in gross or habitual negligent conduct in the prescription of controlled substances.

When any professional collaborative relationship in a psychiatric setting is legally defined by statute as a supervisory relationship, a degree of control by the supervisor over the supervisee is implied that is not present in a collaborative relationship or when a consultant is employed. A collaborative relationship is a relationship between peers or colleagues, each of whom has individual responsibility for the consequences of treatment interventions. A consultant, whose job it is to clarify diagnosis or make treatment recommendations, has no responsibility for the consequences of any ensuing interventions of the consultee based on the consultation.

Supervisory liability includes the notion of *foreseeability*. In agreeing to supervise the APRN, the supervisor is responsible for assessing the APRN's competency. On the basis of this assessment the supervisor can make some judgment about the adequacy of the APRN's clinical knowledge and skills. If the APRN is negligent and the supervisor could have *foreseen* that the APRN was not adequately competent to handle the situation in question, the supervisor is liable. This legal principle would apply to any supervisor-supervisee relationship, regardless of the professions involved.

2. *Civil liability for injury to individual patients.* Another area of liability specific to prescriptive practice is medical malpractice. Patients may bring causes of action for malpractice against prescribers when the prescription of drugs has resulted in reasonably foreseeable injury to the patient.

3. *Criminal liability for violation of federal and/or state statutes regulating the prescription and use of controlled substances.* Abuse of prescriptive authority, prescription forgery, or consumer complaints to the licensing authority are examples of criminal liability. Exposure to criminal action and loss of the practitioner's DEA authorization may occur when professionals either willingly, or as a result of patient manipulation, are engaged in prescribing narcotics in amounts and frequency that would suggest a pattern of drug abuse by the patient. Self-prescribing of narcotics or other drugs or prescribing for family members and close friends is limited in most jurisdictions. Prescribers whose practice is impaired by substance abuse of self-prescribed drugs may face criminal action, loss of DEA prescribing authority, and/or a complaint before state licensing authorities. Legal aspects of advanced practice nursing are discussed in more detail in Chapter 8. It is essential that APRNs take personal responsibility to be fully cognizant of the laws and regulations of the state in which they practice.

BASIC PRINCIPLES OF PSYCHOPHARMACOLOGY ■ PRACTICE

Once APRNs are fully integrated into the role of prescriber, they become accountable for the comprehensive psychotherapeutics of the patients under their care. Sound practice is the basis for continued skill development, for the achievement of favorable patient outcomes, and for insurance against risk of liability. The 11 basic principles of sound psychopharmacology practice that follow can serve as a means for achieving optimum patient care.

Identifying Target Symptoms and Diagnosis

Before prescribing a psychotropic medication, the importance of a comprehensive biopsychosocial assessment cannot be overemphasized as the basis for treatment decisions. This includes the identification of target symptoms to establish a baseline before treatment begins and to monitor the success of treatment. It is also important to monitor changes in the patient's mental status, medical condition, and quality of life (e.g., satisfaction with home and family life, functioning at work, and overall sense of well-being).

Many patients have disorders that are not easily classified, or some patients with a seemingly classic disorder may not respond to a traditional drug. Target symptom and quality of life assessments are especially important when a patient's diagnosis is unclear. They can be the bases for establishing a list of possible diagnoses and "rule out" diagnoses that can be approached systematically. As mentioned earlier in this chapter, rating scales can be extremely useful for these purposes.

To optimize clinical management of complicated illnesses, it is also important to document the baseline mental status and mental status changes over the course of treatment. Particular attention should be given to documenting risk of suicide or violence.

Screening for Medical Problems and Drug Interactions

Medical illness, organicity, or substance use can be responsible for a patient's psychiatric symptoms, and drug interactions can increase the toxicity of prescribed drugs (e.g., nonsteroidal antiinflammatory drugs [NSAIDs] may increase lithium levels) or decrease the effectiveness of a planned treatment (e.g., anticonvulsants can increase the metabolism of tricyclic antidepressants), thereby lowering serum levels.

A patient who is reluctant to share information about himself or herself at the initiation of treatment may be more willing to disclose personal information (e.g., substance use, sexual abuse) as a therapeutic alliance develops. Elderly patients whose mental status is within normal limits at the initiation of treatment may begin to develop symptoms of cognitive impairment or a new medical illness over the course of treatment. A patient with a history of substance abuse who is abstinent at the initiation of therapy may begin to use alco-

hol or drugs again. Therefore these aspects of patient assessment should be reassessed and monitored throughout the course of treatment, particularly if there is an unexplained worsening of symptoms, and appropriate treatment or referral should be arranged.

Obtaining a Detailed History

Obtaining a detailed history of a patient's illness and past pharmacologic treatment may help the APRN understand the nature of the patient's illness, make predictions about the future course, identify comorbidity, avoid "reinventing the wheel" by initiating drug trials that the patient has already failed or been unable to tolerate, or identify drug trials that were inadequate either in terms of dosage or length of time. If the patient has had a successful trial of a particular medication in the past, it would be a very reasonable choice to use that medication again. Questioning the patient and family members, contacting both past and present care providers, and requesting medical records (with the patient's written permission) are all ways to gather valuable data.

Recognizing Signs of Impending Relapse

Even when patients manifest a "garden variety" form of a particular DSM-IV disorder, initial symptom development may differ from patient to patient and may manifest in a particular sequence, either gradually or suddenly. There may also be certain kinds of stressors to which an individual patient may be more vulnerable and that might be more likely than other life events to precipitate a relapse. Being able to recognize both the patient's earliest initial manifestation of illness and potential precipitants can avert a more serious exacerbation. It also allows the practitioner to make timely and less costly interventions.

It is most important that the recognition of early signs of illness be a mutually collaborative effort with the patient, and, if permitted, with family members who, as more objective observers, may be able to identify initial signs of exacerbation or relapse better than the patient. Warning signs can be monitored and reviewed with the patient at each contact.

Forming a Therapeutic Alliance

The therapeutic alliance is arguably the most important determinant of adherence to pharmacologic treatment (Forman, 1993). The dynamics involved in establishing and maintaining an alliance with any patient imply that the involvement of the APRN is as important as the involvement of the patient. A well-developed alliance leads to improved communication, shared decision making, and shared risk.

There are many interventions that can foster the establishment and maintenance of the therapeutic alliance. Chapter 9 describes indicators of a therapeutic alliance as demonstrated by research. These should always be within the context of the APRN's demonstrated empathy, honesty, and respect for the process of engaging the patient in treatment. Before clinical interventions are instituted, the APRN should do the following:

- Assess the patient's knowledge base, experience with treatment and treatment relationships, and readiness to begin therapy.
- Inform the patient about the nature of his or her disorder and about the proposed treatment. This may include written educational materials that are specifically geared to the patient's educational level.
- Address questions that the patient might hesitate to ask.
- Demonstrate expertise to engender trust in the patient, and discuss all reasonable treatment options.
- If permitted by the patient and if appropriate, consider recruiting family members or significant others who are invested in the patient's well being to participate in the treatment process.
- Coordinate care with other providers.

Knowing Well One or Two Drugs Per Class

A thorough working knowledge of one or two drugs in each class is an excellent foundation on which to begin practicing psychopharmacotherapy and upon which to build. A working knowledge includes pharmacokinetic and pharmacodynamic mechanisms, dosages, and side effects. APRNs should discuss side effects with their patients in advance of initiating treatment, and develop a clear idea of which side effects require reassurance, treatment, or discontinuation. They must also learn to differentiate between side effects that may mimic certain symptoms and the symptoms themselves (e.g., neuroleptic induced akathisia may be confused with psychotic agitation).

Administering a Full Trial of New Medication

Inadequate dosing and duration are the main reasons for failure of antidepressant trials in well-diagnosed patients, and this may hold true for other classes of drugs as well (Hyman, Arana, & Rosenbaum, 1995). If a patient's target symptoms do not improve or only improve partially, or if the patient cannot tolerate the medication because of adverse effects after a fully adequate trial, that particular agent can be ruled out or possibly augmented. If, on the other hand, an agent is discontinued before a fully adequate trial has been administered and the drug is considered to be ineffective or only partially effective, it is a missed opportunity.

Keeping Regimens Simple

Keeping regimens and dosing schedules simple will help improve adherence to treatment and avoid additive side effects (Hyman, Arana, & Rosenbaum, 1995). This includes determining the lowest effective dose for any particular stage of a patient's illness. Psychotic disorders and particular dosage requirements often change over time, with higher doses needed in the acute phase than are needed for long-term maintenance (Hyman, Arana, & Rosenbaum, 1995). In the elderly, lower doses are used when initiating treatment, and dosage changes should be less frequent than in younger patients because time for drugs to reach steady state is often prolonged (Salzman, 1998).

Continuing ineffective medications indefinitely and accumulating multiple medications can lead to unnecessary costs and side effects. Adjunctive and combination therapies may be appropriate for certain conditions; however, when medications no longer prove useful to the treatment regimen, it is critical to discontinue them. It may be difficult to determine that a medication has failed unless objective target symptoms have been tracked since the beginning of the trial. For example, if a patient reports no change in a disrupted sleep pattern or in a poor appetite, unless the APRN has established a clear baseline of number of hours of sleep and/or the patient's weight before the initiation of treatment, establishing clear efficacy will be more difficult.

When discontinuing psychotropic medications, it is best to taper dosages slowly to help prevent rebound or withdrawal symptoms. When symptoms do occur during a taper, it is important to distinguish between temporary symptom rebound, which frequently occurs after discontinuing short-acting benzodiazepines and is brief and transient but often severe; recurrence of the disorder (the long-term return of original symptoms); and withdrawal, which is also transient, can be severe, and will be identifiable by the appearance of new symptoms characteristic of withdrawal from the particular drug (e.g., the occurrence of serotonin syndrome as the result of abrupt withdrawal of some serotonin reuptake inhibitors) (Hyman, Arana, & Rosenbaum, 1995).

Being Aware of Financial Costs of Drugs

The guiding principle related to drug cost is *cost-effectiveness*. For example, the least expensive drug may not be the most cost-effective if clinical outcome is not optimal, thus diminishing quality of life, or if the costs of treating side effects offset initial savings. On the other hand, if compliance and safety are enhanced and relapse is minimized, an initially more costly drug may be the most cost-effective choice. Thus a narrow focus on the dollar amount of a drug's cost alone is inadequate. When drugs are equally safe and effective, dollar amount is a valid basis for selection.

Cost containment has led many health plans to prefer generic compounds over proprietary drugs. Are there differences in the therapeutic equivalence between types of generic drugs and between generic versus brand name drugs? The FDA has only required that a manufacturer demonstrate that a given dose of a compound will produce blood levels within 20% to 30% of the proprietary form (Cohen, 1997). Although the use of generic drugs may result in savings, it is important to be aware of this range of equivalency. Patients who are changed from a trade name drug to a generic drug (or vice versa) may respond a little differently. They may report that the medication is a little more or less potent or that a new side effect has appeared. This may also occur after a change in generic manufacturers. Because of the variability among manufacturers, it may be important to know the name of the firm that actually manufactures the drug.

Adhering to Legal and Ethical Standards

APRNs are legally obligated to know the minimal requirements for licensure and regulation in the state in which they practice and are responsible for acting within the scope of practice defined by those laws (ANA, 1994b). The APRN is also legally obligated to ensure that documentation of patient assessment and treatment is included in the clinical record and that it includes the following:

- Identification of target symptoms
- Differential diagnosis and/or comorbidity
- Effectiveness of medications

- Side effects
- Patient education
- Compliance
- Referral of treatment responsibility or consultation
- Patient consent for release of information

Informed consent for pharmacologic treatment must be obtained before prescribing or administering medication. This includes the documentation of a discussion with the patient of risks, benefits, and alternative treatments other than medication and of the patient's understanding and agreement to be treated. Informed consent has become an increasingly important issue in all health care specialties. In psychiatry, however, several key problems may result from the difficulty in evaluating a patient's capacity to understand fully the benefits and risks of the medication prescribed or to interpret the provided information in a realistic way. This issue is particularly pressing in the psychotic or demented patient, and legal guardianship may be needed at times for adequate informed consent. See Chapters 8 and 19 for further discussion about legal and ethical issues.

Another issue related to informed consent is whether the APRN should inform the patient of every side effect listed in the Physicians Desk Reference (PDR, 1998) or merely highlight the most common ones. APRNs need to enter into an open dialogue with all patients regarding the benefits and side effects of medication, even with those patients who are self-taught. Patients who read the PDR, which lists virtually all side effects ever reported in drug trials, even if they were not due to the drug, need to be informed of the relative probability of a side effect occurring. Package inserts now often include tables comparing side effects in patients treated with a given drug with those observed with a placebo. This places these issues in a much better perspective. Giving the patients materials that describe a medication's relative risks can also work well.

A particularly difficult problem involves informed consent of the risk of developing tardive dyskinesia (TD), which effects some 14% of patients maintained on neuroleptic medication for 3 or more years (Schatzberg & Cole, 1991). One approach to dealing with this problem is to inform the patient and/or the family of the risk of TD before prescribing neuroleptics. This may be too anxiety provoking and impractical for the acutely psychotic patient, particularly since TD generally is a delayed onset side effect and there may be a pressing need to medicate the patient quickly. Another approach is to broach the subject after 4 to 6 weeks of treatment, before embarking on long-term or maintenance therapy. Any approach should include the conservative administration of neuroleptics—both in terms of time and dosing, a mutually cooperative attitude regarding the monitoring of patients for the emergence of dyskinetic movements, and a formal documented disclosure informing the patient of the risk of TD.

Another dilemma facing the APRN is whether to prescribe standard drugs for indications that have not been approved by the FDA or to prescribe them at doses that are higher than those recommended in the PDR. Are practitioners at legal risk when they prescribe drugs for nonapproved uses or at higher than recommended doses? The American Medical Association and the FDA have taken the position that the use of any marketed drug for nonapproved indications or at higher dosages for individual patients is within the purview of the clinician (Schatzberg & Cole, 1991). Each clinician must decide whether he or she wishes to assume the risk. If the APRN opts for a conservative approach, he or she will probably encounter patients with treatment-resistant disorders who will require alternative treatments. It may help to seek outside consultation from a more expert psychopharmacologist. Another approach is to explain the scope of the problem to patients, provide them with available published reports on positive benefits, and document this in the record. The record should reflect the basis for the clinical decision and an understanding of the available evidence.

Seeking Consultation

There are many instances during the course of treatment when consultation might be indicated. Consultations are often sought when diagnosis is unclear or when a patient's symptoms have not responded to one or more medication trials. The outcome of an evaluation, initially or during ongoing therapy, may suggest a treatment modality beyond the scope of the APRN's practice or professional expertise. For example, the patient's condition may require the assessment of a primary care or medical specialty provider. Whatever the indication for the consultation, it should be continued for as long as the consultant and the APRN deem necessary, and all recommendations and consequent interventions should be documented in the medical record.

IMPLICATIONS FOR
■ THE FUTURE

In the field of psychiatry, psychopharmacotherapy is progressively becoming the primary modality of treatment for patients with Axis I disorders, and pharmacologic intervention plays a significant role in the treatment of dually diagnosed patients as well. Historically, until the advent of widespread government regulation of pharmacologic agents and the dominance of prescriptive practice by physicians, nurses worked independently of physicians and made recommendations regarding drug therapy in a variety of situations. The current move toward accountability and autonomy in nursing across specialties is resulting in a gradual but progressive acknowledgment of the expanding scope of nursing practice in related legislation. Graduate nursing school curricula and clinical practica continue to evolve to meet this challenge. Prescriptive authority and the skills and knowledge required for the practice of psychopharmacotherapy are necessary tools for the growth of advanced practice psychiatric nursing, and APRNs are well positioned to master this new frontier.

RESOURCES AND CONNECTIONS

WEBSITES

US Food and Drug Administration
  www.fda.gov/opacom/hpnews.html
Psychopharmacology Tips
  UHS.bsd.uchicago.edu/~bhsiung/tips
Mental Health Net Psychopharmacology and Drug References
  www.cmhcsys.com/guide/pro22.htm
RxList - The Internet Drug Index
  www.rxlist.com/
Pharmaceutical Companies on the Web
  griffin.vcu.edu/~gkrishna/pk/pk_company.html
Drug Information
  www.healthtouch.com/level1/p_dri.html

JOURNALS

Psychopharmacology Bulletin
Essential Psychopharmacology
Journal of Clinical Psychopharmacology
American Journal of Psychopharmacology
The Medical Sciences Bulletin

REFERENCES

American Nurses Association. (1994a). *A statement on psychiatric-mental health clinical nursing practice and standards of psychiatric-mental health clinical nursing practice.* Washington, DC: American Nurses Publishing.

American Nurses Association. (1994b). *Psychiatric mental health nursing psychopharmacology project: Task Force on Psychopharmacology.* Washington, DC: Author.

American Psychiatric Association. (1994). *Diagnostic and statistical manual of mental disorders: DSM-IV.* (ed. 4). Washington, DC: Author.

Bailey, K.P. & Snyder, M.E. (1995). The implementation of advanced practice psychiatric nurse prescribers: a comprehensive model. *Journal of the American Psychiatric Nurses Association, 1,* 183–189.

Bailey, K.P. (1996). Preparing for prescriptive practice: advanced practice psychiatric nursing and psychopharmacotherapy. *Journal of Psychosocial Nursing, 34,* 16–20.

Cohen, L.J. (1997). Commonly asked questions about trade name vs. generic pharmaceutical products. *Journal of Clinical Psychiatry, 15,* 2–6.

Forman, L. (1993). Medication: reasons and interventions for noncompliance. *Journal of Psychosocial Nursing, 31,* 23–25.

Greenlaw, J. (1985). Definition and regulation of nursing practice: an historical survey. *Law, Medicine & Health Care, 6,* 117–121.

Hales, A., et al. (1998). Preparing for prescriptive privileges: a CNS-physician collaborative model: expanding the scope of the psychiatric-mental health clinical nurse specialist. *Clinical Nurse Specialist, 12,* 73–80.

Harkless, G.E. (1989). Prescriptive authority: debunking common assumptions. *Nurse Practitioner, 8,* 58–61.

Howard, P.B., & Greiner, D. (1997). Constraints to advanced psychiatric-mental health nursing practice. *Archives of Psychiatric Nursing, 11,* 198–209.

Hyman, S.E., Arana, G.W., & Rosenbaum, J.F. (1995). *Handbook of psychiatric drug therapy.* Boston: Little, Brown & Company.

Moniz, D. (1992). The legal danger of written protocols and standards of practice. *Nurse Practitioner, 17*(9), 58–60.

Olfson, M., Pincus, H.A., & Sabshin, M. (1994). Pharmacotherapy in outpatient psychiatric practice. *American Journal of Psychiatry, 151,* 580–585.

Pearson, L. (1998). Annual update of how each state stands on legislative issues affecting advanced nursing practice. *Nurse Practitioner, 23*(1), 14–66.

Physicians' Desk Reference. (1998). Montvale, NJ: Medical Economics Data Production Company.

Salzman, C. (1998). *Clinical geriatric psychopharmacology* (ed. 3). Baltimore, MD: Williams & Wilkins.

Schatzberg, A.F., & Cole, J.O. (1991). *Manual of clinical psychopharmacology.* Washington, DC: American Psychiatric Press.

Sovner, R., Bailey, K.P., & Weisblatt, R.E. (1990). An HMO psychopharmacology service. *HMO Practice, 4,* 162–166.

Starr, P. (1982). *The social transformation of American medicine.* New York: Basic Books.

Temin, P. (1980). *Taking your medicine: drug regulation in the United States.* Cambridge, MA: Harvard University Press.

Prevention in Mental Health and Substance Abuse Services

NANCY M. VALENTINE and SANDRA J. McELHANEY

■ INTRODUCTION

"An ounce of prevention is worth a pound of cure." Psychiatric nurses learned this lesson at home long before they were confronted with how challenging this might be in practice. In daily life, this concept is difficult enough to apply consistently to personal goals such as eating right, exercising, and getting enough rest. Applied to the field of behavioral health where the continuum of options and interventions can range from learning positive parenting skills, to trying to reduce the incidence of serious mental illnesses, to preventing gang violence, the order of magnitude and associated challenges are much greater.

Clinicians are educated to be astute observers of human behavior and to learn from a combina-tion of life experiences and role models provided by respected mentors. For many, the lessons have been mixed. Unless clinicians developed professionally in a setting that strongly valued prevention and put these principles into practice, it is unlikely that they appreciate the potential that prevention holds for the populations they routinely encounter in either mental health or primary care settings. For many in practice, just the idea of prevention seems like a distant notion in a more ideal world. Psychiatric-mental health nurses value health promotion and disease prevention in practice, but how many actually make this a priority?

Given the emphasis on comprehensive patient care and an appreciation for prevention as a core value in their education, advanced practice registered nurses (APRNs) are in a unique position to foster prevention strategies in the delivery of mental health and substance abuse services. As systems of care are developed, APRNs are becoming more focused on accountability for effective, efficient, and productive outcomes. Nurses practice from a discipline base that values integrated wellness care within a family and community context. They are thus able to develop systems of care in which there are incentives for prevention to flourish. In contrast, medicine has traditionally considered both prevention and cure, but over the past century has focused primarily on cure. Nurses are in a pivotal position to partner with physicians and other providers to balance the continuum of care. Threading prevention throughout integrated systems of care is a function that nurses can assume through leadership within the context of the interdisciplinary team. APRNs can also advocate for having prevention strategies imbedded in practice and reimbursed by insurance and managed care companies.

The purpose of this chapter is to influence the prevention-focused practice patterns of APRNs in psychiatric and mental health care. The topics explored are the need to make prevention a priority in mental health and substance abuse services, the use of prevention as a model for determining program development, the consideration of how prevention research information can be used by nurses in both mental health and primary care settings, and the pivotal role that managed care companies can play in the integration of prevention into their core business values and contracts.

PRIORITIZING THE PRACTICE ■ OF PREVENTION

Engaging in prevention practices may lack the excitement associated with using new technology. Prevention in health care is often left to those with a primary interest in public health matters. This situation is further accentuated in the field of mental health, perhaps as a result of the perceived lack of proven outcomes and the more severe restric-

tions placed on reimbursement for mental health care. Despite the discussion of the need for more emphasis on prevention that has occurred over the past decade, prevention is often relatively low on the list of health care priorities. At best, it seems to be one of those ideal practices considered as an afterthought rather than a driving force in the delivery of care.

Every clinician learns something about prevention in professional training. Consumers also hear about it but often ignore recommended behavior changes hoping that the doctor or medication can solve their problems. Finally, payers tend to think of prevention as an unnecessary "add on" to the cost of a contract in a competitive marketplace. In the busy world of health care delivery, which still subscribes to a medical model of episodic care, an emphasis on prevention is missing. In managed care delivery models, where providers are increasingly allotted specific and shrinking amounts of time to see each patient, there is often no time left in a visit to discuss prevention strategies. Therefore, although there is nearly universal recognition that prevention is important, there is little understanding of what really works. There are minimal incentives to make prevention a priority in the delivery of services, especially when that translates into "what serves the short-term bottom line" (Chapel & Strange, 1997).

To further complicate matters, it is not surprising that in a health care system that has traditionally been financially rewarded for doing more within a disease-focused model of care, there have been few business incentives for marketing prevention. Even for conditions that are known to respond to attention to risk factors and the benefits of rehabilitation, such as coronary artery disease, such intervention programs are mainly excluded from medical insurance reimbursement. As Leaf (1993) notes in calling for a balance between the curative and preventive approaches, " Blue Cross/ Blue Shield and Medicare will pay $30,000 for coronary bypass graft operations and more than $100,000 for heart transplant surgery but not for a $1000 to $2000 rehabilitation program. Medicare specifically eschews reimbursement for preventive measures." With fundamental changes in financing moving to an increasingly market-driven, competitive model where capitation is used to control costs, there may be new incentives emerging for decreasing risk and emphasizing preventive strategies. However, this awareness is evolving slowly.

Given the early stage of development of many managed care arrangements, winning contracts based on price often takes precedence over quality considerations, especially those that can only be measured with a long-term yardstick. "Today, 'lean and mean' wins managed care contracts. In this environment, prevention activities haven't yet proven themselves because the art and science of defining and measuring health outcomes are still in their infancy" (Chapel & Strange, 1997). There are those who forecast that it is difficult to see how a more competitive financing and delivery system will actually be responsive to what Ginzberg (1996) describes as "an order of magnitude change in the public's belated awareness of and responses to the fact that most diseases and illnesses result from their behavior and life styles, not from genes and viruses." Clearly, the culture will need to change among health professionals and the public alike. People will have to accept more responsibility individually for their own health through choices they make and the lifestyles they pursue. They will need to realize that they can no longer engage in whatever lifestyle they wish and then, when illness strikes, expect a pill or operation to erase the adverse health effects of a lifetime of self-abuse. Also, health care providers must avoid perpetuating such misbeliefs.

OVERCOMING PREVENTION ■ BARRIERS

An essential barrier to overcome is the slow transfer of positive attitudes and knowledge of health promotion to the behavioral health field. In the treatment of physical health, the concept as well

as the practice of prevention is more accepted than it is in behavioral health. For example, parents of a new baby experience prevention during the "well baby" visits scheduled periodically throughout the early years of life. During these visits, important disease-preventing immunizations are administered, and even the most harried pediatric providers typically spend at least a few moments educating parents about ways to foster their children's physical and emotional well-being. If such regular well visits were part of the overall approach to health care, there would be ample opportunities to explore potential sources of stress and ill health with patients on a routine basis. Health Maintenance Organizations (HMOs) emulate this model when they schedule regular annual check-ups that include assessment of mental health as well as physical health parameters.

Health outcomes suffer when the sole emphasis is on the treatment of illness in systems of care. Changing the emphasis to include prevention will require fundamental shifts in perspective and attitude for those schooled exclusively in the traditional treatment approaches. However, the potential outcome of fostering improved behavioral health and diminishing the burden of disease should make the exploration of preventive options attractive to all parties.

Ultimately prevention will need to be marketed to all stakeholders including providers, payers, and patients. Providers will need to gain access to the growing evidence base of preventive approaches in mental health. This will require a shift in the way practitioners are trained because there must be some exposure to prevention strategies to prepare for their integration into practice (Greenfield & Shore, 1995). Payers will need to be educated about which prevention strategies yield evidence-based results (French et al., 1996; Hunkeler, Meresman, & Goebe, 1997; Katon et al., 1997) and specific strategies that influence the bottom line (Fox et al., 1996; Morse et al., 1997; Quinivan et al., 1995; Renz et al., 1995; Revicki et al., 1997; Weisner et al., 1996). No matter how efficacious preventive efforts may be, if no one is willing to pay for them, their utility is compromised. Finally, patients will need to be educated about their role and responsibility for their own health status. This is an evolutionary step away from a paternalistic health care system that functioned to foster dependency on the wisdom of the doctor and "the system."

How penetrable are these numerous barriers? The good news is that over the past several decades the concept of prevention has grown within the mental health and substance abuse communities. This interest is based on the recognition and evolving acceptance of the fact that secondary and tertiary treatment interventions are not enough to ameliorate human suffering. A sound public health framework requires that behavioral health problems, like physical health problems, be confronted on all fronts including prevention through strategies such as early intervention, treatment, and rehabilitation.

Incidence and Prevalence of Mental Illness

Recognition of the mind-body connection is fundamental to the discussion of the interface between physical and mental illness (Gabbard, 1997). Although physical and mental illnesses are still categorized primarily as separate phenomena, there is nearly always a strong connection, as illustrated by a study of the association of stress and illness with the common cold. The researchers demonstrated that the rates of both respiratory infection and clinical colds increased in a dose-response manner with the degree of increased psychologic stress (Cohen, Tyrell & Smith, 1991).

Moving into the mental health arena, the statistical results of the United States National Comorbity Survey (which represents an estimation of the incidence and prevalence of psychiatric disorders among a noninstitutionalized population between 15 and 54 years of age) found that the occurrence of behavioral illnesses is greater than previously thought (Kessler et al, 1994). Nearly 50% of re-

spondents reported at least one lifetime disorder, and almost 30% reported at least one 12-month disorder. The most common disorders were depressive episode, alcohol dependence, social phobia, and simple phobia. This morbidity is more highly concentrated than previously recognized in roughly one sixth of the population who have a history of three or more comorbid disorders. What is particularly interesting about these findings is that the majority of people with mental illness never receive treatment of any type. Even among those with multiple diagnoses, less than 50% are treated, which underscores the need for more outreach and research on barriers to treatment as well as prevention.

However, in spite of such reports, mental health and substance abuse issues often get lost in the prevention dialogue. With so much emphasis on and advocacy for paying attention to heart disease, cancer, and accidental or violence-related injuries in the health care media, it is easy to see why mental illness and substance abuse problems are often overlooked. It comes as a surprise to the lay public and often to many health care providers that mental illness creates such serious disabilities. The underlying factors that contribute to this fact are a combination of stigma, lack of information, prejudice against the optimism associated with chances for a cure, and fear of dealing with patients who have the potential for violence.

However, these illnesses are among those that create the greatest degree of mortality and disability worldwide. Murray and Lopez (1996) describe the effects of diseases on the populations of every country. One of the dimensions of the analysis is described as the Years of Life Lost (YLLs), a measure of premature death, especially at younger ages. They have compared the leading causes of YLL known in this decade and project both similarities and changes over the 30-year period between 1990 to 2020. Of the 15 leading causes of YLL, those ranked that have mental health and substance abuse implications include self-inflicted injuries (ranked 12th), violence (ranked 14th), and war (ranked 15th) in 1990. By the year 2020, self-inflicted injuries will be nearly the same (ranked 13th) with violence and war moving up to 11th and 7th place, respectively.

Using a related measure, Disability-Adjusted Life Years (DALYs), a measure of projected years lived with a disability, the conditions associated with mental illness and substance abuse become even more sharply focused as critically important societal problems that contribute to personal, family, employer, and community burden. Of the 15 leading causes of years lived with a disability, unipolar depression is ranked fourth in 1990 and is projected to rise to second place as a leading cause of disability worldwide by the year 2020. Problems in 1990 associated with war (ranked 16th), self-inflicted injuries (ranked 17th), and violence (ranked 28th) will each move up in the list to 8th, 12th, and 14th, respectively by the year 2020, a disturbing upward trend. Of the ten leading causes of disability affecting 472.7 million people worldwide in 1990, five are related to mental health and substance abuse. Depression is at the top of the list with a ratio of 2:1 as compared with the other four. Cumulatively, 103 million people are affected as follows: depression (50.8 million), alcohol use (15.8 million), bipolar disorder (14.1 million), schizophrenia (12.1 million), and obsessive-compulsive disorder (10.2 million), accounting for 22% of the ten leading causes of disabilities worldwide.

From this important study it is evident that the most dramatic effects of mental illnesses are on morbidity rather than mortality. Therefore interventions that focus on reduction in illness are a more sensitive criterion of the success of prevention strategies than reduction of deaths. This understanding is supported by Leaf (1993) who argues that "reduction of morbidity, rather than only extension of life, seems to me to be the logical measure of success of a health care system." Quality of life, not merely survival, becomes a logical objective of increasing the emphasis on prevention.

Contemporary Definition of Prevention

The classic definition of prevention taken from the field of public health includes primary prevention (incidence), secondary prevention (prevalence), and tertiary prevention (disability). This was a model that worked when the etiologies of disease were thought to be more linear in their relationship to disease progression over time. Today, it is known that few illnesses have a single causal agent and that the complexity of risk and protective factors must be considered. A committee of the Institute of Medicine (IOM) of the National Academy of Sciences met to develop a definition of prevention that would consider this knowledge. The outcome of this work was to formulate a new classification system for all of mental health. In this model, the word prevention relates to those interventions targeted to a population before the initial onset of a problem or disorder. Treatment involves screening for existing disorders and offering appropriate standard care, including interventions to prevent recidivism. Ongoing maintenance involves after-care services.

Within this framework, prevention is further classified into three subgroupings: universal, selective, and indicated (Fig. 14-1). *Universal interventions* are offered to everyone in the population regardless of risk (e.g., all children receive immunizations). *Selective interventions* are targeted to individuals who are at greater risk of developing behavioral health problems than the population at large (e.g., teen parents and their children receive special skills training to prevent child abuse). Such risk may be attributable to various combinations of biologic, psychologic, or social factors that are associated with the onset of disorder. Finally, *indicated interventions* are offered to individuals who are identified as being at high risk or experiencing early prodromal symptoms of a disorder (e.g., mothers with postpartum depression and their infants). This model, contrasted with the classic definition from public health that is constructed on a hierarchy, treats all aspects of care equally and

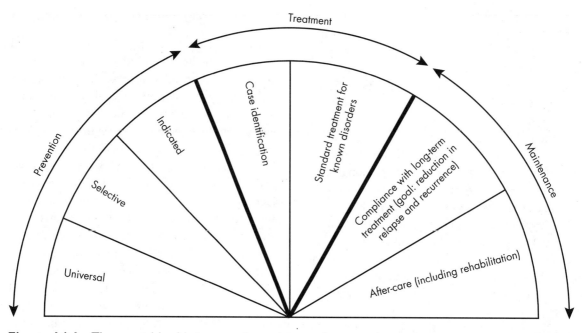

Figure 14-1 The mental health intervention spectrum for mental disorders. From Mrazek, P.J., & Haggerty, R.J. (1994). *Reducing risks for mental disorders.* Washington, DC: National Academy Press.

recognizes that all are important in establishing a complete system of care (IOM, 1994; NMHA, 1986).

Applying this definition of *prevention* to all populations poses interesting questions. An example of these challenges is outlined in a discussion of prevention and early intervention for mental disorders in the elderly. Although the need for universal preventive interventions in later life is apparent, there are few major empiric investigations of such interventions. A review of IOM intervention research programs revealed that most prevention programs are directed at infants, preschoolers, elementary-age children, and adolescents (Mrazek & Haggerty, 1994). The striking absence of prevention research to address the needs of adults and the growing population of elderly is important. In applying the definitions of prevention, the areas for study become apparent. A selective prevention intervention focused on the individual at risk for a mental disorder must be empirically based on research regarding the etiology and course of mental illness. With older adults, research in this area is in its infancy. As such, several areas of priority are suggested. These include understanding individual differences among older adults in responding to the stresses and challenges of late life, categorizing the unique risks, and identifying challenges among the oldest. Indicated prevention focuses on prompt treatment of individuals with a diagnosable mental disorder. For the older adult, it is important to identify the biologic, social, and psychologic markers for risk of mental disorder in late life as well as the optimal combination of biologic, social, and psychologic factors for effective preventive interventions and prompt treatment protocols (Smyer, 1995). Several studies of the course of depression in the elderly are beginning attempts to answer these questions for this population (Alexopoulos et al., 1993; Alexopoulos et al., 1996; Devanand et al., 1996; Martinez et al., 1996; Reynolds et al., 1995).

A PREVENTION
■ INTERVENTION MODEL

In the development of a prevention intervention model, knowledge of the research literature is essential in knowing which areas of inquiry are rich for program development. Although there is a broad array of topics, two categories emerge for targeting populations in need of services:

1. Developmental research focusing on early childhood development and the implications for preventive intervention across the age continuum.
2. A risk model targeting those populations who are vulnerable and therefore able to benefit from intervention.

Although there is blending of the two in some cases, highlights of examples of the relevant literature are reviewed in this context.

Developmental Prevention Research

In the developmental approach, individuals are targeted for preventive intervention based on their stage of life. The premise is that in each stage of life there are developmental challenges that, if positively resolved, lead to overall human growth and positive well-being, and if negatively resolved or left unresolved, can lead to potentially negative outcomes, including poor mental health and substance abuse-related problems. Preventive interventions have been researched and developed for the following age groups: infants, children, adolescents, adults, and the elderly, essentially every group across the lifespan. Of these developmental stages, as already noted, the research to date has placed strong emphasis on the needs of children and adolescents and their adult caregivers.

A review of the literature indicates some interesting examples of the important evidence for preventive interventions using the developmental approach. Beginning with childhood, it is recognized that early observations are critically important and that interventions, whether with the child, family, or child and family together, do

make a difference. For example, troubled family interaction very early in a child's life can predict problems later. This was demonstrated by researchers who observed that child externalizing behavior at 3 years of age was found to be almost monotonically related to chronically troubled family interaction, regardless of whether problem behaviors were reported by mothers, fathers, or day care providers (Belsky, Woodworth & Cormic, 1996). In a longitudinal study from a birth cohort where behavioral observations during the first 3 years of life were empirically tested to determine if there were links to specific adult psychiatric disorders such as anxiety and mood disorders, antisocial personality disorder, recidivism and violent crime, alcoholism, and suicidal behavior, findings suggest some linkages. Undercontrolled 3 year olds were more likely to meet diagnostic criteria for antisocial personality disorder and be involved in crime at 21 years of age. Inhibited 3 year olds were more likely to meet diagnostic criteria for depression at 21 years of age. Both groups were more likely to attempt suicide, and boys in both groups had alcohol-related problems. Controlling for family social class did not change the findings (Caspi et al., 1996). Therefore observing the child's behavior often indicates problems that need to be addressed with the family as a unit.

Following the complex course of behavior development and considering the implications for preventive treatment are illustrated in work done by Henry and colleagues (1996). In a longitudinal study that examined the relationship between family characteristics and degree of violence at later stages of life, they found that family factors were associated with both types of conviction outcomes (both violent and nonviolent), whereas childhood temperament was associated primarily with convictions for violent offenses. Two distinct components of behavioral regulation were identified as operating: 1) social regulation as determined by family socialization; and 2) individual differences in self-regulation. In each of these scenarios, two pathways emerge. In the first, a child who has done well throughout childhood will run into adolescent behavior problems in response to any type of family or environmental disruption. In this case, "acting out" behavior is contained and does not carry over into adulthood. In the second instance of differences in self-regulation, the child who has difficulty early in life, especially in the context of family disintegration, is at risk for early onset of violent offending that carries on into adulthood. The researchers therefore concluded that it is the regulatory characteristics of the child that determine the "shape" that antisocial behavior will take.

The challenge, however, lies in determining which factors make a difference and are therefore able to be influenced through intervention. A multisite, multimodal study of attention-deficit hyperactivity disorder (ADHD), the most common childhood mental disorder, demonstrates the complexity of investigating the multiple factors involved in linking prevention with treatment (Richters et al., 1995). In this study, the methodology was designed to determine which factors contribute to the problem and which interventions are most efficacious. In preparing for the study, Richters and colleagues noted that despite decades of treatment research and clinical practice, there is an insufficient basis for determining under which circumstances and with which child characteristics (comorbid conditions, gender, family history, home environment, age, nutrition and metabolic status, etc.) which treatments or combination of treatments (stimulants, behavior therapy, parent training, school-based intervention) have what effects (improvement, stasis, deterioration) on which domains of child functioning (cognitive, academic, behavioral, neurophysiologic, neuropsychologic, peer relations, family relations) for how long (short versus long term), to what extent (effect sizes, normal versus pathologic range), and why (processes underlying change). This multisite study can contribute prevention and treatment options for this important area based on a sound understanding of the etiology and developmental course of the disorder.

In a related study on male gender and predisposition to conduct disorder (CD), researchers concluded that parental substance abuse, low socioeconomic status, and oppositional behavior are key factors in boys' progression to CD (Loeber et al., 1995). Physical fighting, although not a symptom of oppositional defiant disorder, should be targeted in preventive interventions along with CD symptoms. The researchers also noted that ADHD is implicated in the early onset of CD but not in later onset CD. An example of a treatment intervention that is modeled on a developmental and clinical understanding of CD is the FAST track program that focuses the strategy of preventive intervention for children who are considered high risk when they enter school. Using parent training, home visiting and case management, social skills training, academic tutoring, and teacher-based classroom intervention, the program is designed to promote competence in the family, child, and school and thus prevent conduct problems, poor social relations, and school failure (Bierman et al., 1992). Interventions such as these may potentially prevent longer-term problems such as tobacco smoking, which has been associated with classroom aggression and disruptive behavior among boys as early as in the first grade.

A team of violence researchers (Caspi et al., 1994) considered behavior problems that plague society in a study that asked whether some people are crime prone. They concluded that when negative emotionality (the tendency to experience aversive affective states) is accompanied by weak constraint (difficulty in impulse control), negative emotions may be translated more readily into antisocial acts. In considering gender differences that might relate to aggression and associated disorders, Crick and Grotpeter (1995) rejected the simple explanation that boys are more aggressive than girls (based on physical and verbal aggression models). They developed a model of aggression that they hypothesized to be more typical of girls, referred to as *relational aggression* (behaviors intended to damage another's friendships or feeling of inclusion in the peer group). Results indicated that this type of aggression places females at risk for serious adjustment difficulties since these subjects were significantly more rejected and reported significantly higher levels of loneliness, depression, and isolation relative to their nonrelationally aggressive peers. A related study (Caspi et al., 1993) that explored delinquency among girls examined processes linking biologic and behavioral changes in different school settings during adolescence. This study confirmed previous research that early puberty is associated with behavior problems in girls, although this finding was confined to mixed sex educational settings. The researchers concluded that for the initiation and maintenance of female delinquency, two factors are necessary: puberty and boys. They also noted that biologic rather than chronologic age may be more relevant for understanding behavior.

In considering the role of family in developmental adjustments, two studies highlight the importance of parental issues and interactions. The first focuses on internalizing problems. In this study (Barber, Olsen, & Shagle, 1994), two separate components of parental control were identified that were associated differently with adolescent adjustment difficulties. One component, psychologic control, characterized by intrusive and emotionally manipulative parental behavior, was associated with internalizing problems in young adolescents, such as feelings of loneliness and unhappiness. The other form of parental control identified was behavioral control, characterized by lax rule setting and enforcement and poor parental monitoring of youth whereabouts. Consistent with prior research, behavioral control was associated with externalizing problems in adolescents, such as delinquency and truancy. In a related study (Conger, Patterson, & Xiaojia, 1995) parental stress related to depression was found to be correlated with disrupted discipline practices. These poor discipline practices appeared to provide the direct link with developmental outcomes for a sample of Oregon and Iowa boys.

In the area of violence prevention, there is evidence that suggests that successful efforts to curb violence should begin early in a child's life. Researchers also believe that it is possible to determine early on what predisposing factors play a role in a child's life. Based on a 10-year study conducted by Buka and Earls (1993), three broad areas of risk factors were identified:

1. Child health and neurologic status
2. Early academic skills and success
3. Family functioning and parenting style

The investigators found the following:

- There are established early risk factors for later criminality and violence.
- The established predictors indicate links in a developmental sequence, rather than single causes, leading to violence and delinquency
- Knowledge is necessary in estimating the magnitude of risk resulting from each factor, understanding that these estimates are influenced by a child's gender and the context in which they occur.

As these samples of studies of early developmental issues indicate, preventive intervention is indeed relevant and needs to be considered in an overall approach to delivering quality services.

Vulnerable Populations Prevention Research

The concept of risk suggests that persons included in a particular group are more likely to develop a disorder than those who are not in the group. Examples of risk groups include the following:

- Individuals who are experiencing major life stressors or transitions such as recent job loss, divorce, and bereavement
- Individuals who are suffering from a diagnosed mental health or substance abuse problem or those with chronic physical conditions
- Family members of persons with mental illness and/or substance abuse problems

A review of the literature on risk studies yields a variety of topics of interest and promising potential for application. An example of such preventive strategies related to life stressors includes the JOBS program intervention. This intervention model was designed to provide unemployed participants with social support, job search skills, and inoculation against setbacks as necessary components for enhancing their sense of mastery. The outcomes illustrate an intervention that has proven results, especially for those at risk for increase of depressive symptoms (Vinokur, Price, & Schuly, 1995).

A study of psychopathology among children placed outside their home (Schneiderman et al., 1998) is another example of identification of a population at risk. Knowledge such as this has important implications for the assessment of patients in primary care settings where routine screening for depression, substance use, and other potential psychosocial elements of the health profile is as important as the assessment of all other systems.

Research that deals with risks associated with family members with mental illness and substance abuse includes examples such as the New York High Risk Project, which began in 1971 as a prospective, comparative, longitudinal study of children with one or two parents who had schizophrenia and groups of children whose parents had other or no psychiatric disorders (Erlenmeyer-Kimling & Cornblatt, 1987a; 1987b). The researchers concluded that to develop effective preventive intervention for children at risk for schizophrenia, the next step in high-risk research should entail piloting cognitive behavior therapy methods in this population (especially those found to have deviant attention performance), with evaluations over a 2- to 3-year period to determine the efficacy of such interventions.

An example of research interventions that present opportunities for devising preventive interventions for family members is illustrated by a study of infants of depressed mothers (Field et al., 1996). A sample of infants of these mothers were given a series of massage therapy sessions and matched with a sample of infants exposed to rocking, and the results were compared. The massaged group exhibited greater weight gain, significantly improved emotional responsiveness, sociability, soothability, and greater decreases in urinary stress catecholamines/hormones such as norepinephrine, epinephrine, and cortisol. Studies related to birth complications and the effects on behavior at the point of adolescence (Raine et al., 1994), and the effects of early neuromotor deficits coupled with unstable family environments (Raine et al., 1996) are other examples of attempts to link early experiences of populations at risk resulting from health and family status and the implications for interventions designed to preserve and enhance functional status.

Examples of findings related to individuals with a diagnosed mental or substance abuse problem are illustrated in a study of depressive symptoms as attributable risk factors for first-onset major depression (Horwath et al., 1992). In this study, longitudinal data were used, and adults were interviewed 1 year apart. Persons with depressive symptoms and those with dysthymia were 4.4 and 5.5 times, respectively, more likely to develop a first-onset major depression during the 1-year period than those without such symptoms. The lifetime prevalence rate was 24%. The attributable risk is a compound epidemiologic measure that reflects both the relative risks associated with depressive symptoms (4.4) and the prevalence of exposure to that risk (24%). Attributable risk is a useful measure to determine the burden of risk to the community. In this study, it was determined to be greater than 50%, which means that more than 50% of cases of first-onset depression are associated with prior depressive symptoms. Persons with first-onset major depression were 1.5 times more likely to be female than male and more often to be Hispanic than Caucasian. This is an important finding from a public health perspective since it indicates that depressive symptoms are often unrecognized and untreated, and identification and effective treatment can have important implications for the prevention of major depression.

In another study, the recognition of the high incidence of comorbidity of depression and panic disorder and the relationship between panic disorder and the high rate of suicide suggested the need for a screening mechanism to detect this dual diagnosis (Gorman & Coplan, 1996). Another example is the work of Fawcett and colleagues

(1987) on clinical predictors of suicide in patients with major affective disorders. Their findings suggest that variables related to hopelessness, loss of pleasure, and mood cycling are key and differentiate those who commit suicide from those who do not, despite patient reports of suicidal ideation, current as well as past attempts, and medical severity of prior attempts. The ability to differentiate between complex symptomatology can be important in making treatment decisions and determining the intensity of follow-up care. The investigators also noted that instruments available for assessing current and past suicide attempts are generally very reliable and were recommended to be part of the mental health intake process.

PREVENTION AND MANAGED ■ CARE

The role of prevention within managed care can also be explored as a significant opportunity to improve health. In proposing such an approach, it is with the understanding that managed care companies, like most successful businesses, are driven by the bottom line of profits and attractiveness of the plan to new enrollees or customers. Because of the good public image associated with prevention, it has the potential to attract enrollees, foster an increase in consumer satisfaction, and thus result in greater profitability for the managed care organization. Therefore the goal is clearly one of determining the most efficacious approaches. If effective, researched, and evaluated prevention services are offered, then consumers will receive high-quality interventions that have the potential to avert a range of behavioral health problems.

Having broadly identified the potential scope of preventive mental health and substance abuse services, it is necessary to develop strategies to get managed care companies to value prevention and make it a standing component of the contract. Although it can be argued that initial investments in prevention will pay off in terms of reduced service utilization costs over time, the present reality is that most people who are enrolled in managed care plans will stay with their current plan for only 1 or 2 years. As such, the potential savings for any single company would not be realized unless the standards were that every payer was willing to support prevention. In the latter scenario, it would not matter that subscribers left managed care plan A to enroll in managed care plan B, since all would benefit nearly equally from the pooled investment. Only when high-quality services are provided for the entire continuum will there be a reduction in the incidence, prevalence, and overall costs of mental disorders.

The purchasers of health care services have the opportunity to effect a great change in the health status of this country. They are doing this by broadening the delivery system and incorporating prevention along with treatment and maintenance. Making the change has required several paradigm shifts: from an illness model to a health orientation, from a discrete intervention model to a holistic orientation, and from a focus on individuals to a focus on families and how illness in one member places others at risk. Government-funded programs are directed toward the public's health and are significantly affected by cost shifting from one system to another. Children, for example, who do not receive prevention services for substance abuse often end up in the child welfare and juvenile justice systems, where the long-term costs far outweigh the initial investment in prevention. An example of such cost effectiveness of prevention is illustrated in a study by Olds and colleagues (1993) on the effect of prenatal and infancy nurse home visitation on government spending. Outcomes indicated that for low income families, within 4 years, the cost of the visitation program was totally repaid with a dividend of $180 per family, with savings recovered in less use of Aid to Families of Dependent Children, food stamps, Medicaid, and Child Protective Services.

As a strategy to build consensus among the diverse members of the field of mental health and substance abuse treatment and prevention, the American College of Mental Health Administration (ACMHA) initiated a project entitled Santa

Fe Summit on Behavioral Health, which will meet yearly from 1997 to 2000. The first meeting in 1997 was devoted to outcomes and performance measurement and the domains targeted were prevention, access, process and performance, outcomes, and structure. The framework for incorporating prevention into managed care arrangements (ACMHA, 1997) based on the

consensus of multiple experts and organizations interested in setting standards is outlined in Box 14-1.

Identified themes as to why purchasers should value prevention include the fact that the cost of not providing services and the resulting morbidity are huge, based on the disability analysis discussed earlier. In addition, there is the potential for pre-

---

box 14-1

THE NEED FOR PURCHASERS TO VALUE PREVENTION AND INCORPORATE PREVENTION INTO HEALTH CARE PRIORITIES

Overarching values: The values related to prevention that underlie any system of care that will achieve the purchaser's goal of keeping employees or citizens healthy and productive include the following:

- The system of care, including outcomes, must be operationalized, defined, and evidence-based.
- There must be aggressive outreach in service delivery.
- Access barriers to health must be eliminated.
- Consumers must be involved in a process of self-management and empowerment with an existing partnership between consumers and purchasers in determining policy and individual services.
- Health care should build on the consumers' strengths and increase their potential.
- Children and families should be the highest priority.
- A risk and resilience model should be used in assessment and service delivery.
- A primary goal of service should be to foster healthy life development.
- Health care should be collaboratively linked to other community resources.
- Risk profiling of important populations is necessary. The issue of what is important may vary among purchasers and consumers. Risk factors vary in different populations, but they

should be identified at rates predicted by epidemiologic data.

- Risk populations should be identified as early as possible with screening at key access points in the health delivery system.
- The interventions that are provided should be appropriate. The interventions should be associated with the risk profiles of the enrolled population and should focus on risks amenable to change.
- Wherever possible, the interventions should be based on identified programs, which have a strong evidence base.
- Enrollees with identified high-risk factors should engage in the interventions, receive the full course of the program, and be encouraged to maintain their behavioral changes.
- For those who receive the preventive intervention, there should be an enhanced performance outcome. There should be a reduction of risks and reduction of onset of illnesses in the areas targeted and meaningful to purchasers and customers.
- Provision of these services will affect the management and finance of purchasers. There will be significant resources (dollars and staff) associated with risk profiling, risk reduction, and resiliency promotion. Appropriate staff will need to be hired to provide the services, and they are likely to need additional training.

From ACMHA, 1997.

vention to be cost effective and the possibility that employee productivity for businesses in the commercial marketplace could be increased. Finally, it may also be the right thing to do for the patients being served. Managed care companies can use the risk and evidence-based framework for maintaining and measuring prevention services in managed care as developed by Santa Fe Summit participants. These guidelines (ACMHA, 1997) are outlined in Box 14-2.

ROLE OF THE APRN IN ■ PREVENTION

There are three key areas where the APRN can play a significant role in the transition of the current system of care into one that is focused on prevention: 1) to be knowledgeable about the literature and to search for evidence-based examples of prevention strategies that work, 2) to apply these research findings in practice, and 3) to col-

---

box **14-2**

IMPLEMENTING PREVENTION STRATEGIES IN MENTAL HEALTH AND ADDICTION SERVICES

- The term *prevention* should be reserved for only those interventions that occur before the initial onset of disorder.
- The target disorders or conditions to be prevented and the target populations for the preventive interventions should be identified and selected by the purchasers (i.e., the true payers of the health care plan) in collaboration with the mental health and substance abuse organization. Thus the decisions will ultimately reflect the values of both the purchasers and service providers.
- Only disorders or conditions for which there are known malleable risk and protective factors should be targeted.
- Only conditions for which there are known, science-based, preventive interventions should be targeted.
- Individuals and families should be screened for the occurrence of risk factors that are associated with the first onset of a disorder or condition.
- All those identified through screening as being at high risk for developing a particular disorder or condition must be offered the preventive intervention to prevent that condition. If they accept the offer, the preventive service must be provided.

- Those who provide prevention interventions must be thoroughly trained in the relevant risk assessment tools and in the implementation of each specific preventive intervention that is delivered.
- Process and capacity measures should be documented such as percentage of personnel receiving training, percentage of total enrollees who are informed regarding risk identification, percentage of health care population screened, percentage who use the prevention services, and so on.
- The intermediate performance measures should focus on risk status within the targeted population. Change or lack of change on the targeted risk factors should be documented for each individual and the risk population as a whole.
- The key performance measures should focus on the primary disorder or condition to be prevented. These outcomes are the ultimate targets of the interventions.
- Documentation of the costs of risk assessments and prevention programs should be collected not only for the whole serviced population but also on an individual basis.

From ACMHA, 1997.

lect data on outcomes of these strategies in order to add to the fund of knowledge so that replication of useful interventions can be shared broadly. Although there is much research to be done, there are ample studies available to get started. Applying the framework as outlined by the Santa Fe Summit consensus document allows the APRN to target primarily selective and indicated preventive strategies. Creative approaches can then be devised that consider the setting, appropriate providers, and types of interventions.

Settings

Virtually any setting in which health care, early education, or child development activities occur is potentially suitable for the provision of preventive intervention. Managed care personnel, insurers, and employers need to be encouraged to think about how to creatively expend their resources in a variety of settings where the results can enhance general health and well-being, increase provider productivity, and reduce costs associated with mental health and addiction.

Appropriate Providers

The type of intervention can suggest the appropriate providers. Ultimately, the range of providers should go well beyond the traditional mental health community. Among those cited are providers in obstetrics and gynecology, pediatrics, and primary care, and health department personnel, all of whom could greatly expand the provision of preventive interventions. In addition, staff in a broad range of child care settings (e.g., Head Start and other preschool programs) and educators could be used if appropriately trained in preventive intervention techniques. For example, in a study of outreach interventions for the homeless mentally ill, Jones and Scannell (1997) advise using all available personnel resources, which can include voluntary workers, past users of services, and professional workers, as an alternative to traditional services.

Types of Interventions

Just as there are multiple risk populations for preventive interventions, there are also numerous modalities of intervention to meet the needs of these groups. A range of service providers in various delivery settings offers such interventions. Albee and Gullotta (1996) identified four major groupings of prevention activities, all of which can be suitable for application within managed care.

Education. Education increases knowledge, which is believed to encourage healthy behaviors and discourage unhealthy behaviors. Education can be subdivided into the following:
- Information that informs and enlightens such as books, newsletters, articles, lectures, films, instructional videos, and warning labels
- Anticipatory guidance that forewarns and equips an individual with an understanding regarding some life event, such as childbirth education, home visiting and parenting training, retirement planning, and hospice
- Behavioral feedback that enables an individual to modify behavior such as transcendental meditation, yoga, or biofeedback

Personal and social competency promotion. This grouping includes activities that promote individual and social competency. These are efforts that promote development of cognitive skills, belonging, being valued, and being able to make a meaningful contribution to a group. Most efforts also attempt to improve psychologic states and traits, such as an internal locus-of-control, self-esteem, self-efficacy, and self-concept of ability. Resiliency promotion efforts also fit within this grouping. These efforts can be divided into two groups:
- Social skills training that enables individuals to learn from a specified curriculum and, most importantly, to practice skills in a group, such as interpersonal cognitive problem solving.
- Social skills opportunities that exist in settings such as scouting, 4H, and Boys and Girls Clubs. In one sense, there is not a specified educational

curriculum or practice drills for participants engaged in these programs. In another sense, the actual activities of these programs represented through programming or rank advancement can be viewed as the curriculum.

Natural caregiving activities. This area recognizes the importance of individuals both giving and receiving support and nurturing:

- Indigenous caregiving is an acknowledgment that each of us has a responsibility for our own health and that of our fellow human beings. Mentoring programs such as Big Brothers/Big Sisters and volunteers who deliver meals to the elderly are examples of indigenous caregivers.
- Trained indigenous caregiving recognizes that certain professions or occupations, such as the clergy, teachers, police, bartenders, and others, have significant opportunities to practice these skills. This enables them to go beyond their job descriptions to assist others.
- Mutual self-help groups have formed around life events or experiences to enable individuals to be both the givers and receivers of care. These can be organizations such as Alcoholics Anonymous or electronic list-serves focused on particular areas.

Community organization and systems interventions. These types of activities involve groups of individuals, organizations, and agencies:

- The first phase, community organization, looks to encourage change within a broad social context to reduce ill health and/or promote good health. Examples include the public relations efforts of All-State Insurance several years ago to use its corporate resources and image to promote seat belt use and the installation of air bags in cars, or the Rotary International's efforts to inoculate all children against polio by the year 2000.
- The second phase, systems intervention, looks at fostering institutional practices that reduce ill health or promote good health. Examples of this effort include lower life insurance premiums for nonsmokers, lower car insurance premiums for honor roll students, and special incentives like reduced membership costs to join a health club.

IMPLICATIONS FOR ■ THE FUTURE

The future success of prevention program development depends on the connectivity between the research community and clinicians, payers, and patients. As behavior and interventions are studied and questions about "what works" are answered, there will be greater incentives to use them broadly. For example, if depression screening demonstrates early case finding and routes to early recovery and greater employee productivity, there will be enthusiasm among health plans, employers, clinicians, and patients to adopt this intervention.

A window into the future of prevention is outlined in the recently published report of the National Advisory Mental Health Council workgroup on Mental Disorders and Prevention Research, entitled *Priorities for Prevention Research at NIMH* (1998). The framework suggested for modern prevention science includes the following recommendations:

- Adopt an expanded definition of prevention research.
- Strengthen epidemiologic foundations of prevention research.
- Stimulate preintervention and intervention studies of early childhood risks for adverse developmental outcomes.
- Expand research on depression and anxiety across the life span.
- Refine and advance the empirical basis for conduct disorder prevention research.
- Broaden disorders and populations targeted for prevention research.
- Expand studies on comorbidity prevention.
- Develop a program of preventive services research including prevention policy research.
- Encourage and support long-term follow-up in prevention research.

- Build prevention research capacity especially through training grants.

In addition, the National Institute of Mental Health is fostering the development of scientific leadership in the field, support for cross-institute and cross-agency linkages, and emphasis on the dissemination of prevention research (NAMHC, 1998).

The opportunities for APRNs in psychiatric and mental health care to play a significant role in prevention are available for clinicians, researchers, and educators. The focus on healthy living and quality of life are fueling much of the energy to explore how mental illness can be turned into mental health, and substance abuse can be treated like any other problem, where hope for interventions that make a difference are considered to be just around the corner.

RESOURCES AND CONNECTIONS

PROFESSIONAL JOURNALS

American Journal of Community Psychology
Health Promotion Practice (a journal of health promotion and health education applications, policy, and professional issues)
Journal of Primary Prevention

BOOKS

Haddix, A, et al. (1996). *Prevention effectiveness.* New York: Oxford University Press.

Hegarty, V. (1998). Prevention: the case for evidence-based criteria. *Prevention Notes.* VA National Center for Health Prevention: NCHP.

Issues in children's and family lives: an annual book series. Thousand Oaks, CA: Sage Publications.

Volume 1: Hampton, R.L. (Ed.). *Family violence: prevention and treatment.*

Volume 2: Ryan, B.A., & Adams, G.R. (Eds.). *The family-school connection.*

Volume 3: Blau, G.M., & Gullotta, T.P. (Eds.). *Adolescent dysfunctional behavior.*

Volume 4: Hampton, R.L., Jenkins, P., & Gullotta, T.P. (Eds.). *Preventing violence in America.*

Volume 5: Bloom, M. *Primary prevention practices.*

Volume 6: Albee, G.W., & Gullotta, T.P. (Eds.). *Primary prevention works.*

Mrazek, P., & Haggerty, R. (1994). *Reducing risk for mental disorders.* Washington DC: National Academy Press.

National Mental Health Association. (1995). *The NMHA directory of model programs to prevent mental disorders and promote mental health.* Alexandria, VA: Author.

Preventive Services Task Force. (1996). *Guide to clinical preventive services* (ed. 2). Baltimore: Williams & Wilkins.

CLEARINGHOUSES

National Clearinghouse on Child Abuse and Neglect and Family Violence Information
P.O. Box 1182
Washington, DC 20013
800-FYI-3366
Fax: 703-385-3206

National Committee for the Prevention of Child Abuse
322 S. Michigan Avenue
Suite 1600
Chicago, IL 60604-4357
312-663-3520

National Institute on Aging Information Center
P.O. Box 8057
Gaithersburg, MD 20898-8057
800-222-2225
Fax: 301-589-3014

National Worksite Health Promotion Resource Center
777 North Capitol Street, NE, #800
Washington, DC 20002
202-408-9320 or 202-408-9333
Fax: 202-408-9332

The Ontario Prevention Clearinghouse (OPC)
#1200-415 Yonge Street
Toronto, Ontario M5B 2EJ
416-408-2121
Fax: 416–408-2122

National Mental Health Association Prevention Clearinghouse
1021 Prince Street
Alexandria, VA 22314-2971
703-684-7722

WEBSITES
Centre for Evidence Based Medicine
www.acponline.org/journals/ebm/ebmmenu.htm
United States Preventive Services Task Force
158.72.20.10/pubs/guidecps

References

Albee, G.W., & Gullotta, T.P. (1996). *Primary prevention works*. Thousand Oaks, CA: Sage Publications.

Alexopoulos, G.S., et al. (1993). The course of geriatric depression with "reversible dementia": a controlled study. *American Psychiatric Association, 150*(11), 1693–1699.

Alexopoulos, G.S., et al. (1996). Recovery in geriatric depression. *Archives of General Psychiatry, 53,* 305–312.

American College Mental Health Administration. (1997). *Preserving quality and value in the managed care equation. Final Report of the Santa Fe Summit on Behavioral Health. Report #1.* Pittsburgh, PA: Author.

Barber, B.K., Olsen, J.E., & Shagle, S.C. (1994). Associations between parental psychological and behavioral control and youth internalized and externalized behaviors. *Child Development, 65,* 1120–1136.

Belsky, J., Woodworth, S., & Cormic, K. (1996). *Troubled family interaction during toddlerhood.* Unpublished research NIMH. Human Development and Family Studies.

Bierman, K., et al. (1992). A developmental and clinical model for the prevention of conduct disorder: the fast track program. *Development and Psychopathology, 4,* 509–527.

Buka, S., & Earls, F. (1993). Early determinants of delinquency and violence. *Health Affairs, 12*(1), 47–64.

Caspi, A., et al. (1993). "Unraveling girls' deliquency: biological, dispositional, and contextual contributions to adolescent misbehavior. *Developmental Psychology, 29*(1), 19–30.

Caspi, A., et al. (1996). Behavioral observations at age 3 years predict psychiatric disorders: longitudinal evidence from a birth cohort. *Archives of General Psychiatry, 53,* 1033–1039.

Caspi, A., et al. (1994). Are some people crime-prone? replications of the personality crime relationship across countries, genders, races and methods. *Criminology, 32*(2), 163–195.

Conger, R.D., Patterson, G.R., & Xiaojia, G.E. (1995). It takes two to replicate: a mediation model for the impact of parents' stress on adolescent adjustment. *Child Development, 66,* 80–97.

Chapel, T.J., & Strange, P.V. (1997). Is altruism killing prevention? when health systems take on the role of public health provider. *Health Care Forum Journal, Sept/Oct,* 46–50.

Cohen, S., Tyrell, D.A.J., & Smith, D.P. (1991). Psychological stress and susceptibility to the common cold. *New England Journal of Medicine, 325,* 606–612.

Crick, N.R., & Grotpeter, J.K. (1995). Relational aggression, gender and social-psychological adjustment. *Child Development, 66,* 710–722.

Devanand, D.P., et al. (1996). Depressed mood and the incidence of Alzheimer's disease in the elderly living in the community. *Archives of General Psychiatry, 53,* 175–182.

Erlenmeyer-Kimling, L., & Cornblatt, B. (1987a). The New York High Risk Project: a follow-up report. *Schizophrenia Bulletin, 13*(3), 451–461.

Erlenmeyer-Kimling, L., & Cornblatt, B. (1987b). Implications for prevention intervention from prospective research on children at risk for schizophrenia. In Steinberg, J.A., & Silverman, M.M. (Eds.). *Preventing mental disorders: a research perspective, NIMH monograph.* Rockville, Maryland: National Institute of Mental Health.

Fawcett, J., et al. (1987). Clinical predictors of suicide in patients with major affective disorders: a controlled prospective study. *American Journal of Psychiatry, 144*(1), 135–140.

Field, T., et al. (1996). Massage therapy for infants of depressed mothers. *Infant Behavior Development, 19,* 107–112.

French, M.T., et al. (1996). Healthcare reforms and managed care for substance abuse services: findings from eleven case studies. *Association for Health Services Research Annual Meeting Abstract Book 13,* 141–142.

Fox, M.H., et al. (1996). The use of support groups among pregnant substance abusers: implications for managed care. *Best Practice Benchmarking Healthcare, 1*(2), 89–93.

Gabbard, G.O. (1997). Dynamic therapy in the decade of the brain. *Connecticut Medicine, 61*(9), 537–542.

Ginzberg, E. (1996). The potential and limits of competition in health care. *Bulletin of the New York Academy of Medicine 73*(2), 224–236.

Gorman, J.M., & Coplan, J.D. (1996). Comorbidity of depression and panic disorder. *Journal of Clinical Psychiatry, 57*(Suppl 10), 34–41.

Greenfield, S.F., & Shore, M.F. (1995). Prevention of psychiatric disorders. *Harvard Review of Psychiatry 3*(3), 115–129.

Henry, B., et al. (1996). Tempermental and family predictors of violent and non-violent criminal convictions: age 3 to age 18. *Developmental Psychology 32*(4), 614–623.

Horwath, E., et al. (1992). Depressive symptoms as relative and attributable risk factors for first-onset major depression. *Archives of General Psychiatry, 49,* 817–823.

Hunkeler, E.M., Meresman, J., & Goebe, J.M. (1997). Implementing a new model of care for managing depression in the primary care setting of an HMO: physician training, nurse telephone follow-up, peer support. *Abstract Book Association for Health Services Research, 14,* 8.

Institute of Medicine (IOM). (1994). *Reducing risks for mental disorders: frontiers for preventive intervention research.* Washington, DC: National Academy Press.

Jones, A., & Scannell, T. (1997). Outreach interventions for the homeless mentally ill. *British Journal of Nursing, 6*(21), 1236–1240.

Katon, E., et al. (1997). Population-based care of depression: effective disease management strategies to decrease prevalence. *General Hospital Psychiatry 19*(3), 169–178.

Kessler, R.C., et al. (1994). Lifetime and 12 month prevalence of DSM-III-R psychiatric disorders in the United States: results from the national comorbidity survey. *Archives of General Psychiatry, 51,* 8–19.

Leaf, A. (1993). Preventative medicine for our ailing health care system. *Journal of the American Medical Association, 269*(5), 616–618.

Loeber, R., et al. (1995). Which boys will fare worse? early predictors of the onset of conduct disorder in a six-year longitudinal study. *Journal of the American Academy of Child and Adolescent Psychiatry, 34*(4), 499–509.

Martinez, R.A., et al. (1996). Delusional and psychotic depression in late life: clinical research needs. *The American Journal of Geriatric Psychiatry, 4,* 77–84.

Morse, G.A., et al. (1997). An experimental comparison of three types of case management for homeless mentally ill persons. *Psychiatric Services, 48,* 497–503.

Mrazek, P.J., & Haggerty, R.J. (Eds.). (1994). *Reducing risks for mental disorders: providers for prevention intervention research.* Washington, DC: National Academy Press.

Murray, J.L., & Lopez, A.D. (1996). *The global burden of disease: a comprehensive assessment of mortality and disability from diseases, injuries, and risk factors in 1990 and projected to 2020.* Published by the Harvard School of Public Health on behalf of The World Health Organization and the World Bank.

National Advisory Mental Health Council Workgroup on Mental Disorders Prevention Research. (May, 1998). *Priorities for prevention research at NIMH: a report by the NIMH.* Publication No. 98–4321.

National Mental Health Administration (NMHA). (1986). *The prevention of mental-emotional disabilities update, 7*(3), 2.

Olds, D.L., et al. (1993). Effect of prenatal and infancy nurse home visitation on government spending. *Medical Care, 31,*155–174.

Quinivan, R., et al. (1995). Service utilization and cost of care for severely mentally ill clients in an intensive care management program. *Psychiatric Services, 46*(4), 365–371.

Raine, A., et al. (1994). Birth complications combined with early maternal rejection at age 1 year predispose to violent crime at age 18 years. *Archives of General Psychiatry, 51,* 984–988.

Raine, A., et al. (1996). High rates of violence, crime, academic problems, and behavioral problems in males with both early neuromotor deficits and unstable family environments. *Archives of General Psychiatry, 53,* 544–49.

Renz, E.A., et al. (1995). The effect of managed care in the treatment outcome of substance abuse disorders. *General Hospital Psychiatry 17*(4), 287–292.

Revicki, D.A., et al. (1997). Cost-effectiveness of newer antidepressants compared with tricyclic antidepressants in managed care settings. *Journal Clinical Psychiatry, 58*(2), 47–58.

Reynolds, E.F., et al. (1995). Maintenance therapies for late-life recurrent major depression: research and review. *International Psychologeriatrics 7*(Suppl), 27–39.

Richters, J.E., et al. (1995). NIMH collaborative multisite multimodel treatment study of children with ADHD. I. Background and rational. *Journal of the American Academy of Child and Adolescent Psychiatry, 34,* (8), 987–1000.

Schneiderman, M., et al. (1998). Mental health services for children in out-of-home care. *Child Welfare, 77*(1), 29–40.

Smyer, M.A. (1995). Prevention early intervention for mental disorders of the elderly. In Gatz, M. (Ed.). *Emerging issues in mental health and aging.* Washington, DC: American Psychological Association.

Vinokur, A.D., Price, R.H., & Schuly, R. (1995). Impact of the JOBS intervention on unemployed workers varying in risk for depression. *American Journal of Community Psychiatry, 23*(1), 39.

Weisner, D., et al. (1996). Cost and effectiveness of day hospital vs. traditional outpatient treatment in an HMO chemical dependency program: six month results of a randomized controlled study. *Association for Health Services Research Annual Meeting Abstract Book, 13,* 43.

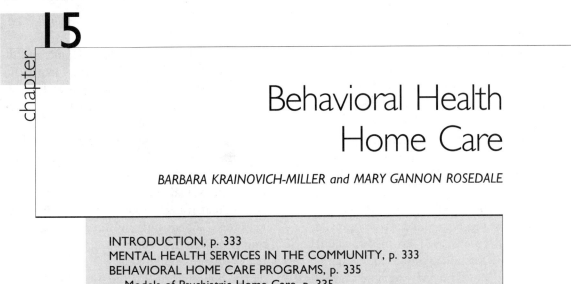

chapter 15

Behavioral Health Home Care

BARBARA KRAINOVICH-MILLER and MARY GANNON ROSEDALE

▪ INTRODUCTION

The purpose of this chapter is to reconceptualize psychiatric home care as a holistic behavioral home care (HBHC) service. A model of HBHC is presented whereby psychiatric-mental health and related physical health care is delivered in the home setting. The target population consists of patients who have a psychiatric diagnosis and exhibit behavior that impedes their ability to function and thus have a need for skilled psychiatric nursing intervention. The goal of this model is to improve the quality of life for people with mental illness by making advanced practice psychiatric-mental health nursing services as accessible, attentive, and effective as possible for patients and their care partners (Haber, 1997a). Economic pressures to provide cost-effective quality services require the creation of systems that flexibly meet the patient needs. In turn, this framework provides more creative treatment modalities aimed at identifying patient strengths and increasing independence while lessening symptoms. The major focus is on creating a system around patients' expressed needs rather than asking patients to fit into an existing or transposed system. The expanded role of the advanced practice registered nurse (APRN) in psychiatric and mental health care can be pivotal in designing home care models that facilitate this population's integration into mainstream communities. The examples offered in this chapter were drawn from a nurse-designed psychiatric behavioral home care agency in which APRNs are key players.

MENTAL HEALTH SERVICES IN ▪ THE COMMUNITY

In the 1960s a new world view held promise that mental illness could be treated better in the community rather than in a mental institution. Deinstitutionalization of the chronically ill, made possible by the new pharmacology of the time, was implemented on a broad scale (Forchuk & Voorberg, 1991). However, for many reasons, the Community Mental Health Centers Act of 1963, amended in 1975 (NIMH, 1992), was unable to implement the type of system that those with serious and persistent mental illness really needed. Although programs were designed with the concepts of primary, secondary, and tertiary prevention, in reality they were based on a medical model with a psychiatric pathology framework. That is, while they used the term *prevention*, the actual focus was on treating the psychiatric patient who was not hospitalized with medications, rather than on providing services that would prevent the individual from becoming hospitalized once again in an institutional setting.

Despite the community mental health movement's good intent, the deinstitutionalization of psychiatric patients took place without the resources to provide community-based services. The movement changed where the psychiatric patient was "housed" but did little to assist the patient with a mental illness to become a functioning individual in the community. Not only were there inadequate facilities for those discharged from state hospitals, but the communities themselves had attitudes that were unaccepting of those with mental illness because of the stigma attached to mental illness. Many of the younger people experiencing mental illness were not welcomed by their home communities, which contributed to a growing number of homeless individuals with mental illness (NIMH, 1992).

Currently the majority of those with mental illness, including those who are severely and persistently mentally ill, reside at home with their families and/or significant others (i.e., their caregivers). Reengineering efforts, such as shorter hospitals stays and other managed care initiatives to curtail continued escalating medical costs while providing primary care services, have contributed

to the need for home care services (Haber & Billings, 1995). This is particularly true for patients with mental illnesses, especially those with severe and persistent mental illness (SPMI) (Dee, van Servellen, & Brecht, 1998).

Medicare will cover psychiatric home care services if the patient has an active psychiatric diagnosis and all of the following:

- Has been evaluated by a physician
- Is reevaluated by the physician every 60 days
- Requires skilled nursing intervention by a trained psychiatric nurse
- Meets home bound status

Home bound status for the psychiatric patient means that the patient's psychiatric illness prevents him or her from leaving the home and partaking in usual activities of daily living in the community, as well as seeking psychiatric services. The following patient characteristics are associated factors for justifying homebound status:

- Confined by severe depressive signs and symptoms of anergia or anhedonia
- Confined by severe anxiety that impairs ability to leave home
- Confined by perceptual and/or cognitive deficits resulting from impaired judgment and self monitoring skills
- Confined to bed/nonambulatory
- On restricted activity
- Severely dyspneic on exertion
- Unable to negotiate stairs

Examples of skilled nursing services for the patient with an active psychiatric illness include 1) conducting a comprehensive assessment, 2) performing a venipuncture for medication or liver function monitoring, 3) providing psychoeducation, and 4) conducting psychotherapy.

Medicaid is a state-administered form of reimbursement. Each state has its own criteria for eligibility and reimbursement. Third-party payers, private health insurance companies, and managed care organizations adhere to their own rules and regulations in determining eligibility and services for psychiatric patients. Some patients pay directly for psychiatric home care services, and most agencies have a sliding fee scale based on the patient's ability to pay.

BEHAVIORAL HOME CARE ■ PROGRAMS

In the 1990s psychiatric in-patient stays were commonly 7 days or fewer (Stahl, 1995). Since most people with chronic mental illness live with their families, there was a need to create flexible psychiatric treatment programs that did not rely on psychiatric in-patient treatment models (Adams, 1994). The programs had to be relevant and easily accessible to the consumer of these services.

Models of Psychiatric Home Care

There are several models of psychiatric home care (Backlar, 1997; Becker et al., 1996; Bigelow, McFarland, & Olson, 1991; Hauenstein, 1996; Kates et al., 1997; Peterson, Drone, & Munetz, 1997; Polivka, Kennedy, & Chaudry, 1997; Wasylenki et al., 1997). One example is the Summit Model (Peterson, Drone, & Munetz, 1997). It was designed to provide services for the severely and persistently psychiatrically impaired individual using intensive case management teams. The psychiatrist provides the clinical leadership for the interdisciplinary treatment team (ITT). The ITT consists of approximately 10 case managers, a registered nurse (RN), a counselor, and representatives from residential, vocational rehabilitation, and partial hospitalization services. Patients are assigned to various ITTs based on individualized assessment of patient service needs by the social worker. The RN on the ITT is not an advanced practice nurse. The case managers, who are not RNs, have varied educational backgrounds (e.g., some have a master's degrees in social work or are licensed counselors, and others are high school graduates with on-the-job experience with those who are severely mentally ill). The case managers carry out a variety of functions such as advocacy,

transporting patients, symptom and medication compliance monitoring, assessment and teaching of community living skills, and provision of information and referrals. Partial hospitalization services are also a part of this model.

According to Peterson, Drone, and Munetz (1997), the future of case management in psychiatric home care depends on the creation of individualized plans of behavioral health care rather than a " 'one size fits all approach'. . . [i.e.,] custom-tailoring of services to fit the individual at each point in his or her [mental] illness and rehabilitation." The authors recommend that if such programs are to be cost and quality effective, the role of case manager is best carried out by the APRN who has the knowledge base and advanced skills to manage a system of care.

The role of the RN as a member of the ITT is a key variable. The model explicated in this chapter suggests that the RN be prepared as an APRN. The APRN is skilled at implementing the strategies outlined in Box 15-1. The APRN is often the "keeper" of the ethics of community psychiatric-mental health care. For example, APRNs use this strategy when they link the expressed needs of patients who have a serious mental illness with the goals of their providers. APRNs are also skilled at sustaining levels of direct communication and contact among the patients, community providers, psychiatrists, non-nurse case managers, and other members of the ITT (Provan, Sebastian, & Milward, 1996).

Effective outreach is conceptualized as a part of an assessment phase of home care programs (Raskin et al., 1996). The following are examples of effective outreach modalities:

1. Assertive community treatment (ACT) teams for high users of psychiatric care, such as high-risk groups who have traditionally been treated in long-term psychiatric facilities
2. Mobile crisis teams, providing expanded behavioral triage services
3. Prevention programs in the primary schools of a community

STRATEGIES FOR IMPLEMENTING SUCCESSFUL PSYCHIATRIC HOME TREATMENT PROGRAMS

- Develop a mission statement reflecting a holistic, interdisciplinary, collaborative mental health care (HICMHC) model rather than a traditional medical model.
- Determine the participating organizations and patient focus, and explicate to each the compatible values of each participating organization.
- Ascertain top administrative and middle manager support from each participating organization for the HICMHC model before program planning.
- Develop and implement standing committee structures to support change efforts.
- Implement formal training to support change among interdisciplinary team members.
- Coordinate information dissemination among all providers and participants.
- Involve all providers in the program's committee structure (e.g., educational session planning).
- Develop and implement standards for research-based practice protocols as well as written documentation among all providers.
- Conduct formal evaluation with providers and participants (e.g., interviews at 3-month intervals).
- Present outcomes to participating organizations and the community at large.
- Provide diverse and flexible employment programs.
- Uphold the ethics of community mental health care.

A review of several models of psychiatric home treatment programs revealed a number of strategies for implementing successful programs. Box 15-1 describes several of these strategies. Central to psychiatric home care programs is the use of some type of case management framework as well as the concept of an interdisciplinary treatment team. Wasylenki and colleagues (1997) believe that using the strategy of educational sessions that focus on team building as well as patient information can make psychiatric home care treatment for individuals with an acute phase of a major mental illness a viable alternative to hospitalization. Therefore the APRN in behavioral home care must be an expert in health teaching for individual teaching sessions as well as for use in the broader concept of psychoeducation. The newer models of psychoeducation embrace both a biologic and psychodynamic explanation of mental disorders and related treatments. The focus is not only on the patient but also on the family and significant others or caregivers on admission and throughout their episode of care, regardless of the setting (Siegmann, & Long, 1995; Krainovich-Miller, 1997).

A model of holistic behavioral home health care for patients with mental illnesses designed by an APRN in psychiatric nursing is described in the next section. The APRN in this model is a master's-prepared RN who has acquired the credential as a certified specialist in psychiatric-mental health nursing through ANA certification as well as the advanced competencies and skills of the nurse practitioner.

Holistic Behavioral Home Care Model

The design of the Holistic Behavioral Home Care (HBHC) Program is based on the strategies outlined in Box 15-1. This program focuses on developing innovative systems and ways of thought and action that promote the interests and ideals of people with mental illness toward greater independence. It draws upon the ten principles listed in Box 15-2 and provides the services listed in Box 15-3. The target population for this program is similar to most psychiatric home care programs across the country (Warner, 1997):

- Newly diagnosed psychiatric patients (either a primary or secondary diagnosis) and their families (significant others)

box 15-2

PRINCIPLES OF HUMANISTIC BEHAVIORAL HOME CARE

1. Services are shaped by the patients and their care partners' expressed needs.
2. There is a program commitment to holistic practice.
3. Care is delivered by forging trusting partnerships with patients, care partners, and providers.
4. Strategies are creative as well as flexible in order to meet patient needs.
5. There is a program commitment to valuing experiential knowledge of all participants.
6. The patient and setting are viewed via a "humanizing" lens.
7. The APRN is a key member for promoting linkages in the continuum of care.
8. There is a commitment to seize the critical teaching moments for patients.
9. Services incorporate outcome-focused, cognitive behavioral interventions.
10. Economic sensitivity includes overcoming financial obstacles to care.

box 15-3

SERVICES OF THE HBHC PROGRAM

Comprehensive in-home assessment
Mental status evaluation
Crisis intervention
Cognitive behavioral therapy
Individual and family counseling
Behavioral modification and contracting
Medication administration, monitoring, and teaching
Health guidance, teaching, and referral
Symptom management
Rest, sleep, and wake activities
Risk factor reduction
Anxiety reduction strategies
Correction of actual or potential environmental safety hazards
Activities of daily living management
Emergency measures
Functional coping strategies
Social skills training
Case management
Accessing and coordination of team and community resources
Supervision of professional and paraprofessional nursing personnel
Vocational training and preparation

From Priority Home Care, New York, NY.

- Previously diagnosed psychiatric patients at risk for re-hospitalization
- Families coping with problems at home
- Homeless individuals and families
- School-age children

The case study presented in Box 15-4 illustrates the type of patient receiving services through the HBHC program.

According to the Health Care Financing Administration (HCFA, 1979) "psychiatrically trained nurses are nurses who have special training and/or experience beyond the standard curriculum required for an RN." Consistent with Medicare criteria (HCFA, 1979), the behavioral health RN is a qualified and experienced APRN (Haber, 1998a). Paraprofessionals who provide services on behavioral health cases are required to be certified as home health aides and to have

satisfactorily completed a behavioral health training course. The standards outlined in this model are consistent with the standards required by the Joint Commission for Accreditation of Healthcare Organizations (JCAHO).

The overall goal of the HBHC program is to preserve and enhance a person's functional position in the home and community. Outcomes are evaluated by patients' demonstrating the following:

- Increased psychologic, social, and occupational functioning as measured by the Global Assessment of Functioning (GAF) Scale (Piersma & Boes, 1997)

box 15-4

CASE STUDY

Bruce, age 51, has emphysema and bipolar disorder, mixed type. He has been receiving home care services from an APRN who coordinated services, including a home health aide and physical therapist in the home. Improvement in Bruce's medication management, mental status, exercise tolerance, ambulation, and use of oxygen and nebulizer are the focus of service. When Bruce reached his maximum level of functioning, Medicare reimbursement ceased, but Bruce continues the home care services on a self-pay basis. He feels that the services of the APRN and home health aid are vital during the months of August and February when the weather threatens his respiratory functioning and he becomes more isolated. The isolation contributes to Bruce's feelings of alienation, and to avoid a depressive relapse, Bruce works with the APRN to manage his anxiety and physical limitations by using a variety of cognitive behavioral techniques, such as challenging his negative thoughts and creating a journal. In addition, the APRN conducts a head-to-toe physical assessment and instructs Bruce in practicing deep breathing and positive visualization to reduce anxiety and promote air exchange.

- Decreased symptom severity as measured by the Brief Psychiatric Rating Scale (BPRS)
- Participation in the least restrictive treatment environment as measured by decreased emergency room visits and hospitalization
- Perception of a therapeutic relationship with a nurse as measured by the Helping Alliance Questionnaire Revised (HAQR)

As illustrated in Box 15-3, the HBHC's program and other home care programs offer a variety of treatment modalities. To some extent psychiatric treatment modalities are essentially the same from setting to setting, and the mandate is to deliver cost-effective quality care. In the home setting the way a service is implemented may change to some degree. Using "what is available in the home setting" becomes a framework for interventions; they need to be practical, individually tailored, and easily demonstrated by or to the patient. For example, a patient may identify that listening to music helps him or her relax. As part of "seizing a teaching moment," the APRN has the patient demonstrate this anxiety reduction strategy by doing the following:

- Identifying his or her anxiety level and assigning a numerical value (e.g., 1 = low and 10 = very high) to an anxiety scale
- Choosing the tape or CD to be played
- Playing the tape or CD for a specified time
- Reevaluating his or her anxiety level using the numerical scale at the end of the musical selection

In this model, case management is viewed both as a treatment modality and as an advocacy role. Often the time spent on these activities is very intensive, yet the time spent is not reimbursable. For example, the APRN needs to become knowledgeable about bilingual and bicultural issues because he or she will be involved with the training and supervision and sometimes even with the hiring of bilingual and bicultural paraprofessionals (Musser-Granski & Carrillo, 1997). Therefore APRNs must learn how to use their time most effectively to bring about needed services. The following objectives must be met to be an effective case manager:

- Act as an advocate for the patient's wishes
- Act as a communication link for care partners
- Integrate all of the services outside of the home care program
- Promote consensus on outcomes among providers and the means for achieving them
- Establish behavioral contracting for all persons involved in care
- Train and supervise paraprofessionals assigned to the caseload
- Assume responsibility for the completeness and appropriateness of all medical record documentation

For example, Bruce's APRN (see Box 15-4) coordinates care among the home health aide, the psychiatrist, the pulmonary specialist, the physical therapist, the attorney, and his brother. This requires multiple phone calls, meetings, and establishing behavioral contracts among the parties as well as ongoing documentation of these communications. Another example to highlight the complexity of the case manager role involves a simple medication change for Bruce. He tells his APRN that his pulmonary specialist increased his Theodur dose. The APRN verifies this information with the pulmonary physician, faxes and sends a written order reflecting the dose change to the physician for signature, informs the psychiatrist of the medication change, incorporates this on Bruce's plan of care, instructs the home health aide to pick up the medication from the pharmacy, and documents this process, including making sure that the original signed physician order is received and placed in Bruce's chart within 1 month.

ADVANCED PRACTICE PSYCHIATRIC NURSING IN ■ HOME CARE

Emerging Role of the APRN in Home Care

Since the 1950s advanced practice psychiatric nurses have had an effect on the care of those requiring psychiatric-mental health services (Peplau, 1991). By the 1990s APRNs had established a credible tradition as providers of mental health services for individuals with mental illnesses (patients) and their families and significant others (caregivers) in in-patient and community mental health settings, as well as in private practice (Billings, 1997) and home care.

A review of the services provided by psychiatric home care programs (see Box 15-3) indicates the need for an APRN as a key member of the interdisciplinary treatment team rather than an RN prepared at the basic level. However, APRNs credentialed as certified specialists (CSs) who enter this area of practice may need to acquire advanced knowledge and practice skills related to physical assessment and psychopharmacology. At present, APRNs who have advanced psychiatric nursing experience as a CS may acquire these additional competencies through post-master's education leading to certification as a nurse practitioner (NP). Several graduate psychiatric nursing programs across the country offer a degree in a combined or blended CS/NP role. This type of curriculum prepares "advanced practice mental health nurse specialists/practitioners to provide primary care and mental health services to adults with physical and mental health problems . . . [it prepares] graduates for certification as both an adult nurse practitioner and as a psychiatric mental health clinical specialist" (Williams et al., 1998). See Chapter 20 for a discussion of role preparation in graduate education programs.

Standards of Care and Performance

APRNs who work in the behavioral home care setting use the nursing process as explicated in the ANA's (1994) psychiatric and mental health nursing standards of care. (See Box 15-5 for the categories of the standards.) These standards of care and professional performance are performed within the context of the principles of psychiatric behavioral home care. They are in concert with the ANA's *Nursing's Social Policy Statement* (1995), *Standards of Community Health Nursing Practice* (1986a), *Standards of Home Health Nursing Practice* (1986b), *Standards of Clinical Practice* (1998), and other major ANA documents.

APRNs in practice must be familiar with these ANA documents, especially the role and function of the advanced practice nurse (ANA, 1994). The ANA's *Standards Related to Community Health Nursing* (1986a) and *Home Health Nursing* (1986b) indicate that their respective standards of care be used in conjunction with other ANA documents. A review of these 1986 documents revealed that although they remain consistent with the basic components of nursing process as explicated in more recent ANA publications, they

CATEGORIES OF STANDARDS OF CLINICAL CARE AND PROFESSIONAL PERFORMANCE

STANDARDS OF CARE

I. Assessment

II. Diagnosis

III. Outcome identification

IV. Planning (selecting therapeutic interventions to achieve outcomes)

V. Implementation (documenting interventions including the following)

  a. Counseling

  b. Milieu therapy

  c. Self-care activities

  d. Psychobiological interventions

  e. Health teaching

  f. Case management

  g. Health promotion and health maintenance

  h. Advanced practice interventions (psychotherapy, prescription of pharmacologic agents, and consultation)

VI. Evaluation (documenting patient attainment or nonattainment of expected outcomes)

STANDARDS OF PROFESSIONAL PERFORMANCE

I. Quality of Care

II. Performance appraisal

III. Education

IV. Collegiality

V. Ethics

VI. Collaboration

VII. Research

VIII. Resource utilization

From ANA, 1994.

do not focus on the advanced practice role of the nurse in these settings. For example, the following are listed as home health care standards (1986b): organization of home health services, theory, data collection, diagnosis, planning, intervention, evaluation, continuity of care, interdisciplinary collaboration, professional development, research, and

ethics. The process criteria explicated for each standard mainly focus on the role of the RN at the basic level rather than the APRN at the advanced level. For example, Home Health Care Standard VI. Intervention lists 12 activities of the nurse generalist (e.g., "administers medically prescribed medications and treatments,") and after the list of nurse generalist activities it states the following: "in addition, the nurse specialist functions as a consultant to the nurse generalist in nursing interventions" (ANA, 1986b). Neither of these documents specifically addresses the role of the APRN in the diagnosis and treatment of the psychiatric population. The tremendous changes in home health care and community health care and the growth in psychiatric home care and managed care require the use of the ANA's latest documents to guide competent advanced practice psychiatric-mental health nursing in the home care setting.

Different aspects of the expanded role of the APRN in psychiatric and mental health care are discussed in several chapters in this book. APRNs in behavioral home care address the primary health care needs of their patients. They must have physical assessment skills and prescriptive authority, as warranted by their credentials and role. Therefore the remainder of the chapter focuses on the other aspects of the APRN role in the delivery of psychiatric home care services.

APRNs working in the psychiatric home care setting quickly realize that their tried and true psychiatric nursing theories, interventions, and assessment skills cannot be automatically transposed to patients in that setting. For example, in the inpatient setting an initial psychiatric nursing history and health assessment may be performed by the psychiatric nurse functioning at the basic level, or an APRN may visit a newly admitted patient as part of the consultative role. It is within the standards of practice for the APRN, in a consultative role, to conduct a psychiatric and physical health assessment as outlined in Box 15-6. The protocol in that situation would usually require the APRN to review documented health assessments performed by the psychiatrist as team leader, as well as other members of the ITT, and

<table>
<tr><td>

box 15-6

COMPREHENSIVE PSYCHIATRIC NURSING ASSESSMENT: BASIC ELEMENTS

Demographic data including religion, race/culture, family, caregivers
Psychiatric diagnosis, medical diagnosis, prognoses
Safety measures
Nutrition and diet
Functional limitations and activities permitted
Mental status
Homebound status
Psychosocial variables
Vital signs and weight
Complete physical examination
Infection control, Universal Precautions
Environmental safety
Orders for services and treatment
Goals and rehabilitation potential
Discharge plan
Clinical findings, nursing diagnosis, summary, interventions, instructions
Patient bill of rights, do-not-resuscitate orders, proxy, advance directive, living will
Risk factors, knowledge deficits
Outcome, response to teaching

</td><td>

box 15-7

OBJECTIVES FOR AN INITIAL PSYCHIATRIC HOME CARE VISIT

1. Complete a comprehensive psychiatric nursing assessment.
2. Administer standard instruments (e.g., Brief Psychiatric Rating Scale) to document mental health status, levels of functioning (e.g., Global Assessment of Functioning), and psychiatric diagnoses (e.g., Beck's Depression Inventory) and to establish baselines for future assessments.
3. Collect data for quality improvement evaluation (e.g., length of stay with home care services, and patient satisfaction with nurse care questionnaire).
4. Review safety issues, environment, and infection control with patient using standard form (e.g., Patient Instruction Check List).
5. Review with patient and secure signatures on authorization and acknowledgment and consent forms.
6. Complete a home health certification and plan of care form (e.g., Form 485).
7. Complete paraprofessional's plan of care that outlines services to be performed by the home health aide.
8. Initiate documentation of the therapeutic alliance (e.g., Nurse Helping Relationship Questionnaire [NHRQ-R]), and leave the tool with the patient.

</td></tr>
</table>

interview the patient in relation to selected aspects of the psychiatric history and/or health assessment. The home care setting requires a comprehensive psychiatric home care assessment using a primary health care framework. The components listed in Boxes 15-6 and 15-7 illustrate the complexity of this initial assessment visit and the need for the skills and competencies of the APRN.

Comprehensive Assessment and Behavioral Home Care Principles

In general, services for patients requiring psychiatric home care are based on the assessment variables outlined in Box 15-6. Although these variables appear similar to those that are assessed in the inpatient psychiatric or community-based settings, the difference lies in the way in which they are assessed. For example, the HBHC model requires that an APRN use the principles of behavioral home health care (Box 15-2) to guide the initial comprehensive assessment, such as paying particular attention to the patient's expressed need. An APRN's first visit to a recently discharged patient diagnosed with schizophrenia would include performing a comprehensive assessment in the home setting as outlined in Box 15-6 as well as conducting other assessments and securing signed documents as indicated in Box 15-7.

The objectives for an initial psychiatric home care visit are outlined in Box 15-7. APRNs are familiar with the Brief Psychiatric Rating Scale (BPRS) and Global Assessment of Functioning (GAF) score. These are common tools in the inpatient setting where they are more frequently used by other health providers. The Nurse Helping Relationship Questionnaire (NHRQ-R) is an example of a tool used for patients to self-report their perception of a therapeutic alliance with the APRN. Consistent with Peplau's (1991) interpersonal theory, NHRQ-R was a tool modified to evaluate the effect of the nurse-patient interpersonal relationship on outcomes. In addition, satisfaction questionnaires are completed by patients as part of an overall quality improvement program, with patient satisfaction as one measure of a positive outcome.

The forms in Box 15-7 are usually completed after the APRN leaves the patient's home. Although these forms were drawn from the HBHC agency, the basic data that are collected and documented do not vary greatly from one psychiatric home care setting to another. Certification regulations as well as Medicare and Medicaid requirements require certain documentation (NAHC, 1994). Documentation in home care, similar to the inpatient setting, is very extensive. However, help may be on the horizon. Hand-held computers with word processing documentation capabilities are being used by several visiting nurse and other home care agencies across the country (Martin, 1998). This may decrease the amount of time spent in writing documentation by hand. Therefore computer skills are a must for the APRN in home care.

Conducting a comprehensive psychiatric assessment. A comprehensive psychiatric assessment (CPA) requires that the APRN conduct an in-depth physical assessment. Other components of personal health and the environment are also assessed extensively (see Box 15-6). This differs to some degree from the inpatient and from the private practice setting. For example, the environmental, safety risk, and infection control areas are assessed in a very detailed manner. Select data are documented on the CPA form, and an additional assessment is conducted using the Patient Instruction Check List. Examples of the type of assessed data are found in Table 15-1. The APRN implements a teaching plan based on the assessed data. The teaching is reviewed with the patient and caregiver and then evaluated. As with other forms of documentation, the Patient Instruction Check List is signed by the APRN and becomes a part of the permanent patient record.

Nutritional assessment is conducted in a similar manner. For example, the HBHC's program must adhere to the requirements of the New York State Department of Health. The State requires that additional documentation be used as well as the standard assessment on the CPA form. These additional data are illustrated by sample items of nutrition in Table 15-2. Upon completion, the APRN determines the score and makes a nutri-

table 15-1

SAFETY, ENVIRONMENT, AND INFECTION CONTROL EXAMPLES: PATIENT INSTRUCTION SHEET	
AREA	**ASSESSMENT**
Safety issues	Patient or caregiver verbalizes knowledge of how to evacuate home in case of fire or other emergency.
Environment	There is running water, electricity, functioning stove, and a refrigerator.
Infection control	Patient or caregiver is instructed in the signs and symptoms of wound infection (e.g., elevated temperature, redness or swelling, drainage) and verbalizes understanding.

tional referral if necessary (e.g., for a patient who receives more than three Bs, more than two Cs, or one or more Ds). A similar method is used for other variables. For example, if extrapyramidal side effects are observed, then the APRN conducts an AIMS Test, determines the score, and intervenes as dictated by the findings. The APRN also uses specialized scales, such as the Hamilton or Beck Depression Scales, to substantiate certain diagnoses. The administration and interpretation of these instruments requires advanced practice skills and training.

Putting principles into practice. Key to completing a CPA in the home setting is activating principle number one. The APRN must recognize the vital nature of asking the simple question "What kinds of things do you need help with?" This gives the APRN entry into the patient's world. In using this principle, the APRN has the opportunity to demonstrate cultural sensitivity. As the APRN walks with the patient through his or her home, this question frames every assessment variable listed in Box 15-6. It is essential that this

---

table 15-2

NUTRITIONAL ASSESSMENT FORM

ASSESSMENT DATA	YES	NO	YES=
Patient has no difficulty eating			A
Patient has lost >20 lb in last 3 months without wanting to			D
Patient had nausea/ vomiting for >7 days			C
Patient uses drugs occasionally			B
Patient has enough money to buy food			A
Score: Total # Bs____ Cs____ Ds____			

From Priority Home Care, New York, NY.

---

principle be included in an orientation program and be reinforced throughout the APRN's practice. The following example illustrates the importance of this principle:

Ted, an APRN experienced in home care, asks Victoria, a 40-year-old woman with chronic paranoid schizophrenia, what kinds of things she needs help with. Victoria responds that she needs a body-guard because she is being followed and stalked by men in her neighborhood. Ted responds that his goal is to help her feel safe. To meet this objective, Victoria agrees to take her Prolixin and to leave her home in the company of Ted. After taking the medication for 2 weeks, Victoria becomes less paranoid and finds herself looking forward to Ted's visits and no longer thinking of herself needing a body guard. Ted's work with Victoria focuses on medication adherence, anxiety reduction strategies, decreasing isolation, and enhancing her social skills.

This vignette illustrates that a traditional nursing technique of giving recognition to a patient's feelings but at the same time presenting reality might be in conflict with principle number one. For example, Ted might have said, "I recognize that you are afraid Victoria, but I do not see anyone following you." However, this response would have invalidated the patient's experience, increased anxiety, and impeded the development of a trusting relationship. By working with the patient's expressed need, Ted was able to bring about a successful outcome.

The special nature of the environmental assessment of a patient in the home was mentioned previously. The following is an example of how this aspect of the CPA is carried out using another principle via a humanizing lens. An inpatient environment is artificial in the sense that the staff takes care to "safety proof" the unit. However, the patient's home environment offers unique assessment information regarding the person's functional abilities and safety risks. Key to completing this aspect of the assessment is activating principle six (Box 15-2). Using a humanizing lens, the APRN views the environment as an outward expression of the person's values, interests, and habits. Giving recognition to these elements facilitates communication. For example, an APRN might notice several photographs on the patient's wall and ask about them. This gives the patient an opportunity to reflect on these past moments and offers an opportunity to talk about important relationships and/or aspects of life. This technique signals to the patient that the APRN is interested in getting to know the patient as a whole person, addresses principle three of "forging" a trusting relationship, and at the same time provides an unobtrusive way for performing cognitive assessment. This example also highlights the nonlinear nature of a comprehensive assessment.

Using communication techniques. Therapeutic communication techniques in the home care setting are slightly different than those in the inpatient setting. The APRN's communication must be based on cues in the patient's environment and accelerate the process of establishing trust. Using this perspective can make the difference in whether the APRN has a successful first visit and subsequent visits. The following scenario may illustrate this point:

An APRN visits a home care patient for the first time and uses basic therapeutic techniques such as introducing herself and explaining her role to help the patient make the transition from the hospital to the home. In addition, she indicates that a health assessment and medication teaching about Clozaril will be included in the visit. Boxes 15-8 and 15-9 illustrate the differences between an APRN approaching this initial encounter from a traditional paradigm versus an HBHC view. Both APRNs in this situation use the same assessment guide yet they derive different nursing diagnoses, interventions, and outcomes. Although Nurse Miller assesses data for a diagnosis of anxiety, her lack of specificity (i.e., moderate anxiety) obviously prevents her from determining that this level of anxiety would prevent the patient from benefiting from her teaching. There are, of course, several variables that contributed to the first APRN's line of communication versus that of the second APRN. Some of the following factors and/or combinations of these factors influenced the first APRN's interaction with the patient and help explain why the principle of setting boundaries and

box 15-8

FIRST EXAMPLE: COMMUNICATION WITH A PATIENT, MS. SMITH, IN THE HOME DURING INITIAL ASSESSMENT

Nurse Miller: "Hello Ms. Smith, I am Nurse Miller. My purpose for visiting you is to help you be more comfortable with your transition from the hospital to your home. I will be teaching you about your medication Clozaril."

Ms. Smith: "That's nice, but I have so much to do. They rushed me out of the hospital, and I really wasn't ready. I can't seem to concentrate."

Nurse Miller: "Are you taking your medication? Let me see it?" (*Preliminary nursing diagnosis:* Anxiety possibly related to not taking medication and/or being discharged)

Ms. Smith: "It's over on the table. I really need to get my laundry done. I don't remember if I took it since I got home."

Nurse Miller: (feeling devalued and concerned about the time pressure) "I think it's really important that I complete my assessment and review your medication now. I see that you are having trouble with taking your medication; that is probably why you can't concentrate."

Ms. Smith: (sits down, looks very distracted, and apparently listens)

Nurse Miller: "It is very important that you take your medication. It will help keep you out of the hospital." (completes teaching, performs health assessments and other tests)

Outcome: Ms. Smith is unable to hear what the nurse says, is annoyed by the nurse's visit, and refuses to let the nurse in on the next visit. She does not continue with the medication and is seen in the emergency department 2 weeks later.

directing which patient needs are to be met at a particular visit did not work in this setting.

1. The APRN was not on her own turf, and she no longer had the "in charge" position of the inpatient setting.

box 15-9

SECOND EXAMPLE: COMMUNICATION WITH A PATIENT, MS. SMITH, IN THE HOME DURING INITIAL ASSESSMENT

Nurse Rose: "Hello Ms. Smith, my name is Nurse Rose, I'm your home care nurse. My purpose for visiting you is to help you be more comfortable with your transition from the hospital to your home. I need to ask you some questions, teach you about your medication Clozaril, and ask you to sign some consent forms. What kinds of things do you need help with?"

Ms. Smith: "That's nice, but I have so much to do. They rushed me out of the hospital, and I really wasn't ready. I can't seem to concentrate."

Nurse Rose: (thinking to herself: "Ms. Smith is distracted and moderately anxious; I need to collect more data") "It sounds like you are having a hard time."

Ms. Smith: "My washing machine is broken, and I have laundry piling up. I don't know what to do."

Nurse Rose: (thinking to herself: "This is not a Clozaril-teaching moment, this is a rela-tionship-building moment. *Preliminary nursing diagnoses*: Impaired home maintenance management and related moderate anxiety) "Let's take a look at this together. Where is the washing machine?"

(During the nursing intervention of assisting the woman in determining the problem with the washing machine [the plug was out of the wall], the patient continues to verbalize her concerns. By attending to the patient's expressed need, the patient's anxiety level is greatly reduced. She feels understood and is eager to show her appreciation for the nurse stepping out of her "professional role.")

Ms. Smith: (After the patient has loaded her clothes in the machine) "Didn't you want to tell me about my medication?"

Outcome: The patient's anxiety was reduced, and problem solving laid the groundwork for their work together. Future visits indicate adherence to medication regimen, and there is evidence that learning took place.

2. Her anxiety level may have been increased because this was her first visit to this patient's home or maybe her first home care visit.

3. The patient's anxiety level may have been increased, and her anxiety was transmitted to the APRN.

4. The nurse may have been feeling the time pressure of her case load for the day (e.g., she had four other new admissions assessments to do as well as five other visits to supervise home health aides and she had already spent a half-hour with this patient and none of her objectives for this visit were completed).

5. She felt devalued by the patient's response to her initial comments about the purpose of the visit.

Experienced APRNs are sometimes surprised to find that they cannot use their unique friendly but professional inpatient or private practice style and be assured of positive patient outcomes with home care patients. A similar reaction has been noted by those new to psychiatric home care.

As a word of caution, these principles, strategies, suggestions, and interventions are not fool proof. Because APRNs are familiar with manipulating various situations for positive patient outcomes, the following APRN story illustrates the need for caution but also the need to develop creative strategies to bring about such outcomes.

An APRN indicates that she has experienced first visits and positive outcomes similar to Nurse Rose's first visit, yet when she returns for the second visit, the patient will not let her in. Therefore she develops the "excuse strategy." She always leaves an umbrella at a first visit to a patient's home. Then, if the patient refuses her entry the next time, she is able to persuade the patient to let her in to retrieve it. By stating to the patient that the umbrella was "left" rather than "forgotten," the basic trust in their relationship is not compromised. Once she is face to face with the patient, she is usually able to elicit why the patient was refusing her visit, intervene accordingly, and bring about a positive outcome.

This illustrates the point that an APRN must keep the focus of any visit on seeing the patient in order to intervene and evaluate outcomes. Although this might seem manipulative or somewhat coercive, the APRN uses this strategy in a caring way and does not force herself on the patient. It also illustrates how powerful the presence of the nurse is in bringing about positive patient outcomes (Peplau, 1991).

The APRN must be an active member of the ITT. Although the previous discussion focused on data collection during an assessment, the APRN is often implementing interventions simultaneously. The following example illustrates the need to articulate these interventions to others:

During an ITT meeting, an APRN reports that Ms. Jones remains depressed, sits at home all day, sometimes watching television, and eats only a small amount when her daughter offers food. The APRN neglects to mention the interventions that she implemented. She then moves on to her next case. Another ITT member interrupts her to suggest several interventions, all within the realm of APRN practice.

In this instance, the APRN should have educated the other team members about her use of advanced practice interventions. All of the clinical standards indicated in Box 15-5, in particular those that reflect advanced practice interventions and outcomes, must be communicated to the ITT members in a clear and succinct manner.

Engaging community support systems. The community support system is a resource of all models of psychiatric home care. It enables persons with mental illness to participate in the community in which they reside. The services that a community provides such as banks, restaurants, clothing stores, religious institutions, schools, su-

permarkets, parks, movie theaters, and so on enable individuals with mental illnesses to live in the real world. The APRN uses this type of system to provide the patient with multiple opportunities for more independent functioning in the community.

Table 15-3 describes therapeutic growth opportunities of community living. These factors are both protective and curative. They help the individual preserve a level of functioning, such as being oriented to time and place, and give opportunities to enhance his or her level of functioning. The premise of these growth opportunities is that patients are actively involved in defining and attaining goals, and all these activities are in concert with the notion of increased independent functioning through problem solving. Motivation is enhanced by its own reinforcement. For example, hunger is a motivating factor for finding food. In the institutionalized setting, the patient is a passive recipient of food. Passivity rather than independence is reinforced. When the patient attends prescribed meal times, he or she misses multiple opportunities for making decisions, such as what time to eat, what to eat, where to buy the food, how much to spend for it, whom to eat with, how to prepare the food, and so on. In the community, the APRN helps individuals access community support systems that foster decision making and having personal and social skills and activities of daily living.

Essential Competencies and Skills of the APRN in Home Care

Box 15-10 lists the essential competencies and skills needed by the APRN. Items 1 through 5 have been discussed previously. These focus on the APRN being an expert clinician with additional physical assessment skills and pharmacology knowledge.

Business savvy. *Business savvy* refers to the APRN's knowledge of economic and financial concepts related to accessing health care delivery services from both the provider and patient

table **15-3**

THERAPEUTIC GROWTH OPPORTUNITIES OF COMMUNITY LIVING

OPPORTUNITY	GOAL
TIME ORIENTATION Patient needs to distinguish weekends from weekdays, mornings from afternoons, and afternoons from evenings.	Patient sets own schedule for activities of daily living (e.g., meals, bathing, dressing, shopping, sleeping) as well as meets scheduled appointments for treatment and/or work.
PLACE ORIENTATION AND NAVIGATION Patient needs to determine where he or she resides in relation to community destinations and be able to establish the route and method of transportation to such destinations.	Patient will be able to do the following: • Read a map or ask for information regarding a bus or subway or other transportation method to a destination such as a treatment facility, grocery or other service stores, and work. • Determine the amount of money needed to secure transportation (e.g., buy token, bus or train ticket, and so on).
ORIENTATION TO PERSON Patient needs to be able to identify himself or herself in a variety of roles rather than just the patient role (e.g., I am now in the: shopper role, commuter role, bank customer role, consumer role, neighbor role worker role, and so on) and be recognized by others in a variety of different roles.	Patient, in answer to the prompt "Tell me about yourself," • Describes his or her identify and functioning through the lens of the different roles he or she occupies. • Discusses being recognized by neighbors, addressed as Mr. or Ms. Smith by sales clerks, and so on.

perspective. This knowledge can be acquired through formal master's courses, onsite continuing education, or through distance learning related to the business of health care. Some APRNs are able to develop their own enrichment program by reading journals such as *Nursing Management*, *Nursing Economics*, *Harvard Business Review*, as well as *The Wall Street Journal* and *The New York Times*. The related skills are best acquired by seeking a mentor knowledgeable in this area. The APRN must be computer literate and able to use various software packages to build and use databases, analyze data and trends, and document treatments and outcomes.

Political savvy. Political savvy is also seen as an essential competency and skill needed to be a "broker" for the patient. The APRN literally is the link between and among providers, patients, and other community resources. For instance, political savvy is demonstrated when the APRN realistically applies leadership and management principles to delegate tasks to paraprofessionals and advocate and negotiate on behalf of the patient for insurance coverage. Box 15-11 lists additional political activities that shape the role of the APRN in the home setting. These types of activities are framed around the APRN's commitment to meeting the patient's expressed needs as a priority and a commitment to being involved beyond the expected "9 to 5" job mentality to secure quality care for psychiatric patients in the home care setting. The persistence of the APRN determines how well these activities

APRN COMPETENCIES AND SKILLS FOR PSYCHIATRIC BEHAVIORAL HOME CARE

APRN must be able to render psychiatric mental health care reflecting the ability to do the following:

1. Reframe psychiatric nursing theory, principles, and interventions to meet patients' expressed needs.
2. Use the ten principles of humanistic behavioral home care outlined in Box 15-2 as a framework for practice.
3. Demonstrate competencies and skills of a certified clinical nurse specialist in psychiatric-mental health nursing to meet the focus of primary care.
4. Demonstrate advanced physical assessment skills in relation to primary care needs of patients.
5. Demonstrate advanced knowledge of psychopharmacology, and exercise prescriptive authority where indicated.
6. Demonstrate business and political savvy.
7. Demonstrate bilingual and bicultural skills.
8. Develop and implement psychoeducation programs for patients and caregivers.
9. Design, implement, and evaluate paraprofessional staff education programs.
10. Design, implement, and evaluate research-based practice protocols and other patient programs.

APRN ACTIVITIES FOR POLITICAL AND ECONOMIC CHANGE

The APRN must be persistent to do the following:
- Influence other providers (e.g., physicians, psychologists, social workers, health care aides) to deliver humanistic quality comprehensive care.
- Build coalitions with patients, caregivers, consumer groups, local politicians, and other health care providers.
- Lobby politicians at the local and state levels to secure emotional and financial support through changes in health care policy and subsequent legislation (e.g., to secure psychiatric patients' rights to care and appropriate insurance reimbursement).
- Use "healthy" manipulation of the health delivery system to secure appropriate patient services.

bring about political and economic change for the patient (Haber, 1997b). Whether acquired through a formal master's curriculum or post-master's certificate program, or through mentors and other creative clinical fellowships, APRNs need the competencies and skills denoted in Box 15-11 to be effective in the home care setting through the delivery of cost-effective quality nursing care. Other chapters in this book describe the managerial, political, legal-ethical, and advocate role of the APRN.

Economic sense. Many of the concepts of Haber's (1997a) emerging paradigm of the delivery of mental health services for 2000 and beyond (Box 15-12) are already evident in the health care delivery system as seen in the examples presented in this book. In particular, economic factors in the form of "payment" for services are the foundation for every aspect of program development and provision of services (Peterson, Drone, & Munetz, 1997). The APRN must view this as a priority; it is critical to helping the patient enter the behavioral health home care system. For example, if a psychiatric home care service receives a referral for a patient with no means of financing services (i.e., no insurance or private funds), from one view this would mean that the patient would not be accepted for service. Using the "rehumanizing" lens, the APRN would approach this "payment" obstacle as a problem to be solved. By reframing this challenge as a system failure to meet the patient's needs, the APRN might broaden the search for a solution by accessing charity care resources, consulting with mental health and nonprofit centers, networking with resourceful colleagues, and advocating for a way to penetrate this closed system. Advocacy means finding a way to make it work, using every possible means to find coverage. Customer service orientation means throwing out the blue collar mentality ("It's 4:30 pm; it's too late to get a nurse."). This approach is another example of the APRN going beyond the minimum standard operating procedures (Box 15-13).

Pragmatically this means that APRNs must recognize their own discomfort with financial issues related to accessing care. It is of course difficult to be pushed outside one's comfort zone. It is hard for a clinically competent APRN to say to others in the field, "I don't know about all this financial stuff. I need help." It is understandable when an APRN first says, "The business of payment for

---

box 15-12

EMERGING PARADIGM: MENTAL HEALTH SERVICES FOR 2000 AND BEYOND

Capitated reimbursement
Managed care
Continuous care
Integrated delivery systems
Community-based services
Primary care
Care (low tech)
Wellness focus (prevention model)
Population-based care
Consumer focus
Egalitarianism
Collaboration
Diversity of providers
Outcomes

From Haber, 1997a.

---

box 15-13

TIPS FOR ENHANCING THE APRN'S PRACTICE IN THE HOME CARE SETTING

1. Embrace the notion that an effective psychiatric home care service redirects the providers rather than the patients through the system.
2. Always ask the patient, "What do you think you need?"
3. Design programs that are creative, flexible, and tailored to the individual.
4. Use the strategy of reframing problem situations for providing services.
5. Expect conflicts that potentially prevent the meeting of patient-expressed needs; view them as obstacles that have solutions.
6. Always wear a rehumanizing lens. It cuts down the glare of the pressure generated by the need to keep cost-effectiveness at the same level while providing quality psychiatric-mental health services.
7. Blend the expert clinician skills of the CS and NP with business and political skills to be a key player in meeting the primary health care needs of individuals with mental illness.

8. Use communication based on cues from the patient's environment to establish trust.
9. Use critical thinking strategies during the diagnostic reasoning process to seize teaching moments.
10. Develop computer literacy skills to design efficient program evaluation and documentation methods.
11. Use political strategies to bring a new paradigm of home care services to patients and caregivers.
12. Develop alliances with consumer mental health groups to provide cost-effective quality care to patients.
13. Keep up with Medicare, Medicaid, and other health insurance and managed care regulations.
14. Cultivate the quality of persistence as a needed characteristic of forging relationships with patients, caregivers, health care providers, and other political and business groups.

care is not my concern." Acknowledgment of this discomfort will enable him or her to seek the necessary knowledge regarding financial issues to access this fragmented system more easily. This will in turn enable the APRN to apply critical thinking skills to these financial issues that are often the barrier to accessing care for patients. Once critical thinking skills are reframed in this manner, they enable the APRN to produce and implement creative solutions.

Healthy manipulation. Another concept to be reframed is the use of manipulation. APRNs need to think of the process as "healthy manipulation" of individuals in the health care system who by their nature, role, or job title have become barriers to meeting patients' needs. Appropriate use of business and political savvy skills enables the APRN to use healthy manipulation. APRNs must acknowledge that there is economic opportunity in partnering with people who have political clout. Some APRNs may be shocked by this notion. Others in the field who are concerned with the idea that patient and system conflicts are inherent in managed care programs may question this type of intervention (Padgett, 1998). However, partnerships, whether between or among patients, care givers, or providers, are the only realistic way that patients' expressed needs can be met. If the expressed needs of the patient and their caregivers are kept as the focus, then the concerns voiced by Padgett will be addressed. For example, an APRN may need to "unbundle" services when working with a managed care company. The APRN might think that the optimal care for the patient is to provide ongoing nursing visits and supplemental home health aide hours for a short period of time. However, the managed care provider may require the APRN to "unbundle" the usual services of a particular critical pathway (i.e., the APRN may need to negotiate specific goal directed services such as one medication visit or one family intervention visit rather than all the desired services). This is an example of minimizing potential conflicts as well as manipulating health care system variables. In essence it is a win-win situation.

APRNs should expect to have some difficulty accessing services for their patients. An APRN who does not reframe may think, "Why do I keep hitting my head against a brick wall. Why doesn't everyone think the way I do?" The reframing strategy in this case is to say, "What can I do to help people think the way I do?" This simple technique can save the APRN from many bruises and disappointments. Of course, this requires the use of strategies related to business and political savvy, which may thrust the APRN without such skills, once again, into the discomfort zone. However, this too can be reframed, and in so doing, the APRN will feel more comfortable and in control. Once this occurs, the highly developed critical thinking skills used so easily with clinical decisions will bring forth flexible and creative strategies to meet the patient's expressed needs.

Alliances with consumers. The APRN must develop alliances with consumer groups. The work of consumer mental health groups such as the Alliance for the Mentally Ill—Family Alliances for the Mentally Ill (AMI-FAMI) demonstrate how political activities can be used in a positive way to bring the attributes of the new paradigm into place. For example, federal legislation and expanded Community Support Program (CSP) funding arose from a consumer advocate lobby to combat stigma, gain control over treatment, and take an active role in developing systems for care.

The consumer movement rose from the ashes of failed deinstitutionalization and the community mental health moment. In 1979, approximately 100 self-help groups combined to form the National Alliance for the Mentally Ill (NAMI). This movement has grown to include over 1200 local and state affiliates with about 170,000 members.

The State Comprehensive Mental Health Services Plan Act of 1986 greatly expanded the role and influence of consumers. It required that each state mental health planning council be composed of a balanced number of consumers of mental health services and their family members (NIMH, 1987). In effect, consumers were no longer token representatives or passive recipients of mental health services. They would no longer accept the label of "treatment resistant"; they had come to the table with the goal of redefining treatment.

The Protection and Advocacy for Mentally Ill Individuals Act (1986) established the first federally funded advocacy program for each state and specified that advisory boards include 50% representation of patients and families.

The Americans with Disabilities Act (1990) provided protection from discrimination in employment for persons with mental disabilities. This protection prevented prospective employers from asking if a person ever had a mental disability and required employers to make reasonable accommodations for qualified people with mental disabilities. The inclusion of people with mental disabilities in the ADA federal initiative resulted from the vigorous lobbying and empowerment of mental health consumers. APRNs must not only be aware of the NAMI movement but must form active alliances with this emerging power base. This type of collaborative relationship is necessary to design programs that meet the needs of psychiatric patients and their families or significant others. This type of relationship becomes a strong political voice for the creation of appropriate health policy that will support the delivery of mental health services in the home.

IMPLICATIONS FOR THE ■ FUTURE

Historically, the chronically mentally ill population was given custodial care in state hospitals. Those patients who returned to the community were expected to partake in community mental health centers such as day treatment and partial hospitalization programs. However, the principles of planning for psychiatric treatment neglected an essential treatment: home care. Most patients with psychiatric illness return home to live with their families, and this home base is the ideal locus for care. Rather than asking patients to fit into existing structures that promote dependence, social incompetence, stigma, the sick role, ongoing relationships with institutions, symptomatic be-

havior, and a low level of functioning, the holistic behavioral home care model suggests that individually tailored treatment plans be brought to the patient. So the question becomes, "Who is the ideal practitioner to bring this care?" The APRN is the answer.

The wave of the future is the combined CNS/NP role. Currently, some APRNs have both the CS and NP credential; however, few actively practice as psychiatric NPs (i.e., they have not established collaborative practices with psychiatrists [where mandated] and they do not actively prescribe medications in accordance with their respective state's nurse practice act or legislation) (Haber, 1998b). However, if APRNs are to participate as key players in meeting the primary health care needs of individuals with mental illnesses, then they must embrace the challenges of the nurse practitioner role, especially that of exercising prescriptive authority. In addition, the APRN of the future must incorporate the business, computer, and political skills previously described to continue to create models of psychiatric home care that meet the needs of consumers.

RESOURCES AND CONNECTIONS

ORGANIZATIONS AND PROFESSIONAL ASSOCIATIONS

National Association for Home Care
201-547-3540
www.nahc.org

Association for Ambulatory Behavioral Healthcare
703-836-2274
Email: aaph@pie.org

American Federation of Home Health Agencies
301-588-1454

American Hospital Association Society for Ambulatory Care Professionals
312-422-3000
Fax: 312-422-4577

American Association for Continuing Care
202-857-1194

National Alliance for the Mentally Ill (NAMI)
703-524-7600
www.nami.org

American Psychiatric Nurses Association (APNA)
202-857-1133
www.apna.org

Home Health Care Nurses Association
850-474-8869

National League for Nursing (NLN) CHAP
800-669-9656 or 212-363-5555

References

Adams, T. (1994). The emotional experience of caregivers to relatives who are chronically confused—implications for community mental health nursing. *International Journal of Nursing Studies, 31*(6), 545–553.

American Nurses Association. (1986a). *Standards of community health nursing practice.* Washington, DC: Author.

American Nurses Association. (1986b). *Standards of home health nursing practice.* Washington, DC: Author.

American Nurses Association. (1994). *A statement on psychiatric-mental health clinical practice and standards of psychiatric-mental health clinical practice.* Washington, DC: Author.

American Nurses Association. (1995). *Nursing's social policy statement.* Washington, DC: Author.

American Nurses Association. (1998). *Standards of clinical nursing practice.* Washington, DC: American Nurses Publishing.

Americans with Disabilities Act. (1990). *Public Law 101–336.* Washington, DC: US Government Printing Office.

Backlar, P. (1997). Ethics in community mental health care: can we bridge the gap between the actual lives of persons with serious mental disorders and the therapeutic goals of their providers? *Community Mental Health Journal, 33*(6), 465–471.

Becker, D.R., et al. (1996). Job preferences of clients with severe psychiatric disorders participating in supported employment programs. *Psychiatric Services, 47*(11), 1223–1226.

Bigelow, D.A., McFarland, B.H., & Olson, M.M. (1991). Quality of life of community mental health program clients: validating a measure. *Community Mental Health Journal, 27*(1), 43–55.

Billings, C. (1997). Psychiatric-mental health nursing: 2000 and beyond. In Haber, J., et al. (Eds.). *Comprehensive psychiatric nursing* (ed. 5). St. Louis: Mosby.

Dee, V., van Servellen, G., & Brecht, M. (1998). Managed behavioral health care patients and their nursing care problems, level of functioning, and impairment on discharge. *Journal of the American Psychiatric Nurses Association, 4*(2), 57–66.

Forchuk, C., & Voorberg, N. (1991). Evaluation of a community mental health program. *Canadian Journal of Nursing Administration, 6,* 16–20.

Haber, J., & Billings, C.V. (1995). Primary mental health care: a model for psychiatric-mental health nursing. *Journal of the American Psychiatric Nurses Association, 1,* 154–163.

Haber, J. (1997a). Delivery of mental health service. In Haber, J., et al. (Eds.). *Comprehensive psychiatric nursing* (ed. 5). St. Louis: Mosby.

Haber, J. (1997b). Policy and politics: a 1997 legislative preview. *Journal of the American Psychiatric Nurses Association, 2*(6), 219–220.

Haber, J. (1998a). Policy and politics: making sense of the new medicare reimbursement laws. *Journal of the American Psychiatric Nurses Association, 4*(2), 67–68.

Haber, J. (1998b). Personal communication.

Hauenstein, E.J. (1996). Testing innovative nursing care: home intervention with depressed rural women. *Issues in Mental Health Nursing, 17*(33), 33–50.

Health Care Financing Administration (HCFA). (1979). *Medicare home health manual. HCFA-Publication Number 11-T273, rev 3/95,* Washington, DC: USDHHS.

Kates, N., et al. (1997). An in-home employment program for people with mental illness. *Psychiatric Rehabilitation Journal, 20*(4), 56–60.

Krainovich-Miller, B. (1997). Health teaching. In Haber, J., et al. (Eds.). *Comprehensive psychiatric nursing* (ed. 5). St. Louis: Mosby.

Martin, K. (June 30, 1998). Personal communication.

Musser-Granski, J., & Carrillo, D.F. (1997). Clinical care update: the use of bilingual, bicultural paraprofessionals in mental health services: issues for hiring, training, and supervision. *Community Mental Health Journal, 33*(1), 51–60.

National Association for Home Care. (1994). *Basic statistics about home care 1994.* Washington, DC: Author.

National Institute of Mental Health (NIMH). (October, 1987). *Toward a model plan: administrative document in response to Public Law 99–660, Title V. The state comprehensive mental health plan act of 1986.*

National Institute of Mental Health (NIMH). (1992). Caring for people with severe mental disorders: a national plan to improve services. *Schizophrenia Bulletin, 18,* 559–696.

Padgett, S.M. (1998). Dilemmas of caring in a corporate context: a critique of nursing case management. *Advances in Nursing Science, 20*(4), 1–12.

Peplau, H.E. (1991). *Interpersonal relations in nursing: a conceptual frame of reference for psychodynamic nursing.* New York: Springer.

Peterson, G.A., Drone, I.D., & Munetz, M.R. (1997). Diversity in case management modalities: the Summit model. *Community Mental Health Journal, 33*(3), 245–250.

Piersma, H.L., & Boes, J.L. (1997). Brief reports: the GAF and psychiatric outcome: a descriptive report. *Community Mental Health Journal, 33*(1), 35–41.

Polivka, B.J., Kennedy, C., & Chaudry, R. (1997). Collaboration between local public health and community mental health agencies. *Research in Nursing and Health, 20,* 153–160.

Provan, K.G., Sebastian, J.G., & Milward, H.B. (1996). Interorganizational cooperation in community mental health: a resource-based explanation of referrals and case coordination. *Medical Care Research and Review, 53*(1), 94–118.

Raskin, R., et al. (1996). A model for evaluating intensive outpatient behavioral health care programs. *Psychiatric Services, 47*(11), 1227–1232.

Siegmann, R.M., & Long, G.M. (1995). Psychoeducational group therapy changes the face of managed care. *Journal of Practical Psychiatry and Behavioral Health, 1*(1), 29–36.

Stahl, D.A. (1995). The pulse of managed care in 1996 and beyond. *Nursing Management, 27*(4), 16–17.

The Protection and Advocacy for Mentally Ill Individuals Act. (1986). *Public Law 99–319*, Washington, DC: US Government Printing Office.

Warner, R. (1997). Response to "A home-based program for the treatment of acute psychosis." *Community Mental Health Journal, 33*(2), 163–165.

Wasylenki, D., et al. (1997). A home-based program for the treatment of acute psychosis. *Community Mental Health Journal, 33*(2), 151–162.

Williams, C.A., et al. (1998). Toward an integration of competencies for advanced practice mental health nursing. *Journal of the American Psychiatric Nurses Association, 4*(2), 48–56.

Acute Care and
Crisis Management

ANNE BATEMAN

■ INTRODUCTION

Acute mental health care has evolved, not from careful rational planning, but as a response to chaotic shifts in the health care system at large. During the current transformation to managed mental health care systems, acute mental health services in the private and public sectors have to respond to the demand to reduce inpatient bed days and to stabilize individuals in the community. As a consequence, emergency psychiatric services for the acute care of mental illness and crisis

have adopted the basic principles of managed care: efficiency and cost-effectiveness.

Within the emerging managed mental health care systems, advanced practice registered nurses (APRN) and other providers must contend with a variety of factors that affect the services they provide, including systems issues, the therapeutic process itself, and patient outcomes. Patient characteristics, access to available services, and utilization patterns have changed since the advent of managed care (White et al., 1995). Today there are pressing needs resulting from the increased

355

number of patients in special populations, including children, the elderly, individuals with HIV/AIDS, the homeless, the severely and persistently mentally ill, individuals with dual diagnosis, the uninsured, and the underinsured. The managed mental health care system often seems to be structured with minimal consideration of the complexities related to the precipitants of the psychiatric emergency situation (White et al., 1995). These complexities pose a high risk to the patient and to the APRN who seeks to manage the psychiatric crisis in a therapeutic way. However, as with any major change, there is opportunity. For the APRN, there is the opportunity to develop a scope of practice that meets the needs of the patient and family during various crisis stages, even when the system may be limited.

HISTORICAL CONTEXT OF EMERGENCY ■ PSYCHIATRIC SERVICES

Early Development of Services

In 1963, the Community Mental Health Centers Act in the United States mandated that the care and treatment of the mentally ill shift from the institution to the community. The result was the establishment of community-based outpatient and residential programs specifically designated for those with a chronic mental illness. In the development of this system of care, emergency services were identified as one of the essential components of a comprehensive community-based system of care (Geller, 1991).

The intention of this approach to treatment was to improve the quality of patient care through a supportive and therapeutic network of comprehensive care in the community. The general assumption was that the well-being of the mentally ill was to some extent influenced by the social context within which they lived. More specifically, derivations of social theory state that the success of the reintegration of the mentally ill into society is affected by the attitudes of the primary care provider, family members and significant others,

as well as the general public (Bateman, 1995). As deinstitutionalization progressed, the role of the emergency psychiatric service was to provide rapid intervention at the onset of psychiatric decompensation and psychosocial crisis to avoid unnecessary acute hospitalization (White et al., 1995).

Bassuk (1980) and Ellison, Hughes, and White (1989) described the initial role of the emergency psychiatric service as supportive and an alternative to structured therapy and day treatment. The manner in which these services have been perceived and used has evolved from that of a supportive "after hours" link to the system of care to a clearly delineated point of entry to the larger network of managed psychiatric services.

In the four decades since the development of community-based services for public sector institutionalized patients, significant quantitative and qualitative shifts in both the role and structure of emergency psychiatric services have taken place. For example, the volume of emergency psychiatric service patient visits has doubled and the acuity level has increased by over 50%. In addition, staffing has shifted from mental health workers prepared at the baccalaureate level to master's-prepared clinicians. Community-based services, which have been thrust into the forefront of psychiatric care for patients in both the public and private sectors, now provide a critical prescreening function for patient access to and diversion from the broad spectrum of managed psychiatric services (Segal, Watson, & Akutsu, 1996).

Influence of Managed Care on Services

During the evolution of the health care system, the characteristics of individuals who seek emergency psychiatric service have changed somewhat in terms of a greater diversity of special populations. In the premanaged care era, the average patient was either "the walking wounded" or "the walking wounder." Individuals sought treatment because they were experiencing psychologic and often physical pain. Some were referred by the police, family, or other service provider because they were at risk of dangerous behavior directed at themselves or another individual in the community.

Today, with the inception of the managed care initiative, individuals seek treatment or are referred to the emergency psychiatric service for similar reasons; however, now the evaluation is a mandated step in the process rather than the patients' choice. This means that patients treated in both the public and private sectors must be prescreened by a designated team before gaining access to certain levels of care, including inpatient, detoxification treatment, and certain types of outpatient care such as intensive day treatment. Although this process varies from state to state (e.g., Massachusetts has had managed Medicaid psychiatric services since July 1993), plans have begun to initiate federally funded managed Medicare for a variety of services and coverage programs.

Managed care service providers in both the public and private sectors now contract in a competitive process for emergency psychiatric services that include much of the original focus of evaluation, assessment, referral, and diversion from inpatient level of care. The mandated "screening" at the designated emergency psychiatric service is a mixed blessing for both inpatient and outpatient providers. On the positive side for the inpatient facility, the patient who has been prescreened arrives on the unit with a comprehensive assessment and insurance authorization, saving the admitting staff a great deal of time. On the downside, there is fierce competition for inpatient psychiatric patients. The inpatient facility must develop collegial relationships with the emergency psychiatric service to facilitate admissions, unless the unit is the designated receiving facility (Nicholson et al., 1996).

For the outpatient facility there is now a more clearly designated site to refer the acute and difficult to manage individual, whereas in the past the outpatient clinician would often be faced with a struggle in the process of referring to the emergency psychiatric service. The expectation was that the outpatient clinician was responsible for the management of the crisis situation and that the emergency psychiatric service was only used as a last resort. Often the public sector emergency psychiatric service would not accept the privately insured individual because of limited resources and an inability to bill for these services. The message was "take care of your own patient since that is what you get paid to do." Now, even with the less acute admission referral, the patient must be "prescreened" before the admission will be approved by the third-party payer managing the patient's insured care. Not only does this process add time to the standard admission as well as the acute admission, the outpatient clinician is also faced with the possibility that the screening service will rule out the need for an admission and the patient will be diverted to a less restrictive level of care. The result has been a continued struggle about clinical roles and responsibility, often with the patient in the middle of the conflict.

As struggles abound in the process of integrating managed mental health care into service delivery, the system today resembles that of the early days of deinstitutionalization: rapid reduction in access to inpatient services often with the risk of compromising quality care and patient safety (Kane, 1995). As in the earlier days of state and federal mandates to reduce the number of inpatient events, managed care providers are now forced to limit access to inpatient care.

Early research in the area of emergency psychiatric services has primarily focused on nonclinical issues. Although the setting has the potential to provide a rich environment for treatment outcome research, until the mid-1990s the majority of research concentrated on broader systems issues, such as referral patterns, admission decisions, and outcomes driven by the payer source.

Some current research has considered issues such as access to outpatient services for individuals and families in crisis and assessment and treatment of acute psychosis in the emergency psychiatric service (Bateman, 1995; Schwartz & Hughes, 1996; White et al., 1995). In these studies, patient characteristics and the type of service provided are discussed. The average patient was male (52.9%); single or divorced (71.2%); currently experiencing some type of relationship difficulty; with past or present substance abuse (73.1%); unemployed (88.6%) with a long history of work related difficulties; receiving state funded primary insurance (64.6%); with a presenting problem of depression (20.9%), suicide attempt or ideation (55.8%), psychotic behavior (39.85), and aggression (19.9%). Approximately 40% of the patients were admitted to an inpatient unit (public sector, 43.2%), while the remainder were stabilized in the emergency psychiatric service and discharged to home or a diversion program with outpatient follow-up as indicated. As was the case in the early years of emergency psychiatric services, patients were equally self-referred and referred by police and others.

It is important that the APRN clearly understand the role of emergency psychiatric services in relation to the scope of practice. Positive outcomes in the referral process are the direct result of a collaborative relationship with the emergency psychiatric service (Segal, Watson, Akutsu, 1996). The example in Box 16-1 describes an intervention used by an APRN, as the clinical director of an emergency psychiatric service, and the staff of a referring agency.

EMERGENCY PSYCHIATRIC
■ SERVICE DELIVERY

Program Models and Methods

Models and methods of emergency psychiatric service delivery encompass a broad spectrum. The primary goal of the emergency psychiatric service has been to provide rapid intervention and stabilization intended to avert unnecessary inpatient psychiatric hospitalizations. The traditional model and method has varied little since the early inception of the emergency psychiatric service. The services usually include crisis intervention, psychiatric assessment, mobile outreach, acute holding or crisis stabilization beds, and medical evaluation. Traditional emergency psychiatric ser-

box 16-1

APRN INTERVENTION BETWEEN EMERGENCY PSYCHIATIC SERVICE AND REFERRING AGENCY

As the clinical director of the Emergency Mental Health Service (EMHS), it was the responsibility of the APRN to intervene when there was a struggle between a referring agency and the EMHS staff. The APRN provided consultation and training to the various community agencies, including the police, nursing homes, and residential programs. She made visits to better understand the environment from which the referrals came, such as the residential program that had as many as 30 residents being supervised by two paraprofessional staff. However, these training sessions for community-based staff and the EMHS staff did not reduce the difficulties, particularly after hours when fewer managerial staff were available.

As an acute intervention, the APRN implemented a plan with the director of one of the residential sites to hold several staff meetings "on the road" at each other's site. This plan was intended to accomplish two goals: 1) to familiarize staff with the environment from which the resident was being referred and 2) to provide an opportunity for the staff to get to know one another. In addition, during the shared meetings, the APRN and the staff would review situations that had recently occurred. The staff began identifying shared issues, such as delays in transportation and overcrowding. As a proactive measure, new staff made site visits as part of their orientation. Overall, this process helped the EMHS staff and the residential staff understand the issues related to the referral process, and they were able to solve problems more effectively.

vices have multidisciplinary crisis staff who may or may not be trained on an advanced level. Their method focuses more on crisis intervention where the patient would be stabilized at the time of the crisis and referred for follow-up services or to another more intensive level of care. These models may involve 24-hour on-site and/or on-call staff reporting to an APRN or other master's-prepared clinician located in a free-standing mental health clinic or residential program. If a physician is involved in the process, it is often by telephone. Some emergency psychiatric services are located in acute hospital settings, where the intervention is provided by the resident psychiatrist, APRN, or staff drawn from the psychiatric inpatient unit. In facilities with no onsite psychiatric services, the evaluation is conducted by the physician in the emergency room, and the designated offsite emergency psychiatric service is consulted. At this point either the patient is referred to the emergency psychiatric service or the clinician comes to the emergency room to complete the assessment and provide recommendations for referral and disposition.

Another effective model includes a process of managing the less acute, or "urgent care," patient outside of the emergency setting. In this model, the APRN sees the patient in crisis within 4 hours of the request for services. Urgent care is usually provided within the outpatient clinic by clinical staff who are scheduled to have one or two urgent care appointments as part of their regular case load. In most outpatient psychiatric clinics, there is little difficulty filling these time slots, particularly when there is a collaborative relationship with the area emergency psychiatric service. Some settings provide an urgent care group psychotherapy, which is an effective way to meet the needs of several patients in crisis while conserving limited clinical resources. Providing urgent services in both individual and group modalities benefits the clinic, payer, and payer source by increasing consumer satisfaction.

Environmental Factors

The model of service provided differs from community to community and from state to state and is molded by numerous environmental factors,

some of which are discussed in this chapter. Mandates from public and private payer sources have forced emergency psychiatric service to expand services to include such specializations as the following:

1. Clinicians trained in the evaluation and assessment of children and adolescents
2. Substance abuse clinicians
3. Mobile outreach
4. 24- to 48-hour crisis stabilization
5. Rapid access to face-to-face evaluation in 1 hour or less

The emergency psychiatric service is now required to have physician availability 24 hours per day, and the evaluating clinician is required to be trained at an advanced level. In this environment, the APRN, psychologist, social worker, and master's-prepared mental health counselor function in similar roles, each bringing his or her own specialization to the clinical intervention. The APRN brings advanced practice knowledge and skills related to psychobiologic and psychosocial dimensions of the individual. The combination of competencies and holistic approach is invaluable given the increase in medical comorbidity in this population (Schwartz & Hughes, 1996).

As with much of the health care delivery system today, the expectation for enhanced services has not been met with additional resources. The emergency psychiatric service has been expected to do more with less. Many psychiatric service providers have been forced to contract with outside vendors for segments of the emergency component to remain fiscally solvent. Ironically, changes in service delivery have not emerged from clinical need but more often from resource availability. The goal of "avoiding inpatient hospitalization at all costs" becomes more difficult with current mandates that limit access to outpatient services (Segal, Watson, & Akutsu, 1996).

Family Effect on Service Delivery

The evolution of psychiatric services has been driven by two major forces: managed care mandates from a variety of different payer sources and family members. All aspects considered, families have had the greatest effect on the delivery of inpatient care and emergency psychiatric services (Geller, 1991).

From the early days of the community mental health movement, families have worked to change the scope of treatment for those with chronic mental illness and mental retardation. Their efforts led to expanded federal legislation and the process of deinstitutionalization. These families, many uniting in local and state chapters of the National Alliance for the Mentally Ill, decried long waits for services, lengthy hospitalizations, problems with access to services after-hours, and a lack of family inclusion in treatment planning (Segal, Watson, & Akutsu, 1995). For example, a poignant family problem ensued when the families caring for a mentally ill member were subjected to humiliation by the necessity of involving police to assist with transporting their family member to the emergency psychiatric service.

Families lobbied for mobile outreach services in their community as a method of intervention that would minimize the involvement of the police. Mobile services were designed to provide a rapid response to a mental health crisis in the setting where the crisis is occurring. The goal of the mobile service was to stabilize the crisis onsite and avoid the necessity of transporting the individual to the emergency psychiatric service (Bassuk, 1980; Engleman et al., 1998; Hoult, 1996). However, the families' frustration has continued because many programs providing mobile outreach request police back-up as a safety precaution when responding to a private residence. Mobile outreach may not always meet the needs of the family whose desire is the removal of the problematic member from the home in a quiet and humane manner. Their desire may be in conflict with the mandated goal of mobile outreach, which is to stabilize the individual in the community setting whenever possible (Hoult, 1996).

This discrepancy in conceptual understanding of mobile services highlights a broad misconception of the role and responsibility of emergency psychiatric service as a whole. The public, family, store proprietor, police, residential, or outpatient program usually wants the individual with the problem removed and hospitalized, while the service is under mandate to avoid hospitalization. The result is that few are satisfied with the delivery of services by the emergency psychiatric service. The emergency psychiatric service has the largest number of complaints of any hospital or community-based mental health program in part because of the confusion in role expectation (Gold Award, 1997).

This lack of understanding has been a long-standing burden for the emergency psychiatric service: to remove and hospitalize goes against the mandate; to intervene, stabilize, and not hospitalize dissatisfies consumers and families (the customers of the service). The APRN needs to anticipate problematic situations and take a proactive stance in the organization's internal and external customer education about the role of the emergency psychiatric service. Providing a rapid response to complaints in an open and nondefensive manner is a key responsibility for the APRN to ensure effective service delivery and positive consumer outcomes.

Functions of Clinical Staff

Urgent or *acute care, crisis intervention,* and *crisis management* are synonymous terms in emergency psychiatric service. Any combination of these services will be provided depending on the scope of the service delivery. The goal of the service is to provide rapid intervention at the onset of the crisis, taking into consideration all aspects of the individual's lived experience, including the biopsychosocial concerns. This intervention is intended to assist the individual with returning to the pre-crisis level of functioning or better. The process of crisis intervention has the ability to assist the individual with gaining insight into the precipitating events and behaviors and to improve problem solving and coping ability.

Emergency psychiatric service staff are primarily prepared as master's-level clinicians, although some programs may have mental health workers to assist the clinician. Different disciplines function in complementary roles on the emergency psychiatric service team depending on the program model. The psychiatric clinical nurse specialist (APRN) and the physician provide advanced-level patient assessment; psychopharmacologic evaluation; and supervision of the registered nurse, allied health professionals, and mental health workers. The registered nurse, social worker, psychologist, and counselor provide evaluation, assessment, stabilization, and referral of individuals and families in accordance with the program protocols. The registered nurse also provides a physical assessment as part of the evaluation. In some models, after the initial assessment, the psychiatric resident or staff psychiatrist further evaluates the patient. Referral and disposition result from this multidisciplinary intervention.

Unique to the nurse at any level of practice are assessment skills. The nurse is trained on the basic level to provide an assessment that considers the holistic needs of the individual, family, and others significant to the situation. This assessment encompasses the biopsychosocial, cultural, and spiritual realms of the patient's lived experience. In an emergency, the true aspects of why the patient is in crisis may have little to do with the circumstances that resulted in the request for services at the time.

With the changing expectations of the emergency psychiatric service resulting from the influences of managed care, there has been a shift in staffing patterns to a more independent, advanced-level clinician. In this model, the APRN effectively provides an independent assessment without the necessity of further consultation at the time of the emergency. The APRN brings a holistic perspective to patient evaluation and treatment that is an important part of this model. This method of service delivery can be more cost effective and timely than the previous multilevel, often redundant evaluation by several providers (Perrault, 1996). However, this model has not been embraced by every hospital administration, and some emergency departments mandate that every patient be seen by a medical physician at the time

of the emergency visit. In situations where medical intervention is not indicated, the patient is then subjected to additional wait times and costs. Over time, managed Medicaid and Medicare regulations will require changes in the practice of multiple evaluations from the perspective of cost and patient satisfaction.

ACUTE CARE AND
■ CRISIS MANAGEMENT
Stages of Crisis

The APRN uses acute care interventions and crisis management to guide an individual and family through an emotionally and physically traumatic event. The methods involve using problem-solving skills aimed at regaining equilibrium. Problem solving is a structured process where each step is contingent upon the results of the previous step. In his classic formulation, Caplan (1964) describes four developmental stages of crisis:

- There is a rise in tension with discomfort as the stress and tension continues.
- There is an increased discomfort as coping skills are unsuccessful and the stress continues unresolved.
- The stress initiates internal stimuli, and the individual mobilizes internal and external resources in an attempt to reduce the discomfort. The problem is either redefined, or the individual gives up the effort of goal attainment.
- Without resolution, the stress and tension increases, and the individual experiences disorganization and further decompensation.

Every attempt is made to stabilize and regain equilibrium. Aquilera (1994) discusses the balancing factors that contribute to the return to equilibrium and states that strength or weakness in any of these factors could precipitate a crisis or contribute to resolution. These factors include the following:

- Perception of the event
- Situational supports
- Coping mechanisms

When the individual perceives the situation to be overwhelming and is unable to use the usual coping skills and systems of support effectively, the stress and discomfort continues to escalate. As a result, the individual is unable to regain balance without significant external intervention.

Caplan (1964) reported that left without intervention, the crisis situation will resolve in 4 to 6 weeks. However, there continue to be residual negative effects resulting from the unresolved issues associated with the loss, and the individual is unable to move beyond or adjust to the changes.

As Fig. 16-1 demonstrates, the effects of the crisis tend to recycle repeatedly until the cycle is broken. With each cycle the individual struggles to regain equilibrium but becomes less and less able to function, relying on regressed behavior and thought processes while the ineffective coping mechanism only complicates the situation. With intervention the individual experiences a decrease in the negative psychobiologic symptoms. As equilibrium is regained and the patient moves towards

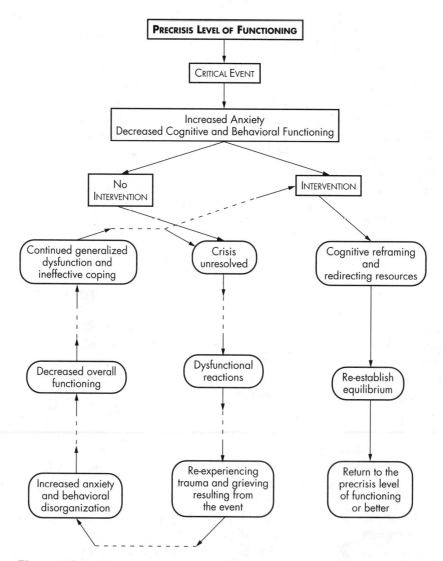

Figure 16-1 Conceptual model for acute care and crisis management.

stabilization, new insights are acquired that will help improve coping and general level of functioning.

APRNs can conceptualize the process of acute care and crisis management as depicted in Fig. 16-1. They use interventions to interrupt the cycle of further loss of equilibrium with physical and emotional distress and aid the patient in resolution of the crisis. Through crisis intervention there is often personal growth leading to the potential for an improved level of functioning.

Critical Incident Stress Debriefing

Critical incident stress debriefing (CISD) is a valuable community service provided by some emergency psychiatric services. CISD is a method of intervention that is effective in situations where a major stressor has affected a group of individuals in stressful occupations, such as first responder personnel (i.e., police, fire, ambulance) (Mitchell & Bray, 1990). The goal is to provide intervention close to the onset of the crisis with the intent of reducing the long-term effect of the event for those in highly stressful occupations. Recently, the model has been applied to whole communities after a disaster or traumatic event that has affected various groups of individuals, such as mass homicides in schools or restaurants or environmental disasters.

The CISD team is composed of specially trained volunteers from various professions, including, police, fire department, ambulance, school, hospital, and emergency psychiatric service staff. A debriefing is scheduled within 24 to 48 hours of a "bad call" that involved the injury or death of a police or ambulance partner, death of a child, or multiple casualties resulting from accident, acts of nature, or violent events. The Federal Emergency Management Agency (FEMA) is able to send CISD teams to work with survivors and rescue personnel. During such tragic events, CISD teams across the country may be put on alert for possible deployment to assist the teams on site.

A CISD involves four to six CISD team members who conduct the session in a structured process as pictured in Fig. 16-2, which shows the levels of emotional intensity experienced during the debriefing by the participants. The goal is to provide rapid intervention as soon as is practical after the incident. Upon request, the team is activated and the individuals involved in the incident are assembled at a designated location, usually a school or hospital conference room. Each person is invited to share his or her thoughts, feelings, and perceptions of the event. An effort is made to clarify any misconceptions about the facts of the incident. The team emphasizes validation of feelings and provides education about the physical and emotional effects of acute and prolonged stress. After the completion of the debriefing process a second session is scheduled if indicated. Anyone in need of more intensive intervention is referred for individual psychotherapy.

CLINICAL CASES IN EMERGENCY ■ PSYCHIATRIC SERVICES

Regardless of the emergency psychiatric service model and method, the clinical issues remain similar. Patients are in varying degrees of emotional and often physical pain. They are depressed, anxious, and often agitated, angry, and hostile. Relationship issues are often most prevalent. Family members or significant others may accompany the patient and mirror the emotional and cognitive behavioral responses expressed by the patient. More than 60% of the time, substance use or abuse is a major factor affecting the immediate situation. The APRN must be able to manage the multiple issues that accompany the patient's primary complaint (Bateman, 1995; Schwartz & Hughes, 1996; White et al, 1995).

First Time Use of Emergency Psychiatric Services

Marcia is a 19-year-old single African-American female who has come to the emergency psychiatric

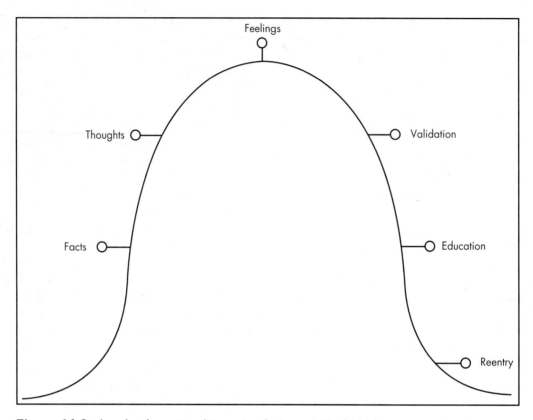

Figure 16-2   Levels of emotional intensity during a critical incident stress debriefing. (Adapted from Mitchell, J., & Bray, G. [1990]. *Emergency service stress.* Englewood Cliffs, NJ: Prentice Hall.)

service for the first time. She is brought to the emergency room by her girlfriend who reports that Marcia has become increasingly depressed over the last week after midterm exams. Marcia feels that she did not do as well on her exams as she could have because she was having trouble sleeping. She reports feeling less and less like herself since she started attending a small college 1 year ago. She is worried about her grades and her ability to do the course work. In spite of her worrying, she has been getting straight As and probably scored well on her midterms.

During the evaluation Marcia appears sad and cries easily. She reportes feeling sad and lacking energy since she left home to begin her freshman year. She indicates that her family is very happy and excited about her being at college and that she does not want to let them down by not doing well. She indicates that she feels she might need help in coping with all the changes she has been experiencing. She denies being suicidal, stating that she could never consider hurting herself because it is against her religion.

The APRN who conducts the evaluation identifies the neurovegetative signs of decreased sleep, loss of appetite, difficulty concentrating, and sleep disturbances. The APRN diagnoses unspecified situational depression. The APRN prescribes an SSRI medication, and a follow-up visit is scheduled for a psychopharmacologic evaluation in 3 weeks. Upon completion of the evaluation, Marcia is referred to the urgent care clinic with an appointment for the next morning. In addition, a referral is made to the Young Adult Transition Group. Marcia is discharged with her girlfriend.

This case shows the advantage of having an APRN in the emergency psychiatric service. The APRN is able to conduct a complete evaluation, assessment, and referral, as well as provide the psychopharmacologic evaluation and prescribe the appropriate medication.

Repeated Use of Emergency Psychiatric Services

The community mental health clinic is familiar with Chris, a 39-year-old single Caucasian male, although he does not attend regular programming He drops in several times a week, usually just to sit in the Friendship Coffee and Snack Shop. He used to come more often when smoking was allowed in the building, but now he visits less frequently. Sometimes he buys something from the thrift clothing shop. At least once during the week he talks with his case manager just to check in and is usually doing "just fine."

In the past 20 years since he was diagnosed with schizophrenia, undifferentiated type, Chris's days have been spent "dropping in" on most of the experiences of his life. He has stopped visiting his sister who works all day. Both his parents died when he was much younger and hospitalized most of the time. There is no other family. He is proud of his two-room efficiency apartment and the fact that he is not in a group home with "all those other people who have so many problems." He likes to be home before it gets dark so he can watch television and feel safe.

Chris takes his medication and keeps to this routine every day, except on the first Friday of the month when the Social Security check arrives. On that Friday night, the laughter and noise of the crowd at Jesse's Bar and Grill are very inviting, and the fish and chips there are the best he has ever had. He usually takes a walk over to the bar to have supper and a beer.

The emergency psychiatric service has extensive experience with Chris as well. The staff knows that he is likely to come in around the beginning of the month after he receives his check. This time when he arrives, escorted by the police after drinking for several days, he has been physically assaulted and exploited financially. He is grossly intoxicated, paranoid and delusional, physically disheveled, and uncooperative. The emergency plan for Chris has been in place for several years now. The team has a clear plan to manage his behavior. He is given his usual medications and is started on a benzodiazapine regimen to manage alcohol withdrawal symptoms. He is assisted with his personal care and placed in the crisis stabilization bed for re-evaluation in 24 hours. When his condition stabilizes within 48 hours, he is cleared for discharge.

This case is a typical scenario in the current mental health service delivery system. In prior years, without an intervention of crisis stabilization by emergency psychiatric services, Chris would have been readmitted to the acute inpatient unit where he might have decompensated and required an admission of several weeks. In this case, with a specifically designated crisis plan, inpatient admission was averted and the patient was returned to the community more rapidly. Therefore the outcome is considered positive in that it demonstrates the effectiveness of an integrated system of treatment for a severely and persistently mentally ill individual, with a preplanned crisis plan that avoids an admission and lengthy hospitalization. Follow-up and treatment of Chris's issues that precipitated the crisis will be managed by primary providers of his integrated treatment plan.

ROLES OF THE APRN IN EMERGENCY ■ PSYCHIATRIC SERVICES

The APRN in psychiatric-mental health has become a valuable member of the emergency psychiatric service team. The advanced skills that APRNs bring to service delivery have proven to be effective in the current managed care environment (Perrault, 1996). Crisis intervention and brief psychotherapies are the mainstay of their practice. Some APRNs also function in the role of nurse practitioner (NP), incorporating the knowledge and competencies of a primary care provider. Other APRNs work collaboratively with primary care NPs to manage some patients' specialized needs. (See Chapter 20 for a discussion of these roles.) In addition to the role of clinician, the APRN is effective as nurse manager, consultation-liaison nurse, and case manager. Each of these roles requires the expertise to function independently while engaging in interdisciplinary collaboration. Table 16-1 lists some of the major functions of the APRN in different roles.

APRNs have special training to provide psychopharmacologic assessment and psychotherapy in a variety of therapeutic modalities. They may also have prescriptive authority depending on state regulations and their type of clinical practice. The combination of comprehensive interventions has

the advantage of maintaining continuity of care for the individual, family, and service. The APRN in the emergency psychiatric service has an understanding and awareness of the community service options available to the individual and family in crisis and can be effective in facilitating access to the necessary resources. For example, the APRN would provide the initial assessment in the emergency service and determine that brief problem-focused psychotherapy is indicated. The patient would be scheduled for several follow-up visits for therapy and evaluation with the APRN through individual and/or group urgent services.

COORDINATED USE OF EMERGENCY ■ PSYCHIATRIC SERVICES

Jane is a 27-year-old married Caucasian female who has been receiving mental health services for the last 12 years. She has a primary diagnosis of borderline personality disorder with post-traumatic stress disorder and a chronic rheumatologic disorder, nonspecific, since her first admis-

table 16-1

ROLES OF THE APRN IN EMERGENCY PSYCHIATRIC SERVICES

CLINICIAN	NURSE MANAGER	CONSULTATION-LIAISON	CASE MANAGER
Nursing assessment	All roles of APRN clinician by choice or role design; PLUS	All roles of APRN clinician by choice or role design: PLUS	All roles of APRN clinician by choice or role design; PLUS
Psychologic assessment			
Psychopharmacologic assessment	Unit management: scheduling, budgeting, project planning, implementation, and quality improvement	Inter-unit and department clinical interface	Management of cases: including clinical, social, and system considerations
Psychotherapy			
Medication prescription			
Referral	Inter-intra unit organization interface		

sion. She lives with her husband and their 3-year-old daughter. Jane has above average intelligence and has completed a graduate degree in education, although she has never worked in her chosen field. She has been frequently hospitalized for self-abusive behavior, usually cutting, although she has had one severe overdose that left her unresponsive and on a respirator for 5 days several months after the birth of her daughter. She has extensive scarring on her abdomen and inner thighs. She reports intermittent alcohol abuse, which usually results in a several-day binge and cutting behavior. Her husband's work requires him to be out of town frequently. She is careful not to use alcohol unless he is home and available for their daughter.

Her family of origin has a history of both depression and substance abuse. She is an only child. Jane reports being sickly as a child who had to spend long periods of time away from home in the hospital when, she states, her mother would not come to visit. Her father visited her, often several times a day, usually while he was intoxicated. Jane also reports what she calls "weird loving" from her father from as early as she could remember. Shortly after Jane was born, her mother became ill and spent most of her time in bed. Jane cannot remember a time when her mother did anything other than have meals with the family.

Jane reports feeling lonely and afraid most of her childhood. She had few friends and states that the kids at school often made fun of her because she was shy and quiet. She describes two special girlfriends, both of whom moved away, and Jane never talked to them again. When Jane was in high school her mother began taking her to see her therapist because her mother felt there was something wrong with her. When she was a senior, Jane started seeing her own therapist who became ill and stopped seeing her after 1 year of treatment. Over the years Jane has worked with two other therapists, one who moved to another state and another who just stopped seeing her and did not return her phone calls.

The results of difficult terminations have exacerbated Jane's issues of abandonment and trust. In spite of this she remains the "good patient," never late, compliant, and cooperative with her treatment plan. However, she is very provocative at times and states that she always wants to die. On occasion she would leave her therapy session without incident and go directly to the emergency psychiatric service, having superficially cut herself on the way.

After a stretch of frequent parasuicidal behavior resulting in almost weekly admissions, an interdisciplinary team of her clinicians develops a plan. Together they present it to Jane, her husband, and her parents. The team consists of her individual therapist, her two group therapists, her psychopharmacologist, staff from the inpatient and day treatment units and the emergency psychiatric service, and her primary physician and rheumatologist. The focus of the plan is to provide Jane with a safety net of interventions that will be followed by all of the team of clinicians to minimize splitting and to ensure a consistent response to her many behavioral responses. For example, she cannot go to the emergency psychiatric service until she first talks to her primary therapist. Since most of her hospitalization stays are brief, she will be admitted to the holding unit for 48 hours and then be reevaluated for hospitalization. She can request an inpatient admission; however, she is allotted only 10 inpatient days per contract period. This means that she must use the days judiciously. In any situation she has to be able to contract for safety.

Psychodynamically this plan is intended to provide Jane input and control over the course of her care with a consistent, responsive system of clinicians in whom she can begin to develop trust. Providing her with more than one focus for her primary care is intended to minimize the recapitulation of her childhood abandonment issues. From a systems perspective this plan that includes Jane, all of her care providers, and her family will reduce the frustration of a single clinician's feeling solely responsible for her safety.

Over the first 6 months of this plan Jane requires one stay in the holding unit and her parasuicidal behavior is reduced to less that once per month. In the second 6 months she is able to keep herself safe, and although she occasionally calls, she does not come to the emergency psychiatric service. Each time that she calls, the plan is reinforced and discussed with her. This plan reduces episodes of parasuicidal behavior by 50% and inpatient admissions by 100% in the first 12-month period.

APRNs are frequently engaged as therapists with patients such as Jane. This case study demonstrates how the emergency psychiatric service, as part of a comprehensive treatment plan, can effect positive outcomes for complex patients receiving care in a multiservice system of care.

IMPLICATIONS FOR
■ THE FUTURE

The managed care movement is affecting the emergency psychiatric service in ways that have been described. However, the issues of safety, responsibility, and accountability need to be mentioned. As the area of responsibility and decision making about the clinical needs of patients becomes shared and more diffuse, patient safety becomes an issue. Service cutbacks, downsizing, and merging—all attributed to managed care—may contribute to the increased potential for violence on the service unit (Carroll & Morin, 1998). Acting-out and physically aggressive patients are forced to come into the emergency psychiatric service, an environment where fewer staff are available to assist in behavioral management. The risk for violence in the emergency psychiatric service is greater for patient and staff alike (White et al., 1995).

Who is ultimately responsible for positive as well as negative patient outcomes: the clinician or team of clinicians evaluating the patient, or the managed care provider who considers the clinical information as reported by others? The burden of safety, responsibility, and accountability lies with the clinical team of the emergency psychiatric service. Upon completion of the evaluation and assessment, the clinician must advocate for the patient and whatever encompasses the clinical indication for intervention and disposition.

The APRN has a crucial role on the team, with several aspects to the role including that of independent clinician, educator, and leader. The APRN in this role has the opportunity to guide the other members of the clinical team, the patient and significant others, and the managed care provider through the process of the emergency psychiatric service. In addition, the APRN as the team leader can improve service delivery on the administrative level.

RESOURCES AND CONNECTIONS

ASSESSMENT TOOLS

DSM-IV (1994)
Beck Depression Inventory (Beck and Steer, 1984)
Hamilton Rating Scale for Depression (HSRD) (Hamilton, 1960)
Global Assessment of Functioning (American Psychiatric Association, 1994)

ORGANIZATIONS

American Orthopsychiatry Association
330 Seventh Avenue, 18th Floor
New York, NY 10001
212-564-5930
Fax: 212-564-6100
www.amerortho.org

American Psychiatric Nurses Association
1200 19th Street, N.W., Suite 300
Washington, DC 20036
202-857-1100
Fax: 202-429-5112
www.apna.org

Health Resource Center on Domestic Violence
Family Violence Prevention Fund
383 Rhode Island Street, Suite 304
San Francisco, CA 94103-5133
1-888-Rx-ABUSE
www.fvpf.org/health/health@fvpf.org

National Alliance for the Mentally Ill
200 N. Glebe Road, Suite 1015
Arlington, VA 22203-3754
703-524-7600
www.NAMI.org

Emergency Services
www.mentalhealth.org/emerserv/GUIDECC.HTM

References

American Psychiatric Association. (1994). *Diagnostic and statistical manual of mental disorders* (ed. 4). Washington, DC: Author.

Aquilera, D. (1994). *Crisis intervention: theory and methodology* (ed. 7). St. Louis: Mosby.

Bassuk, E. (1980). The impact of deinstitutionalization in the general hospital psychiatric ward. *Hospital and Community Psychiatry, 31,* 623–27.

Bateman, A. (1995). The experience of barriers to mental health care access for individuals and families [abstract] *Journal of the American Psychiatric Nurses Association, 1*(6), 202.

Beck, A., & Steer, R. (1984). Internal consistencies of the original and revised Beck Depression Inventory. *Journal of Clinical Psychology, 40,* 1365–1367.

Caplan, G. (1964). *Principles of preventive psychiatry.* New York: Basic Books.

Carroll, V., & Morin, K.H. (September/October, 1998). Workplace violence affects one-third of nurses: survey of nurses in seven SNAs reveals staff nurses most at risk. *American Nurse,* 15.

Ellison, J., Hughes, D., & White, K. (1989). Frequent repeaters in a psychiatric emergency service. *Hospital and Community Psychiatry, 40*(3), 250–260.

Engleman, J., et al. (July, 1998). Clinicians decision making about involuntary commitment. *Psychiatric Services, 49*(7), 941–945.

Geller, J. (1991). Any place but the state hospital: examining assumptions about the benefit of admission diversion. *Hospital and Community Psychiatry, 42*(2), 145–162.

Gold Award. (November, 1997). Linking mentally ill persons with services through crisis intervention, mobile outreach, and community education, Project Response, Mental Health Services West, Portland Oregon. *Psychiatric Services, 48*(11), 630.

Hamilton, M. (1960). A rating scale for depression. *Journal of Neurology, Neurosurgery, and Psychiatry, 12,* 56–62.

Hoult, J. (1996). Mobile crisis service. [letter]. *Psychiatric Services, 47,* 46.

Kane, C.F. (1995). Deinstitutionalization and managed care: deja vu? *Psychiatric Services, 46,* 883–884, 889.

Mitchell, J. & Bray, G. (1990). *Emergency service stress.* Englewood Cliffs, NJ: Prentice Hall.

Nicholson, J., et al. (1996). The consequences of managed care on child inpatient dispositions from an emergency mental health service. I. Impact on utilization. *Psychiatric Services, 47,* 1344–1350.

Perrault, J. (July, 1996). Mobile crisis team nursing. *Nursing Spectrum.*

Schwartz, N., & Hughes, D. (1996). Assessment and treatment of acute psychosis in a psychiatric emergency service. *Essential Psychopharmacology, 1*(2).

Segal, S., Watson, M., & Akutsu, P. (1996). Quality of care and use of less restrictive alternatives in the psychiatric emergency service. *Psychiatric Services, 47,* 623–627.

White, C., et al. (1995). Factors associated with admission to public and private hospitals from a psychiatric emergency screening. *Psychiatric Services, 46,* 467–472.

Working with Families

VICTORIA S. CONN and DIANE T. MARSH

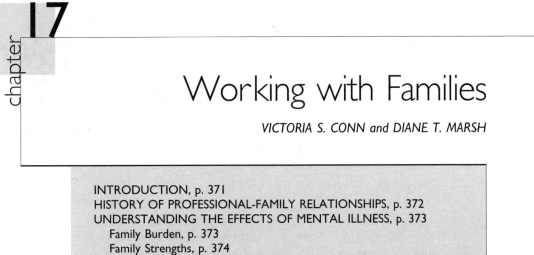

■ INTRODUCTION

When the first generation of advanced practice psychiatric-mental health nurses graduated from their training programs in the 1950s, new winds were blowing in the mental health field that shaped mental illness as a family phenomenon and made families, not individuals, the focus of treatment (Peplau, 1975). Today the prevailing winds still shape mental illness as a family phenomenon, but the focus has shifted from the family's presumed effect on mental illness to the adverse effect of mental illness on the family. This chapter identifies families as a population at risk for serious stress-related problems and calls upon advanced practice registered nurses (APRNs) in psychiatric and mental health care to work collaboratively with them to reduce their burden and facilitate positive adaptation.

Maurin and Babich were in the vanguard of forward-thinking nurse leaders who anticipated advanced practice roles for APRNs a decade ago. As Maurin (1989) observed, "Nursing is just now beginning to attend to the impact of mental illness on families and to understand their perspective." Similarly, Babich (1991) noted, "For some mental health professionals, this requires a broadening of conceptual frameworks to view the family's dynamics as a response to coping and adaptation rather than as the cause of the patient's problems."

Nursing responded appropriately during the 1990s, the "Decade of the Brain," as professional attention turned away from family pathogenesis models of mental illness and toward neurodevelopmental models. With backing from the Center For Mental Health Services, a series of continuing education programs reintroduced APRNs to their biologic roots and taught them new skills in psychopharmacology. Concurrently, the national mental health advocacy organization National Alliance for the Mentally Ill (NAMI) promulgated the message that families who had long been considered "part of the problem" should now be made "part of the solution" as partners in treatment.

This was not an easy transition for nursing because the mindsets of some of the most influential nursing leaders had been formed in an earlier era when patients were objects to be cared for, and their families were considered impediments to that end (Taylor, 1994). Nevertheless, when the Coalition of Psychiatric Nursing Organizations convened in 1992 to revise the Standards of Psychiatric-Mental Health Clinical Nursing Practice (ANA, 1994), collaborative treatment planning with family caregivers was incorporated under Standard VI. Collaboration.

HISTORY OF PROFESSIONAL-FAMILY ■ RELATIONSHIPS

The nature of professional-family relationships has varied over time according to the assumed etiology of mental illness and the degree of contact between the two groups. For example, during the asylum period, when professionals and families had little contact with one another and mental illnesses were attributed to the interaction of heredity and societal conditions, professional attitudes toward families were nonadversarial and distant. Not until the ascendancy of psychoanalysis did professional perspectives on families become pernicious, and even then the effect on families was negligible. Although the "schizophrenogenic mother" was prominent in the psychiatric literature, families did not read the literature, and they did not often come into contact with psychiatrists because treatment focused on the individual to the exclusion of the family. For these reasons, professional-family relationships in the late 1940s and into the 1950s are best described as adversarial and distant. This mode lasted until the era of deinstitutionalization brought professionals and families into relationships that were adversarial and close.

When deinstitutionalized patients went home to their unprepared families (and inadequate community services), many suffered relapses. In accordance with the prevailing assumptions about families, the relapses were taken as evidence that the home environments were countertherapeutic (Wynne, Bernheim, & Wynne, 1990). As Lefley (1996) has discussed, this assumption spurred the investigation of theories that emphasized the "double bind" (Bateson et al., 1956), "schismatic" and "skewed" marital relationships (Lidz, Fleck, & Cornelison, 1965), and communication deviance (Wynne et al., 1977).

Graduate students in psychiatric-mental health nursing were among those who learned to recognize and analyze disturbances in ongoing family systems and to contribute to the development of a new treatment for schizophrenia called *family therapy*. Families initially welcomed family therapy because it was described to them as a method of addressing family problems, the resolution of which would benefit the patient. Some families later described family therapy as "adding insult to injury," but they were willing to be wrong if it would help their children. In the mid-1950s, Muuray Bowen initiated a project that involved hospitalizing entire families for periods up to a year. The theoretical outcomes were later described by Bowen enthusiasts as analogous to the outcomes of Darwin's 5-year voyage on the H.M.S. Beagle. Darwin "suddenly" saw evolution, as Bowen "suddenly" saw the family as an emotional unit (Kerr & Bowen, 1988). Most families did not share this enthusiasm, but they deferred to the experts. For example, James Howe, a father of two sons diagnosed with schizophrenia, said, "We paid $450 an hour to be told we caused our sons' illnesses. Our mouths dropped open, and we were a little incredulous, but what did we know? They were the experts" (McClory, 1986).

When NAMI was organized in 1979, the founding members wanted most to improve mental health services. However, a second major objective was to reduce iatrogenic burden by challenging existing theory and practice about families. The NAMI agenda also included the support of biologic research. Samuel Keith, who headed schizophrenia research at the National Institute of Mental Health (NIMH) in the 1970s, predicted that brain research would eventually remove the onus from families for causing mental illness. Keith (1997) empathized with the families' dilemma: "Families were four times punished: blamed for causing the illness, forced to watch the deterioration of their loved one, excluded from treatment plans, and required to pay for such treatment."

Within 10 years, thanks to the expanding research budget, more scientific information about the brain was generated than ever before. As Keith predicted, family attributions of mental illness became the exception rather than the rule. Nursing leaders now envision collaborative and close relationships with families and with family advocacy organizations. These partnerships are expected to endure in the future. To make this vision a reality, psychiatric-mental health nurses must include among their competencies an empathic and research-based understanding of the effects of mental illness on families.

UNDERSTANDING THE
■ EFFECTS OF MENTAL ILLNESS
Family Burden

Mental illness brings about such significant changes in people's lives that many families count time in terms of before and after its advent. The burgeoning literature on this topic has generated two basic concepts: family burden and family strengths. *Family burden* is defined as the overall level of distress experienced by the family in response to the illness. Researchers make a further distinction between *objective burden,* which refers to practical problems such as paying medical bills and enduring day-to-day hassles, and *subjective burden,* which refers to the family's affective responses to the illness.

It is sometimes said that objective burden must be experienced to be believed. Newcomers to family support groups often express relief at finally being able to speak openly about things that the uninitiated might find incredible. The following examples of objective burden were recorded during family interviews in two states:

1. *Difficulties accessing treatment:* "I called the mental health center and told them my girl was seeing demons. I begged, 'Why don't you give her a phone call or send her a postcard and ask her to come in?' It's been 3 weeks, and she hasn't gotten a phone call or a postcard" (Conn et al., 1986).

2. *Bizarre behaviors:* "My son locked himself in his bedroom for 9 months. My brother walked around outdoors in his pajamas telling the neighbors that we were trying to poison him" (Conn et al., 1986).

3. *Unexpected responsibilities:* "We are going to have an illegitimate grandchild whose mother has schizophrenia. Guess who is going to raise this child" (Conn et al., 1986).

4. *Encounters with the law:* "Our son wanted to go see Jimmy Carter because he was a Christian and might be able to help him with his problems, so he went to the White House and signed himself in as a mental patient. The first we knew of it was when the FBI and the SWAT team arrived at my place of business" (Marsh, 1992).

In the mid-1980s, the editor of a mental health newsletter reported that American families were the primary caregivers of their ill relatives much of the time and caregivers of last resort all of the time (Pepper & Ryglewicz, 1986). This is still a fairly accurate statement in spite of the creation in the past 15 years of a system of case management services that theoretically frees families from their unofficial case management duties: confronting housing authorities, fighting for entitlements and insurance coverage, investigating new medications, transporting relatives to services, and rescuing them from the criminal justice system.

Subjective burden refers to the cascade of powerful feelings that families experience in response to the illness. Sometimes families compare their experience with walking through a minefield when, at any moment, an explosion may be set off. The first feeling, however, is general disbelief. Mental illness is the last thing the average family expects. Disbelief sometimes becomes entrenched as denial, which is the family's way of protecting itself from the minefield. Families usually try to normalize their relative's emerging symptoms for as long as possible, but eventually something happens to dissolve that illusion.

The whole family was together for Christmas, and after dinner Sandra went for a walk by herself. Two hours later, she was back at the door with a policeman, who told us, "This young lady says her father is trying to kill her." That was the breaking point that told us something was terribly wrong with Sandra (Roberts, 1986).

The breaking point for Jo Anne Hinckley came with a phone call from *The Washington Post* informing her that her son had shot Ronald Reagan (Hinckley, Hinckley, & Sherrill, 1985).

Once the tragedy is acknowledged, a common reaction is anger. Often, the safest target for anger is oneself (expressed as guilt or depression) or one's spouse. Blaming one's spouse is a very common response in parental bereavement and stems not only from the need for an object for one's anger but also from the failed expectation that the partner should understand and provide necessary emotional support.

Fear is another inescapable emotion. Families are often afraid *for* their loved ones, and sometimes afraid *of* them. Although dangerousness and violence are greatly exaggerated by the media, families have valid reasons for fearing violence when their ill relatives are refusing treatment (or being unsuccessfully treated) or when they are at the same time abusing drugs or alcohol. E. Fuller Torrey (1995) has compared the family's experience of living in fear of a family member with living in a special circle of Hell:

The ambivalence inevitably felt by the family members (after an incident of violence) is formidable; fear and love, avoidance and attraction, rest uneasily side by side. Afterwards, no matter how well the patient gets, no matter how much time elapses, the memory of the past assault or violence never fully recedes.

Subjective burden also includes intense feelings of grief, anxiety, and uncertainty, as the following parents convey:

1. *Grief*: "In the dark soul of the night, I grieve for all of us: for the anguish of the past and the present and for the uncertainty of the future. Most of all, I grieve for my son and for his lost hopes and dreams" (Marsh, in press).
2. *Anxiety*: "When I meet his former classmates who are now working, finishing graduate degrees, or married, I am always aware that these things are not possible for him, just the same as someone would feel had their son died. Yet this is a mourning without end because, of course, Gary is not dead. He is very much still with us, seemingly eternally 13 years old" (Willick, 1994).
3. *Uncertainty*: "At the time of our son's diagnosis and in the many months following, I was overwhelmed with fright for him and full of anxiety, guilt, and self-doubt. The intensity of my emotional response led me to fear that all along I had never known who I was and that indeed I must have contributed to the serious impairment of my child's mind" (MacGregor, 1994).

Family Strengths

Although this chapter emphasizes family needs, the omission of family strengths would be misleading, because families have the potential to respond to the catastrophe of mental illness with resilience, rebounding from adversity and prevailing over the circumstances of their lives. Clinicians may unwittingly overlook family strengths by forming their impression of families prematurely on the basis of stereotypes. Moreover, families are often encountered for the first time in crisis situations when they may appear to be clinically disturbed but in fact are informationally and sleep deprived. If an APRN expects, on the basis of past training, to see a "dysfunctional" family, it is possible to mistake normal reactions to abnormal situations as pathologic. For example, a father's "dazed" expression might be taken for "disinterest," and the erratic behaviors of a mother who is beside herself with worry might be misconstrued as "overinvolvement." Even when the family as a whole is in shock, it is worth the effort to seek out the member with the best shock absorbers who may be able to speak and act for the others. As one family member asserted, "I can now say that, like that old aluminum foil ad, I am 'oven-tempered for maximum strength'" (Marsh & Dickens, 1997).

■ MITIGATING FAMILY RISK

While acknowledging that families often develop adaptive strategies on their own, this chapter recommends nursing strategies for mitigating family risk. Given the revival of interest in prevention that has accompanied managed care, secondary prevention strategies that were proposed in the 1960s by community psychiatrist Gerald Caplan (1964) are receiving fresh exposure, including crisis counseling, grief work, education, and support networks. Among Caplan's target populations for preventive services were people experiencing or witnessing natural disasters such as fires or floods and families witnessing the terminal illness of a loved one. A current list would include the victims and witnesses of terrorist attacks and hijackings, as well as families witnessing the mental illness of a loved one.

We in the family movement contend that the impact of mental illness is a shattering, traumatic event in the life of a family, that we have suffered the loss of those precious to us, that we struggle daily with the calamities of relapsing and incurable illnesses. We believe that families of people with serious mental illnesses certainly qualify as a population under emotional siege. In other words, we think that families are ideal candidates for secondary intervention strategies (Burland, 1996).

Family members (with the exception of spouses) are vulnerable on two counts: genetically

and as a result of exposure to traumatic experiences. Spouses are free of genetic risk, but they share in the risk for stress-related physical and mental problems: hypertension and stroke; depressive and anxiety disorders; addictions to tobacco, alcohol, and drugs; and the undermining of relationships and careers.

Stuart Nursing Prevention Paradigm

The Stuart Nursing Prevention Paradigm, which incorporates the four-step nursing process, was designed to be used in a goal-directed way to decrease the incidence of mental illness and to promote mental health (Stuart, 1998). The model presented here has been adapted for use by psychiatric-mental health nurses with families (and individual family members) dealing with mental illness:

1. *Assessment*. Identify the population at risk (e.g., families exposed to mental illness) and the stressor that precipitates maladaptive responses (perceived family burden associated with the manifestations of the relative's illness) weighed in balance against family resources (family resilience and external support system).
2. *Planning*. With input from family members, generate a Family Action Plan (or an Individual Action Plan for a given family member) to decrease stress, increase resilience, and access supports in order to promote positive adaptation.
3. *Implementation*. In collaboration with the family, implement the plan.
4. *Evaluation*. Determine the plan's effectiveness in terms of short- and long-term goals for family adaptation and self-defined family satisfaction.

Until recently, mental health professionals most often worked with families in the context of family therapy. However, as discussed previously in this chapter, using family therapy with a family that is reeling from the effects of mental illness is as inappropriate as asking family members still floating on debris after a flood to analyze their reasons for opting to live in a flood plain. Family advocates are not alone in their opposition to family therapy for these populations. The Schizophrenia Patient Outcomes Research Team (PORT) Treatment Recommendations state unequivocally that family therapies based on the premise that family dysfunction is the etiology of the patient's schizophrenic disorder should not be used (Lehman et al., 1998).

Fortunately, there is a viable alternative to family therapy: family consultation. This intervention can be offered on a one-time, intermittent, or continuing basis. Table 17-1 illustrates the differences between the two modalities. Family consultation as practiced by mental health professionals has much in common with the consultation services offered by architects and financial planners. Just as families consult architects about their dream house, or financial planners about their nest eggs, families consult a mental health professional functioning as a family consultant for help in creating a Family Action Plan for dealing with mental illness.

Effective consultation with families who are under extreme stress requires excellent listening skills, the ability to communicate simply and clearly, and the humility to check frequently with the family to be sure that the communication remains germane to their self-defined needs for assistance. It also requires an appreciation and knowledge of families' cultural diversity. Psychiatric nurses at the basic level can function as family consultants who make use of various interventions (counseling, support, education, skills training, and referral to support and advocacy groups), whereas APRNs can provide psychoeducation and clinical interventions (psychotherapy, and when legally permitted, psychopharmacology).

Family education is consistent with the health teaching nurses traditionally do with patients and families dealing with diabetes or heart disease. The application of this important function to patients with mental illness and their families is also mentioned in Chapter 18. In response to the scarcity of educational programs offered by professionals, NAMI has developed a family education program. In many states, psychiatric nurses can refer families to NAMI's Family-to-Family Education Program, which consists of twelve $2\frac{1}{2}$-hour sessions that are team taught by trained family members.

table 17-1

COMPARISON OF FAMILY THERAPY AND FAMILY CONSULTATION

	FAMILY THERAPY	FAMILY CONSULTATION
Paradigm	Family dysfunction	Family competence
Professional role	Therapist	Consultant
Family role	Patient	Consultee
Mode	Authoritarian	Collaborative
Focus of intervention	Family system	Family agenda
Goal	Reduced dysfunction	Enhanced coping
Outcome measure	Patient improvement	Family satisfaction
Communication	Often partially concealed	Open, direct, and complete
Family status	Part of patient's treatment plan	Part of patient's treatment team
Place in family action plan	Often sole family service	One component of service plan

From Marsh, in press.

Referral to support groups is another effective intervention that has a long history in the substance abuse field, predating its adoption in mental health. Names and phone numbers of contact persons for NAMI affiliates in any geographic area are available by calling the toll-free number: 1-800-950-NAMI. The number is often busy, but callers can leave a request on the machine, along with their name and address. It is a good idea to request lists of local affiliates; NAMI's Resource Catalogue (books, posters, and videos); and information about NAMI's website. Psychiatric-mental health nurses are welcome to join NAMI and to attend local and national meetings to learn from families about their experiences with mental illness and to let families know that help is available from psychiatric-mental health nurses. Although families just starting their journey with mental illness have a compelling need for support, most families farther down the road become involved in advocacy. This transition is easily made in NAMI affiliates, where advocacy is regarded as the final stage in family adaptation. Winning a fiercely fought battle for a group home or persuading advertisers to withdraw a stigmatizing ad are activities that, in addition to their intended purpose, help restore lost self-esteem, inspire hope, and in some measure compensate for irreparable losses.

Family psychoeducation is sometimes spoken of interchangeably with family education, but the two approaches have very different philosophic roots. *Family education* was originated by Agnes Hatfield, a professional in the field of education and a founding member of NAMI, based on a needs assessments conducted among families dealing with mental illness. In contrast, *family psychoeducation* is an outgrowth of family therapy and was developed after research conducted in England in the early 1970s showed that certain caregiver behaviors (criticism, hostility, and overinvolvement) labeled *expressed emotion* were associated with increased rates of relapse. Psychoeducation teaches caregivers to modify these behaviors and to improve their basic communication and problem-solving skills to accommodate the special needs of individuals with the core information-processing deficits associated with serious mental illness. Nurses involved in psychoeducation are usually part of a multidisciplinary, institution-based rehabilitation program. Most such programs last between 9 months and 1 year and include a segment on "joining with" or "engaging" the family, followed by sessions on mental illnesses as brain disorders, information and skills related to the management of medication and other treatments, and class exercises and homework assignments on communication and problem solving skills. Elements of a psychoeducation plan are included in Box 17-1.

Randomized clinical trials have repeatedly demonstrated that family interventions that provide some combination of illness education, support, problem solving training, and crisis intervention, in combination with appropriate pharmacotherapy, reduce 1-year relapse rates from a 40% to 53% range to a 2% to 23% range. This is strong evidence for the benefits of family psychoeducation for patients. The evidence for its positive effects on other members of the family is less compelling but has been called "suggestive" (Lehman et al., 1998).

Psychotherapy and psychopharmacology are other useful interventions for a significant minority of family members whose needs go beyond support, education, and skills. Neither psychotherapy nor medication should be considered first-line interventions for family members. However, either modality may offer a valuable resource for those family members whose preexisting mental health problems have been exacerbated by the stress of caregiving or for those who have developed significant reactive problems such as depression, anxiety, or substance abuse.

RISK FOR INDIVIDUAL ■ FAMILY MEMBERS

Although the levels of genetic risk for mental illness associated with various degrees of relationship are available and widely used for genetic

box 17-1

ELEMENTS OF A PSYCHOEDUCATION PLAN

SIGNS AND SYMPTOMS	THERAPEUTIC STRATEGIES
Natural course of the illness	Adaptive coping responses
Possible etiologies	Potential compliance problems
Diagnostic tests and measures	Early warning signs of relapse
Treatment options	Indicated lifestyle changes
Expected treatment outcomes	Balancing needs and taking care of oneself
Medication effects and side effects	

From Sundeen, 1998.

counseling, significantly less information is available about psychosocial risk. The 1994 Institute of Medicine Report on Reducing Risks For Mental Disorders acknowledged that this area is understudied:

Schizophrenia in a family member can become a risk factor for stress-related disorders in other family members. The degree to which caregiver burden is linked with the development of stress-related problems such as depression, irregular sleeping and eating patterns, aggravated health problems, increased use of alcohol and tranquilizers, marital strain, and irritability is not known. However, it has been found that the levels of psychologic distress of family members who care for a person with schizophrenia are about twice the level expected in the general population (Mrazek & Haggerty, 1994).

Existing studies suggest that caregiving conveys a risk for stress-related mental and physical disorders. An epidemiologic survey of mental health in Florida revealed that anxiety, depression, and psychosocial dysfunction were significantly higher for respondents who had a family member with mental illness than for those who did not. The level of reported anxiety and depression was twice as high, and the level of psychosocial dysfunction was three times as high (Arey & Warheit, 1980).

In a study of mental illness in the families of mental health professionals, Lefley (1987) found that 38% of the sample reported an adverse effect on their physical health, with mothers and siblings being the most often affected. Other studies have also identified caregiver burden as primarily a women's issue. For example, in a 1986 study of family burden in Georgia, 80% of the caregivers were women (Francell, Conn, & Gray, 1988). As Patricia Gray (1990) has discussed, society's devaluation of "women's work" can add a second layer of low self-esteem and depression among the mothers, daughters, sisters, and wives who commit large segments of their lives to caring for relatives with mental illness.

Parents

To augment knowledge about the long-term effects of family burden on family health, a Wisconsin research team that included an APRN in psychiatric and mental health care studied the relationship between subjective burden and maternal health in a sample of mothers whose adult children had schizophrenia (Greenberg et al., 1993). In this sample, burdens associated with stigma and worries about the future were significant predictors of maternal physical health.

The reverse of this situation is one in which children have a parent with mental illness. Although this risk has long been acknowledged, many such children and adolescents receive no preventive services, nor do their mothers receive help in parenting. One study showed that the children of single mothers were especially vulnerable because their mothers were least able to fulfill supportive parenting roles (Carpentier et al., 1992).

An NIMH-funded study in Detroit is currently addressing deficiencies in knowledge about the parenting experiences of women with mental illnesses (Mowbry, 1998). The 379 mothers in this study are subject to multiple stressors in addition to their mental illnesses. For instance, most had incomes below the poverty level and many reported deaths in the family, personal injury, and physical illness. Although 90% were linked with mental health professionals, only 17% indicated that they could turn to their mental health professional for "support and advice as a mother" (Mowbry, 1998). Often, mothers with mental illness refrain from mentioning their children to mental health professionals because of their well-justified fear that the children will be taken away from them (Nicholson, Sweeney, & Geller, 1998). Psychiatric nurses who come across to these mothers as trustworthy and willing to work with them around parenting issues are providing valuable services both to these mothers and to their children.

Offspring and Siblings

Personal accounts written by adult offspring reflect the adverse consequences of the failure to provide preventive services in a timely fashion:

I recall clearly the feelings of guilt, fear, anger, grief, and mistrust. I now understand how they affected my life. Why did my father's mental illness affect me so? Because mental illness becomes a family illness, regardless of who carries its symptoms. It reaches out and scars the life of each family member. No one walks away unaffected (Marsh & Dickens, 1997).

The timing of the relative's illness is a crucial variable. If it occurs when offspring or siblings are children, their acquisition of basic trust and attachment may be affected, as well as academic and interpersonal skills. If they are adolescents at the time, there may be problems with emerging sexuality, career planning, and separation from the family of origin (Marsh, in press). Sometimes emotional responses and practical considerations combine to create indecision and ambiguity. For example, young adults who are ambivalent about leaving home may feel pressured to stay in order to help with the caregiving. Likewise, these family members may avoid making a long-term commitment to a life partner as they wait for someone willing to accept an in-law with a mental illness.

In a study of 30 adult siblings conducted in Iowa, nurse researchers found a significant adverse relationship between effects of the mental illness and the health of the "well" sibling (Lively, Friedrich, & Buckwalter, 1995). The schizophrenia of their brother or sister had a reported effect on mental health for two-thirds (66%) of the participants and on physical health for 20%. When describing how their mental health was affected, participants expressed fear of getting mental illness, an impaired sense of self, and sadness and stress. The well siblings, whose average age was 37, admitted to having poor health habits such as lack of exercise and overeating, which they connected with the stress of living with their relative's illness. All participants in the Iowa study experienced grief over the "lost" brother or sister they once knew. In contrast to the grief after the death of a family member, siblings experience chronic, unending grief. The researchers recommended the following actions on the part of psychiatric nurses:

1. Take the initiative to open up communication because siblings need to talk with empathic professionals who understand their point of view.
2. Provide siblings with information and education because this allows the anxiety-producing stimulus to be reappraised, thereby increasing the chance of effective coping.

3. Develop crisis strategies that siblings can easily access to help them deal with suicide threats and attempts, as well as verbal and physical aggression against themselves.
4. Offer stress-reduction methods such as relaxation techniques.
5. Refer siblings to support groups specifically for siblings or for siblings and offspring.

In an intensive study of 14 adult siblings of persons with schizophrenia, Gerace, Camilleri, and Ayres (1993) identified three distinct patterns in the subject's approach to the siblings' illnesses: collaborative, crisis oriented, and detached. One subject in the collaborative category explained how she shared caregiving responsibilities with her mother and her husband:

My mother and I take turns. When one of us gets burned out the other one deals with it. We talk about everything and discuss the alternatives. And my husband is just as much a fighter for my sister and my mom and me. He has just been such a source of support. He can go to my sister and talk sense into her in situations when she is angry at my mother and me (Gerace, Camilleri, & Ayres, 1993).

In one family, the crisis-oriented involvement was well documented during the researcher's visit to a male sibling's home. The telephone rang and the sibling took a call from his father, who needed help because the ill brother was screaming and throwing dishes on the floor, and the mother was crying. After he dealt with the situation by talking individually with each family member, this sibling cried openly and told the researcher that such calls occurred several times a week.

Siblings categorized as "detached" were only relatively detached. They were still involved in housing, finances, and interactions with care providers, but they tried to keep their direct involvement with the ill brother or sister to a minimum. Some appeared to be trying to ease themselves out of the situation because of the high cost to their own growth and well-being. In a study of adult siblings and offspring conducted by Marsh and Dickens (1997), more than three-quarters (77%) of participants had sought psychotherapy. The percentage was even higher (90%) among those who were both siblings and

offspring, and among those who were 10 years of age or younger at the onset of their relative's mental illness. Almost all rated the therapy as helpful, although one participant cited the "very poor grasp of mental illness" among clinicians (Marsh, in press).

Marsh and Dickens pointed out that few of the adult siblings and offspring they studied had any kind of services available to them when they were growing up. Had their concerns been addressed during their childhood and adolescence, perhaps their need for therapy in adulthood would have been less compelling. Box 17-2 shows clearly that

box **17-2**

CONCERNS OF ADULT SIBLINGS AND OFFSPRING

Caregiving for their relative (94%)
Family disruption (83%)
Difficulty balancing personal and family needs (81%)
Sense that their own needs had not been met (79%)
Feelings of helplessness and hopelessness (75%)
Poor self-esteem (75%)
Guilt feelings (74%)
Psychic numbing (70%)
Problems trusting (69%)
Problems with intimacy (69%)
Sense of growing up too fast (67%)
Personal depression (66%)
Chronic sorrow (64%)
Sense of unfulfilled potential (64%)
Need to be perfect (63%)
Grieving process (63%)
Sense of abandonment (61%)
Identity problems (59%)
Fear of violence (57%)
Social isolation (54%)
Fear of suicide (52%)
Effect on personal choices (51%)
Difficulty separating from their family (51%)

Percentages refer to those participants who experienced this illness-related concern at least sometimes. From Marsh & Dickens, 1997.

siblings and offspring live under a cloud of problems. Psychiatric nurses committed to diagnosing and treating human responses to actual or potential health problems need look no further.

Spouses

Although an estimated 35% to 40% of people hospitalized for mental illness are discharged to live with their husbands or wives, and close to half a million persons are constantly exposed to their partner's mental illness, spouses are underrepresented in the family burden literature. However, the spousal burden is considerable.

My husband's schizophrenia is like a third member in our marriage. It is always there. Even with medication, we still deal with his paranoia, his isolation, and his need for my full attention on a daily basis (Marsh, in press).

In a study of couples in England that included a depressed member, researchers found that nearly half of the spouses had come to think of their partners as another child in need of supervision (Fadden, Bebbington, & Kuipers, 1987). Not surprisingly, these couples experienced elevated rates of separation and divorce. Despite valiant attempts to uphold vows to remain faithful "in sickness and in health," many well spouses reluctantly leave the marriage. Three years after the NAMI state affiliate in Alabama made a video about "successful coping" when mental illness invades a family, all the marriages depicted in the video had dissolved. On the other hand, Penny and Fred Frese, who produced a video called *Living With Schizophrenia: A Love Story,* remain together. Dr. Fred Frese, a psychologist who serves on the NAMI Board of Directors, frequently speaks about the adaptation necessary to live in the world of CNPs (his acronym for Chronically Normal Persons) and credits his wife for her role in keeping him organized and functional.

When the durability of the marriage becomes an issue in therapy or consultation, it is usually advisable to assume a neutral stance while assisting spouses to examine their options. Some spouses have complained that therapists too quickly jump to the conclusion that reluctance to divorce is a sign of codependency.

Every single one of us [in the support group] has been told by therapists that we should get a divorce. If we don't get a divorce, there must be something wrong with us. We must be codependent, or on a power trip, etc. That is painfully common" (Marsh, in press).

Ultimately, after making up their minds, some spouses will need help to remain in the marriage, and others will require assistance to leave. Family therapist Edie Mannion (in press), who with family member Marilyn Meisel offers spouse coping skills workshops at the Training and Education Center (TEC) Network in Philadelphia, has described spouses as the "ultimate acrobats." While walking on a highwire of moral dilemmas, they are juggling a host of roles, feelings, and questions If they contemplate divorce, they may worry about precipitating their partner's relapse or even suicide. If they remain in the marriage, they may lose their personal identities in the everyday struggle to play multiple roles in the family without the help of the partner.

In *Crazy Love,* one of the few books about the spousal experience, author Phyllis Naylor (1977) tells of borrowing money to pay for her husband's treatment in a private hospital only to discover after his discharge that he only pretended to relinquish his delusional system to gain his freedom. When Naylor finally left the marriage, it was with great ambivalence:

No matter how thoroughly one insists that a relationship is over, it is never quite ended. No matter how much one wants to begin life anew, the past is never quite forgotten. No matter how strongly I had promised to remain detached, my heart cried out when I saw him, wept for him and for all that he might have been, for what we could have had together" (Naylor, 1977).

In addition to their personal needs, spouses often require assistance in helping their children cope with their parent's mental illness. Marsh (in press) suggests that spouses can benefit from professional assistance in the following areas:

- Learning to explain mental illness to their children
- Assuring the children that they are not to blame

- Encouraging children to discuss their feelings and concerns
- Reinforcing their participation in activities (Scouts, sports, hobbies)
- Providing special comfort in times of distress
- Promoting compassion and respect for the ill parent
- Offering suggestions for answering questions from peers

IMPLICATIONS FOR ■ THE FUTURE

This chapter identifies families as people at risk for stress-related disorders and calls on APRNs to help mitigate this risk. The following vignettes portray RNs and APRNs reaching out to families in the diverse settings in which nurses will be working in the new century.

Nurse-Operated Clinic

Helen Jordan, APRN, obtained her master's degree in psychiatric nursing from a graduate program that taught her the value of family caregiving for the patient, as well as the subjective and objective cost of caregiving for the family. Consequently, she has incorporated these values into the management of a nurse-staffed psychiatric treatment/rehabilitation center located in a state that allows appropriately prepared psychiatric-mental health nurses to practice independently. In this clinic, family assessment modeled on the Stuart Nursing Prevention Paradigm is as much a part of the admission procedure as patient assessment. The resultant Family Action Plan, at a minimum, calls for family caregiver participation along with patients in a multiple-session educational program aimed at illness management and for health maintenance within a treatment context that takes into account the needs of the whole family. Jordan is now developing outcome measures, which she plans to incorporate into a controlled study in order to demonstrate the cost effectiveness of the family-focused treatment used by the clinic.

Office-Based Practice

Janet Brown, APRN, who has an office-based practice of psychotherapy, treats many patients who incidentally are family members of persons with serious mental illnesses. For example, the wife of a couple being seen for marriage counseling has a brother with schizophrenia, and a young woman who consulted Brown because she has trouble maintaining romantic relationships had a mother who was in and out of psychiatric hospitals all during her childhood. Thanks to her extensive reading about the effects of mental illness on siblings and offspring, Brown knows that these bits of family history are relevant to the concerns that brought her patients into therapy. She adjusts her treatment approach accordingly. After experiencing the satisfaction of helping several persons in this way, Brown decides to expand her practice by identifying herself as a consultant to family caregivers as well as a psychotherapist. In preparation, she joined NAMI and attends national and local meetings to learn about the needs of family members and to make families aware of the services provided by psychiatric nurses. (To her surprise, she finds that families are not very well informed about the competencies of APRNs.)

Other Community Settings

Because of the prevalence of mental illness in the population, family members can be found in all community settings. Indeed, NAMI estimates that approximately one out of five families is affected by mental illness. However, these families are easily overlooked because they often refrain from speaking openly about their ill relatives. For example, Emily Jones, who is an APRN working in a school-based primary care program, is unaware that the child referred to her for truancy problems has a mother suffering from schizophrenia. That information does not appear in the school records and will only come out after Emily has established a relationship of trust with another family member, possibly the grandmother.

For the same reason, Don Rude, RN, BSN, who works as a staff nurse at an elder care center while studying for his master's degree in psychiatric nursing, does not know at first that the wife who visits his patient with Alzheimer's disease goes home to a 23-year-old daughter who has been diagnosed with bipolar disorder but refuses medication. Rude learns of the wife's additional caregiving responsibilities only after he takes time to talk with her during visiting hours. She is appropriately grateful for his support; for the book he loans her, *When Someone You Love Has Mental Illness* (Woolis, 1992); and for a referral to a local NAMI support group. Wanting to repay him for his kindness, she volunteers to be a participant in the research on family caregiving that Rude is undertaking for his master's degree.

Dorothy Major, RN, BSN, who directs an intensive case management team serving 25 individuals with serious mental illness, encourages the recipients of intensive case management services to sign confidentiality waivers allowing her to talk with their families. Major, who has a brother with mental illness, looks upon families as an extension of the caregiving network provided by the case management team. She not only makes herself available for consultation regarding day-to-day caregiving issues but also invites families to participate in "medication rounds" that she offers for case managers to supplement their meager backgrounds in psychopharmacology. The family participation is not passive. In addition to acquiring new knowledge, family members are encouraged to share their experientially based knowledge with case managers.

Faculty Practice

Margaret Conners, APRN, PhD, teaches an introductory course in psychiatric-mental health nursing to undergraduates at a school affiliated with a medical center that has a large schizophrenia research program. With the collaboration of the researchers, she has converted some unused space into a Family Resource Center for the families of patients who are participating in research protocols. Connors has equipped the center with books, journal articles, and videos on mental illness and uses it for informal contacts with families, as well as for scheduled "Ask The Nurse" sessions and weekly family education classes. The students in the introductory course participate in the operation of the Family Resource Center under Connor's supervision, and each student arranges with a family for their collaboration in writing a term paper on "Coping With Mental Illness: The Family Perspective." Connors is convinced that the faculty practice serves three useful purposes: 1) provides families with needed support and information, 2) increases the family's motivation to encourage their relatives to participate in research, and 3) provides an interesting and nonthreatening field experience for students that may influence them to select psychiatric nursing for advanced study and future practice.

RESOURCES AND CONNECTIONS

ORGANIZATIONS

National Alliance for the Mentally Ill
200 N. Glebe Road, Suite 1015
Arlington, VA 22203
703-524-7600

National Depressive and Manic Depressive Association
730 N. Franklin Street, Suite 501
Chicago, IL 60610
312-642-0049

BOOKS

Amenson, C.S. (1998a). *Schizophrenia: a family education curriculum.* Pasadena, CA: Pacific Clinics Institute.

Amenson, C.S. (1998b). *Schizophrenia: family education methods.* Pasadena, CA: Pacific Clinics Institute.

Hatfield, A.B. (1990). *Family education in mental illness.* New York: Guilford.

Lefley, H.P., & Wasow, M. (Eds.). (1994). *Helping families cope with mental illness.* Newark: Harwood Academic.

Miklowitz, D.J., & Goldstein, M.J. (1997). *Bipolar disorder: a family-focused treatment approach.* New York: Guilford.

Mueser, K.T., & Gingerich, S. (1994). *Coping with schizophrenia: a guide for families.* Oakland, CA: New Harbinger.

Mueser, K.T., & Glynn, S.M. (1995). *Behavioral family therapy for psychiatric disorders.* Boston: Allyn & Bacon.

Wasow, M. (1995). *The skipping stone: ripple effects of mental illness on the family.* Palo Alto, CA: Science & Behavior Books.

VIDEOTAPES

The Bonnie tapes. (1997). (a) *Mental illness in the family;* (b) *My sister is mentally ill;* and (c) *Recovering from mental illness.* Contact Mental Illness Education Project videos, Hohokus, NJ.

Breaking the dark horse. (1994). Writer's Group/Trident Productions, Inc.

Mental illness: the family story. (1997). Pittsburgh: Alliance for the Mentally Ill of Southwestern Pennsylvania.

WEBSITES

help! A Consumers' Guide to Mental Health Information
www.icomm.ca/madmagic/help/help.html

Georgia Mental Health Network
www.mcg.edu/resources/mh/index.html

Mental Health Education Page: Removing the Stigma of Mental Illness
www.metrolink.net/~jquimby/mh.htm

Mental Health InfoSource
mhsource.com

Mental Health Net
www.cmhcsys.com

Wing of Madness: General Mental Health Sources
members.aol.com/depress/genment.htm

Alliance for the Mentally Ill/Friends and Advocates of the Mentally Ill
www.nami-nyc-metro.org

Family Caregiver Alliance
www.caregiver.org

National Alliance for the Mentally Ill
www.nami.org

National Depressive and Manic-Depressive Association
www.ndmda.org

National Mental Health Association
www.nmha.org

Suicide Awareness/Voices of Education (SAVE)
www.save.org

References

American Nurses Association. (1994). *Statement on Psychiatric-Mental Health Clinical Nursing Practice and Standards of Psychiatric-Mental Health Clinical Nursing Practice.* Washington, DC: American Nurses Publishing.

Arey, S., & Warheit, G.J. (1980). Psychosocial costs of living with psychologically disturbed family members. In Robins, L.N., Clayton, P.J., & Wing, J.K. (Eds.). *The social consequences of psychiatric illness.* New York: Brunner/Mazel.

Babich, K.S. (1991). The concept of discharge planning. In Babich, K.S., & Brown, L. (Eds.). *Discharge planning.* Thorofare, NJ: SLACK Press.

Bateson, G., et al. (1956). Toward a theory of schizophrenia. *Behavioral Science, 1,* 251–264.

Burland, J. (1996). *Alliance for the mentally ill provider course.* Burlington, VT: Vermont Alliance for the Mentally Ill.

Caplan, G. (1964). *Principles of preventive psychiatry.* New York: Basic Books.

Carpentier, N., et al. (1992). Burden of care of families not living with young schizophrenics. *Hospital and Community Psychiatry, 43,* 38–43.

Conn, V.S., et al. (1986). *Families' perspectives of Georgia's State Mental Health System: results of focus groups in 8 catchment areas.* Atlanta, GA: Georgia Department of Human Resources.

Fadden, G., Bebbington, P., & Kuipers, L. (1987). Caring and its burdens: a study of the spouses of depressed patients. *British Journal of Psychiatry, 151,* 660–667.

Francell, C.G., Conn, V.S., & Gray, D.P. (1988). Family perceptions of burden of care of chronic mentally ill relatives. *Hospital and Community Psychiatry, 39,* 1296–1300.

Gerace, L.M., Camilleri, D., & Ayres, L. (1993). Sibling perspectives on schizophrenia and the family. *Schizophrenia Bulletin, 19,* 637–647.

Gray, D.P. (1990). The challenge of caring for the chronically mentally ill. In Nottingham, J., & Nottingham, J. (Eds.). *The professional and family caregiver: dilemmas, rewards, and new directions.* Americus, GA: Georgia Southwestern College Press.

Greenberg, J.S., et al. (1993). Mothers caring for an adult child with schizophrenia: the effects of subjective burden on maternal health. *Family Relations, 42,* 205–211.

Hinckley, J., & Hinckley, J.A., with Sherrill, E. (1985). *Breaking points.* Grand Rapids, MI: Zondervan Press.

Keith, S.J. (1997). Working together. *The Journal of the California Alliance for the Mentally Ill, 8*(3), 9–10.

Kerr, M.E., & Bowen, M. (1988). *Family evaluation.* New York: Norton.

Lehman, A.F., Steinwachs, D.M., & the Co-Investigators of the PORT Project. (1998). At issue: translating research into practice: the Schizophrenia Patient Outcomes Research Team (PORT) Treatment Recommendations. *Schizophrenia Bulletin, 24,* 1–10.

Lefley, H.P. (1987). Impact of mental illness in families of mental health professionals. *Journal of Nervous and Mental Disease, 175,* 613–619.

Lefley, H.P. (1996). *Family caregiving in mental illness.* Thousand Oaks, CA: Sage.

Lidz, T., Fleck, S., & Cornelison, A.R. (1965). *Schizophrenia and the family.* New York: International Universities Press.

Lively, S., Friedrich, R.M., & Buckwalter, K.C. (1995). Sibling perception of schizophrenia: impact on relationships, roles, and health. *Issues in Mental Health Nursing, 16,* 225–238.

MacGregor, P. (1994). Grief: the unrecognized parental response to mental illness in a child. *Social Work, 39,* 160–166.

Mannion, E. (in press). The ultimate acrobats. *The Journal of the California Alliance for the Mentally Ill* [special spouse issue].

Marsh, D.T. (1992). *Families and mental illness: new directions in professional practice.* New York: Praeger.

Marsh, D.T. (in press). *Serious mental illness and the family: the practitioner's guide.* New York: Wiley & Sons.

Marsh, D.T., & Dickens, R.M. (1997). *Troubled journey: coming to terms with the mental illness of a sibling or parent.* New York: Tarcher/Putnam.

Maurin, J.T. (1989). The family experience of mental illness. In Maurin, J.T. (Ed.). *Chronic mental illness: coping strategies.* Thorofare, NJ: SLACK Press.

McClory, T. (1986). History of NAMI. *WAYS, 1,* 16–18.

Mowbry, C.G. (1998). Coping with motherhood and mental illness. *NAMI Advocate, 19*(5), 12–13.

Mrazek, P.J., & Haggerty, R.J. (Eds.). (1994). *Reducing risks for mental disorders: frontiers for preventive intervention research.* Washington, DC: Institute of Medicine, National Academy Press.

Naylor, P. (1977). *Crazy love.* New York: Signet Books.

Nicholson, J., Sweeney, E.M., & Geller, J.L. (1998). Mothers with mental illness. I. The competing demands of parenting and living with mental illness. *Psychiatric Services, 49,* 635–649.

Peplau, H. (1975). Foreword. In Smoyak, S. (Ed.). *The psychiatric nurse as a family therapist.* New York: Wiley & Sons.

Pepper, B., & Ryglewicz, H. (1986). Issues for advocacy. *TIE-Lines, 3*(2), 4–7.

Roberts, S. (1986). *Worst of two worlds: a personal account of a daughter's illness.* In Conn, V. Unpublished personal accounts.

Stuart, G. (1998). Mental health promotion. In Stuart, G., & Laraia, M. (Eds.). *Principles and practice of psychiatric nursing* (ed. 6). St. Louis: Mosby.

Sundeen, S. (1998). Psychiatric rehabilitation. In Stuart, G., & Laraia, M. (Eds.). *Principles and practice of psychiatric nursing* (ed. 6). St. Louis: Mosby.

Taylor, C. (1994). Editorial. *Archives of Psychiatric Nursing, 8*(5), 289.

Torrey, E.F. (1995). *Surviving schizophrenia: a manual for families, consumers and providers* (ed. 3). New York: HarperCollins.

Willick, M.S. (1994). Schizophrenia: a parent's perspective: mourning without end. In Andreasen, N. (Ed.). *From mind to molecule.* Washington, DC: American Psychiatric Press.

Woolis, R. (1992). *When someone you love has a mental illness.* New York: Tarcher/Perigee.

Wynne, L.C., Bernheim, K.F., & Wynne, A.R. (1990). Key issues for training in family therapy with long-term, seriously mentally ill patients and their families. In Lefley, H.P. (Ed.). *Clinical training in serious mental illness* (USDHHS Pub. No. ADM 90-1679). Washington, DC: US Government Printing Office.

Wynne, L.C., et al. (1977). Schizophrenics and their families: research on parental communication. In Tanner, J.M. (Ed.). *Developments in psychiatric research.* London: Hodder & Stoughton.

chapter 18

Consumer Advocacy

PHYLLIS M. CONNOLLY

■ INTRODUCTION

This chapter provides definitions of advocacy from the literature, consumer, and family perspectives. Advocacy needs of consumers and families are identified as well as system level advocacy. The importance of advocacy today is discussed. The role of advocacy within the domains of advanced nursing practice and the skills and competencies are identified. The role and importance of patient advocacy organizations is explained. Outcomes of advocacy and barriers to advocacy are explored. Advice from consumers and families is provided.

In this chapter, persons with serious mental illness are designated as "consumers" rather than "patients" or "clients." The emphasis on the consumer of mental health services is congruent with the empowerment models and concepts of recovery, rehabilitation, wellness, and self-control of symptoms.

ADVOCACY IN
■ ADVANCED PRACTICE
Definitions of Advocacy

Advocacy is defined as "active support as of a cause, idea or policy" (Berube, 1985). *To advocate* is to speak in favor of, recommend, argue for a cause, support, or defend. Bandman and Bandman (1995) define *advocacy* as "giving support and protection to a specific person in need." A stronger statement was expressed by DeFries (1993) asserting that mental health professionals have a professional obligation to diagnose, treat, and ad-

387

vocate. Furthermore, he argues that mental health professionals need to vigorously challenge the status quo and should not accept unrealistic limitations on resources placed by government agencies. He also asserts that mental health professionals should reject programs that are politically expedient and promote preventive services that are cost effective at the expense of treatment services. Last, he urges all mental health professionals to challenge quiescent peers to join in advocacy efforts. Individuals, families, professionals, groups, communities, systems, schools, institutions, and society all need advocacy at various times.

Advocacy is an integral and dynamic component of nursing practice. The core values of nursing—a person-centered focus, active patient/consumer involvement in matters of self-determination, and independence of choice and decision making in matters of health, illness, rehabilitation, and recovery—form the very context for advocacy. Box 18-1 lists the structural support for nursing advocacy.

The *Code for Nurses* established by the American Nurses Association specifically defines the nurse's relationship to the client as one of an advocate (ANA, 1985). Code 3 states that "the nurse acts to safeguard the client and the public when healthcare and safety are affected by the incompetent, unethical, or illegal practice of any person" (ANA, 1985). It is the principle of autonomy (always placing the person at the center of decision making) along with the principles of beneficence (doing good), nonmaleficence (avoiding harm), veracity (telling the truth), confidentiality (respecting privileged information), fidelity (keeping promises), and justice (treating people fairly) that all support the value of respect for persons (Bandman & Bandman, 1995). This is clearly stated in ANA Code 1: "The nurse provides services with respect for human dignity and the uniqueness of the client, unrestricted by considerations of social or economic status, personal attributes, or the nature of health problems" (ANA, 1985).

There are no rights without advocacy. Band-

Box 18-1
SUPPORT FOR NURSING ADVOCACY

- ANA Standard V Ethics: The psychiatric-mental health nurse's decision and actions on behalf of clients are determined in an ethical manner (American Nurses Association, 1994).
- ANA Code 1: The nurse provides services with respect for human dignity and the uniqueness of the client, unrestricted by considerations of social or economic status, personal attributes, or the nature of health problems (ANA, 1985).
- ANA Code 3: The nurse acts to safeguard the client and the public when health care and safety are affected by the incompetent, unethical, or illegal practice of any person (ANA, 1985).
- ANA Code 11: The nurse collaborates with members of the health professions and other citizens in promoting community and national efforts to meet the health needs of the public (ANA, 1985).
- Protection and Advocacy for the Mentally Ill Individuals Act, 1986
- Americans With Disability Act, 1990
- Quality First: Better Health Care for All Americans, 1997

man and Bandman (1995) discuss the three reasons why there are no rights without advocacy: 1) rightholders may not always be in a position to defend their rights, whereas other persons may be; 2) there are no rights without claims effectively made on behalf of such rights; and 3) the right to claim is not necessarily vested in a rightholder alone. Others can and have made claims on behalf of those whose rights have been ignored or violated (Bandman & Bandman, 1995). Often, this is the case for persons with psychiatric or mental health problems.

The document on standards for psychiatric-mental health clinical practice (ANA, 1994), which was developed by the ANA Council on Psychiatric and Mental Health Nursing, the American Psychiatric Nurses Association (APNA), the Association of Child and Adolescent Psychiatric Nurses, and the Society for Education and Research in Psychiatric-Mental Health Nursing addresses the nurse's function as a client advocate. One of the measurement criteria of Standard V. Ethics is as follows: "the psychiatric-mental health nurse's decision and actions on behalf of clients are determined in an ethical manner" (ANA, 1994). According to the rationale provided for this standard, the psychiatric-mental health nurse engages in therapeutic interactions and relationships promoting and supporting the healing process.

Clearly, advocacy is a nursing intervention and an essential component of psychiatric-mental health nursing. Although nursing has always viewed the nurse as an advocate, various social policies, especially those instituted as part of the mental health movement in the 1970s, have increased society's attention to the need for advocacy. As a result, states developed both advocacy programs for patients and grievance procedures, which made it possible for patients to express their views about their treatment. In 1986, the Protection and Advocacy for the Mentally Ill Individuals Act required that all states designate an agency that would be responsible for maintaining the rights of people with mental illnesses. In more recent legislation, the Americans with Disabilities Act (ADA) passed in 1990 offers protection for over 43 million Americans with physical or mental disabilities from discrimination in public services, jobs, and accommodations. Although the ADA is the most extensive legislation yet to afford protection for those eligible, many do not use the protection it offers because of the ongoing stigma related to disclosing a mental illness. Also, according to a recent study (Wasserbauer, 1996), the majority of psychiatric nurses surveyed did not have the knowledge about the ADA to act

as advocates for their patients. Only a few gave patients information related to ADA. Wasserbauer (1997) provides a comprehensive description of the ADA and the need for advocacy for persons with mental disabilities emphasizing the barrier that stigma still plays. The consumer movement, self-help, and empowerment models (Fisher, 1994; Fisher, 1995; Segal, Silverman, & Temkin, 1995a) have not only increased the need for advocacy by the nurse and the need for families to advocate for themselves and their loved ones but have also taught consumers how to advocate for themselves and others.

Key informants of consumers and family members were asked to offer their definitions of *advocacy*, which appear in Box 18 2. Several consumers and family members provided their perspectives about advocacy for this chapter. Through the mail, 24 individuals (family members and consumers) received the APNA brochures *Advanced Practice Registered Nurses in Psychiatric and Mental Health Care* and *Mental Health Care: A Consumer's Guide* and a survey developed by the author to elicit relevant information for this chapter. These people were considered experts (i.e., actively involved in key advocacy organizations). Some hold or held leadership positions. Nine completed the surveys. Their definitions provide the advanced practice registered nurse (APRN) in psychiatric-mental health nursing with some insight into what some consumers and families believe about advocacy.

Need for Advocacy

Many factors contribute to the need for advocacy today including a managed care environment, continuous efforts to cut costs, increased complex care and use of related technology, more options for psychotherapeutic medications, and a shift in treatment setting from institutions to the community and, in some cases, into the criminal justice system. Additional factors are related to changes in treatment approaches: for example, using

box 18-2

CONSUMER AND FAMILY DEFINITIONS OF ADVOCACY

- Speaking out and working towards justice for a population of persons with severe mental illness who have been discriminated against in American society.
- Becoming educated and assertive in the area you are dealing with in order to be effective in promoting changes in treatment, housing, and whatever issues are important to the person or group for which you are advocating.
- Politicking, educating, negotiating, and using proper tools to get your needs or your group needs met.
- Someone who protects the rights of individuals and fights for parity in insurance coverage, for housing, or in the workplace under ADA guidelines either as caregiver or just before the legislature.
- A go between who knows the system and will advise you.
- A fight for rights to not be harmed, hurt, abused, harassed, and to have choice.
- To act voluntarily on behalf of an individual or class of people in order to obtain needed services for those people or to bring about changes that will benefit them.
- Ensuring that consumers' rights are protected at all times and that they receive access to quality care and having professionals who really care about clients and family.

box 18-3

IMPORTANCE OF ADVOCACY TODAY

- Managed care environment
- Emphasis on reducing cost
- Increased complexity of care
- Increased use of technology
- Increased medication efficacy
- Shifts in treatment settings
- Changes in treatment approaches
- Recognition of role of rehabilitation
- Disability view versus disease view
- Effectiveness of psychosocial interventions
- Recognition of need for chronic care
- Emphasis on recovery
- Interest in wellness
- Increased use of self help models

box 18-4

ISSUES NEEDING ADVOCACY

Stigma
Discrimination
Inadequate resources
Cultural diversity
Homelessness
Supported education
Parity
Managed care
Confidentiality standards
Compromised rights
General medical care

psychiatric rehabilitation principles, disability analysis, and psychoeducational approaches (Palmer-Erbs & Anthony, 1995; Palmer-Erbs et al., 1996); an increased recognition of the effectiveness of psychosocial interventions (Corrigan & Garman, 1997; Falloon, Coverdale, & Brooker, 1996); and an acknowledgement of the need for chronic as well as acute care. Finally, an emphasis on recovery, wellness (Fisher, 1994; Moller & Murphy, 1997), and self-help (Cham-

berlin, 1995; Segal, Silverman, & Temkin, 1995a) all increase the need for advocacy for persons with mental illness and mental health problems. Box 18-3 lists the reasons why advocacy is important today.

Box 18-4 lists the many issues needing advocacy today. Three of those issues—discrimination, stigma, and general medical health care—are discussed. Discrimination and stigma are the most critical issues for advocacy. Many consumers report that the stigma of mental illness is a greater burden than the illness itself. To study these issues further, the National Alliance for the Mentally Ill (NAMI) commissioned a survey using their newsletter, *The Advocate,* and their internet site (for an electronic response), as well as distributing the survey through the NAMI Consumer Council (Wahl, 1997). The survey of 1301 people with serious mental illnesses from 49 states revealed that one in three had been turned down for a job for which they were qualified because of a psychiatric label. Half of the consumers reported that they often overheard friends, coworkers, and mental health professionals make hurtful or offensive comments about mental illness. More than one in five had been turned away from volunteer services because of their brain disorder. The ages of the participants ranged from 12 to 94, 56% were female, 80% were Caucasian, 66% attended or completed undergraduate or graduate education. About 26% of the participants were married, and 47% were not employed but had worked before. Their diagnoses included bipolar disorder (25%), schizophrenia (19%), major depression (15%), schizoaffective disorder (5%), multiple diagnoses (14%), unknown (18%), and other (5%). Only 15% had never been hospitalized. The average number of hospital admissions was 5.9. About 61% were living independently at the time of the study, 17% lived with parents or another family member, and 12% lived in semi-independent arrangements (Wahl, 1997). This was not a random sample, reducing the generalizability; it was limited to those who had some connections with NAMI, and participants were not ethnically diverse. The survey's value lies in the fact that the information was provided by the consumers; the perceptions of the persons with mental illness were missing from most of the previous studies (Fink & Tasman, 1992; Wahl, 1995).

General medical care presents another major issue needing advocacy. For persons with brain disorders, mortality rates are twice that of the general population; 50% have known medical disorders, and 35% have undiagnosed medical disorders (Jeste et al., 1996). Most importantly, one in five persons with a brain disorder has a medical problem that may be causing or exacerbating their psychiatric condition (Felker, Yazel, & Short, 1996). In a study sponsored by NAMI, 33% of the 552 consumers reported their physical health status as fair or poor (Uttaro & Mechanic, 1994). In primary care practices, anxiety disorders, depression, and substance abuse are among the most frequently misdiagnosed disorders (NIMH, 1993).

Jeste and colleagues (1996) reported in their literature review that people with schizophrenia may have increased risk of cardiovascular disorders including myocardial infarction and coronary artery disease when compared with the general population. In a study by Viner, Waite, and Thienhaus (1996) of 166 people who were examined during emergency admissions for a hospital inpatient psychiatric unit, 56% had cardiac or pulmonary problems. The sample included persons with a mental disorder, a dual diagnosis of mental disorders and substance abuse, and substance abuse only. In the group with substance abuse alone, 78% were diagnosed with either HIV infection or AIDS. According to Jeste and colleagues (1996), studies in the 1970s and 1980s found a positive association between non–insulin-dependent diabetes mellitus and schizophrenia. It is unclear whether it is related to schizophrenia or secondary to neuroleptic use, which may cause glucose intolerance.

Practice Domains and Advocacy

Benner's original work (1984) identifies seven domains of nursing practice that describe the process of clinical judgment:
1. Helping role
2. Administering and monitoring therapeutic interventions and regimens
3. Effective management of rapidly changing situations
4. Diagnostic and monitoring functions
5. Teaching-coaching function

6. Monitoring and ensuring the quality of health care practices

7. Organizational and work role competencies

Her initial research was carried out with expert clinicians, most of whom were not master's-prepared clinical nurse specialists (CNSs). She later went on to describe the CNS who has both the experience and advanced educational preparation, identifying competencies under each domain.

Benner's work shows that several of the identified domains incorporate advocacy into the role of the advanced practice nurse. The clearest examples are found in the competencies of the helping role: providing emotional and informational support to patients' families, counseling, teaching, mediating, and working to build and maintain a therapeutic community (Benner, 1984). Relevant competencies under the teaching-coaching function were identified as timing, capturing the patient's readiness to learn, and assisting patients to integrate the implications of illness and recovery into their lifestyles. Additionally, under the domain of organizational and work-role competencies, some of the relevant competencies related to advocacy include maintaining a flexible stance toward patients, technology, and bureaucracy.

Benner's work was expanded by Fenton and Brykczynski (1993), and the consulting role domain was identified. This domain includes competency in providing patient advocacy by sensitizing staff to the dilemmas faced by patients and families seeking health care, an important area for psychiatric-mental health nurses. Their work identifies the need for making the bureaucracy respond to patients' and families' needs. This is also emphasized by Price (1995) who states that the consultant advocates by addressing both the patient's problems and the staff's reaction. Clearly, families ask for this type of advocacy (Francell, Conn, & Gray, 1988; Winefield & Harvey, 1994). In the NP role, Brykczynski identifies the domain of management of patient health and illness status in ambulatory care settings, consolidating Benner's domains of diagnostic and monitoring function and administering and monitoring therapeutic interventions and regimens. Operating specifically in the domain of managing the consumer's health and illness status assists in decreasing the gap between recognizing and meeting the health care needs of persons with brain disorders, thus supporting the APRNs role of advocacy (Felker, Yazel, & Short, 1996; Jeste et al., 1996; Uttaro & Mechanic, 1994).

Skills and Competencies for Advocacy

Listening skills are a critical component for the nurse when advocating for patients and families. Although active listening is a skill that should be developed for basic practice, it is probably one of the least developed of the basic nursing skills. Additional competencies and skills necessary for the APRN to effectively advocate are self-confidence, assertiveness, negotiation, and collaboration skills, specifically to work in interdisciplinary teams (Connolly, 1995; Palmer-Erbs et al., 1996). Communication skills—"the manner in which staff make treatment suggestions, how well staff listen, and the level of respect shown in an interaction greatly influence consumers' perceptions of what is helpful [and] caring versus pushy and coercive" (Luckstead & Coursey, 1995)—are also imperative for advocacy work. Physical assessment skills are essential considering the amount of undiagnosed health care problems, comorbidity, and high mortality rates (Jeste et al., 1996; Felker, Yazel, & Short, 1996). Additional competencies are needed to complete mental status assessments and, more specifically, to determine patient competency to make treatment decisions. Skills in crisis intervention, case management, acting as a change agent, and teaching are all critical for effective advocacy. These skills and competencies are listed in Box 18-5.

Teaching and coaching may be one of the primary nursing strategies for advocacy. The APRN teaches staff through direct education and during consultations, addressing both the patient's problems and the staff's reaction (Price, 1995). Advocacy is also achieved through sharing information about patients and families during reports, patient conferences, and staff meetings. Using analogies

box 18-5

SKILLS AND COMPETENCIES NEEDED AT THE ADVANCED LEVEL

Empathetic listening
Self-confidence
Assertiveness
Negotiation
Collaboration
Communication
Physical assessment
Mental status assessment
Crisis intervention
Case management
Change agency
Teaching

is an effective teaching strategy when advocating for patients. Giving patients and families unconditional positive regard and role modeling are valuable forms of teaching others.

Teaching consumers, families, and other health care providers is yet another way to promote advocacy. The ability to advocate was one of the most frequently reported gains for almost 200 participants over a 2-year period after completing a 12-week course based on a wellness approach to relapse prevention (Connolly, Kelly, & Stokes Chen, 1997). The course was modeled after the Moller and Murphy (1997) Three R's Program. The three R's refer to relapse, recovery, and rehabilitation. A wellness framework is applied to facilitate an actualized level of wellness for people with chronic neurobiologic disorders. The goals of the course included teaching patients and families ways for achieving a level of wellness, which assists them in managing symptoms, preventing relapse, and hospitalization. The recovery stage is evident when symptoms are under control. The rehabilitation stage occurs when symptoms are in the background and the people are increasing integration into community life, thus improving the quality of their lives. Teaching is appropriate in both the recovery and rehabilitation stages. The course content includes information about the na-

ture and course of serious mental illnesses, medications and medication management, effective treatments, identification of symptom triggers, coping with activities of daily living, and developing a healthy lifestyle. The course is unique in that it combines consumers, families, students, and providers (including case managers) from an ethnically diverse community in the same class at the same time discussing and addressing the same issues. These are the needs identified by both families and patients in several studies (Uttaro & Mechanic, 1994; Winefield & Harvey, 1994). The results of a 2-year outcome study in the state of Washington of the Moller and Murphy model (1997) using an epidemiologic, controlled-case study design with 176 clients demonstrated a 93.5% decrease in hospital days and an associated estimated savings of $1,086,800.

PATIENT AND FAMILY NEEDS ■ FOR ADVOCACY

Needs of the Consumer

One way to determine areas for advocacy is to determine needs and evaluate whether those needs are met. A study by Uttaro and Mechanic (1994) of 552 consumers contacted from a national sample of 1722 NAMI families between October, 1990 and March, 1991 examined the relationship between the intensity of services received and reported unmet needs for role restoration. One assumption of the study was that recovery and normalization depended on restoring role functioning, specifically roles related to work, satisfactory intimate and social relationships, and involvement in meaningful activities. Fifteen areas were identified to determine if there was a perceived need for help, if the person was receiving the help, and if the person wanted more help. The study findings identified that the areas with the highest levels of unmet needs were keeping busy, recognizing and controlling symptoms, maintaining friendships and intimate relationships, and controlling anger. According to the researchers, there was a positive relationship between depressive symptoms and unmet role needs, which may indicate that depressive symptoms may either contribute to role difficulties or be a product of them. The researchers also suggested that unmet role needs were more important for younger patients.

One major implication of this study is derived from the finding that unmet needs related to role restoration were found among those receiving services, not just those who had severe symptoms or those not receiving any services. There is a need to evaluate and address the patient's response to illness whether or not the symptoms meet the diagnostic criteria for depressive illness. One limitation of the study is the lack of randomness and ethnic diversity. The study does demonstrate that APRNs need to advocate for programs that are effective in restoring role functioning.

Glass (1995) reported on the revisions made to a patient satisfaction questionnaire and the subsequent results of implementing the questionnaire by involving focus groups of patients from a private, nonprofit psychiatric hospital. The results indicated that a caring staff, explanations of treatment, privacy, patient and family involvement in treatment, and involvement in groups and classes were the satisfaction measures considered most

important by the patients. Patients' perceptions of having a better sense of control after treatment was another significant finding in this study. Again, these are all relevant areas for APRNs to consider for advocacy. Box 18-6 contains a list of consumers' needs for advocacy.

In developing this chapter, consumers were asked for examples of advocacy that they received from APRNs in psychiatric and mental health care. These can be found in Box 18-7.

---

box 18-6

CONSUMER ADVOCACY NEEDS

Restoring role function
Recognizing and controlling symptoms
Keeping busy
Maintaining friendships and intimate relationships
Controlling anger
Caring staff
Explanations about treatment
Information regarding medications, side effects, and interactions
Privacy
Involvement in treatment
Information regarding achieving a level of wellness

---

box 18-7

FAMILY MEMBERS' EXAMPLES OF ADVOCACY PROVIDED BY THE APRN

- One of the instructors from the university and I have established a wonderful relationship wherein we have arranged for family members to have $2\frac{1}{2}$ hours to speak with student nurses during their psychiatric rotation.
- The advanced practice psychiatric nurse asked the family member to give permission to share information; this helped to keep the family member in touch with the consumer and to know that the consumer was safe.
- Advocacy helps because it reduces the stigma and prejudice against families and, indirectly, [against] my family.
- The nurse observed my daughter for a week and made holistic recommendations for recovery ... this helped me with information and safe recommendations for a subject that I had no background to pull from.
- A well-known psychiatric mental health nurse was cited as an advocate for families through her presentations before psychiatrists and mental health service administrators. She advocates for use of new medications and better services for consumers.
- Instructional workshops given by an advanced practice nurse; when we took the classes for the client and family (it) really answered many concerns and built confidence that we could manage this dreadful illness.

Needs of the Family

Neurobiologic disorders (schizophrenia, bipolar disorders, and major depression), which affect approximately five million adults in America, are the most stigmatized and feared of any chronic illnesses. One in ten Americans experience some disability from a mental illness in any given year. Families play a major role in the support and care of their mentally ill member (the majority of persons with neurobiologic disorders live with their families), increasing the need for collaboration and for psychoeducational programs, which support and prepare families. Family involvement leverages scarce public mental health service resources by helping the family become part of the service delivery team. It also directly benefits family members, allowing them to feel empowered and relieved of some of the burden they may have been carrying.

Families' perception of burden of care for their relatives was researched by Francell, Conn, and Gray (1988) with 86 family caregivers, most of whom were parents. Results from this study identified several areas of family burden. One area of burden was crisis situations, especially after 5 PM or on weekends, and anger over being referred to law enforcement agencies. Another area of burden was "weariness and frustration related to their long-term roles as patient advocates and case managers" (Francell, Conn, & Gray, 1988). The family caregivers reported difficulties in accessing entitlement programs because of lack of information and resources or from the bureaucratic policies and negative attitudes of some agency personnel. Inadequate community resources was cited as a major contributor to their perceptions of burden and lack of information about diagnoses, current treatments, availability of community resources, and effective strategies for managing the illness. There was also a specific need for information on medication and side effects.

Families were frustrated by the lack of continuity of care in medical therapy, treatment approaches, and record keeping. Some reported that, because of poor security at state mental hospitals, their relatives left without permission and often "drifted from place to place throughout the country" (Francell, Conn, & Gray, 1988). Many experienced difficulty in obtaining information about their relative's diagnosis, treatment plans, and medications because of the implementation of various laws.

The recommendations from the Francell, Conn, and Gray (1988) study were increased family education, inclusion of the family in treatment decisions, changes in current mental health laws, redirection in professional training, and the development of mobile crisis teams. These findings are consistent with numerous other studies including a study by Winefield and Harvey (1994) who identified the needs of family caregivers of persons with chronic schizophrenia. The researchers studied 121 family caregivers in South Australia who had been caregivers for an average of 14 years. These caregivers expressed a need for support of earlier professional intervention in episodes of illness, information about how to lobby politicians for resources, and information about schizophrenia. The caregivers also wanted more information about how families could cope with disturbed behavior, more meetings with the patients' doctor, better supervised accommodations, more day programs in their own area, and better education of police. Clearly, these are all areas that the APRN not only could advocate for but also could provide. Box 18-8 contains a list of families' needs.

Family members surveyed for this chapter were also asked to give an example of advocacy by an APRN. To help set the context for the question, participants were given the APNA brochures *Advanced Practice Registered Nurse in Psychiatric and Mental Health Care* (APNA, 1997a) and *Mental Health Care: A Consumer's Guide* (APNA, 1995). One person responded that, as far as she knew, "no advanced practice psychiatric nurse ever advocated for me in the context of the treatment of either my daughter or my husband." Box 18-9 contains the examples provided by the other family members. One parent felt that an instructor's

box 18-8

FAMILIES' NEEDS

- Assistance during crisis situations
- Information on entitlement programs, resources, community resources, medications, side effects, and interactions
- Strategies for managing the illness
- Respect
- Inclusion in treatment decisions
- Earlier interventions
- Assistance in coping with disturbed behavior
- More meetings with the doctor
- Better supervised housing
- More day programs in their area
- Education of police
- Referrals to NAMI
- Consultation rather than therapy

box 18-9

CONSUMERS' EXPERIENCES AND RECOMMENDATIONS

EXAMPLES OF ADVOCACY

- When my managed care organization wanted to change my therapist, I was able to continue with my present provider.
- The nurse provided advice and consultation for me to advocate for myself.
- By knowing the mental health law, I was able to choose to take medication or not, and stay out of the hospital, and go to a client run center.

RECOMMENDATIONS FOR IMPROVED ADVOCACY

- Help other health professionals who [have] gotten sick.
- See to the consumer's rights for choice.
- Be assertive with colleagues, administrators, physicians, and others on behalf of consumers.

WHEN ADVOCACY IS NOT NEEDED

- Whenever I am present and can speak for myself; otherwise, advocate in all forums at all times.
- When I am able to do it for myself.
- Only when [the] client is restored to some semblance of control or in recovery, being compliant (taking meds, under treatment, etc.).
- When I indicate that this assistance is not wanted.

willingness to advocate was demonstrated by having family members participate in the education of nursing students, increasing the students' understanding of the family's experience of mental illness.

Another question in the survey asked how the APRN could be more helpful to families. Box 18-10 contains the responses to that question. A more expanded response gave a detailed example of lack of advocacy and having "been rebuffed" when attempting to get nurses to make changes. As a result of this experience this family member recommended that "nurses could at minimum be open to talking to families and should insist on having this role."

Needs of Children

Meeting the needs of children of parents with mental illness is an important area for advocacy. Parents have a duty and responsibility for the safety of their children. This becomes even more of an issue during chaotic times (e.g., during a relapse of the parent). Parents need to be taught

to have a plan for those times, one which includes moving the children to a safe place. Children's needs must be met, and stability must be provided. They need to be educated about their parent's mental illness in terms that they can understand and should be assisted in seeing the affected parent or family member as a person with an illness (Spiese, 1996). Marsh (1996) suggests construc-

WAYS IN WHICH APRNs CAN BE MORE HELPFUL TO FAMILIES

- As a whole group, be more visible as partners and advocate for families.
- Get in touch with the family immediately.
- Educate other nurses in academic nursing programs.
- Attend some of the AMI meetings [and] Journey of Hope educational classes, and become even more informed about the family perspective.
- Do not just tell the family to let go—assist them in ways to do so or to stay involved if appropriate.

tive escapes for children such as, art, music, and sports. She also points out the value of spiritual faith. A family support program in Iowa (Murty, 1996) teaches parents to have a crisis plan, provides support to all the family members, includes information on basic growth and development as well as parenting skills, and helps them obtain resources needed to keep the family together. Examples of resources that were arranged were a visiting nurse for assistance with health and medication issues, a homemaker, independent living skills trainers, assistance with managing finances, transportation, child care, and activity programs for children and adolescents. While advocating for the children of parents with mental illness it is important to treat the parents and their relationships with their children with respect (Nicholson, 1996). Parents and their offspring need to be involved in service development and service planning. Special advocacy needs arise when providing services to mothers in jail (Osborne, 1995). Finally, school counselors are recognized advocates for students, and therefore APRNs need to provide education for school counselors. School counselors need to provide training for school staff regarding children's needs. They can act as a liaison for

services within the school and the mental health system (Swartz & Little, 1996).

■ SYSTEM LEVEL ADVOCACY

ANA Code 11 addresses the role of nursing advocacy in the community and for the nation. Collaboration is the key component. "The nurse collaborates with members of the health professions and other citizens in promoting community and national efforts to meet the health needs of the public" (ANA, 1985).

Primary Health Care Model

A primary mental health care model proposed by Haber and Billings (1995) provides an excellent focus for advocating for the health care system changes that families and consumers have already requested (Fisher, 1994; Francell, Conn, & Gray, 1988). The model advocates for continuous and comprehensive services for the "promotion of optimal mental health, prevention of mental illness, and health maintenance, and includes the management (treatment) of and/or referral for mental and general health problems" (Haber & Billings, 1995). The primary mental health care model specifically includes the function of patient advocate and identifies the APRN as the "change agent by assuming a leadership role in collaboration with intradisciplinary and interdisciplinary colleagues to define and shape the nature of change" (Haber & Billings, 1995).

Nurses are in an excellent position to advocate for changes in the mental health system, either from within the system or from outside the system. For example, recognizing the physical health care issues, the mortality rates twice that of the general population (Jeste et al., 1996), the fact that one in five has a medical problem that could be causing or exacerbating the psychiatric condition, and the documented instances of self-reports of poor health status (Uttaro & Mechanic, 1994), there is ample justification for including physical assessments during mental status evaluations in the emergency department. Most people with psychiatric emergencies will be seen in an emergency department first before being transferred to a psychiatric unit or hospital (Viner, Waite, & Thienhaus, 1996).

Legislative Activities

APRNs can advocate through legislative activities, specifically through their professional specialty organization, the APNA. The APNA provides a structure for such advocacy through its Legislative Task Force. The APNA's annual legislative agenda is implemented through a legislative network of APNA members from each state (APNA, 1997b). One example of the effectiveness of such advocacy was the inclusion of clinical nurses specialists (CNSs) and nurse practitioners (NPs) in the Balanced Budget Act of 1997, Public Law 105-33. As a result of the new bill, since January 1998, CNSs and NPs have been eligible for Medicare Part B coverage and direct payment in both rural and urban areas. This means that if the service would be covered under Medicare Part B if provided by a physician, it will be covered when provided by a NP or a CNS. This new legislation increases patient access to CNSs and NPs, thus increasing quality cost-effective care for all eligible recipients.

ANA Code 9 also refers to nurses' advocacy role at the systems' level: "The nurse participates in the profession's efforts to establish and maintain conditions of employment conducive to high quality nursing" (ANA, 1985). Nurses advocate for quality care for patients when upholding the Standards of Practice and the Code for Nurses. Because of specific conditions of employment, patient advocacy frequently puts nurses' continued employment at personal risk (Bandman & Bandman, 1995). In some institutions, nurses are not allowed to inform family members of a patient's diagnosis, medications, or treatment plan because of interpretations of confidentiality laws. When faced with the dilemma of 1) preparing a family for a patient's discharge by providing the information

needed to support the patient's reintegration into the family and the community, and 2) upholding the institutional policies, which prohibit providing such information, nurses may place their jobs in jeopardy. See Chapter 19 for further discussion about confidentiality.

Consumer Advocacy Organizations

Support and advocacy for families are available through the NAMI and its 1140 state and local affiliates. The NAMI was started in 1979 when a group of families came together for support. Today the NAMI is the leading advocacy organization in the nation. It is a grassroots, family, and patient self-help, support, and advocacy organization dedicated to improving the lives of people with severe mental illnesses. The NAMI's members also include mental health professionals. The NAMI has been effective in educating the public about mental illness, advocating for research, and championing legislative issues on national, state, and local levels. One of its more recent successes has been the legislation of the Domenici-Wellstone partial parity amendment to prevent discrimination against people with brain disorders.

APRNs should be acquainted with the various consumer advocacy organizations and should consider joining the NAMI at the state or local level. Working with organized and recognized consumer advocacy groups increases the likelihood of maximizing change in the mental health system as well as the health care system. It also increases sensitivity and knowledge of family and consumer needs and concerns. Fairweather (1980) argues that the mental health bureaucracy maintains the status quo and that change to the status quo must come from professional groups and organizations. Professionals need to tell families about the NAMI. Johnson (1995) believes there is a need for a worldwide family organization, possibly linking the 35 nations that already have such organizations. He believes that families need to know what rehabilitation is and that there should be a friend for every family. He argues for better community services—residences, social clubs, transportation, vocational and rehabilitation programs, and supported work. He also argues for a new kind of professional, one who embraces consultation rather than therapy with families.

In addition to the NAMI, the National Mental Health Association (NMHA) is another example of an effective advocacy organization. The Carter Center, with the efforts of Rosalyn Carter, works specifically on mental health policy through annual symposia. There are several consumer organizations through which consumers, families, and APRNs can bring about system change. Organizations of former patients who often refer to themselves as "survivors" or consumers or clients are prevalent throughout the country and the world. The APRN may work collaboratively with the organizations, hold membership, conduct collaborative research, serve on an advisory board, or provide consultation, again, acting in an advocacy role. A list of mental health advocacy organizations, internet addresses, and resources are found in the Resources and Connections section of this chapter.

■ CONSUMER AS ADVOCATE

The APRN will encounter a challenge in preparing consumers to advocate for their own needs. The nurse's role is as teacher, coach, and mentor for the consumer. Consumers achieve increased self-efficacy and self-esteem as they experience change that has come about through their own efforts—the consumer is empowered. This has been reported as a positive outcome in long-term studies (Moller & Murphy, 1997) specifically on empowerment (Segal, Silverman, & Temkin, 1995a, 1995b), reports about consumer-run self-help organizations (Chamberlin, 1995; Marshall, 1995; Rogers, 1995; Temkin, Silverman, & Segal, 1995), and individual accounts of the value of consumers as advocates (Francell, 1996). The APRN will be challenged to collaborate with and integrate the consumer nonprofessional into helping fellow consumers (peer counseling) in their care. Work-

ing with consumer nonprofessionals in roles such as peer specialists improved communication between case managers and consumers involved in a 2-year study (Felton et al., 1995).

The APRN may also encounter the health professionals who are mental health consumers. The consumer professional is one who is a consumer and seeks education and degrees that may be in the area of mental health. Some are already mental health professionals or professionals in other disciplines before the onset of their mental illness. They appreciate effective communication and collaboration skills of the APRN (Francell, 1996; Lehman, 1995). Some consumers seeking careers in mental health may "need to be actively recruited into professional training and into professional positions" (Chamberlin, 1995). There are many examples of awakening and recovery described by Lefley (1996) that result in major contributions to human-kind. Among those is Kay Jamison, a psychologist with bipolar disorder whose book, *An Unquiet Mind: A Memoir of Moods and Madness,* is used by consumers and professionals around the world.

Consumers and families provided advice for nurses in advanced psychiatric-mental health nursing specifically for this chapter (Box 18-11). A mother who is an APRN details her advice in Box 18-12; she emphasizes the need for advocacy through professional organizations. Another mother's sage advice explicitly cites conditions for effective advocacy. Clearly, there is a request for collaboration and thorough assessment of difficulties in adhering to the treatment plan. Her full response is found in Box 18-13.

■ OUTCOMES OF ADVOCACY
Empowerment

One patient outcome of advocacy is empowerment. It is a process through which patients obtain resources on multiple levels to enable them to gain greater control over their environment (Segal, Silverman, & Temkin, 1995a). Patients gain new resources or competencies such as the

box 18-11

ADVICE FROM CONSUMERS AND FAMILIES

- Learn cultural competence.
- See to the patient's rights and choices.
- Believe what they say.
- Be a resource.
- Help them negotiate a complex service system.
- Be available to family.
- Embrace the family as part of your nursing role.
- Advocate strongly with legislators and managed care administrators.
- Become familiar with the literature on family burden.
- Be aware of the paranoia and stigma.
- Protect anonymity.
- Attend educational classes that include consumers and family members.
- Ask the consumer and/or family member if they want you to advocate for them.
- Keep them informed of their rights (since the patient/client is often informed by others).
- Find out what their needs are and where you can assist, especially in areas of education, resources, and stigma.
- Know about the local AMI.

box 18-12

ADVICE FROM A MOTHER WHO IS AN APRN

You should advocate strongly with legislators and managed care administrators for roles for yourself in the community care of persons with serious mental illnesses. Your education has prepared you well to serve these people, yet in fact nurses are under-represented among community staff. As states close hospitals and move patients into community settings, nurses should follow the patients (just like the money). However, this will not happen if nurses themselves do not join families and consumers in advocating for quality community services. (By the same token, nursing organizations must form alliances with one another.)

In seeking alliances with families and family organizations, advanced practice psychiatric-mental health nurses and their organizations should take the initiative. Remember, many families do not know what APRNs are or what they are supposed to do. Many families have never experienced advocacy by APRNs. On the contrary, they may have experienced being rebuffed. Psychiatric-mental health nurses may have to do some homework to learn how to work with families if their previous training has not prepared them to perceive of families as partners.

As far as advocating for family members within the context of their relative's treatment or rehabilitation, become familiar with the literature on family burden and seek out family members to discuss with them what their needs are in relation to their relative's illness. You cannot effectively advocate for family members unless you understand their needs, and you cannot rely on what you may have been taught in graduate school about the needs of families.

capacity to help others, group leadership skills, and organizational leadership abilities. Empowerment is also "related to the concepts of self-efficacy, self-esteem, and the sense that positive personal change can come about through one's own efforts" (Segal, Silverman, & Temkin, 1995a).

A recent study (Rogers et al., 1997) conducted to develop a scale measuring the patient-defined construct of empowerment identified five factors: self-efficacy and self-esteem, power and powerlessness, community activism, righteous anger, and optimism-control over the future. The study's findings also indicated that empowerment was re-

box 18-13

MOTHER'S ADVICE FOR THE APRN

Be knowledgeable of all persons involved in the area you wish to advocate for. Many times people advocate for the mentally ill to professionals without talking to the mentally ill or the family member. Many times the professionals make decisions concerning the treatment or care plans without talking with the mentally ill person or the family member. They often indicate that a person is noncompliant with treatment without finding out the real reason for missed appointments (e.g., not taking medications or having a defiant attitude). Find out the reason before making judgment calls. Psychiatric-mental health nurses who are advanced in their field *must* attend educational classes that include consumers and family members. Only in this way can they truly be all encompassing in their advocacy.

lated to quality of life and income but not to age, gender, ethnicity, marital status, education level, or employment status.

Fisher's Empowerment Model of Recovery is based on principles that emerged from the experiences of patients in recovery and in the independent living movement (Fisher, 1994). According to Fisher (1994), the principles of the empowerment model are as follows:

- Hope
- Personhood
- Achievement of self-defined goals
- Choices
- The opportunity for consumers to speak for themselves
- Peer support (consumer run services)
- An end to discrimination
- Self-control of symptoms
- Well-being
- Liberty and freedom
- Healing from within

These principles are all congruent with nursing's values, the *Code for Nurses,* as well as the *Standards of Practice,* which support advocacy efforts. Advanced practice nurses must understand these principles to gain a better perspective of advocacy within the empowerment model. In this model, the major barriers to recovery from disabilities are in the attitudinal and physical environment rather than within the individual. The model emphasizes both choice in control of services by those using the services and a basic belief that "it is possible to be a whole, self-determining person and still have a disability" (Fisher, 1994).

Effective Care

Effective care is a primary outcome of advocacy (Arntzen et al., 1995). Decreased stigma and increased empowerment also result from effective advocacy (Segal et al., 1995a, 1995b). Advocacy achieves cost savings by eliminating bureaucratic, attitudinal, insurance, and legal barriers, specifically when APRNs have increased access to patients (Baradell, 1994; Connolly, 1995). As a result of advocacy, quality of care increases, family burden is decreased, rehabilitation is faster (Palmer-Erbs & Anthony, 1995), and individuals experience increased functioning (Connolly, 1995; Rogers et al., 1997; Segal et al., 1995) and support for the human spirit. Advocacy leads to increased quality of life and more effective case management (Felton et al., 1995), improved health care (Connolly, 1995; Haber & Billings, 1995), and patient satisfaction (Connolly, 1995; Pickett et al., 1995). Finally, advocacy results in improvement in the mental health care system (Fisher, 1994). Box 18-14 contains a list of outcomes of advocacy.

■ BARRIERS TO ADVOCACY

Old paradigms often prevent nurses from advocating effectively for patients (Conn, 1997; Sills, 1995). Mental health professionals educated in

18-14

OUTCOMES OF ADVOCACY

Effective care
Appropriate care
Decreased stigma
Empowerment
Cost savings
Quality care
Decrease in family burden
Emphasis on rehabilitation
Increased functioning
Effective managed care
Improvement in the mental health care system

outdated family theories, which explained mental illnesses such as schizophrenia as a result of dysfunctional communication, are not able to advocate for effective care (Conn, 1998; Francell, Conn, & Gray, 1988; Marsh, 1996). Lack of collaboration with patients and families is a further barrier to advocacy (Conn, 1997; Francell, 1996; Francell, Conn, & Gray, 1988; Palmer-Erbs & Manos, 1997). Myths such as increasing compliance with drug treatment can singularly affect rehabilitation outcome, professionals can accurately predict rehabilitation outcomes, or there is a positive relationship between the outcome and the cost of the intervention (Palmer-Erbs & Anthony, 1995) may prevent appropriate advocacy. Issues around confidentiality and privacy act as one of the major barriers for families as advocates (Conn, 1998). Co-optation between advocates and staff in mental health departments may act as a barrier. Professional avoidance of involvement with politics is yet another barrier (DeFries, 1993). Lack of a culturally competent system of care also prevents effective advocacy (Campinha-Bacote, 1994; Choi, 1995).

Personal and professional value conflicts may interfere with successful advocacy (Bandman & Bandman, 1995) as well as loss of focus. Treatment sites focusing exclusively on either medical problems or psychiatric problems tend to contribute

to poor advocacy (Felker, Yazel, & Short, 1996). Advocacy for incarcerated persons presents inherent conflict between the correction perspective (primarily to punish) and the mental health perspective (primarily to understand). There is a fine line "between the requirements of security, health care, and client advocacy" (Peternelji-Taylor & Johnson, 1995).

Some examples of barriers to advocacy are as follows:

- Impaired brain functioning of the patient, preventing an accurate history and incomplete examinations
- Patients' severe symptoms and "free choice" (Lucksted & Coursey, 1995)
- Inappropriate services, substance abuse, lack of knowledge, and concerns over boundaries
- Lack of continuity of care, lack of managed care, poor record keeping, and insufficient education of police (Winefield & Harvey, 1994)
- Lack of information on diagnosis, current treatments, medications, resources, symptom management, and relapse (Palmer-Erbs & Manos, 1997)
- Confusion over legal rights, adversarial positions because of mandated advocacy, and concerns over people in paid advocacy positions
- A lack of understanding of mental illnesses, attitudes, and the physical environment (Fisher, 1994)
- Confusion over empowerment and staff control (Starkey et al. 1997)
- Advocating for a patient, in some cases, could put the nurse's job in jeopardy (Bandman & Bandman, 1995)
- Stigma (Conn, 1997; Fisher, 1994; Wahl, 1997)

IMPLICATIONS FOR
■ THE FUTURE

There is a need for advocacy and the presence of the APRN in psychiatric-mental health nursing who is recognizable to families and consumers (Connolly, 1998). Advocacy for access to the services of an APRN is still one of the biggest challenges both within the profession of nursing and interprofessionally. There is a need to decrease stigma within nursing as well as other disciplines. Advocating for more long-term research focused on women and ethnically diverse populations specifically during the first episode is a priority. APRNs need to advocate for culturally competent care as well as a culturally competent system of care. APRNs will be challenged to increase their functioning as coaches, mentors, and consultants to patients and families, as well as continually assessing levels of satisfaction with care. Advocating for primary care in all settings so as to identify psychiatric problems in any health care setting and to identify the physical health care problems for those receiving services in mental health care settings is a challenge for APRNs. Increasing access through legislative and political activities to achieve parity in health care insurance coverage, housing, and the work place will continue to be a major challenge. Furthermore, APRNs need to advocate for changes in confidentiality and privacy laws that place patients at risk and prevent basic communication between caregivers, providers, and patients and their families. Additional challenges will be met in restoring the role of parent to persons with mental illness while balancing the safety and needs of their children. Forensic nursing may offer the most challenges based on the inherent conflict between the correction perspective and the mental health perspective and the increasing number of mentally ill who are incarcerated. It will take knowledge, strength, courage, and commitment to speak for those who cannot speak for themselves, to go beyond just safeguarding patients, and to advocate for the quality of life of the patients who participate in and receive psychiatric nursing care.

Resources for advocacy are available and accessible. The APRN needs to become familiar with and evaluate the information found on various websites and resource centers as well as the legislative mandates. The APRN needs to assist families and consumers in accessing the information, evaluating the information, and encouraging them to use the resources. "It is only through the joint efforts of the professional and the consumer, united for the purpose of bringing about reform that reform will actually take place" (Fairweather, 1980).

Acknowledgments

I would like to thank the following individuals who gave permission to use their comments, and I would like to publicly acknowledge their time and detailed responses to the questions posed: Victoria Conn, RN, MSN, The National Alliance for the Mentally Ill; Paolo Del Vecchio, Consumer Affairs Specialist, Center for Mental Health Services; Claire Griffin-Francel, APRN, CNS-PMH, Southeast Nurse Consultants, Inc. and Georgia Alliance for the Mentally Ill; Vernon S. Montoya, California Network of Mental Health Clients; Darlene Prettyman, RN, CCDN, Second Vice President, California Alliance for the Mentally Ill; Sharon Roth, RN, BSN, MA, Vice President, The Alliance for the Mentally Ill of Santa Clara County; Katherine S. Salazar; and Patricia Van Damm.

RESOURCES AND CONNECTIONS

RESOURCE CENTERS

Advocacy: American Self-Help Clearinghouse
  201-625-7101

American Psychiatric Nurses Association
1200 19th Street, NW, Suite 300
Washington, DC 20036
202-857-1133
Fax: 202-223-4579
Email: APNA@dc.sba.com

Association for Children's Mental Health
800-782-0883

The Carter Center
One Copenhill
Atlanta, GA 30307
404-420-5155
Fax: 404-614-3737

CMHS Consumer Affairs
Center for Mental Health Services
5600 Fishers Lane; Room 13-103
Rockville, MD 20857
301-443-2619 or 800-345-0981

Center for Patient Advocacy
CPR: National Coalition for Patient Rights
405 Waltham Street, Suite 218
Lexington, MA 02173
800-846-7444
Email: patientadv@aol.com

Center for Psychiatric Rehabilitation, Boston
  University
930 Commonwealth Avenue
Boston, MA 02215
617-353-3549
Fax: 617-353-7700

Consumer Bill of Rights
Box 2429
Columbia, MD 21045-1429
800-732-8200

DART Program
Depression Awareness, Recognition, and Treatment
  Program
National Institute of Mental Health
800-421-4211 or 312-443-4140

Freedom From Fear
308 Seaview Avenue
Staten Island, NY 10305
718-351-1717
Fax: 718-667-8893

International Association of Psychosocial
  Rehabilitation Services (IAPSRS)
10025 Gov. Warfield Pkwy.
Columbia, MD 21044-3357
410-730-7190
Fax: 410-730-5965

KEN, National Mental Health Services, Knowledge
  Exchange Network
PO Box 4240
Washington, DC 20015
800-789-2647
Fax: 301-984-8796
Email: ken@mentalhealth.org

National Alliance for the Mentally Ill (NAMI)
200 N Glebe Road, Suite 1015
Arlington, VA 22203-3754
703-524-7600
Email: frieda@nami.org

National Clearinghouse on Family support and
  Children's Mental Health
800-628-1696

National Depressive and Manic Depressive Association
730 North Franklin Street, Suite 501
Chicago, IL 60610
800-82-NDMA or 312-642-0049
Fax: 312-642-7243

National Empowerment Center
20 Ballard Road
Lawrence, MA 018543
800-POWER-2-U
Fax: 508-681-6426
Email: POWERTWOU@aol.com

National Mental Health Association
800-969-6642

National Mental Health Consumers' Self-Help
  Clearinghouse, CMH
311 South Juniper Street, Suite 1000
Philadelphia, PA 19107
800-553-4539

National Research and Training Center on
  Psychiatric Disability
104 South Michigan Avenue, Suite 900
Chicago, IL 60603-5901
312-422-8180
Fax: 312-422-0740

National Resource Center on Homelessness and
  Mental Illness
800-444-7415

National Stigma Clearinghouse
275 Seventh Avenue, 16th Floor
New York, NY 10001

Obsessive Compulsive Foundation
800-639-7462

Recovery, Inc.
802 North Dearborn Street
Chicago, IL 60610
312-337-5661
Fax: 312-337-5756

WEBSITES

APNA website www.apna.org

Ask Noah About Mental Health
www.noah.cuny.edu/mentalhealth/mental.htm

Center for Psychiatric Rehabilitation
www.bu.edu/SARPSYCH

Center for Mental Health Services (SAMHSA)
www.samhsa.gov/cmhs.cmhs.htm

Emergency Services
www.mentalhealth.org/emerserv/GUIDECC.htm

Healthier You: Mental Health Consumer Information
www.mhsource.com/healthieryou.htm

KEN Knowledge Exchange Network, NMHS: http://
www.mentalhealth.org

The Journal, CAMI www.mhsource.com

Mental Health Statistics
www.mentalhealth.org/mhstats

National Alliance for the Mentally Ill (NAMI)
www.nami.org

National Depressive and Manic-Depressive Association www.ndmda.org

National Panic/Anxiety Disorder News
www.npadnews.com

National Mental Health Information Resources
www.coolware.com/health/joel/mhealth.html

Psychiatric Survivors' Guide
harborside.com/home/e/equinox/welcome.htm

Psych Central, Suicide Helpline
www.grohol.com/helpme.htm

Patient Advocacy Numbers: InfoNet
www.infonet.welch.jhu.edu

Recovery Inc. www.recovery-inc.com

WellnessWeb
www.wellweb.com/preview/zpre.htm

References

American Nurses Association. (1985). *Code for nurses with interpretive statements.* Kansas City, MO: Author.

American Nurses Association. (1994). *A statement on psychiatric-mental health clinical nursing practice and standards of psychiatric-mental health clinical nursing practice.* Washington, DC: American Nurses Publishing.

American Psychiatric Nurses Association. (1995). *Mental health care: a consumer's guide* [Brochure]. Washington, DC: Author.

American Psychiatric Nurses Association. (1997a). *Advanced practice registered nurse in psychiatric and mental health care* [Brochure]. Washington, DC: Author.

American Psychiatric Nurses Association. (1997b). *The American Psychiatric Nurses Association grassroots guide to advocacy.* Washington, DC: Author.

Arntzen, B., et al. (1995). CRF: early experiences at Sacramento's consumer run crisis residential program. *The Journal of the California Alliance for the Mentally Ill, 6*(3), 35–36.

Bandman, E., & Bandman, B. (1995). *Nursing ethics through the life span* (ed. 3). Norwalk, CT: Appleton & Lange.

Baradell, J. (1994). Cost-effectiveness and quality of care provided by clinical nurses specialists. *Journal of Psychosocial Nursing, 32*(3), 21–24.

Benner, P. (1984). *From novice to expert: excellence and power in clinical nursing practice.* Menlo Park, CA: Addison-Wesley.

Berube, M. (Ed.). (1985). *The American heritage dictionary* (ed. 2). Boston: Houghton Mifflin.

Campinha-Bacote, J. (1994). Cultural competence in psychiatric mental health nursing: a conceptual model. *Nursing Clinics of North America, 29*(1), 1–9.

Chamberlin, J. (1995). Rehabilitating ourselves: the psychiatric survivor movement. *International Journal of Mental Health, 24*(1), 39–46.

Choi, J. (1995). Can self help work in Asian cultures? perhaps. *The Journal of the California Alliance for the Mentally Ill, 6*(3), 60–61.

Conn, V. (1998). The family's view of the continuum of care. In Stuart, G., & Laraia, M. *Principles and practice of psychiatric nursing* (ed. 6). St. Louis: Mosby.

Connolly, P. (1995). Transdisciplinary collaboration of academia and practice in the area of serious mental illness. *Australian and New Zealand Journal of Mental Health Nursing, 4*(4), 168–180.

Connolly, P. (1998). President's message: making our work visible. *Journal of the American Psychiatric Nurses Association, 4*(2), 24A-28A.

Connolly, P., Kelly, J., & Stokes Chen, S. (1997). *Maintaining consumer satisfaction: a follow-up survey to the 12 week consumer/family education course.* Unpublished manuscript. San Jose State University.

Corrigan, P., & Garman, A. (1997). Considerations for research on consumer empowerment and psychosocial interventions. *Psychiatric Services, 48,* 347–351.

DeFries, Z. (1993). A call to advocacy. *Hospital and Community Psychiatry, 44,* 101.

Falloon, I., Coverdale, J., & Brooker, C. (1996). Psychosocial interventions in schizophrenia: a review. *International Journal of Mental Health, 25*(1), 3–21.

Fairweather, G. (1980). Implications of the Lodge Society. *New Directions for Mental Health Services,* (7) 89–97.

Felker, B., Yazel, J., & Short, D. (1996). Mortality and medical comorbidity among psychiatric patients: a review. *Psychiatric Services, 47,* 1356–1363.

Felton, C., et al. (1995). Consumers as peer specialists on intensive case management teams: impact on client outcomes. *Psychiatric Services, 46,* 1037–1044.

Fenton, M., & Brykczynski, K. (1993). Qualitative distinctions and similarities in the practice of clinical nurse specialists and nurse practitioners. *Journal of Professional Nursing, 9*(6), 313–326.

Fink, P., & Tasman, A. (Eds.). (1992). *Stigma and mental illness.* Washington, DC: American Psychiatric Press.

Fisher, D. (1994). Health care reform based on an empowerment model of recovery by people with psychiatric disabilities. *Hospital and Community Psychiatry, 45,* 913–915.

Fisher, D. (1995). National Empowerment Center: recovery through self help. *The Journal of the California Alliance for the Mentally Ill, 6*(3), 8–9.

Francell, E. (1996). My role as a consumer-provider: challenges and opportunities. *Journal of Psychosocial Nursing, 35*(1), 29–31.

Francell C.G., Conn, V., & Gray, D.P. (1988). Families' perceptions of burden of care for chronic mentally ill relatives. *Hospital and Community Psychiatry, 39,* 1296–1300.

Glass, A. (1995). Identifying issues important to patients on a hospital satisfaction questionnaire. *Psychiatric Services, 46,* 83–85.

Haber, J., & Billings, C. (1995). Primary mental health care: a model for psychiatric-mental health nursing. *Journal of the American Psychiatric Nurses Association, 1*(5), 154–163.

Jeste, D.V., et al. (1996). Medical comorbidity in schizophrenia. *Schizophrenia Bulletin, 22,* 413–430.

Johnson, D. (1995). Families and psychiatric rehabilitation. *International Journal of Mental Health, 24*(1), 47–58.

Lefley, H. (1996). Awakenings and recovery: learning the beat of a different drummer. *The Journal of the California Alliance for the Mentally Ill, 7*(2), 4–6.

Lehmann, R. (1995). My experiences as a consumer and as a practitioner within the mental health system. *The Journal of the California Alliance for the Mentally Ill, 6*(2), 25–27.

Lucksted, A., & Coursey, R. (1995). Consumer perceptions of pressure and force in psychiatric treatments. *Psychiatric Services, 46,* 146–152.

Marsh, D. (1996). Meeting the needs of offspring. *The Journal of the California Alliance for the Mentally Ill, 7*(3), 56–57.

Marshall, L. (1995). Self help: the challenges of clients helping themselves. *The Journal of the California Alliance for the Mentally Ill, 6*(3), 25–27.

Moller, M., & Murphy, M. (1997). The three R's rehabilitation program: a prevention approach for the management of relapse symptoms associated with psychiatric diagnoses. *Psychiatric Rehabilitation Journal, 20*(3), 42–48.

Murty, S. (1996). Can a support program for families make a difference? two teenagers share their experiences. *The Journal of the California Alliance for the Mentally Ill, 7*(3), 60–62.

National Institute of Mental Health. (1993). *Health care reform for Americans with severe mental illness: report of the National Advisory Mental Health Council.* Rockville, MD. NIMH.

Nicholson, J. (1996). Services for parents with mental illness and their families. *The Journal of the California Alliance for the Mentally Ill, 7*(3), 66–68.

Osborne, O. (1995). Jailed mothers: further explorations in public sector nursing. *Journal of Psychosocial Nursing, 33*(8), 23–28.

Palmer-Erbs, V., & Anthony, W. (1995). Incorporating psychiatric rehabilitation principles into mental health nursing. *Journal of Psychosocial Nursing, 33*(3), 36–44.

Palmer-Erbs, V., et al. (1996). Nursing perspectives on disability and rehabilitation. In Anchor, K. (Ed.). *Disability analysis handbook: tools for independent practice.* Dubuque, IA: Kendall/Hunt.

Palmer-Erbs, V., & Manos, E. (1997). New thoughts on promoting collaborative partnerships with consumers, survivors, and family members. *Journal of Psychosocial Nursing, 35*(1), 3–5.

Peternelji-Taylor, C., & Johnson, R. (1995). Serving time: psychiatric mental health nursing in corrections. *Journal of Psychosocial Nursing, 33*(8), 12–19.

Pickett, S., et al. (1995). Factors predicting patients' satisfaction with managed mental health care. *Psychiatric Services, 46,* 722–723.

Price, N. (1995). The role of the consultation-liaison nurse: caring for patients with AIDS dementia complex. *Journal of Psychosocial Nursing, 33*(8), 31–34.

Rogers, J. (1995). Community organizing: self-help and providing mental health services. *Journal of the California Alliance for the Mentally Ill, 6*(3), 41–43.

Rogers, S.E., et al. (1997). A consumer-constructed scale to measure empowerment among users of mental health services. *Psychiatric Services, 48,* 1042–1047.

Segal, S., Silverman, C., & Temkin, T. (1995a). Characteristics and service use of long-term members of self-help agencies for mental health clients. *Psychiatric Services, 46,* 269–274.

Segal, S., Silverman, C., & Temkin, T. (1995b). Measuring empowerment in client-run self-help agencies. *Community Mental Health Journal, 31*(3), 215–227.

Sills, G. (1995). Breaking free. *Journal of the American Psychiatric Nurses Association, 1*(3), 73–75.

Spiese, V. (1996). And what do we tell the children? *The*

Journal of the California Alliance for the Mentally Ill, 7(3), 50–51.

Starkey, D., et al. (1997). Inpatient psychiatric rehabilitation in a state hospital setting. *Journal of Psychosocial Nursing, 35*(1), 10–15.

Swartz, R., & Little, C. (1996). Schools: a resource for offspring. *The Journal of the California Alliance for the Mentally Ill, 7*(3), 63–65.

Temkin, T., Silverman, C., & Segal, S. (1995). Making self help work. *The Journal of the California Alliance for the Mentally Ill, 6*(3), 4–5.

Uttaro, T., & Mechanic, D. (1994). The NAMI consumer survey analysis of unmet needs.*Hospital and Community Psychiatry, 45,* 372–374.

Viner, M., Waite, J., & Thienhaus, O. (1996). Comorbidity and the need for physical examinations among patients seen in the psychiatric emergency service. *Psychiatric Services, 47,* 947–948.

Wahl, O. (1995). *Media madness: public images of mental illness.* New Brunswick, NJ: Rutgers University Press.

Wahl, O. (1997). *Consumer experience of stigma: results of a national survey.* Washington, DC: George Mason University.

Wasserbauer, L. (1996). Psychiatric nurses' knowledge of the Americans with Disabilities Act. *Archives of Psychiatric Nursing, 10,* 328.

Wasserbauer, L. (1997). Mental illness and the Americans with Disabilities Act: understanding the fundamentals. *Journal of Psychosocial Nursing, 35*(1), 22–26.

Winefield, H., & Harvey, E. (1994). Needs of family caregivers in chronic schizophrenia. *Schizophrenia Bulletin, 20,* 557–566.

Ethical Perspectives and Issues in Advanced Practice Nursing

PATRICIA A. MURPHY and DAVID M. PRICE

■ INTRODUCTION

Ethics is integral to advanced practice psychiatric-mental health nursing. This chapter explores why and how this statement is true, identifies a range of conceptual tools and other resources for "doing ethics," and discusses some of the leading issues in contemporary psychiatric-mental health nursing.

What do we mean by *ethics*? In the university or library, ethics is a branch of philosophy that examines the basis for claims about what is right, good, or obligatory. In nursing and other professional disciplines, ethics is an integral dimension of what one does: deciding, defining, directing, recommending, guiding, helping, assessing, prescribing, and planning. Ethics is not as much a body of knowledge as an activity; ethics is *doing* something. It is *thinking* about what one should do rather than reflexive doing. It is thoughtful doing and responsible acting. Thus defined, ethics is obviously not optional for any professional person. One cannot be a nurse, physician, schoolteacher, or police officer and not do ethics (Aroskar, 1995). Anyone with large, important responsibilities and significant scope for decisions about how to fulfill those responsibilities must necessarily make choices about what is preferable or most important. Any truly responsible professional makes many delicate decisions about the boundaries of his or her responsibility. Such exercise of judgment is essential to the concept of "professional."

In general, higher levels of training, certification and expectation are associated with a wider scope of responsibility and levels of increasing complexity. This means that advanced practice registered nurses (APRNs) in psychiatric and mental health care can expect that they will be confronted with more challenging ethical dilemmas and that they will be expected to deal with those dilemmas more directly and independently.

It would be misleading, however, to think that emergent, clinical dilemmas—"Oh my God! What should we do about him?!"—are the sole indication for thoughtful doing, for responsible action. APRNs are leaders who set and disseminate standards, define good practice, determine priorities, and direct care (Cassidy, 1998). Each of these leadership activities is ethical behavior in that it involves judgments and statements about what is right, good, proper, essential, or most important.

FUNCTIONS OF ETHICS
▪ IN THE PROFESSION

APRNs, individually and collectively, do ethics as a part of several distinct functions. Ethical deci-

sions by APRNs are expressed in several different ways, each with its own contribution to the profession and to patients. The role of ethical reflection is illustrated in the following four professional functions: 1) regulation, 2) definition, 3) leadership, and 4) dilemma resolution.

Formulating Minimal Standards (Regulatory Function)

When APRNs participate in a standard setting, they are doing ethics. Regulations or standards seek to establish either minimal expectations to which someone will be held accountable or to conform behavior to a predetermined pattern in circumstances where standardization is thought to be important. Standards range from the legally established regulations discussed in Chapter 8, to research protocols, to local, institutional rules for summoning a security officer, to a journal article that argues for widespread adoption of a new practice (Hassmiller, 1991). It is a mistake to assume that the unromantic work of regulation formulation is without far-reaching ethical significance. Regulations organize and structure social relations. Anything that defines who may do what to whom under what conditions is ethically significant.

Clearly, any nurse may do ethics in this way. However, with the expanded roles and graduate-level education of the APRN comes a significantly increased expectation of and scope for thoughtful action that functions to regulate professional behavior. For example, a group of APRN educators and practitioners developed the scope and standards of practice for psychiatric-mental health nursing (ANA, 1994). APRNs also serve as members of state boards of nursing or provide consultation about the regulations that govern basic and advanced nursing practice.

Defining the Profession (Definitional Function)

The first task of any profession is to present itself as a service to the public and to other professionals. Even old and well-established professions do this; newer and rapidly changing professions do it very deliberately and self-consciously. This function is typically expressed most formally in a code of ethics or a mission statement. The importance of moral categories in the self-definition of professionals of all kinds is made clear through such documents. Establishing a committee to draft a mission statement or a code of ethics is among the first acts of a newly organized, professional group. Such a code becomes one of the foundational documents that guides strategic planning and is appealed to as members argue about organizational positions, directions, and emphases (Cassidy, 1998).

As advanced practice nursing is still relatively new and evolving, individual APRNs need to seize opportunities to define and differentiate themselves. In their informal attempts at professional self-presentation, they will use ethical terms to distinguish themselves from other practitioners. That is, they will use the language of responsibility and values, of good ends and preferable means. When they do ethics in this way, the function of ethics is to define their role and purposes and to communicate to others the ideals against which they are willing to have their behavior measured.

When a physician subscribes to the Hippocratic ideal of putting the patient's welfare first or when a nurse pledges to provide care with respect for human dignity and uniqueness of the patient, this is different from promising to obey the law or to follow protocol stipulations (Schyve, 1996). Rather, it is a statement about what it means to be a member of one's chosen profession. It is a statement of intention to be guided by the highest, noblest, and most robust definitions of responsibility and not merely the minimal expectations of the regulatory overseer.

Setting Priorities (Leadership Function)

What is most important, urgent, or indicated at any given moment is a kind of moral decision. When the focus of these decisions is on organizations or systems as opposed to the priority

setting that individual APRNs do in the ordinary course of their work, it is an essential part of the expectations for leaders (Cassidy, 1998; Hofmann, 1996).

Whether in the workplace or in the professional organization, leadership entails setting priorities. Mission statements, annual goals, position papers, and budget guidelines are all ways in which an organization selects certain ends, purposes, or programs for special emphasis. Whether in their mental health care agencies or in the American Psychiatric Nurses Association (APNA), when APRNs single out some goals or programs as especially important, even if temporarily so, they are doing ethics. The function of these ethical decisions is distinct from standard setting or the articulation of ideas, although its main purpose is the same: to discern and communicate what professionals should do.

Solving Clinical Problems (Dilemma Resolution Function)

APRNs do ethics when they resolve uncertainty or conflict about how to behave in concrete clinical situations (McDonald, 1994). When thinking about ethical decision making in the health care professions, this function comes to mind first.

Putting it last in a list of the functions of ethical deliberation serves as a reminder of the inevitable (and intended) influence of standards, ideals, and professional emphasis on choices and behavior in the midst of each work day (Davis et al., 1997). It might be said that ethical deliberation in all its functions culminates in and finds its ultimate justification in the thoughtful and responsible choices of an individual APRN doing his or her job on any given day. However, it is also true that the best rule making, the most authentic articulation of professional ideals, and the most appropriate priority setting will grow out of direct involvement in practice. All functions of ethical deliberation within the profession are mutually enhancing. The best practice is exemplified by those APRNs whose ethical discernment serves all of these functions over time.

PROFESSIONAL VIRTUES
■ FOR APRNS

Like other professions, nursing has defined itself largely in moral terms. The American Nurses Association (ANA) *Code for Nurses* (1985) sets out a series of statements that embody the virtues of nursing or the ethical ideals by which American nurses have said they are prepared to be held accountable.

The *Code* speaks in a modern voice, with verbs rather than adjectives or adverbs carrying the punch: "The nurse safeguards . . ."; "The nurse maintains . . ."; "The nurse exercises . . ." Nevertheless, these statements are clearly not meant to describe what nurses *actually* do (sociology), but what nurses *should* do (ethics). The *Code* sets out ideal behaviors or professional virtues.

Some people express impatience with consideration of ideals and virtues, preferring the more concrete categories of enforceable regulations and specific behaviors such as competencies that can be objectively and reliably measured. However, as argued in the previous section, there is an important distinction between the regulatory function and the definitional function of practical ethics. The two functions cannot be subsumed into either one without serious consequences. An ideal without specific applicability is merely decorative; specificity without roots in basic purpose is empty and meaningless. It has been said that ideals are like stars to the sailor: even if one cannot reach them, they provide direction. Clinical navigation (protocol writing, quality management, performance improvement, "best practices," etc.) entail skills that the APRN acquires through specialized education and supervised experience. However, clinical navigation cannot work or at least is not obvious that it is working if the ideals do not shine with sufficient clarity to maintain a sense of direction. The professional virtues (moral ideals) of nursing emerge clearly from the *Code*.

Respect for Persons

Unconditional respect for the dignity of persons is the virtue or ideal intended to be primary in all that modern American nurses think about their role. Respect is the attribute of nursing expressed in the first two statements of the *Code* (ANA, 1985):

1. The nurse provides services with respect for the dignity of man, unrestricted by considerations of nationality, race, creed, color, or status.
2. The nurse safeguards the individual's right to privacy by judiciously protecting information of a confidential nature, sharing only that information relevant to his care.

The special applicability of this most basic of nursing virtues is explored in a later section devoted to prominent issues in psychiatric-mental health nursing. Here it is important to note that, of all illnesses, psychiatric illnesses are among the most stigmatizing (Goffman, 1963). Accordingly, a statement that the nurse respects the patient despite social attributes, personal behavior, or the nature of his or her health problems has particular meaning for the APRN. That the *Code* gives priority to this attribute suggests, in a way, that APRNs can appreciate uniquely that respect for persons is the foundational principle of modern nursing.

A duty to maintain confidentiality is an ancient idea in health care ethics (Beck, 1990). No code of ethics in the recorded Western history fails to include confidentiality among the expectations that health care workers lay upon themselves. It is ordinarily stated in terms of a self-evident obligation or, as here, in the more modern sense of a duty reciprocal to a right of the patient. In either case, the obligation to maintain confidentiality is rooted in the more elemental notion of respect for persons. This duty takes on special relevance since recent changes in the organization of health care, and especially changes in information technology, have posed complex problems for those committed to the ideal of confidentiality. See Chapter 3 for a discussion of ethical dilemmas in information technology.

The second statement in the *Code* has particular applicability for APRNs. An APRN's patients are apt to have information in their health care record that both they and the community regard as especially sensitive. Thus, while APRNs share with other nurses an equal obligation to "judiciously protect information of a confidential nature," the patients of APRNs may be especially subject to harm from breaches of confidentiality (Beck, 1990). Moreover, APRNs are frequently in the uncomfortable and delicate position of having to make hard choices about the limits of the duty of confidentiality. Later in this chapter, dilemmas of confidentiality are shown to be among the most characteristic and perennial of clinical problems in advanced practice psychiatric-mental health nursing.

Advocacy

Advocacy is the virtue that most clearly distinguishes modern American nurses from their nursing ancestors. The earlier ideal for nursing emphasized the military virtues of loyalty to the institution and faithful obedience to the orders of superiors (Roberts, 1983). At a rate that seems maddeningly slow to nursing reformers but has been actually very rapid in cultural terms, the legal virtue of advocacy has become a leading metaphor for what it means to be a professional nurse (Winslow, 1984).

The *Code* expresses this moral ideal in blunt and uncompromising language:

3. The nurse acts to safeguard the patient when his care and safety are affected by incompetent, unethical, or illegal conduct of any person.

Given the vulnerability of so many psychiatric patients and the prevalence of personal and institutional prejudices against those with behavioral disorders, this nursing virtue has particular significance for APRNs (Liaschenko, 1995). The APRN's patients are at risk of mistreatment at many levels by individuals, communities, institutions, and governmental systems. Since every nurse is called to be a vigilant and vigorous advocate, this attribute has significance for APRNs that is rivaled only by their pediatric and geriatric counterparts who also care for very vulnerable populations.

Competence and Clinical Responsibility

The *Code* is brief, almost terse, in its insistence about the virtue of competence:

4. The nurse maintains individual competence in nursing practice, recognizing and accepting responsibility for individual actions and judgments.

The APRN has challenges beyond those of the registered nurse (RN) in the basic level of practice with respect to the maintenance of competency. The amount of mastery expected of an APRN is not the most challenging aspect of this moral ideal, despite how daunting the shear volume of learning might seem in preparing for and implementing the role. Rather, the principal challenge is to keep up with the dynamic nature of the field, incorporating new concepts and technologies, and gauging the implications of societal and cultural forces (Davis et al., 1997). Moreover, unlike the basic level nurse, the APRN may not rely on an employing hospital or other agency to share responsibility for recognizing developments, providing requisite in-service education, and certifying updated competencies.

The *Code* is a bit more explicit about the related ideal of assuming responsibility for judgments about one's own competence and the competence of coworkers:

5. The nurse uses individual competence as a criterion in accepting delegated responsibilities and assigning nursing activities to others.
6. The nurse participates in research activities when assured that the rights of individual subjects are protected.

The complexity of modern health care institutions with its specialization, multidisciplinary teams and dizzying rate of change, compounded by reengineering and faster "throughput" in response to cost-containment pressures, makes this ideal increasingly problematic for almost all nurses (Renz & Eddy, 1996). Those APRNs who manage quality improvement or education for large or small systems of care will have particular responsibility to equip nurses to handle the very worrisome contemporary pressure to accept or delegate nursing tasks when it is uncertain that they match individual competencies. As the impetus for evidence-based practice in psychiatric and behavioral health care gains ground, issues about appropriate delegation for effective assessment and intervention, data collection and analysis, and policy formation and evaluation will increasingly come to the forefront (Boyle & Callahan, 1995).

Professional Responsibility

The *Code*, in common with most of its professional counterparts, emphasizes that nurses have a responsibility to serve and enhance the profession (Aroskar, 1995). The operative verb is "participate":

7. The nurse participates in the efforts of the profession to define and upgrade standards of nursing practice and education.
8. The nurse, acting through the professional organization, participates in establishing and maintaining conditions of employment conducive to high-quality nursing care.
9. The nurse works with members of health professions and other citizens in promoting efforts to meet health needs of the public.

The leaders of organized nursing have touted the benefits of active membership in two ways: (1) membership in the nurse's professional organizations is an obligation; and (2) such membership nourishes the nurse's professional self. Actually, the top positions in organized nursing are disproportionately filled by those with advanced degrees and leadership roles within nursing agencies and nursing education. Part of this phenomenon is explained by the need of those in leadership positions to network with peers beyond the confines of their own practice settings. Also, by virtue of their leadership positions (which require advanced credentials), these leaders have the autonomy and resources to devote time and energy to professional organization activities. As suggested previously, leaders must interact with, learn from, and draw energy from persons and enterprises outside their immediate situation. Otherwise they will not be leaders in deed but only in title.

Thus APRNs will characteristically need to become and remain active in their professional organizations. They will do so because they recognize that taking an active part is professionally responsible. They will also do it because it is intrinsically rewarding and professionally sustaining.

Social Responsibility

Despite the dominant emphasis on respect and advocacy for the individual patient, the *Code* ends by articulating a final virtue:

10. The nurse refuses to give or imply endorsement to advertising, promotion, or sales for commercial products, services, or enterprises.

Social responsibility is an attribute or ideal that the nursing profession shares with other professions but which nursing has particularly emphasized in recent years. APRNs, like other thoughtful citizens and health care advocates, have increasingly come to see health care as a community resource to be shaped to common purposes (Aroskar, 1995). The costs associated with many health care resources beg for widespread sharing of the financial burden. Moreover, there has been enormous public investment in everything from health professional education to the development of prosthetic devices to tax-exempt status for hospitals. All of these factors suggest that the public's health is the public's business to an extent unique in American history (Fuller, 1995).

The ANA, many state nursing associations, the APNA, and most of the other specialty organizations became more politically active and more politically effective during the waning years of the twentieth century. This was partly a function of increasing sophistication and partly a function of opportunity as health care issues have moved toward the top of the national political agenda. The fundamental difference is that nurses and nursing, prominently including psychiatric-mental health nursing, have come to understand that concerted, organized, communal efforts are required to ensure health care that is accessible, affordable, effective, and accountable. See Chapter 7 for further discussion of nursing's political activism as social responsibility.

■ ETHICAL ANALYSIS

When faced with ethical problems, whether in policy or in day-to-day clinical work, the conscientious APRN seeks help to ensure the best outcomes. The term *ethical analysis* means simply careful and systematic efforts to figure out what one should do in a particular situation. There is a variety of resources potentially available to any professional with serious, responsible intentions. "Conscientious," "serious," and "responsible," are necessary qualifiers here. Many people, including several mental health professionals, will choose to respond to their own moral discomfort by denial and avoidance. "It's not so bad," "It's not my job," and "It's just the way things are" are all ways of deflecting responsibility. Resources for ethical analysis are only useful for those who own their responsibility and seek to discharge it with optimal competence and care.

There are several ethical theories in common use among health professionals, although few health professionals probably think of themselves as operating out of an "ethical theory" or using an "analytic method." Such terms mean there are different ways to approach the resolution of an ethical problem. If an APRN characteristically goes about the resolution of a dilemma in a particular, deliberate, reasoning way, he or she is employing an analytic method (Davis et al., 1997).

Virtue Ethics (Role-Based Analysis)

One approach to ethical reasoning is by way of professional virtues, or roles (Husted & Husted, 1991). Virtue ethics is the approach espoused in the *Code for Nurses*. The approach may be seen most clearly by considering the following case example:

The caring, but distraught parents of your teenage patient are seriously considering placing him in a boot camp school/treatment program to deal with his acting out behavior. They say that they are "at wit's end" and that neither outpatient psychotherapy nor special education resources nor short-term hospitalization has "worked." The boy still uses illicit drugs, lies, steals and engages in dangerous behavior. Unhappy and probably depressed, the boy would almost surely resist this placement. He has not been told that his parents intend to drive him there and leave. You know little about programs of this sort, but are generally skeptical of their "extreme" methods. You are especially troubled that your patient is apparently about to be forcibly detained in a treatment program that he has had no part in choosing.

Analysis of this case situation by reference to the virtues of nursing would surely prompt a series of pertinent questions such as those posed in Box 19-1. Thoughtful answers to these questions, if not the questions themselves, should further illuminate the dilemma and lead the APRN closer to a best answer to the practical question, "What should I do?" The essence of virtue ethics is that, after classifying what are the applicable virtues, the APRN uses those concepts as the analytic categories or language tools to examine the specific situation. The aim is always to discern what it means in this concrete instance to be "virtuous"

---

box 19-1

QUESTIONS TO POSE IN VIRTUE ETHICS ANALYSIS

Based on the clinical example of a dilemma with a teen-age boy and his parents, the APRN might ask the following questions:

1. What does it mean, in this instance, to respect my patient's human dignity and uniqueness?
2. How should the fact that he is 15 years old and dependent affect the implications of "respect?" Specifically, does respect oblige me to disclose to a 15 year old his parents' plan?
3. Aside from any applicable legal requirements, do his parents have the right to effectively "commit" him? How does respect for *their* dignity figure in?
4. What do I have to learn in order to competently assess whether an immoral or illegal act is about to happen?

(i.e., what it means to fulfill an APRN's responsibilities).

Clearly, virtue ethics is very close to a role-based analysis in which the nurse essentially asks, "What does it mean to be a good nurse?" As demonstrated previously, the *Code* is cast in this format, outlining in a series of descriptive statements the characteristic behaviors of the "good," or ethical, nurse. That this role description is markedly different, although not necessarily contradictory, from what the APRN would hear from the human resources manager when inquiring about a posted nursing position, or what nurses would read in the Nurse Practice Act of their state, illustrates that there are a number of ways to describe a role. When describing a role in moral terms, as in the *Code*, the APRN forms a basis for doing ethics (i.e., for figuring out how to behave in a specific clinical instance or how to write a rule to guide behavior of nurses in a health care agency).

Principle-Based Ethics

The analytic method that is probably most widely recognized among health care workers is sometimes called *principlism*. It is so widely recognized largely because of the popular text *Principles of Biomedical Ethics,* first published in 1979 by Thomas Beauchamp and James Childress and reprinted many times (Beauchamp & Childress, 1994). This accessible volume proposes that any problem in health care ethics be dissected and examined in terms of four basic principles: autonomy, beneficence, nonmaleficence, and justice.

Autonomy refers to the idea that health professionals should respect others, especially in that highest expression of personhood, decisions about how one should live one's own life. All of what is embraced by such concepts as self-determination, liberty, personal dignity, privacy, and the right of informed consent is caught up in this principle of autonomy. The principle of *beneficence* refers to the notion that health professionals should aim to help others, seeking the optimal balance of benefit over burden and putting the patient's welfare first. The principle of *nonmaleficence* means that one should avoid wronging others and protect them against harm from other persons or forces. "Harm" in this senses does not refer to the unavoidable mutilations of surgery or the pain and distress of a child's vaccination; it refers to doing unwarranted surgery or overcharging for the vaccination. The principle of *justice* refers to treating patients fairly, ensuring each patient his or her due, and distributing scarce resources equitably.

The appeal of principlism has been due in significant part to the fact that its analytic categories can be used by people whose arguments are otherwise quite disparate: *deontologists,* who seek to define the right action by reference to abstract duties or rights, and *consequentialists,* who prefer to calculate which alternative actions are most likely to yield desired outcomes. Although recourse to principles will not bridge the gap between the proponents of these two ethical approaches, it does provide some common language. Moreover, most Americans, including most health professionals, seem to mix deontologic and consequentialist reasoning when offering justification for their ethical decisions. For example, an APRN arguing in favor of disclosure to the 15 year old, whose parents are trying to manipulate him into admission to an alternative school or treatment center, might plausibly appeal to the parents on the basis of both the "right to know" using a concept of inalienable human dignity (deontologic reasoning) and a prediction that withholding information will erode trust and undermine therapeutic relationships (consequentialist reasoning).

Relational Ethics

Bolstered by the seminal work of Gilligan (1982) and others who have argued that women tend to perceive and solve problems in ways different from most men, a newer kind of ethical deliberation has emerged, often labeled *feminist ethics* (Tong, 1989). This methodology departs from traditional dependence upon objectivity, deductive reasoning, and linear analysis. Instead, the person seeking to understand a situation pays particular attention to relationships. "The situation" is thought to *be* the relationships—affectional relationships, power relationships, historic or traditional relationships, gender relationships, class relationships, ethnic or belief-system relationships, and so on. This theoretical orientation is the basis for an "ethics of caring," which has particular reference to nursing (Gadow, 1988; Rafael, 1996).

Referring again to the 15-year-old boy whose parents may send him away to a remote program for adolescents with severe behavior problems, using this method of discerning what to do, the APRN would concentrate on the relationships:

- The parents say, "we are at the end of our rope." What does this mean about their interaction with their son and with each other?
- Is there trust between the APRN and the boy? What kind of trust is there? On what is it based?
- Is the boy's psychologic distance from his parents a function of anger, self-protection, indifference, or something else?
- What does the boy expect from adults in authority? What would he like?

In pursuing this way of understanding (note that "analyzing" might be regarded as an inappropriate word by proponents), the APRN makes no recourse to abstract principles nor to predictions about reaching ultimate goals. Further, this method includes the moral actor in the situation under study rather than seeking an objective vantage point. In the relational approach to ethical reflection, the concept of a disinterested observer is not only *not* valued but is regarded as pretentious and unreal.

Awareness of an ethical problem often begins as a subjective sense of moral dis-ease, regardless of the APRN's preferred analytic method (Forchuk, 1991). The relational approach versus the principle-based approach is more accommodating of the role of feeling and intuition in the APRN's efforts to discern "the right thing to do." A few theorists have taken the concept of "moral sensing" beyond the level of that initial discomfort that is often the first indication of an ethical prob-

lem. However, none seem to suggest that a focus on the subjective and interpersonal aspects of moral decision making obviates the relevance of rational thinking.

It can seem that the virtue-based, principle-based, and relationship-based methods are all too removed from the concrete and particular and thus are of little help in the context of everyday advanced practice nursing. Unfortunately, some academic proponents, more interested in pushing their method than helping practitioners, have unwittingly fostered the impression that ethics is for philosophers and scholars. In fact, frontline practitioners can make good use of ethical theories, provided that they attend carefully to social context and are flexible enough to draw on various theories (Mohr, 1995).

■ ETHICS IN THE LITERATURE

One of the most remarkable phenomena of recent health care history is the enormous explosion of written material about ethics. In the 1970s, a gifted and motivated professional could have kept abreast of what was appearing in English-language journals and trade books on the subject of health care ethics and health policy. By the 1990s, that was impossible. A similar proliferation is apparent in the number of conferences devoted wholly or in significant part to health care ethics and health policy.

In general terms, the printed resources can be grouped under three headings: ethics literature, standards and guidelines, and "clinical" literature. No attempt is made here to survey or catalog these resources but merely to briefly characterize each major category of potentially useful literature to APRNs seeking to be responsible decision makers.

The proliferation of books and articles that deal exclusively and professionally with ethical issues in healthcare is truly impressive, a metaphor for the complexity and perceived importance of these issues at the end of the twentieth century. No library contains it all; no individual could manage to keep up with it all.

Every APRN should own at least one general text in health care ethics or, perhaps, nursing ethics. It may also be good discipline to subscribe to, or otherwise regularly browse in, at least one ethics journal. A few such basic resources are listed in the Resources and Connections section of this chapter. *Medline* and other literature databases catalog many health care ethics and health policy journals. A search with virtually any descriptor plus "ethics" will yield from a few to a flood of citations. When accessing such large electronic catalogs, APRNs must be careful to distinguish between serious ethical reflection and opinion pieces unfettered by scholarly rigor or even fairness.

The prevalence of practice guidelines is another signal phenomenon of modern health care. The adoption of managed care, as well as the more general increase in all manner of system complexities, has spurred demand for written standards of care. Everything from the *Code for Nurses* to position statements on specific practice issues promulgated by specialty organizations, prestigious institutions, or government panels can be placed under the heading of "Standards and Guidelines." Such documents are powerful tools of education, local policy formulation, and clinical dispute resolution. Standards and guidelines can also be used as a justification for professional practice with resentful coworkers and distressed patients and families. See Chapter 12 for a further discussion of practice guidelines.

There is much ethical reflection embedded in books and articles whose main focus is not explicitly "ethical." This text is an example of the characteristic, modern practice of including contributions explicitly on ethics in a volume that is not "a book about ethics." Similarly, many issues of standard nursing and medical journals include articles by professional ethicists or by practitioners with considerable expertise in ethics.

Again, APRNs must appreciate that not everything that appears on the computer screen to be ethical analysis will prove, on closer examination, to be careful, thoughtful, scholarly, and balanced.

High-quality, peer-reviewed journals generally publish high-quality, peer-reviewed ethics articles. In any case, only a critical reader can distinguish when an article with an ethically intriguing title is not matched by ethically rigorous content.

ETHICS COMMITTEES AND ETHICS CONSULTANTS

Resources for the resolution of ethical programs include face-to-face consultation as well as a variety of methods or ways of thinking and kinds of printed materials. Again, there is a variety of such "people resources" potentially available to an APRN in search of help with ethical dilemmas.

Almost everyone begins with a trusted coworker close at hand. "Let me run something by you" or "What do you think we should do when this (situation) happens?" are common ways of eliciting such informal consultation. The ready availability of peers for this kind of assistance with ethical dilemmas is an important consideration for most professionals as they evaluate work environments. Many ethical uncertainties resolve after conversation with a thoughtful and perhaps more experienced colleague. However, when such "curbstone" consultation is not sufficient (i.e., when the distress and disequilibrium of conflict or uncertainty is not dissipated by such first-line helpers), conscientious professionals go into search mode: Who knows about these things? Where is there a specialist with whom I can talk?

APRNs who work in academic medical centers or large, integrated systems can usually find their way to a professional ethicist. Although no accurate accounting exists, there are hundreds of individuals in North America who make their living as scholars and advisors on issues in health care ethics. Some of them are nurses; most of them are at least generally knowledgeable about and sensitive to nursing concerns. Some, perhaps many, are markedly generous with their time and attention to another professional serious about figuring out "the right thing to do," even when that professional is from another institution. APRNs would be well advised to make a point of knowing who in their geographic area and who in their specialty area might fill this description.

Ethics committees are increasingly prevalent in hospitals, nursing homes, hospices, and other health care institutions (Christopher, 1994). An ethics committee is a multidisciplinary, standing panel of persons that represents the ultimate consultative resource in many institutions (Fost & Cranford, 1985). Classically, ethics committees are available for assistance with the toughest of cases and the most problematic of policy questions. Most will conduct educational programs in response to needs uncovered in the course of case review and policy formulation.

Ethics committees do not act like appellate courts, taking over the resolutions of disputes that persist after lower-level intervention. Rather, ethics committees are advisory bodies to be used by first-line clinicians who retain their ethical and legal responsibility for the troubling situation. The authority of an ethics committee is the "moral authority" that attaches to any person or group that will take on and stick with hard, sometimes uncomfortable issues with no other reward than the intrinsic satisfaction of helping (Blake, 1992). Ethics committees proceed with equal attention to the reliability of information; to the perceptions, beliefs, and feelings of the principles; and to the mission of the institution (Felder, 1996).

APRNs should assess the adequacy of ethics consultation resources in their own or affiliated health care agencies (Povar, 1991; Van Allen, Moldow, & Cranford, 1989). Box 19-2 lists questions to assess the adequacy of an institutional ethics committee. If the local ethics committee has no APRN among its active membership, or if the psychosocial disciplines are inadequately represented on the committee, an APRN should investigate the process for volunteering to serve or being appointed (Oddi & Cassidy, 1990). Good ethics committees are always personally and professionally rewarding. The best ones are enjoyable learning experiences (Price, 1995).

---

box 19-2

ASSESSMENT OF AN ETHICS COMMITTEE

To assess the adequacy of an ethics committee, APRNs might ask the following questions:

- What is the mission or purpose of the ethics committee?
- Who are its members and how are they chosen?
- How often does the committee meet?
- Does the committee do case consultation?
- How do the best nurses and physicians regard this service?
- Do they use it?
- How is the service accessed?
- What are the provisions for evaluation or quality improvement?

■ SELECTED ISSUES

APRNs encounter ethical dilemmas many times every day. "What should I say to her?" "How should we deal with behavior like this?" "What's fair in this situation?" "Does my responsibility extend to *that*?" Any time a conscientious APRN is uncertain, confused, or conflicted about a "should" question, that is an ethical dilemma deserving of serious attention.

The following survey of ethical issues in psychiatric nursing is neither exhaustive nor situation specific. Many issues that involve staff in turmoil may not be represented here. If so, it would be a mistake to conclude that a specific issue is not an "ethical" dilemma for APRNs. The issues briefly discussed here inevitably lack the rich detail and immediacy of their expression in particular settings. A general characterization of any issue unavoidably glosses over both elaborations and complications that would be essential to a full presentation of that issue as it demonstrates itself in an actual situation. Given this caveat, a discussion of ethical issues that occur commonly in psychiatric settings is presented.

Determinations of Decisional Capacity and Suicide Risk

APRNs are often involved in efforts to decide whether a patient has lost the capacity to make his or her own decisions (Davis et al., 1997). *Capacity* is a clinical determination in which physicians and nurses are frequently and properly involved. *Competency,* on the other hand, is a judicial determination in which clinicians have an advisory role only (Fletcher, 1997).

A judgment of decisional incapacity may have significant, even dramatic, consequences for the patient. It can mean that a patient goes for a procedure that he or she has been refusing. It can mean being transferred from one care setting to another. It can mean physical or chemical restraints. It can mean that all the really important decisions about the patient's care now are conducted outside his or her hearing. In short, determinations of decisional capacity or suicidal intent are ethically significant decisions (Davis et al., 1997). Moreover, the policies and procedures that define how and by whom, after what kind of process, and with what kind of review those decisions are made are very important, very powerful ethical decisions.

Consider the following case from the records of the ethics consultation service at a private urban, not-for-profit hospital:

Lydia is a 59-year-old African-American woman with a 20-year history of diabetes and a 2-year history of repeated acute care admissions for chronic renal failure, congestive heart failure, diabetic retinopathy, and leg ulcers. After a series of failed grafts, the toes on her right foot were amputated. After attempted laser surgery, she lost one eye and most vision in the other. She was depressed. Worry about memory loss 1 year ago prompted a mini-mental examination on which she scored 24/30.

Earlier this year, Lydia was brought to the emergency department by her family after a change in mental status. She was found to be oriented to person but not to time and place. Diagnosed with end-stage renal disease, she was started on dialysis. Because of her worsening peripheral vascular disease, she had a below-the-knee amputation of her right leg.

A few months later, Lydia was back in the emergency department with complaints of shortness of breath while watching television and undergoing dialysis. A computerized tomography (CT) scan revealed multiple small

strokes. After a short hospitalization, Lydia was discharged, only to reappear in the emergency department later that same day. Her family reported that she was depressed and talking about suicide. When questioned, Lydia said that she wanted to commit suicide by taking pills or shooting herself. She did not have access to a gun. She was readmitted, this time to the psychiatric floor.

In the "psych" unit, nurses were concerned that Lydia may have been placed there inappropriately. They noted her significant medical problems that required extensive physical nursing care. Also, they assessed the suicide potential of this blind, nonambulatory patient as being low. After 1 week in the psych unit, during which Lydia was taken from the unit to her dialysis treatments three times, the psychiatric consultation-liaison APRN contacted the hospital's ethics consultant. The consultant met with Lydia, her husband, the primary care nurse, and the social worker. That same day, two psychiatrists had signed commitment papers, while acknowledging that Lydia retained capacity to make medical decisions. The commitment was put on hold pending a multidisciplinary care planning meeting the next morning.

The patient, the social worker, the primary care nurse, the APRN, the psychiatrist, and Lydia's nephrologist attended the conference. In the presence of all, Lydia acknowledged that she did not want to go on living in her present state of debilitation and diminished quality of life. She would end her life if she were able. When the ethics consultant asked Lydia why she did not simply refuse continued dialysis, it became clear that she did not realize that that was an option. The nephrologist was asked to explain in detail what would happen if Lydia were to quit dialysis. Thus assured that refusing continued dialysis was entirely within her control and that the ensuing pathway to death would be nearly painless and peaceful, Lydia clearly stated her wish to discontinue treatment. A do-not-resuscitate (DNR) order was discussed. The effect of the decision upon her husband and others was explored. Throughout this meeting, Lydia was attentive and appropriately responsive; all present acknowledged that she had made an autonomous and informed decision. Moreover, nobody present expressed any doubts when Lydia, asked if she still wanted to kill herself, said that she would not do that now that she knew that she would be allowed to discontinue dialysis.

Later that day, Lydia was transferred to a medical floor with DNR orders and the discontinuation of dialysis. Lydia told her husband about the plan. He was supportive. A few days later, Lydia was discharged in the care of her husband and a hospice.

Any patient who presents in the emergency department saying that she wants to kill herself is likely to end up in a secure psychiatric unit. At the very least, an APRN or MD will be summoned to make an assessment and recommend disposition. Lydia was indeed suicidal. Although her disabilities suggest that effective suicide prevention might have been afforded on a medical floor, she was admitted to the psychiatry service. There is no real ethical dilemma to this point. The dilemma arose the next day in the mind of an experienced APRN who was confronted with a patient with significant medical problems and a not insignificant but easily manageable psychiatric problem. The APRN was unable, over several days, to convince the unit psychiatrists that Lydia's placement was suboptimal. She felt that the physicians were unwilling to seriously consider her arguments and that they were stuck in the box of the common rule that "suicidal patients belong in 'psych'."

Partly to resolve the ethical impasse with her colleagues, and partly because of a growing sense that she was missing a relevant piece of the puzzle, the APRN called for an ethics consultation. The ethics consultant was able to quickly reframe the issue in a way that led to a prompt resolution. The ethics consultant's complementary knowledge base and theoretical orientation included a perspective in which Lydia's statement that she wished to die was not construed as "suicidal," but rather as a value statement about life with a heavy burden of chronic disease and disability. This alternative perspective also suggested that health professionals, rather than having an obligation to restrain her, were obliged to honor and facilitate Lydia's intent. This is the "something" that the APRN sensed that she was "missing." As the ethics consultant explained, American public policy explicitly holds that refusing life-sustaining treatment is distinct from suicide. The issue had been framed initially in terms of suicidal intent because that is the way the patient had presented herself in the emergency department. It had remained that way because professionals tend to cling to their most familiar conceptual frameworks, even after there is an indication that they may be misapplied or otherwise inadequate.

In Lydia's case, the distinct questions of decisional capacity and suicidal intent became compounded, as they often are, by the medical providers. Lydia's nephrologist needed considerable reassurance that neither her emotional history ("depressed") nor her contemporaneous wish to die were sufficient bases to disenfranchise her as a decision maker. The two psychiatrists who signed Lydia's commitment papers, although apparently missing (or at least choosing not to explore) the distinction between suicide and refusal of treatment, nevertheless made clear that, although a danger to herself, Lydia retained decisional capacity. By acknowledging and underscoring this distinction, the psychiatrists kept open a crucial conceptual door that permitted those with caring, energy, and imagination to forge a positive resolution.

Determinations of decisional capacity are routinely made by internists and surgeons. They call upon the services of APRNs and other mental health professionals only when there is significant doubt or dispute about whether the patient lacks capacity. Not infrequently, a medical or surgical provider is confused, not only by the clinical evidence, but also about the concept of capacity. There may be references in the chart to the patient's orientation or ability to perform memory tasks or even "serial sevens." APRN consultants who find such evidence of misunderstanding can turn it into opportunities to teach the concept that the most discriminating test of a person's capacity to make a decision is the decision process itself.

Consent

Not all issues of consent are reducible to questions of capacity or "Who decides?" As the case of Lydia clearly illustrates, ethical problems arise when patients misperceive the range of options open to them. When such misperceptions are held to be a consequence of a provider's failure to properly inform, there may be a legal as well as ethical breach (Salgo v. Stanford, 1957). In any case, it should be clear that, quite apart from any real or suspected decrement in the patient's capacity for choice, a choice made without consideration of applicable options is a flawed choice. Of all the elements of informed consent, the requirement for explicit disclosure of alternatives may be the one most often missed.

In consultation-liaison psychiatry, the APRN may have to confront some of the inappropriate alternatives proposed by frustrated medical, surgical, pediatric, and obstetric colleagues. They may be aware that the psychiatric armamentarium has such tools as commitment, but they forget about the legal constraints on commitment and gloss over the distinctions between voluntary and involuntary commitment. Frustrated by a patient's behavioral problems, nonpsychiatric health professionals may expect that "psych" will be a ready ally in the case of psychotropic medication or physical restraint (Strumpf & Tomes, 1993). Occasionally, mental health professionals are summoned only after such ill-conceived, unethical, and perhaps illegal efforts have been ordered or actually implemented, often with the consent of inadequately informed family members.

Heading off or interrupting implementation of restraints and psychologic manipulation that is naive, uninformed, or contrary to applicable policy can require delicate handling. In the process, the consultant seeks to decrease embarrassment of professional colleagues and family members and increase their understanding and cooperation. A team meeting focused on devising a comprehensive plan of care for a difficult patient can serve the twin objectives of reconsidering an ill-fated intervention and articulating overall goals or strategies with buy-in by all the principals (Fisher, 1995).

An intriguing subtopic in consent for psychiatric treatment is the development of advance directives for mental health treatment. Modeled after advance directives for care at the end of life, an advance directive for mental health care is a contingency statement prepared by a person with decisional capacity in anticipation of a possible (or expected) future period of decisional incapacity. The maker of the advance directive seeks to 1) register consent or refusal of such invasive treatments as electroconvulsive therapy (ECT),

antipsychotic medications, or restraints; 2) specify the conditions under which these interventions would be acceptable; and 3) appoint the person or persons authorized to consent on his or her behalf. Such psychiatric advance directives enjoy neither the popularity nor (except in a handful of states) the legal status of advance directives for end-of-life care. Nevertheless, many conscientious mental health providers favor such formal declarations as guidance to professionals and family caregivers concerned with respecting patient autonomy (Backlar & McFarland, 1996).

The authenticity of such an advance directive, and hence its moral force, would be strongest when the maker has already lived through a major depression or other illness, has received a variety of treatments, and once stabilized, has stipulated how he or she wishes to be treated in another similar bout. In such circumstances, the APRN could have reasonable confidence that the consent or referral was "informed." Still, psychiatric illnesses tend to be different, in many important respects, from the conditions addressed in end-of-life advance directives. They are not as simple, predictable, or subject to palliation.

Unlike most living wills, which refuse all manner of life-prolonging treatment while asking for liberal comfort care, psychiatric advance directives are typically employed to refuse *particular* modalities (e.g., ECT) or to elect aggressive treatment by any means thought to be medically indicated (Etzel & Kjervik, 1998). In common with the more familiar end-of-life directive, the most useful function of an advance directive for psychiatric care may be the designation of a trusted individual to make decisions when and if the maker is unable to do so. Particularly in instances in which the maker's preferred proxy is other than his or her next of kin, formal appointment is advisable. Regardless of the legal status of written instructions for psychiatric care decisions, all states provide for durable powers of attorney for health care, which take effect when the maker becomes unable to make or communicate health care decisions. Chapter 8 provides more information about the legal process and implications.

QUESTIONS REGARDING A PSYCHIATRIC ADVANCE DIRECTIVE

The APRN might ask the following questions before acting on a signed psychiatric advance directive:

- Has the patient lost his or her capacity to make decisions?
- If so, does he or she nonetheless retain some capacity to contribute to, or be involved in, the decision making?
- If so, how?
- What do his or her general directions mean in these circumstances?
- Are my biases distorting my reading of his or her wishes?
- Do I need help interpreting these wishes?
- How sure is sure enough?

As with the more familiar end-of-life directives, the presence of written directions, while helpful, does not obviate the need for ethically sensitive judgment on the part of professionals and surrogates. Box 19-3 poses questions an APRN might ask regarding the implementation of a psychiatric advance directive.

Stigma of Diagnoses and Treatment

When celebrities or opinion leaders go public about their own psychiatric illness, such openness tends to normalize, demystify, and destigmatize psychiatric maladies (Styron, 1990). Both research evidence and common sense suggest that anything that decreases the shame and avoidance associated with mental illness may facilitate timely treatment and lessen the burdens of the illness itself. On the other hand, APRNs and other mental health workers have powerful incentives to conspire with patients and families to continue the hiddenness of psychiatric diagnoses and psychiatric treatment. Stigma is a reality. Disclosure has had social and economic consequences for many patients (Goffman, 1963). Both legal restraints and a commit-

ment to secondary prevention require APRNs to minimize the effects of societal attitudes and overt discrimination (Trexler, 1996).

This sensitivity to stigmatization may lead some APRNs to do several things that risk violation of other obligations. That is to say, attempts to avoid possibly harmful labeling may involve APRNs in moral conflict. If the APRN were reluctant to label a patient with a stigmatizing diagnosis like schizophrenia or borderline personality and tried to withhold the diagnosis from the patient and his or her family, the APRN might be breaching the duties of full disclosure, honesty, and informed consent. Expressed in consequentialist terms, avoidance of the emotional and social trauma of labeling runs up against the danger of increasing frustration, anger, and mistrust in a patient or family unable to know what is wrong. Although a common concern in the past, a greater emphasis on psychoeducation techniques and the view of family members as partners in the treatment process have largely diminished the likelihood of this type of disclosure dilemma (Trexler, 1996).

However, sensitive to the threat of discrimination born of ignorance and prejudice, mental health professionals may be tempted to "fudge" on particularly stigmatizing diagnoses in reports or billing documents. When the signs and symptoms of two disorders overlap, it may be tempting to write down the least stigmatizing diagnosis, even when clinical judgment inclines the practitioner in the opposite direction. It is hard to be, at the same time, a disinterested scientist and a passionately involved therapist-advocate.

Analogous dilemmas arise in determinations of "dangerousness," a stigmatizing label that conscientious professionals are properly reluctant to apply without substantial cause (Mulvey, 1994). The difference is that a designation of dangerousness ordinarily has the practical effect of protection for the patient or others, perhaps including the APRN doing the labeling.

It should be clear from this brief discussion that simple statements and absolutist rules will be of little help to conscientious APRNs struggling to do the right thing when they are acutely aware of the persistent stigmatization of mental illness and behavioral differentness. On one hand, openness is the ultimate enemy of stigma; on the other hand, openness carries immediate risks for particular patients. Only careful thinking on a case-by-case basis will yield any confident answers to the inevitable and concrete dilemmas posed by patients with mental illness who are subject to pervasive prejudice.

Confidentiality and Disclosure

No obligation of health professionals is so universal and ancient as the obligation to keep confidences. However, no obligation seems harder to observe in practice, perhaps especially in the contemporary practice environment (Marwick, 1996). Computerized patient records, the entirely proper demands of accountability to institutional and third-party payers, modern notions of teamwork, and the growing prevalence of integrated systems of care all conspire against the privacy of individuals and families. Some clinician-ethicists have even concluded that confidentiality is an antiquated concept (Siegler, 1982).

APRNs and other mental health professionals are acutely aware of the role of confidentiality in building and maintaining a therapeutic alliance (Beck, 1990). In some instances, no therapy is possible without the patient's confidence that the therapist will maintain rather strict confidentiality. Often, the patient's concern about a breach of confidentiality is person-specific: "my mother would kill me," or "my husband must not find out."

Mental health professionals, like some other health workers, spend considerable time and effort encouraging their patients to let down their walls of secrecy. The reasons are many: the patient's healing requires participation of family, the secrecy is itself part of the patient's maladaptive behavior, secrecy is destructive of important social relationships, or disclosure is of direct and material benefit to someone else. Efforts by APRNs to persuade their patients to relax strict confidentiality are not evidence of disregard for confidentiality. Such efforts honor the concept.

APRNs also honor the obligation when they struggle with decisions about whether they should breach confidentiality (Smithy-Bell & Winslade, 1994). The demands of confidentiality often collide with demands of the patient's own good or with an urgent need to be fair toward another. (In terms of "principlism," these are described, respectively, as conflicts of autonomy with beneficence, and autonomy with justice.) An APRN caught in such a dilemma shows respect for confidentiality, not by slavish adherence to an absolute rule, but by 1) beginning with a presumption that APRNs should respect confidentiality, and 2) setting a high standard for arguments that the presumption should be overcome in any particular circumstance.

This is the sort of rigorous case-by-case analysis required by the famous Tarasoff (1979) rule for resolution of confidentiality dilemmas arising from the countervailing claims of another's safety. In the Tarasoff decision, California's highest court set out criteria for determining when the duty to warn might overwhelm the duty to maintain confidence. (See Chapter 8 for an explication of this legal guidance.) For present purposes, it is sufficient to observe that the legal duty requires the same kind of critical thinking that would be entailed were the obligations of confidentiality and warning "merely" ethical obligations.

To acknowledge that APRNs will have occasions when breaches of confidentiality are justified is to suggest another ethical question. How should a responsible APRN behave when he or she resolves to breach confidentiality? In particular, should the APRN tell the patient what he or she intends to disclose? A moment's reflection will make clear that this is a moral question distinct from the question about whether breaching confidentiality is justifiable.

Every experienced APRN will be able to think of some instances in which the best resolution would be to keep from the patient that a breach has occurred. Nonetheless, most modern clinicians probably subscribe to the view that disclosure should be the norm. Although the modern moral preference for disclosure has none of the antique patina of the duty of confidentiality, it is probably fair to say that many health professionals, particularly younger ones, regard it as a prima facie duty. That is to say, many approach uncertainty or conflict about questions of disclosure in much the same way they would approach dilemmas of confidentiality: they should start out by presuming that full disclosure is ethically required. Again, like confidentiality, the duty to disclose is an important and authoritative rule, but not an absolute one. It is what lawyers call a *rebuttable presumption* (i.e., if the presumption is to be overcome in particular cases, the burden of showing why belongs to those favoring nondisclosure).

Divided Loyalties in Managed Care

Threats to confidentiality are among the complaints heard from mental health providers about managed care (Biblo et al., 1996). Implicit in the term *managed* is the concept that end-point providers are accountable to a process of review for the appropriateness of the care provided (Boyle & Callahan, 1995). Such review requires that fairly detailed information about diagnosis and about the progress of treatment flows from the therapist to relatively remote persons and mechanisms. Not just therapeutic collaborators and supervisors, but also people called "gatekeepers" and "case managers," must routinely learn about and sometimes discuss information traditionally kept relatively private.

Although the rule of confidentiality is still observed regarding disclosure to persons with an alleged "need to know," the numbers and types of such persons are significantly enlarged in managed care systems (Applebaum, 1996). So marked is this phenomenon that some psychotherapists refuse to participate in any managed care programs, and some others feel obliged to warn their patients about the threat to confidentiality that accompanies any attempt to seek reimbursement from managed care plans (Boyle & Callahan, 1995).

Critics of managed care also contend that health care professionals have incentives to do less for their patients (Finnerty & Pinkerton, 1993). It is claimed that with managed care comes a conflict of interest, a new inducement to make therapeutic judgments conditioned by money. Such critics tend to gloss over the distinction between doing more and doing better. They also fail to acknowledge that previous payment systems undoubtedly skewed professional judgments in the direction of providing unneeded and perhaps harmful care. In any case, APRNs have justifiable concerns about *any* organizational scheme that systematically disrupts the nurse-patient relationship.

Proponents of managed care claim that its influences *improve* care by bringing diagnosis and treatment more nearly in line with nationally recognized standards of care (Millenson, 1997). They contend that by funding only that care that conforms to accepted "best practices," managed care will systematically lift quality as well as avoid waste. There is some evidence to support these claims, although as long as there is a correlation between amount and cost, those whose job it is to contain costs will seek to limit the amount of care. In any case, the advent of managed care has brought a fierceness of cost competition from which the mental health care industry was once relatively immune.

Finally, some APRNs are finding entrepreneurial opportunities in managed care. Ironically, but not surprisingly, APRNs are becoming independent practitioners as physicians are increasingly employed under contract by hospitals and other corporate entities. The principal challenges to nurses in independent practice may be other than what they usually think of as issues of professional ethics. Nevertheless, such nurses will share in the moral burden (and concomitant moral authority) of those who bear unique responsibility for the care of patients.

For APRNs in private practice, whether as independent therapists or consultants or case managers, professional judgment will have a direct effect upon personal income in a way quite different from that of salaried employees, particularly shift workers. As entrepreneurs in a managed care environment, financial success involves satisfying both patients and payers. Most APRNs will manage to do that nearly all the time. However, there will be times when a commitment to patient welfare will require vigorous advocacy and some risk of alienating the managed care company. On the other hand, independently practicing APRNs will have to resist the demands of some patients to "game" the managed care company or to do things that the APRN regards as of little, if any, value. Conscientious APRNs should have "the courage of their convictions" whether or not they work for a salary. However, the cost of conscientiousness is theoretically higher for those whose livelihood is immediately dependent upon customer satisfaction. In view of this, managed care regulations provide some protection against provider dismissal for reasons of cost. Despite what may be rather positive attitudes toward managed care, a conscientious APRN in independent practice will be sensitive to his or her inherently divided loyalties (Cassidy, 1998).

Salaried APRNs in the managed care era will also feel the pressure of cost containment, sometimes even magnified by institutional forces. Whether or not an APRN's role explicitly includes case management, the institutional drive to hold down costs can be more or less relentless (Mohr & Mahon, 1996). Even if not an acknowledged criterion of job performance, efficiency has become a foreground concern as never before. *Efficiency* is a dynamic term, pointing to a balance of input and output. By contrast, cost containment is a unilateral, unidimensional notion and does not contain within it a reference to work accomplished. APRNs, as professional leaders and institutional managers, must both promote quality care and be fiscally responsible. It is a matter of balance, of optimizing and seeking a high return in patient

benefit for each unit of resources expended. Thus decisions in pursuit of efficiency are always ethical decisions (Price, 1998).

The advent of managed care has spurred interest in long-term outcomes as the appropriate measure of effectiveness. Many health care professionals, in and out of the mental health field, have been surprised—and sometimes a little embarrassed—to realize how many therapeutic interventions have been widely adopted on the basis of very little or very inconclusive evidence of long-term efficacy, let alone long-term cost-effectiveness. APRNs and other mental health leaders more concerned with the people's health than filling hospitals or promoting a treatment modality welcome the increasing demand for and availability of outcome measures (Applebaum, 1996). Although health care leaders, regulators, and payers have been satisfied with good process ("Is it well done?" or "Is it done by well credentialed people?"), managed care has pushed for results ("Does it help the patient in the long run?") Although the impetus for this change in the way quality is measured has been prompted by concern for cost containment, it may also be seen as an opportunity to reform health care by reasserting its ethical roots: the patient's benefit comes first (Potter, 1996; Renz & Eddy, 1996). Further discussion of managed care and clinical outcomes is presented in Chapters 2 and 12, respectively.

Whistle Blowing

To begin, the dilemma of whistle blowing involves a conflict between the values of loyalty and protection of others (Bosek, 1993). Once that conflict is resolved, a secondary conflict often comes into sharp focus: the conflict between doing one's duty toward others and the duty of self-protection (Polston, 1999). APRNs may differ from most nurses in respect to these dilemmas. On one hand, APRNs are much more able than most nurses to influence institutional decisions or to effectively challenge the choices of other clinicians. On the other hand, a higher level of education and a broader scope of responsibility may mean for many APRNs an increased awareness of problems potentially in need of exposure.

Properly applied, *whistle blowing* means more or less open disclosure of a dangerous practice when such disclosure would likely interrupt a pattern detrimental to patient care or the public good (DiMotto, 1995). Whistle blowing is at least embarrassing and perhaps seriously harmful to the person or corporate entity whose policy or practice is uncovered. Whistle blowing may also be directly or indirectly costly for the whistle blower, despite public or institutional rules prohibiting retaliation. Whether a whistle blower is regarded as a hero or a "rat" typically depends on the politics or social position of the beholder.

In any case, decisions about whether or how to blow the whistle on an illegal, immoral, or incompetent practice will be among the hardest decisions that any professional is likely to make. To protect oneself and innocent coworkers and to be effective, a prospective whistle blower should first undertake a careful ethical analysis along the lines outlined in Box 19-4 (Price & Murphy, 1983).

Occasions for whistle blowing in mental health have involved insurance fraud: "padded" bills, charges for services not rendered, deceptive advertising, falsifying diagnoses to qualify for higher funding, and dumping patients regardless of condition once benefits have run out. Other indications for whistle blowing are systematic overtreatment or mistreatment: excessive medica-

---

box 19-4

A GUIDE TO WHISTLE BLOWING

- **What is the dangerous practice?** Write it down. Be precise, concrete, and specific. Avoid editorializing; put just the facts. (If your answers seem vague, whistle blowing may be inappropriate.)
- **Who exactly is endangered? How?** Specifically, how would blowing the whistle protect those at risk? (If you cannot specify who is in danger and how your whistle blowing would remove the danger, whistle blowing is probably not indicated.)
- **Check your facts.** Seek verification from others. Document. Remember: if you are wrong, everybody gets hurt and nobody benefits.
- **Question your own credibility.** Assess yourself and your motives. If your motives are self-serving or if you are not generally regarded as competent, reliable, and honest, your disclosure may be dismissed or discounted.
- **Find support.** Recruit at least one trustworthy advisor or confidante. Have this person critically and objectively review all the prior steps. If the foregoing analysis supports blowing the whistle, you would be well advised to proceed with the process.
- **Go through channels.** The point of justifiable whistle blowing is to get results, not to make a splash and not to punish. You should aim to get effective action at the lowest possible level. If it proves necessary to "go public," the whistle blower's credibility will be greater if he or she first tried to get action on the inside. **Exception:** if the offensive practice poses an immediate and serious threat, you might be justified in choosing the quickest and surest route.
- **Be open.** Anonymous whistle blowing tends not to be effective. Moreover, taking responsibility enhances professional stature.
- **Be persistent.** Once the whistle is blown, you are obliged to see it through. The whistle blower should make clear his or her commitment to press for action until the improper practice is stopped.

tion, useless therapy, abusive treatment, threats or other coercion to detain voluntary patients, unnecessary hospitalization, and treatment without standard assessment or planning (Mohr, 1995).

Mohr (1995) studied the behavior of psychiatric nurses (including a few APRNs) in a series of for-profit hospitals in Texas cited for widespread fraud and abuse. Her findings suggest that, despite truly anguishing distress on the part of nurses at what they experienced and resignations by some, most nurses were constrained from doing the right thing by a variety of factors including financial self-interest in the face of potential job loss and the apparent unresponsiveness at all levels of administrative and regulatory redress. By virtue of conflicting organizational and professional ideologies and a nursing tradition of oppressed behavior (Roberts, 1983), the nurses in this situation were constrained from acting independently to defend their professional principles and advocate for their patients. Mohr (1995) also observed that corporate wrongdoing and the appropriate responses of nurses to it is a subject in need of more, and more open, discussion.

Right to Treatment

Whether all citizens should have guaranteed access to basic health care is one of the primary public issues at the turn of the twenty-first century (Fuller, 1995). It is a policy issue, a legal issue, an economic issue, and a political issue. At bottom, however, it is an ethical issue: Am I my brother's keeper? Do we have a claim on each other, by virtue alone of our common membership in the American family, to share each other's basic health care burdens? Traditionally, the public and political answer to those questions has been "no."

Increasingly, voices are heard arguing that "new occasions teach new duties" and that circumstances have changed in ways that are morally relevant (Wagner, Austin, & Von Korff, 1996). In particular, these voices point to the related facts that modern America has become rich and that modern health care has become enormously ex-

pensive. In the meantime, it might be observed, partial government guarantees like Medicare and Medicaid helped dismantle the traditional system of charity care, which, in any case, was not well suited to contemporary needs.

APRNs, while pressing individually and as a group for "right action" on the broad questions of public policy, also have an opportunity for advocacy on behalf of individuals and patient communities (President's Advisory Commission on Consumer Protection, 1998). How an APRN feels and how strongly he or she feels about patients' rights issues will inevitably make a practical difference in that APRN's behavior when confronted by a patient whose access to urgently needed care is frustrated. Since many APRNs will be positioned to encounter underserved individuals, it behooves each one to carefully consider the crucial question of whether access to basic health care is something that all citizens should have as a birthright (Dougherty, 1992).

In our current system, access to health care is largely a matter of contractual agreement rather than community covenant, except for the categorical coverage afforded to the old (Medicare) and the poor (Medicaid). The rest of the population is party to health care contracts that people buy individually or through their employers or unions, or they are parties to no contract at all and thus potential objects of the community's charity.

To the extent that managed care shifts responsibilities for care to enrollees, including the responsibility to assess limitations on and access to care, there is reason for special concern among mental health professionals. APRNs may become involved in their patients' choices at the point of health plan enrollment. Both choices among plans and choices regarding treatment options within plans pose particular problems in managed mental health care. This is obviously true for persons with mental disorders that tend to impair judgment. It is also, but more subtly, true of everyone else. Most people seem to readily contemplate the risk of devastating somatic illness while thinking of mental illness as something that happens to other people. This phenomenon helps explain why so many people are shocked when they discover how little their health plans (whether indemnity or managed care) allow for psychiatric care. APRNs alert to this reality can think about ways to protect patients and communities against the harmful consequences of judgments impaired by illness or by the sort of denial practiced by most people.

Research

Several chapters of this book are devoted to research, including the social purposes and professional stakes for APRNs in current and future mental health investigations. These are topics heavy with ethical implications for Americans and for mental health professionals (Silva, 1995). In this chapter, however, the discussion of research is limited to the actual conduct of mental health research in clinical settings and its implications for the behavior of APRNs working in those settings.

A mere generation ago, well within the memory of nurses and physicians still practicing, it was common for patients (and others) to be involved in research studies without their informed consent (Beecher, 1966). Most, but not all, of such studies were relatively benign. Most of those who designed, funded, or implemented such studies were honest, caring health professionals horrified by the monstrous excesses of the Nazi era. However, they did not perceive anything inherently wrong with placebo-controlled clinical trials conducted without the full knowledge of subjects who were also their patients.

It has now been years since such research was allowed. Federal regulations, tied to reimbursements without which few universities or health care institutions could survive, have mandated practices and oversight mechanisms that make outlaws of investigators who do not adhere to very strict procedural safeguards. The regulations extend to all manners of research using human subjects. *Research* is defined broadly to include all systematic observation intended to extend generalizable knowledge. The regulations embrace behavioral, as well as biomedical, investigation (Code of Federal Regulations, 1985).

A key feature of the system of procedural safeguards is the requirement that each proposed research project using human subjects be approved by an Investigational Review Board (IRB). Most large hospitals and virtually every university nursing or medical school has one. APRNs, even those with no ambition to pursue careers in research, might well consider a term of service on an IRB. It can be a very interesting and professionally growth-producing experience.

Despite being hemmed in rather tightly by federal regulations, IRBs vary considerably in the rigor of their reviews and the robustness of their interpretation of their mandate (Institute of Medicine, 1989). The best of them inquire deeply and imaginatively into the proposed studies brought before them, insisting not only on relative safety and provisions for truly informed consent but also on scientific merit. As one long-time IRB member was fond of saying to colleagues who balked at IRB inquiry into features such as experimental design and statistical adequacy, "No research, however benign, is ethically approvable if it is methodologically or conceptually flawed. If it cannot answer the questions it purports to be interested in, there is no justification for even taking up the time of our patients."

As diligently as an IRB may conduct its reviews, few, if any, are able to monitor the implementation of the study protocols to ensure that they are actually conducted in the form that they were approved. Any confidence about that is based on trust in the integrity of investigators and the conscientiousness of their clinical colleagues. While the reported incidence of flagrant research fraud or wholesale violation of subject safety provisions is very small, it is reasonable to expect that, in research as in other endeavors, corners do get cut, sometimes at the expense of subjects and in violation of the terms of IRB approval.

APRNs are obligated to uphold high standards of research integrity (Silva, 1995). This obligation is derived from several, more basic duties:

- Obligation to protect patients who are current or prospective research subjects

- Obligation to protect the public health, which is dependent, in part, on properly conducted research
- Obligation to protect and promote the integrity of psychiatric nursing (and the healing professions in general)
- Obligation to maintain the clinical setting as a therapeutic environment

To be optimally prepared to fulfill this obligation to uphold high standards of research implementation, there is no substitute for first-hand involvement in the conduct or management of actual investigations. An APRN need not be a "researcher" to participate in research or to review research on an IRB. Such experience helps those whose primary vocation is clinical to be better consumers of research and better sentinels against ethical breaches, intended or accidental, by those who do studies involving their patients. Chapter 33 provides further discussion of the APRN role in clinical research trials.

IMPLICATIONS FOR ■ THE FUTURE

To be an APRN in psychiatric-mental health care is to be ethically robust. That means being not only a moral person, but one who thinks carefully about what it means to be good and moral. The world of mental health care is too complex, too variable, and too much in flux for clinicians' behavior to be guided entirely by abstract rules or measured reliably by static truths (Renz & Eddy, 1996). Especially those who teach and lead must be prepared to think about "should" questions as surely as about other kinds of questions (Biblo et al., 1996). Ethical discernment and ethical analysis are basic competencies for APRNs. Continuing development of those basic competencies throughout the APRN's career is a reasonable expectation of a professional.

The eight issues selected for explication in this chapter comprise only a partial list of the ethical challenges facing APRNs at the dawn of the twenty-first century. Rapid system change will undoubtedly soon pose additional issues presently unseen and alter the face of those now familiar. Through it all, APRNs will struggle to define and redefine what it means to be conscientious in the particular circumstances of their time and place. In those efforts, they will be guided by, but not enthralled by, nursing's traditions.

American nursing is markedly different than it was at the middle of the twentieth century, not merely or even most importantly in its technologic sophistication or educational advancement, but in its ethical self-definition (Arosker, 1995). Nursing was always an ethical enterprise, defining itself by its moral commitments. *Modern* nursing, while standing firm on some traditional commitments, has rearranged some others. While faithfulness to patients is a constant, nurses have come to see faithfulness as entailing vigorous advocacy when necessary. Being a "team player," always important to the self-understanding of nurses, is now seen in a different light. Teamwork now is understood to require the collaboration of differently trained professionals rather than a division of labor between those who direct and those who follow directions (Husted & Husted, 1991).

Such reevaluation will continue in psychiatric-mental health nursing as elsewhere. APRNs are expected to be in the vanguard of that evolution. They must discern the ethical requirements for advanced practice nursing's role in mental health knowledge, technology, and practice and critically evaluate specific proposals for what it means to be an ethical APRN.

RESOURCES AND CONNECTIONS

BASIC TEXTS

Ahronheim, J.C., Moreno, J., & Zuckerman, C. (1994). *Ethics in clinical practice.* Boston: Little, Brown, & Co.

Bandman, E.L., & Bandman, B. (1995). *Nursing ethics: through the lifespan* (ed. 3). Stanford, CT: Appleton & Lange.

Benner, P., Tanner, C., & Chesla, C.A. (1996). *Expertise in nursing practice: caring, clinical judgment, and ethics.* New York: Springer Publishing.

Drane, J.F. (1993). *Clinical bioethics*. Kansas City, MO: Sheed and Ward.

Fletcher, J.C. (1997). *Introduction to clinical ethics* (ed. 2). Frederick, MD: University Publishing Group.

Husted, G.L., & Husted, J.H. (1991). *Ethical decisionmaking in nursing*. St. Louis: Mosby.

JOURNALS

Bioethics Forum
Business and Professional Ethics Journal
Ethics
Hastings Center Report
Journal of Business Ethics
Journal of Mass Media Ethics
Journal of Medical Ethics
Kennedy Institute of Ethics Journal
Nursing Ethics
The International Journal of Applied Philosophy
The Journal of Clinical Ethics
The Journal of Law, Medicine, and Ethics
The Journal of Medicine and Philosophy

ETHICS CENTERS

American Nurses Association
Center for Ethics and Human Rights
600 Maryland, SW, Suite 600
Washington, DC 20024
800-274-4ANA

American Society for Bioethics and Humanities (ASBH)
4700 West Lake Avenue
Glenview, IL 60025-1485
(847) 375-4745
Fax: 847-375-4777
Email: info@asbh.org
Website: www.asbh.org

American Society of Law, Medicine, and Ethics (ASLM&E)
765 Commonwealth Avenue, 16th floor
Boston, MA 02215
617-262-4990

Kennedy Institute of Ethics
National Reference Center for Bioethics Literature
Georgetown University
Washington, DC 20057-1065
202-687-3885 or 800-MED-ETHX
Website: guweb.georgetown.edu.nrcbl

References

American Nurses Association. (1994). *A statement on psychiatric-mental health clinical nursing practice and standards of psychiatric-mental health clinical nursing practice*. Washington, DC: American Nurses Publishing.

American Nurses Association. (1985). *Code for nurses with interpretive statements*. Kansas City, MO: Author.

Applebaum, P. (1996). Managed care and the next generation of mental health law. *Psychiatric Services, 47*, 27–28, 34.

Aroskar, M.A. (1995). Envisioning nursing as a moral community. *Nursing Outlook, 43*(3), 134–138.

Backlar, P., & McFarland, B.H. (1996). A survey on use of advance directives for mental health treatment in Oregon. *Psychiatric Services, 47*(12), 1387–1389.

Beauchamp, T.L., & Childress, J.F. (1994). *Principles of biomedical ethics* (ed. 4). New York: Oxford University Press.

Beecher, H. (1966). Ethics and clinical research. *New England Journal of Medicine, 274*(24), 1354–1360.

Beck, J.C. (Ed.). (1990). *Confidentiality versus duty to protect: foreseeable harm in the practice of psychiatry*. Washington, DC: American Psychiatric Press.

Biblo, J.D., et al. (1996). Ethical issues in managed care: guidelines for clinicians and recommendations to accrediting organizations. *Bioethics Forum, 12*(1), MC3-MC24.

Blake, D. (1992). The hospital ethics committee and moral authority. *HEC Forum 4*(5), 6–8.

Bosek, M.S. (1993). Whistle blowing: an act of advocacy. *Medical Surgical Nursing, 2*(6), 480–482.

Boyle, P.J., & Callahan, D. (1995). Managed care in mental health: the ethical issues. *Health Affairs, 14*(3), 7–22.

Cassidy, V.R. (1998). Ethical leadership in managed care. *Nursing Leadership Forum, 3*(2), 52–57.

Christopher, M.J. (1994). Integrated ethics programs: a new mission for ethics committees. *Bioethics Forum, 10*(4), 19–21.

Code of Federal Regulations, Title 45, Part 46 (Protection of Human Subjects) pursuant to the Public Health Services Act of 1985, as amended.

Davis, A.J., et al. (1997). *Ethical dilemmas and nursing practice* (ed. 4). Stamford, CT: Appleton & Lange.

DiMotto, J. (1995). Whistle blowing: seven tips for reporting unsafe conduct. *Nursing Quality Connection, 4*(4), 8, 12.

Dougherty, C.J. (1992). Ethical values at stake in health care reform. *Journal of the American Medical Association, 268*(17), 2409–2412.

Etzel, B., & Kjervik, D. (1998). Advance decision making for psychiatric care. *Journal of Psychiatric Mental Health Nursing, 5*(1), 63–67.

Felder, M. (1996). Can ethics committees work in managed care plans? *Bioethics Forum, 12*(1), 10–15.

Finnerty, J.J., & Pinkerton, J.V. (1993). Ethical considerations of managed care. *Obstetrical and Gynecological Survey, 48,* 699–706.

Fisher, A. (1995). The ethical problems encountered in psychiatric nursing practice with dangerous mentally ill patients. *Scholarly Inquiry of Nursing Practice, 9*(2), 193–208.

Fletcher, J.D. (1997). *Introduction to clinical ethics* (ed. 2). Frederick, MD: University Publishing Group.

Forchuk, C. (1991). Ethical problems encountered by mental health nurses. *Issues in Mental Health Nursing, 12*(4), 375–383.

Fost, N., & Cranford, R.E. (1985). Hospital ethics committees: administrative aspects. *Journal of American Medical Association, 253,* 2687–2692.

Fuller, M. (1995). More is less. increasing access as a strategy for managing health care costs. *Psychiatric Services, 46,* 1015–1017.

Gadow, S. (1988). Covenant without care: letting go and holding on in chronic illness. In Watson, J., & Ray, M. (Eds.). *The ethics of care and the ethics of cure: synthesis in chronicity.* New York: National League of Nursing.

Gilligan, C. (1982). *In a different voice: psychological theory and women's development.* Cambridge, MA: Harvard University Press.

Goffman, E. (1963). *Stigma: notes on the management of spoiled identity.* Englewood Cliffs, NJ: Prentice Hall.

Hassmiller, S. (1991). Bringing the patient self-determination act into practice. *Nursing Management, 22*(2), 29–32.

Hofmann, P.B. (1996). Hospital mergers and acquisitions: a new catalyst for examining organizational ethics. *Bioethics Forum, 12*(2), 45–48.

Husted, G.L., & Husted, J.H. (1991). *Ethical decision making in nursing.* St. Louis: Mosby.

Institute of Medicine (1989). *The responsible conduct of research in the health sciences.* Washington, DC: National Academy Press.

Liaschenko, J. (1995). Ethics in the work of acting for patients. *Advanced Nursing Science, 18*(2), 1–12.

Marwick, C. (1996). Medical records privacy, a patient rights issue. *Journal of the American Medical Association, 276*(23), 1861–62.

McDonald, S. (1994). An ethical dilemma: risk versus responsibility. *Journal of Psychosocial Nursing, 32*(1), 19–25.

Millenson, M. (1997). *Demanding medical excellence: doctors and accountability in the information age.* Chicago: University of Chicago Press.

Mohr, W.K. (1995). Multiple ideologies and their proposed roles in the outcomes of nurse practice setting: the for-profit psychiatric hospital scandal as a paradigmatic case. *Nursing Outlook, 43*(5), 215–223.

Mohr, W.K., & Mahon, M.M. (1996). Dirty hands: the underside of marketplace health care. *Advances in Nursing Science, 19*(1), 28–37.

Mulvey, E.P. (1994). Assessing the link between mental illness and violence. *Hospital and Community Psychiatry, 45*(7), 663–668.

Oddi, L.F., & Cassidy, V.R. (1990). Participation and perception of nurse members on the hospital ethics committee. *Western Journal of Nursing, 12*(3), 307–317.

Polston, M.D. (1999). Whistleblowing: does the law protect you? *American Journal of Nursing, 99*(1), 26–31.

Potter, R. L. (1996). From clinical ethics to organizational ethics: the second stage of the evolution of bioethics. *Bioethics Forum, 12*(2), 3–12.

Povar, G.J. (1991). Evaluating ethics committees: what do we mean by success? *Maryland Law Review, 50*(3), 904–919.

President's Advisory Commission on Consumer Protection and Quality in the Health Care Industry (1998). *Quality first: better health care for all Americans.* Washington, DC: U.S. Government Printing Office.

Price, D.M. (1995). Ethics committees and nurses. *Journal of Nursing Law, 2*(1), 57–64.

Price, D.M. (1998). Doesn't everyone want an efficient nurse? *Journal of Nursing Law, 5*(1), 51–55.

Price, D.M., & Murphy, P.A. (1983). How and when to blow the whistle. *Nursing Life, 3*(1), 50–54.

Rafael, A.R. (1996). Power and caring: a dialectic in nursing. *Advances in Nursing Science 19*(1), 3–17.

Renz, D.O., & Eddy, W.B. (1996). Organizations, ethics, and health care: building an ethics infrastructure for a new era. *Bioethics Forum, 12*(2), 29–39.

Roberts, S. (1983). Oppressed group behavior: implications for nursing. *Advanced Nursing Science, 5*(7), 21–30.

Salgo v. Leland Stanford, Jr., University Board of Trustees, 317 p. 2d 170 at 181 (1957).

Schyve, P.M. (1996). Patients rights and organizational ethics: the Joint Commission perspective. *Bioethics Forum, 12*(2), 13–20.

Siegler, M. (1982). Confidentiality in medicine—a decrepit concept. *Journal of American Medical Association, 307,* 1518–21.

Silva, M.C. (1995). *Ethical guidelines in the conduct, dissemination, and implementation of nursing research.* Washington, DC: American Nurses Publishing.

Smithy-Bell, M., & Winslade, W. (1994). The impact of law on privacy, confidentiality, and privilege in psychotherapeutic relationships. *American Journal of Orthopsychiatry, 64*(2), 180–193.

Strumpf, N.E., & Tomes, N. (1993). Restraining the troublesome patient: a historical perspective on the contemporary debate. *Nursing Historical Review, 1,* 3–24.

Styron, W. (1990). *Darkness visible: a memoir of madness.* New York: Random House.

Tarasoff v. Regents of the University of California, 17 Cal. 3d 425, 131 Cal. Rptr. 14, 551 P. 2d 500 (1979).

Tong, R. (1989). *Feminist thought: a comprehensive introduction*. Sydney, Australia: Allen and Unwin.

Trexler, J.C. (1996). Reformulation of deviance and labeling theory for nursing. *Image: Journal of Nursing Scholarship, 28*(2), 131–135.

Van Allen, E., Moldow, D.G., & Cranford, R. (1989). Evaluating ethics committees. *Hastings Center Report, 19*(5), 23–24.

Wagner, E.H., Austin, B.T., & Von Korff, M. (1996). Organizing care for patients with chronic illness, *Milbank Quarterly, 74*(4), 511–544.

Winslow, G.R. (1984). From loyalty to advocacy: a new metaphor for nursing. *Hastings Center Report, 14*, 32–40.

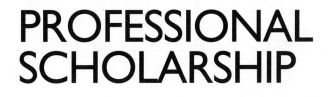

unit THREE

PROFESSIONAL
SCHOLARSHIP

20

Graduate Nursing Education for Advanced Practice

CAROLE A. SHEA

■ INTRODUCTION

Graduate education in nursing is the foundation for advanced practice. Although there is still debate about entry into nursing at the basic level, there is consensus that practice at the advanced level requires a master's degree (AACN, 1994; Camilleri, 1997). As of 1998, certification for advanced practice in psychiatric and mental health nursing requires a master's degree in nursing. Despite these stipulations, there is still considerable variation in the programs that offer graduate education to prepare the advanced practice registered nurse (APRN) for psychiatric and mental health care. The call for new roles has spawned curricula and teaching methods that offer the prospective graduate nursing student choices in content emphasis, role preparation, and practice opportunities. However, with choice comes uncertainty about such things as the "right" program; the best way to learn; practical matters of location, cost, and convenience; and employment possibilities after graduation.

Graduate education encompasses master's de-

437

grees, post-master's certificates, doctoral degrees, and post-doctoral training programs. This chapter describes the evolution of graduate nursing education—primarily master's degree programs for advanced practice—in the changing academic environment, compares master's program curriculum models for advanced nursing practice in psychiatric and mental health care, and discusses academic issues related to futuristic practice.

EVOLUTION OF GRADUATE
■ NURSING EDUCATION

The purpose of university education is to transmit, generate, discover, and apply knowledge through undergraduate and graduate programs for the benefit of society (Boyer, 1990; Krahenbuhl, 1998). The transmission and application of knowledge that is broad in scope is the goal of most undergraduate programs. These programs grant associate degrees (e.g., A.S. is Associate of Science in nursing) and bachelor degrees (e.g., B.S.N. is Bachelor of Science in Nursing), which span technical, liberal arts and sciences, and professional education. At the graduate level, the primary emphasis is on the generation and discovery of new knowledge through research and scholarship within a discipline. Graduate education includes master's and doctoral degrees, as well as non-degree post-master's and post-doctoral studies. The master's degree has many designations, for example, Master of Science (M.S.), Master of Arts (M.A.), Master of Business Administration (M.B.A.), and Master of Science in Nursing (M.S.N.). There are also several designations for doctoral degrees, such as Doctor of Philosophy (Ph.D.) in a discipline (e.g., psychology or nursing), Doctor of Education (Ed.D.), Doctor of Public Health (Dr.P.H.), Doctor of Nursing Science (D.N.S. or D.N.Sc.), Doctor of Medicine (M.D.), Juris Doctor (J.D.), and Doctor of Nursing (N.D.). The Ph.D. is the standard degree program for creating an academic scholar who generates and discovers knowledge. The M.D., J.D., and N.D. degrees prepare individuals for basic practice in a

profession; they are considered a first professional degree, not an advanced or research degree, even though they are titled "doctor."

Originally, the master's degree was intended to prepare those who had a bachelor degree with in-depth knowledge of the special content, skills, and methods necessary for teaching. Today the focus has expanded beyond pedagogy to encompass master's-degree programs that have several goals. They are stepping stones to doctoral programs in many fields; terminal degree programs for professional career advancement; apprenticeship programs that emphasize "doing" in science and professional practice under the watchful guidance of a professor, preceptor, or mentor; and community-centered programs emphasizing critically thoughtful social action (Redman & Ketefian, 1997). Given their well-defined purpose and specialized content, master's-degree programs in the professions tend to focus more on the generation and application of advanced knowledge on the cutting edge rather than the discovery of new knowledge. The master's degree in nursing is the necessary credential for advanced clinical practice.

Doctoral degree programs follow the tradition of the nineteenth-century German model of education. This model purposes to expand the scientific knowledge base of a discipline through the graduate student's theoretical study in a defined area and investigation of original research, with oversight and mentorship by a senior theorist or scientist. The scientific method is considered paramount to generate theory and discover knowledge. Most of the scientific breakthroughs that characterize the twentieth century owe their discovery to the rigorous study and research training scholarly scientists receive in traditional Ph.D. programs. The advanced *professional* doctoral programs (e.g., D.N.S., Dr.P.H., and Ed.D.) also rely on the scientific method and rigorous research training, but they tend to investigate different subject matter (e.g., psychosocial rather than neurophysiologic phenomena; problems of a clinical rather than theoretical nature) and use a wider variety of research methods (quantitative and qualitative) (Downs, 1989; Grace, 1983). They generate research that has more direct applicability to the field than "pure bench science," which may have no immediate utility. In nursing there are doctoral programs that grant Ph.D. degrees as well as D.N.S. or D.N.Sc., Ed.D., and N.D. degrees. Doctoral preparation is essential for the roles of nurse researcher and academic educator. It may also be required for some positions in executive nursing service, consultation, and health policy.

In the first half of the twentieth century, the basic education of nurses was conducted primarily in training hospitals where nursing students were responsible for providing all patient care. As a consequence, service took precedence over their nursing education. When students finished their apprentice-model training, they took positions as graduate nurses outside of hospitals in private homes and community agencies. Therefore there was a dearth of well-educated nurses employed in general hospitals (Hanson, 1991). Training in a clinical specialty, for instance in psychiatric nursing or public health nursing, occurred after graduation by immersion in nursing practice in that specialty area rather than through a formal program of study (Christman, 1992).

Without the foundation of baccalaureate preparation in nursing, there was little thought about graduate-level education for specialized clinical practice. The first master's degree program for nurses was instituted at Teachers College of Columbia University in the early 1920s to prepare graduate nurses for the functional roles of teachers and administrators. Teachers College of Columbia University and New York University created the first doctoral programs for nursing in the 1930s, granting Ed.D. degrees. In part these programs were a response to the rapid proliferation of hospital nursing schools, which needed teachers, supervisors, and administrators educated beyond the basic level. In part they were an attempt by the nursing leadership to upgrade the teaching of nursing and to improve the professional status of nursing (Camilleri, 1997; Hanson, 1991).

The emphasis on functional preparation persisted until the first master's program for clinical preparation, which happened to be in psychiatric nursing, was designed by Peplau at Rutgers University in the early 1950s. (The first *clinical* doctoral nursing program, developed at Boston University in the early 1960s, also focused on psychiatric nursing.) Peplau's program prepared psychiatric nurses for clinical practice at an advanced level, with a primary emphasis on psychosocial theories, advanced nursing, and psychotherapy skills. Psychiatric nursing was a logical choice for the first master's program for several reasons.

1. Psychiatric nursing was a specialty that had not been included in the basic nursing curriculum; it required "post-graduate" training, which generally took place in large state or private mental hospitals.
2. Peplau had developed a theoretical basis for advanced psychiatric nursing practice, which was published in 1952, gaining wide acceptance in nursing.
3. The federal government supported psychiatric nursing with funds to train psychiatric nurses.
4. There was a shortage of psychiatric physicians after World War II and the Korean conflict that opened the door for psychiatric nurses with advanced education and training.

The model of advanced clinical education soon spread to other clinical specialties. Since then, master's programs have grown exponentially in number and clinical specialty areas. The various foci of clinical specialties and emphases on functional role preparation continue to wax and wane in reaction to the health care needs of society and the demands of the marketplace for advanced practice nurses (Christman, 1992; Huston & Fox, 1998; Redman & Ketefian, 1997).

FORCES FOR CHANGE ■ IN EDUCATION

Graduate education in general, and master's programs in particular, evolve within the context of major trends and shifts in priorities of the larger society. Nursing programs must respond also to the directives of the profession. At the close of the twentieth century, such trends as an information-based society, service-driven economy, globally-accessed technology, and the aging and culturally-diverse population, have exerted strong influences on the curriculum and type of degree programs that are developed by faculty members and supported by students, employers, and the public at large. Institutions of higher learning must also grapple with the rapid pace of change itself. This presents special challenges to offering programs that are both pertinent to the contemporary needs of the academic disciplines and the democratic society yet relevant for future needs and the professional career advancement of graduates of these programs.

Pressures for Academic Reform

The world of academia is undergoing sweeping changes similar to those experienced in the health care arena (Huston & Fox, 1998). The public's expectations for accessible, affordable, and effective quality education have led to an academic reform movement (Bok, 1992). Criticisms that question the basic purpose and value of a college education for the average citizen have been levied against institutions of higher learning (Krahenbuhl, 1998; Shea, 1995). Some of the questions the university must address to maintain the confidence and continued support of the public are as follows:

1. How can individuals, families, and tax-paying citizens afford to send a student to college, given soaring tuition costs that continue to outpace other economic indices? Where is the value-added of a college education in terms of outcomes? What are the alternatives to a costly college-based education?

2. Is the primary mission of the university to teach students or to conduct research? What is the appropriate balance among a) the goals for teaching, research, and service to the outcomes of educating citizens; b) advancing knowledge and science; and c) producing qualified workers for the future?

3. Are curricula up-to-date and teaching methods appropriate for today's students? Are the subjects too broadly representative or too narrow in focus? Are the faculty members accepting of alternative viewpoints or constrained by traditional doctrines? Is the university investing in technology for the future? Are the faculty members investigating fundamental innovations in their teaching methodologies?

4. Are the university and its individual faculty members guilty of fraudulent research practices? Are research findings deceptive or false? Have research funds been mismanaged? Are ethical standards ignored? Are there conflicts of interest between researchers and funding sources? If so, how can the public be reassured that strong policies and corrective measures are now in place?

5. What is the blueprint for the future? If the university is the "think tank" for society, is it keeping ahead or merely keeping pace with changes in major industries and institutions? Has its vision expanded to include the trend toward globalization and a world without boundaries? Does it support research that seeks to solve the toughest issues such as dwindling resources, environmental pollution, racism, family violence, genocide, poverty, infectious disease, and genetic alteration?

These questions are being debated at all levels of higher education and at intersecting points with other social and commercial institutions. The pressures to transform higher education are having a dramatic effect on the university's traditional mission, operating systems, faculty members, and students. The centuries-old values and mission embodied in the concept of "ivory tower" are not only outmoded but impossible to sustain in today's fast paced, technology driven, culturally diverse society. Taking its cue from the business world, the university is seeking a new paradigm that will fit with an emphasis on *learning*, not teaching

(Denning, 1996; Skiba, 1997). With learning as its organizing principle, the university must concern itself with product orientation (productivity measures and education outcomes, not the teaching process), customer satisfaction (student-centered focus, not faculty-centered), and quality improvement (measures of value-added and excellence, not merely meeting accreditation standards). Denning (1996) has made forecasts that threaten the existence of the university in its present form:

- Students will form learning communities to study one subject in depth at a time.
- The on-campus classroom and faculty office will be replaced by extensive use of the Internet and information technologies creating a "virtual campus" to locate, disseminate, and coordinate information and communication among students, faculty members, employers, and other interested parties.
- Programs of study will be developed to meet specific requests of customers (e.g., adult students, professionals, employers, special interest organizations) leading to degrees, certificates, and other forms of educational validation not available currently.
- Graduates will need to carry a portfolio of experiences and competencies that indicate proficiency and expertise, not beginning levels of knowledge and competency.
- Students at all levels of learning will be active participants in the study of complex problems to learn first hand, through research, about innovation and discovery.

A new paradigm that will bridge the best of academic tradition and innovation is elusive, however. Change is even harder to mandate in the university than in health care, which has more features of an industry than a venerable institution. Unlike modern health care, which is only about 150 years old, higher education dates back to the medieval centuries; it is steeped in philosophies, values, customs, and practices that have stood the test of time for many generations. Furthermore, with the lessons learned recently from the health care system's tumultuous unplanned

move to an economic model in a managed-care environment (Gabel, 1997), there is an understandable reluctance to rapidly convert the traditional university to a modern, more commercial service model.

Nursing Education Reform

Nursing education has not been exempt from the reform movement (Shea, 1995). As in the past, social and professional forces helped put the latest curriculum revolution in motion. Huston and Fox (1998) discuss ten health care market trends that have far-reaching implications for nursing education. The social trends and major effects on nursing are as follows:

1. *Growth of the health care labor force.* Nursing is projected to be one of five occupations with the largest number of new jobs; however, nurses will need to have a career orientation that acknowledges the need for life-long learning to take full advantage of this trend.
2. *Economics as a driving force.* Nurses need to understand health care as "big business" and become well-versed in the language, customs, and strategies of the financial aspects of their own practice and health care delivery in general.
3. *Continued movement of health care away from hospitals.* Nurses need to deliver services that address the common health problems representative of people as a whole, as well as the acute, specialized needs of severely ill individuals in community-based settings.
4. *Growth of managed care.* Nurses must provide services that are population- and evidence-based, cost-effective, and competitively priced, and they must be competent providers and advocates of quality patient care.
5. *Changing demographics—the aging populace.* Nurses need a comprehensive knowledge of gerontology and the related competencies to meet the complex needs of the rapidly growing number of elders in various clinical and community settings.

6. *Changing demographics—increasing multiculturalism.* Nurses from many cultural backgrounds must be recruited and retained in nursing to match the ethnically-diverse patient population so that cultures can be maintained, interchanged, and bridged, thereby improving the delivery of culturally competent health care.

7. *Profound information and technologic growth.* Nurses need to maintain their "high touch" focus even as they become very proficient in the use of many "high-tech" information and communication systems, to build interpersonal expertise for an era that holds the potential for ever-increasing levels of stress and social isolation.

8. *Nursing's lack of involvement in political change.* Nurses need to become active participants and leaders in professional organizations, policy-making ventures, and political networks to enable health care legislation that supports nursing values.

9. *Replacement of registered nurses with unlicensed assistive personnel.* Nurses need to delegate care safely and effectively and to demonstrate with clear evidence the need for and contribution of professional nursing care to improved patient outcomes.

10. *Increasing complexity.* Nurses need to become critically thinking, independent decision makers and life-long learners to continue to have a positive effect on the health of individuals, families, and communities.

Nurse educators have become cognizant of these trends and are working to revise the curriculum, update the learning process, and devise new clinical learning opportunities in the community. Both undergraduate and graduate programs are beginning to reflect an increased emphasis on health promotion and disease prevention, population-based care, cultural competence, ethical-legal considerations, management and delegation, and service delivery in the managed-care environment and community-based settings (Dyer et al., 1997;

Pullen et al., 1994; Shea, 1995; Williams et al, 1998).

Market forces are not the only factors causing a wholesale change in nursing education. As mentioned previously, the impetus for educational reform has come from within nursing and the health care system itself. Curriculum revision has been strongly encouraged by professional organizations, private foundations, and federal agencies that have a vested interest in the education of nurses and other health professionals. Paralleling health care market reform in the 1990s, several reports were issued that called for a redirection of nursing and health professions education toward a community-based, primary health care model (AACN, 1996; ANA, 1991; NLN, 1993; NONPF, 1995; Pew Health Professions Commission, 1993; SERPN, 1996).

The community-based, primary health care model is not meant to be simply a change in the venue where services are delivered or a single focus on one type of care or specialty area (Pullen et al., 1994; Shea, 1995). Rather, it is intended to be a change in the world view of health care. It is the product of a novel synergy between the disciplines of community health and primary care that is distinct from either one and more than the sum of their parts. In the area of service, it means that health care providers will partner with community residents to define important health problems, develop culturally-appropriate treatment plans, and deliver competent care within community settings such as health care clinics, schools, homes, churches, day care centers, and other community agencies (Pullen et al., 1994). In education, the model proposes a different underlying philosophy about the teaching and learning of health professions students, which emphasizes critical thinking, problem-based learning, interdisciplinary teams, health promotion and disease prevention interventions, and concepts such as family, culture, community, partnership, and compassionate care (Kaufman, 1985; Matteson, 1995; Shea, 1995).

In nursing, the American Nurses Association (ANA, 1991) started the revolution with its *Agenda for Health Care Reform*, which presented nursing's part in creating a system that would provide accessible, affordable, cost-effective, quality health care for all. The National League for Nursing (NLN, 1993) followed with its vision for nursing education that would increase the number of diverse providers (especially APRNs), faculty members, administrators, and researchers prepared to deliver community-based, community-focused health care with a renewed interest in health promotion and disease prevention. The American Association of Colleges of Nursing (AACN, 1996) specified the essential components of all master's education programs to ensure consistency of preparation for advanced practice as nurse practitioners (NPs), clinical nurse specialists (CNSs), certified nurse midwives (CNMs), and certified registered nurse anesthetists (CRNAs). The National Organization of Nurse Practitioner Faculties (NONPF, 1995) delineated curriculum guidelines and set the required specialty program standards for preparing NPs. The Society for Education and Research in Psychiatric-Mental Health Nursing (SERPN, 1996) published its position statement on *Educational Preparation for Psychiatric-Mental Health Nursing Practice* and established guidelines for the core content, psychiatric-mental health nursing content, and clinical skills to be taught in undergraduate and graduate nursing programs. (See the SERPN education guidelines in Appendix F.)

The Pew Charitable Trusts Fund, the Robert Wood Johnson Foundation, and the W. K. Kellogg Foundation commissioned studies and structured major funding programs to help devise new ways to educate health professionals for the transforming health care system. These private foundations did not specify curriculum content or teaching methods for educational programs, but they advocated an additional set of competencies to support the clinical and technical skills traditionally taught to graduates. For example, the Pew Health Professions Commission (1993) recommended that health professionals should be able to do the following:

- Emphasize health and participate in primary health care delivery.
- Use teaching and counseling interventions to promote and maintain the health of individuals, families, and communities.
- Include individuals, families, and communities in the decision-making processes affecting their health and the treatment of illness.
- Demonstrate understanding and appreciation of cultural diversity and a commitment to working with underserved and vulnerable populations.
- Understand the need for and participate in interdisciplinary teams to deliver comprehensive care.
- Develop a deep understanding and appreciation of the community's role in the health of its individuals, families, and institutions.

The Kellogg Foundation funded programs that proposed to educate nursing and medical students together using interdisciplinary models for teaching and learning primary health care in partnership with communities (Matteson, 1995; Pullen et al., 1994). The Robert Wood Johnson Foundation concentrated on supporting the medical education of generalist physicians in primary health care rather than physicians in the medical specialties.

The most profound alteration called for by the professional groups and the foundations was the shift in the balance toward increasing the supply of primary care providers, with a concomitant decrease in specialty care providers. The U. S. Department of Health and Human Services (USDHHS) Division of Nursing responded by implementing the Congress-approved funding priorities to support nursing programs that provide master's education in primary care, particularly in medically underserved areas. This source of funding (and the need to remain competitive with other programs in their region) led to an immediate expansion of new and continuing NP master's-degree programs and the development of non-degree certificate programs for master's-prepared CNSs who were seeking to become NPs. Market studies reinforced this trend with projections of a shortage of NPs in underserved urban and rural areas and high–managed-care states (AACN, 1998; Buerhaus & Staiger, 1997). The move to master's education for NPs in primary care was augmented further by the promulgation of professional clinical standards, licensure regulations for advanced practice, and certification requirements. By the mid-1990s, of the 306 master's programs in nursing, 199 had NP programs with the majority of the NP students in the family nurse practitioner track (NLN, 1997). By 1995, 52.3% of all master's students were enrolled in NP programs (NLN, 1997). In its *National Sample Survey of Registered Nurses*, the Division of Nursing (1997) found that 44% of all APRNs practicing in 1996 were prepared as NPs.

Despite the increase in the number of master's programs and the graduation rate of APRNs (9261 master's students graduated in 1995 [NLN, 1997]), overall only 6% of America's 2.5 million RNs are prepared as APRNs (Division of Nursing, 1997). Yet projections call for about 25% of the total nursing workforce to be APRNs (Christman, 1992). Where will these nurses come from? In 1995, 1516 basic nursing programs graduated 97,052 RNs, with 32.2% having bachelor degrees, 60.5% with associate degrees, and 7.2% with diploma certificates (NLN, 1997). Even with the marked decline in hospital schools of nursing, the long-term legacy of nursing education as a byproduct of hospital service rather than a component of higher education, of nursing as a culture of craft orientation (i.e., skill-based) rather than professionalism (i.e., knowledge-based), has resulted in the minority of RNs holding a bachelor degree (Camilleri, 1997). This in turn limits the number of RNs who are eligible to seek preparation as APRNs in master's programs. Therefore the importance of recruitment, retention, and graduation of nurses at the bachelor level cannot

be ignored in any discussion of graduate education. All of the arguments and inducements to seek nursing as a promising and rewarding career must be vigorously promoted by nurse educators, service administrators, and the professional associations through a variety of media to attract the best and the brightest nurses and facilitate their career mobility (Buerhaus, 1998; McCloskey & Grace, 1997).

Christman (1992) charges that the nursing profession has been studied extensively by those within and outside the profession but that nursing has not used the data to plan for deliberate change and growth to new heights as a professional scientific career. The promise for remedying this dilemma resides in the transmission, generation, discovery, and application of knowledge about advanced clinical practice within institutions of higher learning. This is where planning, implementation, and evaluation can take place systematically in collaboration with service partners and other stakeholders in graduate nursing education.

MASTER'S EDUCATION FOR ■ ADVANCED PRACTICE

Education for advanced nursing practice is based at the master's level of graduate study. The nursing curriculum for master's-degree education has followed a somewhat typical pattern: some combination of a general core of courses, a set of theory and practicum specialty courses, and role preparation courses (Harper, 1996). However, in terms of consistency among programs, the "devil is in the details" as the familiar saying goes. The length of master's programs varies from 9 months to more than 2 years, with some requiring full-time study only, and others allowing full-time or part-time study. The number of credits (semester or quarter hour) varies, with most programs having 36 semester or 48 quarter hour credits. The curriculum core varies in content and comprehensiveness, with some programs having most of their credits allocated to the core and some having almost all allocated to the specialty. The specialty component varies in content and depth, even in programs within the same specialty area. The amount of clinical time in the practicum varies from none in some specialties to more than 1000 hours in others. Clinical placements, the methods for securing them, and the means for precepting students vary according to available clinical resources and sites, as well as the teaching philosophy of the program. The role preparation varies according to function and specialty, with some programs preparing students only for the clinician role, only for a functional role, or requiring both clinical and functional role preparation. Costs vary greatly depending on the type of program and institution (public or private university). In short, there has been no standard curriculum and no consistency in the educational preparation for advanced nursing practice at the master's level (Burns et al., 1993).

With federal and state legislators instituting regulations for advanced practice in the 1990s, (see Chapter 7), there was a renewed determination to address the consistency of master's education in nursing. However, because master's education for advanced clinical practice prepares RNs for different specialty roles—NPs, CNSs, CNMs, and CRNAs—it is necessary to balance the need for standardization with flexibility to meet emerging and persistent societal health care needs and the standards of nursing specialties.

Essential Curricular Components

Consensus about a master's curriculum was achieved among nursing educators through a series of regional conferences held under the aegis of the AACN to identify the key educational components for advanced clinical practice. *The Essentials of Master's Education for Advanced Practice Nursing* (AACN, 1996), which emerged from these conferences, outlined a curricular framework that is intended to guide the design and evaluation of master's programs for all advanced practice nurses. The curriculum has three components (AACN, 1996):

1. *Graduate nursing core.* Foundational curriculum content deemed essential for all students who pursue a master's degree in nursing regardless of specialty or functional focus.
2. *Advanced practice nursing core.* Essential content to provide direct patient/client services at an advanced level.
3. *Specialty curriculum content.* Those clinical and didactic learning experiences identified and defined by the specialty nursing organizations.

Fig. 20-1 depicts the relationship of the curriculum components to the specialty roles for advanced nursing practice. *The Essentials* document describes the content areas of the graduate nursing core and the advanced practice nursing core components. The content areas are listed in Table 20-1. There is a definition and a set of competencies for each content area that the graduate must achieve. Since the areas are broadly defined, it is expected that each master's program will customize the content to meet its mission and address particular student population needs and the health care issues of its geographic region. The document does not describe the content of the third component, the specialty curriculum content. It stipulates that the specialty organizations will define and describe the content and competencies for the specialty. In the wake of *The Essentials* document, many specialty organizations, including psychiatric nursing associations, have worked to establish guidelines and criteria for their constituents.

There has been no study to date to determine the extent to which contemporary master's programs have adopted the AACN curricular framework. In the future, data may be available from the Commission on Collegiate Nursing Education, a separate subsidiary of the AACN, which evaluates bachelor's and master's programs through its process of accreditation.

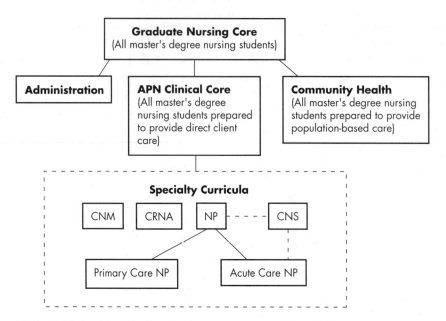

Figure 20-1   Model of master's nursing curriculum. (From the American Association of Colleges of Nursing. [1996]. *The essentials of master's education for advanced practice nursing.* Washington, DC: Author.)

Specialty Curricular Content and Competencies

The content and competencies for education in advanced practice psychiatric-mental nursing are derived from the statement and standards of clinical practice in the specialty (ANA, 1994a) and the position statements of the professional organizations such as the APNA, SERPN, the Association for Child and Adolescent Psychiatric Nursing (ACAPN), the International Society of Psychiatric Consultation-Liaison Nurses (IPCLN), and the National Nursing Society on Addictions (NNSA). The psychiatric nursing organizations have collaborated to define curriculum guidelines and competency standards for psychiatric-mental health specialty education.

Today's master's curriculum must embody the biopsychosocial paradigm (Abraham, Fox, & Cohen, 1992; Johnson, 1998) and the components of a primary mental health care model (Dyer et al., 1997; Haber & Billings, 1995) to be considered among the cutting edge programs. It must include content and competencies recommended for the expanded clinical functions of the APRN in psychiatric and mental health care (ANA, 1994a; APNA, 1997; Williams et al., 1998) and address special issues such as primary mental health care (SERPN, 1997), psychopharmacology and prescriptive practice (ANA, 1994b), and the managed behavioral healthcare environment (ANA, 1997). Specialty curriculum content with related competencies specific to advanced psychiatric-mental health nursing is presented in the *Education Guidelines* developed by the SERPN (1996). See the Appendix for a list of the essential psychiatric-mental health nursing content and clinical skills.

When the specialty content and competencies are combined with the graduate nursing core and advanced practice core components, the result is a curriculum that is both comprehensive in terms of advanced nursing practice and in-depth at an advanced clinical level in the specialty of psychiatric-mental health nursing. This education is put into practice as master's-program graduates implement the role of the APRN. For further description of the advanced roles and functions of the APRN, see Chapter 1. Also, many chapters in this book

table 20-1

AACN ESSENTIAL GRADUATE NURSING CURRICULUM ELEMENTS

COMPONENT	CONTENT
Graduate nursing core	Research
	Policy, organization, and financing of health care
	• Health care policy
	• Organization of the health care delivery system
	• Health care financing
	Ethics
	Professional role development
	Theoretical foundations of nursing
	Human diversity and social issues
	Health promotion and disease prevention
Advanced practice nursing core	Advanced health/physical assessment
	Advanced physiology and pathophysiology
	Advanced pharmacology
Specialty nursing content	To be developed by specialty organizations

Adapted from AACN, 1996.

present examples of how the APRN implements the advanced clinical practice role in a variety of situations and settings with different patient populations.

Post-Master's Certificate Programs

Post-master's certificate programs are designed for RNs who already have a master's degree in nursing and are seeking academic preparation to meet eligibility requirements for national certification in a specialty (Payne & Baumgartner, 1996). There are several purposes of post-mas-

ter's certificate programs. Nurses with a master's degree enroll in a certificate program for the following reasons:

• To add advanced clinical preparation to their original functional role preparation (e.g., a nurse administrator CNS becomes a psychiatric-mental health CNS).

• To change their original clinical specialization to another clinical area (e.g., a critical care CNS becomes a psychiatric-mental health CNS).

• To combine knowledge, skills, and role functions within their specialization with those of another (e.g., a psychiatric-mental health NS becomes a psychiatric-mental health NP).

Certificate programs may be offered as formal education programs carrying college credits or as continuing education programs with contact hours. In credit-bearing certificate programs, the curriculum is composed of a combination of advanced practice nursing core and specialty didactic and practicum courses. In fact, many programs offer the same courses to both master's-degree and certificate students. Post-master's students earn graduate course credits and receive a certificate (not a master's degree) in the specialty area upon completion of the program. When certificate programs are embedded in master's programs, they benefit from the accreditation scrutiny that the master's programs undergo. Certificate programs offered as continuing education should be approved by an accrediting agency such as the American Nurses Credentialing Center.

Nurses seeking advanced practice preparation through certificate programs should examine the programs carefully. Post-master's programs should not be confused with other types of certificate programs offered as staff development and continuing education, for example. There is little consistency among these "free-standing" certificate programs in terms of the content, number of contact hours, length, clinical requirements, faculty expertise, and so on. Also, nurses seeking preparation for certification should bear in mind that national certification for advanced clinical practice in a specialty requires academic preparation in a master's program or post-master's certificate program within a school of nursing that grants graduate-level academic credit. However, nurses who espouse a life-long learning philosophy and are pursuing professional development may well benefit from approved continuing education certificates and other contact-hour programs, depending on their individual learning needs and career goals. See Chapter 21 for further discussion of continuing education.

CURRICULUM MODELS FOR PSYCHIATRIC-MENTAL ■ HEALTH NURSING

Model of the Clinical Nurse Specialist Curriculum

Since their inception, most master's programs in psychiatric-mental health nursing have educated CNSs who are skilled in the direct and indirect care of the those with mental health problems and serious mental illness (Dyer et al., 1997). The CNS's stock in trade is psychotherapy in the direct care of individuals, groups, families, and communities. CNSs are also prepared for indirect care in the roles of educator, manager, consultant, and researcher. To prepare for their multiple roles, CNS students take courses that emphasize psychobiologic and psychiatric theories of human behavior of individuals, groups, and families. Most programs include courses on neuroscience and psychopharmacology. CNS students also study clinical diagnosis and treatment of psychiatric illness, community mental health, the consultation process, program planning and evaluation, research methods, ethical-legal issues, and management and organizational development. The specialty curriculum is a combination of theoretical content and supervised or precepted practicum experiences. To meet certification requirements, most programs structure a sequence of 16-hour/week practicum of direct clinical care in which the students carry a caseload of patients over time and participate in agency-sponsored learning activities and clinical supervision.

The practice of CNSs is recognized through state nursing practice acts and federal legislation. Many CNSs have become leaders in the profession as clinicians, administrators, educators, policy makers, researchers, and consultants with national and international reputations. Thus master's programs have successfully met the challenge to provide competent providers of mental health services and to advance the profession of nursing.

However, with changes proliferating throughout academia and health care, faculty members in graduate education and APRNs in various practice settings are contending with a major controversy: Should advanced practice psychiatric-mental health nurses be educated in the CNS role, the NP role, or a blend of the CNS/NP role? The answers that educators and APRNs give to these questions will determine the future of psychiatric-mental health nursing as a specialty in advanced practice (Dyer et al., 1997; Flaskerud & Wuerker, 1999; Haber & Billings, 1995; Lego & Caverly, 1995; Stuart, 1997; Talley & Caverly, 1994; Tusaie-Mumford, 1993; Williams et al., 1998).

Clinical Nurse Specialist versus Nurse Practitioner Controversy

In their much-quoted article, Fenton and Brykczynski (1993) compared their studies of the practice of CNSs and NPs to define the similarities and differences in these advanced practice roles. Using the same research design, qualitative methods, and conceptual framework in both studies, the researchers observed and interviewed CNSs and NPs in actual practice situations. They defined the domains and competencies of advanced practice based on Benner's work (1984). They concluded that "there is evidence that the findings of both studies have applicability to understanding the differences and similarities between the CNS and the NP and that much of the knowledge, skills, and competencies are *shared depending on the setting and situation*" (Fenton & Brykczynski, 1993). This is one of the clearest statements highlighting the dilemma concerning the roles of the CNS and the NP: essentially the CNS and the NP share most of what they know and do, depending on the context of practice, yet they have separate roles.

Others (Bigbee, 1996; Page & Arena, 1994) have described the development of the roles in terms of history, organizational development, education, goals, patient or client, preceptors, level of prevention services, diagnoses, treatment modalities, employment, and professional dynamics. The most distinctive differences cited between the CNS and the NP are that 1) the CNS spends about equal time in direct care and indirect care, while the NP spends 85% or more time in direct care, and 2) the CNS is employed in a tertiary setting caring for acutely ill individuals and families, and the NP is employed in primary care settings providing care for patients with common health problems. On the basis of these distinctions, many educators and APRNs claim that both roles are inherently unique and should be treated as separate entities, with different educational programs and clinical practice employment (Page & Arena, 1994). Still others argue that the CNS and the NP should be distinct roles because the profession has not advanced to the stage where it can redesign the roles into one innovative role given the current uncertainties of the health care system. For example, practice settings are shifting; there are various reimbursement mechanisms tied to licensure, certification, and roles; there are different state licensure regulations; national health care legislation is constantly changing; public opinion is still somewhat confused in its understanding of advanced practice nursing roles; and nursing specialties seem wedded to their historical titles and functions (Bigbee, 1996; Harper, 1996; Mastrangelo, 1993; NONPF, 1995).

To a great degree these debates were instigated in the mid-1980s when the growth of advanced practice nursing was coming into full-bloom (Harper, 1996). The supply of APRNs prepared in a profusion of specialties could barely meet the demand of a burgeoning health care system that was oblivious to the managed care threat looming on its horizon. The health care system was high-tech and specialty-driven in large medical centers and numerous community hospitals; the attitude was "more care equals better care" (Millenson, 1997). With cost less of a concern, the role of the CNS could be more diffuse and flexible, geared to meeting the needs of an individual institution or patient population. Primary health care was treated as a mission for a few dedicated health professionals working in underserved urban and rural areas. The NP, coming from an educational program that emphasized direct patient care and collaboration with physicians, spent the bulk of the time diagnosing and treating medical problems in ambulatory clinics and community health centers. As such, the distinctions between the two roles—CNS and NP—were marked and well-noted by nurses and other health care providers.

The provision of expert care, staff development, support groups for families and staff, consultation, and patient education that took much of the CNS's time in the 1980s would become expensive luxuries in today's cost-conscious health care agencies. With health care reform, not only the so-called luxuries of indirect care began to disappear, but the role distinctions between APRNs became blurred as all providers had to engage in direct care and services for which they or their institution could be directly reimbursed. Role blurring also occurred among the professions as legislative changes such as prescriptive authority expanded the role of APRNs, making them a cost-effective option to physicians. Other trends such as the general emphasis on health promotion and the shift to community-based care made the content and contextual differences between CNS and NP education much less relevant. As the AACN *Essentials* (1996) document shows, the content areas and competencies in common far outweigh the differences in role enactment. This helps to explain the proliferation of direct care NP and blended CNS/NP roles in acute care and tertiary settings (Payne & Baumgartner, 1996; Shuren, 1996) and the incorporation of population-based care and program planning in the practice of primary care NPs (NONPF, 1995). It also feeds the development of new roles (e.g., case manager, clinical researcher, and corporate nurse), which are proposed as important roles in tomorrow's health care systems (Berger et al., 1996).

Where are psychiatric nurses in this debate? Judging from the literature (Lego & Caverly, 1995 is representative), psychiatric nurses span the full scope of the argument for and against the incorporation of some or all of the NP role and functions into their advanced practice. However, it is a somewhat different argument from their perspective. As the original group of CNSs, many feel they own the title, which has historical significance and public recognition, and are loathe to give it up for the NP title. They are especially proud of their heritage as a specialty that developed in master's programs, not certificate programs as NP education did. Unlike other CNS specialty groups whose practice was weighted toward indirect care, most psychiatric CNSs have devoted their time to providing direct clinical care in their practice of psychotherapy with individuals, groups, families, and couples (Campbell, Musil, & Zauszniewski, 1998). The practice settings of psychiatric CNSs are varied; they practice in health maintenance organizations, behavioral healthcare agencies, community mental health centers, forensic units, addiction centers, private group practices, large mental institutions, academic medical centers, ambulatory clinics, and special schools for children. They provide a broad range of services for individuals across the lifespan and families, groups, and communities. They give specialized care to those who have serious and persistent mental illness and other mental disorders, personality disorders, dependence on drugs and alcohol, or life crises; to special populations such as those who are homeless, incarcerated, or institutionalized in nursing homes; and to those who have medical as well as mental health problems. (See Chapter 1 for a discussion of psychiatric nursing phenomena and the functions of the APRN in

psychiatric and mental health care.) Many practice independently with fee-for-service or third-party reimbursement. Most work in collaborative arrangements with an interdisciplinary team or practice group. In short, they might be said to be exhibiting the major characteristics of the NP's role, except that until very recently, most did not treat physical health problems.

Psychiatric CNSs were proscribed from doing physical assessment and providing other advanced physical health care by the nature of their education and practice, which focused on psychosocial phenomena and mental health problems. Also, their philosophical beliefs about the value of psychiatric methods, such as psychoanalysis, and psychodynamic concepts, such as "transference" and "regression," assumed that physical contact with patients was counterproductive and should be strictly limited (Gutheil & Gubbard, 1993). In the field of psychiatric care, the "no touch" policy was adhered to in an overly rigid fashion by some and overstepped egregiously by others (i.e., sexual assault), with most psychotherapists taking a "hands off" approach to patient contact (Gallop, 1998; Smith et al., 1997). Therefore the idea that an APRN in psychiatric-mental health care could conduct a physical examination of a patient and also engage appropriately in some forms of psychotherapy seemed impossible. However, with the reintroduction of the mind-body connection into psychiatric nursing, there is a better appreciation of the need to make that connection between the APRN and the patient by embracing the biopsychosocial paradigm in practice (Abraham et al., 1992; Caverly, 1996; Dyer et al, 1997; Haber & Billings, 1995; Johnson, 1998; Williams et al., 1998).

In addition to the shifting paradigm, there are two other factors that have influenced the development of NP and CNS roles in psychiatric nursing. There is evidence that 1) many patients seek care for psychiatric problems in primary care settings but are underdiagnosed and undertreated by primary care providers, and 2) the primary health care needs of psychiatric patients are not being addressed adequately within the mental health care system (Dyer et al., 1997; SERPN, 1997; Stuart, 1997; Williams et al., 1998). To address these needs and respond to the call for more NPs in the transforming health care system, many graduate psychiatric nursing programs have developed a psychiatric NP track (see the list of master's programs in Appendix H). The intent of these programs is to prepare a practitioner with advanced education and clinical competence in both primary health care and psychiatric care (Johnson, 1998). The scope of the psychiatric NP's practice is to do the following:

- Provide comprehensive care for the population of patients whose primary diagnosis is a medical illness, with a secondary psychiatric diagnosis or a comorbid psychiatric problem.
- Treat the common physical illnesses of psychiatric patients.
- Monitor the physical and mental health of patients receiving psychiatric treatment from other psychiatric professionals.
- Conduct the initial comprehensive assessment of psychiatric patients.

The educational preparation of the psychiatric NP is based on the graduate nursing core (AACN, 1995), the standard primary care NP content (NONPF, 1995), plus a psychiatric component: mental health promotion, the diagnosis and management of mental illness, psychopharmacology and somatic therapies, and some psychotherapies (Johnson, 1998). The programs vary in length, and most prepare graduates for both the NP and the CNS certification exams. However, graduates are not eligible for the CNS exam until they have completed the required number of supervised hours in the direct care of psychiatric patients after graduating from the program. (They are eligible for the primary care NP exam immediately upon graduation.)

Programs that prepare CNSs also include content related to physical assessment, pathophysiology, pharmacology, health promotion and disease prevention, and diagnosis and management of illness. However, this does not mean that all psychiatric CNSs must fully implement the NP role. In fact, if the CNS were to adopt this comprehensive approach, there would be a danger that the intensive, specialized psychiatric treatment needs of patients with a *primary* diagnosis of mental illness would be neglected or treated only superficially. Patients with a primary psychiatric diagnosis are the mainstay of the psychiatric CNS's practice. Therefore CNSs need extensive knowledge related to psychiatric illness etiology (especially the emerging neuroscience and genetics issues), diagnosis, and treatment. They need sophisticated competencies in therapeutic interventions, particularly in the evidence-based cognitive, behavioral, and interpersonal therapies. Unless there is even more in-depth preparation in the specialty, the negative impact on the CNSs' ability to conduct research and establish evidence-based practice will persist. For example, not a single *nursing* research study met the standard interdisciplinary criteria for inclusion in the formulation of the Agency for Health Care Policy and Research depression guidelines.

In an effort to expose students to both advanced psychiatric specialty care and general primary health care, some psychiatric nursing programs have condensed the specialty component. This is necessary because of constrictions on the overall number of courses and credits that can be offered reasonably, even within an expanded master's program. However, neither CNSs nor NPs can develop the necessary level of competency in specialty practice and research if graduate programs teach "watered down" versions of psychiatric etiology and treatment and offer limited clinical experiences. These educational short-cuts do a disservice to the graduate students, the psychiatric patient, the health care system, and the psychiatric nursing specialty in general.

Graduate programs that prepare NPs fulfill a large portion of the population's need for primary mental health care but will not provide for the specialized needs of the seriously mentally ill. At the same time, programs that teach CNSs only the traditional practice of psychotherapy run the risk of producing graduates who will become underutilized and quickly outmoded, thereby not providing services for psychiatric patients either. The challenge is to continue to develop CNS programs that focus in-depth on the specialty, while teaching the knowledge and skills related to the ability to screen for physical abnormalities, make differential diagnoses of physical and mental illnesses, and use appropriate referral sources for follow-up care.

The expectations held by employers, patients, payers, and other providers for the services of psychiatric APRNs are very high. They want clinicians who know that mental health care must be targeted in its focus and evidence-based in its treatment plan; responsive to the patient's immediate health care needs, however complex; inclusive of the patient's cultural preferences and participation in health care decisions; and consistent with cost-effective and quality measures. To meet these expectations, APRNs have to be prepared to draw upon various theories and interventions and expand role functions, rather than rely on a single approach or orientation to practice. Therefore nursing educators must develop synergistic teaching-learning strategies in a creative curriculum that translates relevant general health care knowledge and skills within the context of the psychiatric nursing specialty.

Model of the Blended Clinical Nurse Specialist/Nurse Practitioner Curriculum

The curriculum for the blended CNS/NP role is comprised of the content for preparation in both the CNS and the NP roles but also includes synthesis courses to learn the blended features of the dual role. See Dyer and colleagues (1997) and Williams and colleagues (1998) for sample curricula. The CNS content focuses on psychobiologic phenomena, diagnosis and management of psychiatric illness, and psychotherapeutic interventions. The NP content focuses on health promotion and disease prevention and the diagnosis, treatment, and management of common physical health problems, with an emphasis on the care of adults or children (i.e., the adult nurse practitioner or the pediatric nurse practitioner). Advanced physiology, pathophysiology, and pharmacology are included. The competencies expected of the APRN who wants to practice in the blended CNS/NP role in mental health are presented in Table 20-2. Examples of successful practice in blended aspects of the CNS/NP role are described in several chapters in Unit Two.

There are several curricular implications of preparing APRNs in the blended CNS/NP role for psychiatric-mental health care. Some intermediate considerations are as follows:

1. Master's programs will have to add courses and credits to accommodate dual preparation, lengthening the program and thereby going against the trend of paring down the number of courses to make master's education more timely and affordable. This may prove to be cost-effective, however, if the graduates are prepared to deliver comprehensive primary and mental health care and function in roles that are not setting-dependent.

2. Territorial battles between CNS and NP faculty members will have to cease so that resources can be used to the best effect and creative programs can be developed to take advantage of new opportunities in the transforming health care system. *Intra*disciplinary curriculum development will have to take precedence. The faculty member's ability and willingness to "think outside the box" should be highly rewarded by both academic and service administrators.

3. There are few faculty members and preceptors who practice in the blended CNS/NP role currently. This inhibits a fast start-up for new programs and will require formal education and extensive cross-training to prepare faculty members and preceptors with the necessary knowledge, skills, and practice experience to be good teachers and role models for graduate students.

4. There are few practice sites that are prepared

table 20-2

COMPETENCIES FOR THE CNS/NP ROLE IN ADVANCED PRACTICE IN MENTAL HEALTH

COMPETENCIES	CORE COURSES	CLINICAL CORE	PSYCHIATRIC MENTAL HEALTH COURSES	ADULT PRACTITIONER COURSES	SYNTHESIS COURSES
1. Integrate theory, practice, and research and apply in clinical practice	1	1	2	1, 2	3
2. Use critical thinking skills	1	2	2	2	3
3. Access and collaborate with community groups			1, 2	2	3
4. Provide care to clients in non-traditional community sites			1, 2	2	2
5. Identify clients at risk for mental health problems			1, 2	2	3
6. Plan and implement intervention strategies for clients at risk			1, 2	2	3
7. Involve client and family in the planning and implementation of care			1, 2	2	3
8. Plan and implement psychoeducational approaches with psychiatric clients and families			1, 2	2	3
9. Perform rapid assessments		1	1, 2	2	3
10. Diagnose and manage common and recurrent psychiatric symptoms or conditions			1, 2	2	3
11. Provide care for psychiatric patients across the continuum of care			1, 2	2	3
12. Apply clinical principles of psychopharmacology		1	2	2	3
13. Screen for physical abnormalities		1		2	3

Note: Undergraduate levels of preparation are assumed across all competencies. Competencies: 1 = introduced; 2 = practiced; 3 = integrated.

continued

table **20-2**

COMPETENCIES FOR THE CNS/NP ROLE IN ADVANCED PRACTICE IN MENTAL HEALTH—cont'd

COMPETENCIES	CORE COURSES	CLINICAL CORE	PSYCHIATRIC MENTAL HEALTH COURSES	ADULT PRACTITIONER COURSES	SYNTHESIS COURSES
14. Perform comprehensive health history and physical examination		I		2	3
15. Perform differential diagnosis of physical and mental illness		I	2	2	3
16. Manage common physical illnesses				I, 2	3
17. Refer clients for physical symptoms or illness when appropriate			I, 2	2	3
18. Identify legal and ethical issues in direct and indirect practice	I		I, 2	I, 2	3
19. Use consultation in regard to identified legal, ethical, and clinical problems			I, 2	2	3
20. Analyze public policy for its impact on mental health	I		I, 2		3
21. Analyze mental health policy for its impact on practice			I, 2		3
22. Develop a contract for a third party provider for the delivery of mental health services			I, 2		
23. Perform cost benefit analysis for psychiatric interventions	I		2		
24. Use intervention research findings in providing care	I		2	2	3
25. Use common assessment and outcome measurement tools	I	I	I, 2	2	3
26. Collaborate with consumer/advocacy groups			I, 2		3
27. Foster wellness and encourage preventive behaviors	I		2	2	3

continued

table 20-2

COMPETENCIES FOR THE CNS/NP ROLE IN ADVANCED PRACTICE IN MENTAL HEALTH—cont'd

COMPETENCIES	CORE COURSES	CLINICAL CORE	PSYCHIATRIC MENTAL HEALTH COURSES	ADULT PRACTITIONER COURSES	SYNTHESIS COURSES
28. Work effectively in teams with other health care professionals	I		2	2	3
29. Provide health care across all segments of the population	I		2	2	3
30. Manage large volumes of scientific and technical information	I	2	2	2	3
31. Maintain documentation of practice activities	I	2	2	2	3
32. Understand and respond to the diverse needs and values of different cultural or ethnic groups in the community	I	I	2	2	3
33. Support the role that service agencies in the community play in meeting health needs			I, 2	2	3
34. Develop programs for aggregates and large populations			I, 2		

From Williams et al., 1998.

to offer training for the blended CNS/NP role. This will call for creativity on the part of teaching faculty members and precepting providers to develop opportunities for sufficient practice in each role and then synthesis of the blended role. Professional staff in the clinical sites will need continuing education to appreciate the new roles and participate actively in the learning process for providers and students.

5. Students who seek the blended CNS/NP role may come with different backgrounds in practice and experience. The fairly standard requirement of 1 to 2 years of inpatient psychiatric nursing experience may be irrelevant or unattainable for some otherwise highly-

qualified students. (See Chapter 1 for a description of the many paths nurses take in psychiatric nursing.)

6. APRNs who are certified as CNSs may have to return to graduate school for additional education to qualify for certification as an NP if they want to be eligible for third party reimbursement and prescriptive authority in the future. Post-master's programs will need to develop a curriculum that does not duplicate prior learning and concentrates on the synthesis of the blended CNS/NP role for this group of learners.

7. Certification for the blended CNS/NP role has yet to be developed. Currently, graduates must sit for two exams: 1) the clinical specialist in

adult or child/adolescent psychiatric and mental health care and 2) the corresponding adult or pediatric nurse practitioner. After much debate in the field, the American Nurses Credentialing Center is in the process of developing a psychiatric nurse practitioner exam. This interim step will require those who want to practice in the blended role to take both the clinical specialist and the nurse practitioner exams in psychiatric nursing.

As with all major changes in a well-established field, developing the blended CNS/NP role as an option for APRNs in psychiatric nursing is proving to be an enormous challenge. However, both educators and practitioners working together can meet the challenge by giving due respect to the traditions of the past, resolving the inconsistencies and inadequacies of the programs and practices of the present, and imagining a future in which the psychiatric APRN can choose a role that fits with his or her career aspirations and the needs of society. Some may choose to be all things to a select group of patients (the CNS/NP) and some may choose to be something special to many patients at different levels of the health care system (the CNS). At this point in the evolution of psychiatric nursing, the profession and the public need both of these alternatives.

CHOOSING THE
■ RIGHT PROGRAM
Program Characteristics

In an ideal world, students could choose a master's program that offers a cutting edge curriculum; is taught by experienced doctorally-prepared and specialty-certified faculty members who use state-of-the-art learning technology and teaching methods; is a partner with excellent clinical facilities that have competent providers and interesting patients; develops research opportunities in a variety of areas; graduates students in a timely way; and has a 100% passing rate on the certification exam and a 90% to 100% employment rate of its graduates in APRN positions in their area of interest

upon graduation. Of course this "perfect" program would include full financial support with tuition remission and a living stipend for its students so they could pursue graduate study full-time.

The only problem with this picture is that it is very far from the real world of graduate education in nursing (Shea, 1994). The realities are as follows:

- Curriculum development is in flux with little or no evaluation data to guide efforts to revise and improve master's programs.
- Not all faculty members are prepared at the doctoral level; many achieved tenure in the era when the master's degree was considered the terminal degree.
- Many faculty members are certified, but schools of nursing must compete with health care services that offer much higher salaries for certified specialists.
- Even when faculty members are skilled in the use of technology, their universities may lag behind in upgrading their systems and technical capacities.
- The competition for clinical preceptors and facilities is unparalleled in the history of nursing education. Some programs force students to find their own clinical placements or require students to take a "time out" from their program until an appropriate placement becomes available. With downsizing and other cost-cutting, some clinical facilities lack a sufficient number of patients or variety of cases to allow students to meet program objectives and certification standards.
- If faculty/student ratios are too high for individual learning needs, the curriculum is outdated, competent faculty role models are absent, or students are compelled to work full-time so that it interferes with their studies, the graduates of such programs may be at risk for failing certification exams.
- Programs that do not pay attention to the demands of the market and produce too many graduates, or produce graduates without the requisite knowledge, skills, and experience,

make it difficult for their graduates to find employment in the areas and at the levels in which they were educated.

- The financing of nursing education has never been adequate, but with the federal government's attention directed to graduate medical education at a time when the balanced budget trims funds for education as a matter of course, there is added concern for graduate nursing education (Aiken, Gwyther, & Whelan, 1996).

Despite these realities, most graduate nursing programs may suffer a few but not all these shortcomings. The most highly rated ones are listed annually in the *U.S. News and World Report* survey. While the reliability of this survey may be questionable, it does seem to reflect the national reputation of programs as rated by faculty members and administrators. However, just knowing which programs have an excellent reputation does not ensure that an aspiring student's dreams for graduate education will come true.

Most nurses enter graduate study at the midcareer stage and have many constraints on their capacity to choose the ideal program for them. Because they are older and more established with family responsibilities and community ties, their geographic mobility is restricted and they are limited to the programs offered within a convenient commuting distance. There are usually many more financial demands for their salary, which compels them to continue working full-time and to consider the least expensive educational alternatives, which may or may not be of good quality. Furthermore, the number of psychiatric nursing programs has diminished as a result of declining enrollments (Stuart, 1997), and there is a geographic maldistribution with more programs located in the southern part of the United States (NLN, 1997). Therefore making a choice to study psychiatric nursing may involve considerable sacrifice in terms of time, travel, effort, and money to enroll in a program that meets both personal and professional objectives. However, because psychiatric nursing programs are striving to remain viable, they are often willing to construct a more individualized program of study to match the student's interests and experience.

Admission Criteria

Admission criteria vary but usually include a combination of the following:

- BSN degree from an accredited program
- Official copy of all college transcripts
- Grade point average of 3.0, or a B average
- Undergraduate statistics course with a passing grade
- Graduate Record Examination (GRE) scores
- 1 to 2 years of nursing experience
- Letters of recommendation from faculty members and employers or superiors
- Goal statement or essay

Many prospective students fit most but not all of the criteria. Depending on the school's philosophy and admission policies, the size and quality of its applicant pool, and its enrolled student body, the admissions committee may be willing to waive one or more of the established criteria or substitute a different criterion in favor of admitting the otherwise eligible student. For example, two criteria that psychiatric nurses might not meet are the BSN degree and high GRE scores. For many years, nurses who were educated in diploma or associate degree programs and worked in psychiatric nursing seemed more inclined to get a bachelor degree in psychology or social work rather than a BSN degree. Their career mobility was challenged only when they applied to graduate nursing school. Some schools will admit these applicants without a BSN degree with the condition that they are required to take additional nursing courses, such as community health nursing or nursing research, because these subjects are likely to be missing from their undergraduate curriculum. In the case of GRE scores, nurses may score relatively low on the GRE (e.g., have a combined score of less than 1500 for the verbal, quantitative, and analytic parts of the exam). Low scores may be the result of memory loss resulting from the passage of many years since they last encountered the subject matter; unfamiliarity with standardized tests; cultural bias of the test; lack of studying for the exam; test-taking anxiety; or poor academic ability. Rather than deny admission, the committee might recommend acceptance on a probationary basis (i.e., full acceptance will be given only after the student has successfully completed 2 to 4 courses in the master's program).

Most programs give more weight to the mature applicant's goal statement and letters of reference. The goal statement should be a well-written essay that conveys the applicant's motivation for graduate study in the specialty area, academic strengths, professional experience, related interests, and community service. It should be written in a clear, concise, and grammatical style with no typographical errors or misspellings. The essay *must* be created using a word processor to indicate at least some computer skills. Since communication is the heart and soul of psychiatric nursing, the essay should demonstrate considerable competence in this area. The reference letters should document the personal essay in an objective and honest way, describing the applicant's strengths and abilities, but not glossing over limitations or weaknesses that may preclude success in graduate school or indicate that the applicant has specific learning needs.

Academic Progression

About 70% of graduate nursing students are part-time students (NLN, 1997) and full-time everything else. Although most master's program are less than 2 years in length for full-time study, students may take up to 5 to 7 years to complete the program. The length of time from matriculation until graduation may be influenced by family needs, financial pressures, personal illness, the demands of full-time work, and many other factors. Faculty advisors encourage their students to make steady progress by taking at least two or more courses per semester or quarter to complete the program in a timely way. This keeps the student eligible for financial aid and ensures that the education will be relevant and useful to the student and future employers upon graduation. Graduation rates (the length of time it takes a student to complete the program after enrollment) influence the reputation and rating of a program. Therefore faculty members and students have a vested interest in academic progression through the program.

One of the potential forces for assisting progression is the availability of peer study groups and mentoring programs. With a large contingent of part-time students, it is often difficult to create a cohort of class peers. Students progress at different rates in the program because they may enter and take courses at different points in the program. Nevertheless, student and faculty efforts to connect around research projects, class group assignments, seminar presentations, interdisciplinary colloquia, clinical practicum groups, and social events represent time well-spent. These are the activities that forge powerful bonds and foster strong professional socialization. They provide an outlet for the inevitable stress that abounds during the seemingly endless round of paper writing and clinical work-ups. They engender an enthusiasm for the subject matter as students discuss and begin to try out psychotherapeutic techniques with one another. Matching the content with the process through self-reflection and peer consultation is an exciting yet protected way to learn a sometimes personally painful subject. As many graduates will attest, the relationships they established in graduate school have outlasted the content that they learned.

After graduation, APRNs have a professional duty to precept, supervise, and mentor graduate nursing students, to give back to their programs some of the benefits they received as a student. The pressures of productivity measures in managed care settings make this very difficult. However, APRNs should recall the essential part their own preceptors played in helping them build a satisfying career. Few other professional activities bring such rewards as successfully passing on the pearls of wisdom, hard-won experience, and passion for the specialty to the next generation of psychiatric nurses in advanced practice.

Doctoral Study

For some nurses, doctoral study is a logical progression in their careers. Their motivation may come from an intrinsic interest in scientific study and research, a desire to emulate an important role model, or the need for a doctoral degree as the required credential for positions in education, research, or administration.

The factors in choosing a doctoral program are similar but not exactly the same as for a master's program. Doctoral students, like master's students, are older and at a mid-career stage; therefore location, cost, and convenience enter the picture. However, there are several important differences:

1. There are only 73 doctoral nursing programs in the United States, with many states having only one or no program (see the list in Appendix I). Therefore, unless the student is living in a large metropolitan area, he or she must be willing to travel to the program or to relocate. However, there are programs that offer distance learning, on-campus weekend programs, and summer-only options.

2. Doctoral programs require the equivalent of several years of full-time study. Usually this includes at least 2 years of full-time coursework and 2 or more years of residency while the student conducts an independent research study and writes the dissertation. Currently, many programs allow part-time study, thereby increasing the length of matriculation, although they may stipulate that the degree requirements must be completed within 7 to 8 years.

3. The cost varies not only according to whether the institution is private or public, but also whether the program has predoctoral traineeships, research and teaching assistantships, and special scholarships to offer. The well-established programs often have the means to offer financial support to their students or may even require that students write grants for support of their study and research.

4. The entrance to doctoral study is very competitive because doctoral programs enroll only a select number of students each year. Doctoral programs are labor-intensive—they require very low faculty-to-student ratios, a close match between the student's scholarly interests and the faculty's established research, and an enduring mentor relationship—and they are resource-limited (e.g., student tuition does not cover the cost of offering the program).

Doctoral programs are not accredited by an external nursing agency or organization (Germain et al., 1994). However, Ziemer and colleagues (1992) found evidence in their study of 44 nursing doctoral programs that the similarity in philosophy and curricula was "striking," despite different degree designations (i.e., Ph.D., D.N.S. or D.N.Sc., or Ed.D.). They suggest that this finding is a result of the dominant effect of university policies, politics, and requirements. All programs, regardless of the type of degree, emphasized research skill development. About 50% of the programs in their study focused on role preparation, with the remainder offering advanced clinical courses or a combination of clinical and role courses. Credit requirements varied widely (39 to 114), but the standard program had 60 credits, with 48 credits in nursing and 12 credits in cognates (other discipline courses) and electives.

The AACN (1993) has established quality indicators that apply to all doctoral programs. The indicators specify in detail the following:

- Characteristics and functions of faculty
- Common curricular elements and program features
- Necessary resources
- Student characteristics and competencies
- Research components
- Comprehensive evaluation plan

The essential curricular elements for doctoral education that are endorsed by the AACN (1993) are listed in Box 20-1.

box

20-1

ESSENTIAL CURRICULUM ELEMENTS FOR DOCTORAL NURSING PROGRAMS

- History and philosophy of science in relation to nursing knowledge
- Current and emerging nursing knowledge
- Methods and processes of theory and knowledge development
- Analysis of and leadership in social, ethical, cultural, economic, and political issues that affect nursing, health care, and research
- Research methods and data analysis techniques
- Progressive, guided, independent research experiences for the student

Adapted from AACN, 1993.

Admission requirements vary by program. Most doctoral programs require a master's degree in nursing, but many will accept a BSN degree in combination with a non-nursing master's degree. Unlike master's programs, which usually specify at least 1 to 2 years of professional experience, there are doctoral programs that do not have previous clinical experience as a requirement. This may be a "non-issue" since very few nurses pursue graduate study directly upon graduation from their bachelor program. However, this trend may be changing as the profession comes to grips with its own aging cohort and the need to recruit nurses at a younger age into graduate study at the master's and doctoral levels.

Academic progression in doctoral programs can be notoriously slow. Most students do well in their coursework, which is structured with substantial peer involvement. However, there are a few points at which progress may be stifled or even stopped. The first point of major tension is the comprehensive examination, a requirement in some programs that precedes admission to being a doctoral candidate. Some students have difficulty synthesizing all they have learned or simply freeze at the prospect of taking exams that have so much importance for their future. Students who anticipate these exams by pursuing their studies and writing their papers in a coherent fashion have much less difficulty.

Once admitted to candidacy, the next obstacle is convening an interested, cooperative, and supportive dissertation committee. The stories are legion about committee members that make it their mission to assert their own views, to the exclusion of any collaborative efforts to produce a quality study. Doctoral candidates are advised to seek the recommendations of their peers and trusted faculty in choosing dissertation advisors. In the event that there is an unsolvable conflict, the student should have recourse to a means of conflict resolution or to a process for changing the composition of the committee.

Many students embark on their dissertation with every expectation of completing the study. However, an often-quoted statistic is that 50% of all doctoral students never finish; they are A.B.D. (i.e., all but their dissertation). There are many reasons why this phenomenon is so prevalent. Some are within the control of the student, and some are not. One of the main distinctions is whether the student invests in the dissertation with the intent that the dissertation is "my life's work," or whether the student sees the dissertation as "a first step in my program of research." In the first case, the student is less likely to complete the study; it is all encompassing, and to finish would be to create a huge psychologic void with no prospect for what would come next. In the second case, the student recognizes that to begin a research journey for life, he or she must take the first step. This student's dissertation is more likely to be realistic in scope, with a well-defined design that suggests the next steps for further research. Obviously, there are many other factors that impact the student's progress in completing a dissertation. However, it is hard to overestimate the importance that the research advisor or mentor plays in making the doctoral study a successful educational and professional experience (Meleis, 1992).

Mentoring

Mentoring is both a rare gift and a professional duty (Trossman, 1998; Vance & Olson, 1998). Without mentoring, careers may fail to thrive and institutions may stagnate. Women need mentors especially, because social institutions still value hierarchy, competition, singular achievement, and colleague recognition for advancement (Wunsch, 1994). Mentors may be sponsors or coaches of younger (or novice) colleagues. Their functions include supplying crucial information, giving the protégé visibility, making arrangements for choice assignments or positions, and teaching the politics of the institution and the discipline. In addition to guidance and support, the mentor should enhance the protégé's sense of identity, competence, and effectiveness within the profession. Mentors may be chosen or appointed, but it is essential that it is a good fit in terms of personal style and academic and professional interests.

The protégé, or mentee, also has duties and responsibilities to receive the full benefits of the mentoring relationship. Wunsch (1994) defines these as "conceptualizing and building a career, setting priorities and using time productively, developing networks, and dealing with senior colleagues." Although she is referring to the role of junior women faculty, these benefits would accrue to graduate students who were paired with a faculty mentor who agreed to work toward these goals.

Although fewer master's programs require a research thesis, engaging in the research process as a novice researcher or working as a research assistant to a senior researcher provides a special opportunity to develop the mentor-mentee relationship. On the doctoral level, conducting research and writing the dissertation are the signature features of the mentor-mentee relationship between the doctoral student and the faculty advisor. The intellectual stimulation of designing a research study and the learning of practical research skills is the foreground for the synthesis of indepth knowledge in a particular area of interest and the discovery of new avenues to enrich professional development. In the background is the sustaining mentor-mentee relationship—challenging, testing, rewarding, and supporting the mentee. This type of experience can also be structured with expert preceptors who use the clinical teaching moment, formal grand rounds, interdisciplinary team conferences, one-on-one coffee breaks, joint authorship of articles on scholarly practice, and attendance at professional conferences to cement the knowledge and skills of advanced practice and scientific research. They put the wheels in motion for the protégé's rewarding career as a highly respected clinician or nurse reseacher.

As graduation nears, the choice of the master's or doctoral program becomes less important. The relationships with faculty, peers, mentors, and patients are what stands out in memories about the experience. If the graduate student has been able to fully participate in the academic rigors and clinical challenges, to reach out to the joys of self-discovery and new friendships, to possess the ideals and the values of a rich and evolving profession, graduate education will be well worth the time, travel, effort, and money that the student spent in becoming a master's-prepared APRN in psychiatric and mental health nursing or a doctorally prepared researcher, educator, administrator, or clinician.

IMPLICATIONS FOR ■ THE FUTURE

In the near future, the most crucial issue is recruitment into the specialty practice of psychiatric nursing. Without an infusion of BSN-prepared nurses into the field, the applicant pool for graduate study will continue to diminish. Stuart (1997) and others have described the factors that influence recruitment. From an educational standpoint, employing the principles of adult learning might go a long way in enticing nurses into psychiatric nursing. According to the andragological theory of Knowles (1978), adult learners may be characterized as self-directed, valuing personal and professional experience, wanting to capitalize on the moment of their readiness to learn, and preferring problem-oriented learning situations (Knowles, 1978). Making programs more accessible, for example through distance learning programs, to more diverse types of nurses (those with no inpatient psychiatric experience or even brand-new graduates from BSN programs) and using creative problem-based case studies instead of lectures and typical clinical supervision seminars may diversify and enliven the specialty (Lewis & Kaas, 1998). While recognizing that there is a fundamental change in today's student who is less willing to respond to the authority of the teacher and the traditional hierarchical faculty-student relationship (Friere, 1991), faculty members must balance a more egalitarian approach with the responsibility to ensure professional education outcomes (Paterson, 1998).

Faculty members will have to confront the challenges posed by Denning (1996) and others who forecast radical changes in what and how students will learn in the future. They will have to conquer their fears and phobias about computers, information technology, distance learning, and their place in a "virtual campus." However, they will be assisted by the next generation of faculty members. As the new faculty members come "on-line," they will bring with them a greater facility with technology and a world view that sees the opportunities and is not limited by the academic traditions of the ivory tower.

Without a significant increase in young clinically-prepared master's graduates, there will be too few viable doctoral program candidates to supply the need for doctorally prepared faculty in psychiatric nursing. This will have a serious effect on the ability to teach and mentor students in the discipline at all levels of education. Also, without a strong cadre of clinically based APRNs, there will not be the researchers needed to build an evidence-based psychiatric practice or to demonstrate the effectiveness of expert practice on psychiatric outcomes.

Partnerships between schools of nursing and clinical agencies in their communities must be developed to ensure that adequate clinical teaching facilities will continue to be available as practice patterns respond to the changes in the health care system. Service must have the opportunity to participate in curriculum development. Consumers and their families should be invited to help plan the curriculum and teach graduate students and faculty members about their perspectives of care, ways of coping, and preferred treatments.

Finally, the CNS versus NP conflict does not have to be resolved in the near future. However, there must be tolerance for both to exist and for the blended CNS/NP role to develop. A premature closure on the issue will stifle what may prove to be an important practice innovation that benefits both mentally and physically ill patients. It is important to recognize that it has taken less than 10 years for the biopsychosocial paradigm to gain acceptance as the foundation of practice. This is a sign that psychiatric nursing is a specialty that understands the change process and is a discipline committed to education and life-long learning.

RESOURCES AND CONNECTIONS

JOURNALS

Advances in Nursing Science
American Academy of Nurse Practitioners
Applied Nursing Research
Clinical Nurse Specialist
Image: Journal of Nursing Scholarship
International Journal of Nursing Studies
Issues in Mental Health Nursing
Journal of American Psychiatric Nurses Association
Journal of Continuing Education in Nursing
Journal of Nursing Education
Journal of Professional Nursing
Journal of Psychiatric and Mental Health Nursing
Nursing and Health Care: Perspectives on Community
Nurse Educator
Nursing Outlook
Nursing Research
Research in Nursing and Health

BOOKS

Bastable, S.B. (1997). *Nurse as educator: principles of teaching and learning.* Sudbury, MA: Jones and Bartlett

Carpenter, D.R., & Hudacek, S. (1996). *On doctoral education in nursing: the voice of the student.* New York: NLN Press.

Chafee, E.E., & Sherr, L.A. (1992). *Quality: transforming postsecondary education.* ASHE-ERIC Higher Education Report No. 3. Washington, DC: the George Washington University, School of Education and Human Development.

Vance, C., & Olson, R.K. (1998). *The mentor connection in nursing.* New York: Springer Publishing.

GUIDES

Annual Guide to Graduate Nursing Education (annual edition) New York: NLN Press. NLN Center for Research in Nursing Education and Community Health
800-669-6959
Email: nlninform@nln.org

Peterson's Graduate Programs in Business, Education, Health, Information Studies, Law & Social Work (annual edition) Princeton, NJ: Author. Peterson's Education Center online at: http//www.petersons.com

Peterson's Nursing Programs (annual edition). Princeton, NJ: Author with the American Association of Colleges of Nursing.
800-338-3282

TESTING AND CERTIFICATION

Advanced Practice Board Certification Catalogue
American Nurses Credentialing Center
800-284-2374
www.nursingworld.org

Commission on Graduates of Foreign Schools of Nursing (CGFNS)
215-349-8767
www.cgfns.org

Graduate Record Examination (GRE)
800-GRE-CALL
www.gre.org

Miller Analogies Test
800-622-3231
National Council of State Boards of Nursing
312-787-6555
www.ncsbn.org

Test of English as Foreign Language (TOEFL)
800-GO-TOEFL
www.toefl.org

WEBSITES

American Academy of Nursing
(www.nursingworld.org/aan/index.htm)
American Association of Colleges of Nursing
(www.aacn.nch.edu)
American Association for Higher Education
(www.aahe.org)
Healthweb Nursing (University of Michigan)
(www.lib.umich.edu/hw/nursing.html)
International Network for Doctoral Education in Nursing (www.umich.edu/-inden/index.htm)
National Academy of Sciences Institute of Medicine (www2.nas.edu/iom)
Pew Health Professions Commission
(www.futurehealth.ucsf.edu/pewcomm.html)
Sigma Theta Tau International Honor Society of Nursing (stti-web.iupui.edu)
The Center for Health Professions, UCSF (www.futurehealth.ucsf.edu)
The W.K. Kellogg Foundation (www.wkk.org)
The National Institute of Nursing Research (www.nih.gov/ninr)
The National League for Nursing (www.nln.org)
The Pew Charitable Trusts (www.pewtrusts.com)
The Robert Wood Johnson Foundation (www.rwif.org)
World Health Organization Nursing and Midwifery (www.who.int/hdp/nur/index.htm)

References

Abraham, I.L., Fox, J.C., & Cohen, B.T. (1992). Integrating the bio into the biopsychosocial: understanding and treating biological phenomena in psychiatric-mental health nursing. *Archives of Psychiatric Nursing, 6*(5), 296–305.

Aiken, L.H., Gwyther, M.E., & Whelan, E. (1996). Federal support of graduate nursing education: rationale and policy options. *Nursing Outlook, 44,* 11–17.

American Association of Colleges of Nursing. (1993). *Indicators of quality in doctoral programs in nursing.* [Position statement.] Washington, DC: Author.

American Association of Colleges of Nursing. (October, 1994). *Certification and regulation of advanced practice nurses.* [Position statement.] Washington, DC: Author.

American Association of Colleges of Nursing. (1996). *The essentials of master's education for advanced practice nursing.* Washington, DC: Author.

American Association of Colleges of Nursing. (February, 1998). With demand for RNs climbing and shortening supply, forecasters say what's ahead isn't typical "nursing shortage." *Issue bulletin*. Washington, DC: Author.

American Nurses Association. (1991). *Nursing's agenda for health care reform*. Washington, DC: Author.

American Nurses Association. (1994a). *A statement on psychiatric-mental health clinical nursing practice and standards of psychiatric and mental health clinical nursing practice*. Washington, DC: American Nurses Publishing.

American Nurses Association. (1994b). *Psychiatric-mental health nursing psychopharmacology project*. Washington, DC: Author.

American Nurses Association. (May, 1997). *Managed behavioral health care curriculum guidelines for psychiatric-mental health and addictions nurses*. Washington, DC: Author.

American Psychiatric Nurses Association. (1997). *Psychiatric-mental health nursing practice*. [Position statement.] Washington, DC: Author.

Benner, P. (1984). *From novice to expert: excellence and power in clinical nursing practice*. Menlo Park, CA: Addison-Wesley.

Berger, A.M., et al. (1996). Advanced practice roles for nurses in tomorrow's healthcare systems. *Clinical Nurse Specialist, 10*, 250–255.

Bigbee, J.L. (1996). History and evolution of advanced nursing practice. In Hamric, A.B., Spross, J.A., & Hanson, C.M. (Eds.). *Advanced nursing practice: an integrative approach*. Philadelphia: W.B. Saunders.

Bok, D. (1992). Reclaiming the public trust. *Change, 24*(4), 12–19.

Boyer, E.L. (1990). *Scholarship reconsidered: priorities of the professoriate*. Menlo Park, CA: Carnegie Foundation for the Advancement of Teaching.

Buerhaus, P.I. (1998). Is another RN shortage looming? *Nursing Outlook, 46*(3), 103–108.

Buerhaus, P.I., & Staiger, D.O. (1997). Future of the nurse labor market according to the health executives in high managed-care areas of the United States. *Image: Journal of Nursing Scholarship, 29*(4), 313–318.

Burns, P., et al. (1993). Masters degree nursing education: state of the art. *Journal of Professional Nursing, 9*, 267–276.

Camilleri, D.D. (1997). Nursing education for the 21st century: old traditions and new challenges. In McCloskey, J.C., & Grace, H.K. (Eds.). *Current issues in nursing* (ed. 5). St. Louis: Mosby.

Campbell, C.D., Musil, C.M., & Zauszniewski, J.A. (1998). Practice patterns of advanced practice psychiatric nurses. *Journal of the American Psychiatric Nurses Association, 4*, 111–120.

Caverly, S.E. (1996). The role of the psychiatric nurse practitioner. *Nursing Clinics of North America, 31*, 449–463.

Christman, L. (1992). Advanced nursing practice: future of clinical nurse specialists. In Aiken, L.H., & Fagin, C.M. (Eds.). *Charting nursing's future: agenda for the 1990s*. Philadelphia: J.B. Lippincott.

Denning, P. (1996). Business designs for the new university. *EDUCOM Review, 31*(6), 20–30.

Division of Nursing, Bureau of Health Professions in the Health Resources and Services Administration. (1997). *National sample survey of registered nurses 1996*. Washington, DC: U.S. Government Printing Office.

Downs, F.S. (1989). Differences between the professional doctorate and the academic/research doctorate. *Journal of Professional Nursing, 5*, 261–267.

Dyer, J.G., et al. (1997). The psychiatric-primary care nurse practitioner: a futuristic model for advanced practice psychiatric-mental health nursing. *Archives of Psychiatric Nursing, 11*, 2–12.

Fenton, M.V., & Brykczynski, K.A. (1993). Qualitative distinctions and similarities in the practice of clinical nurse specialists and nurse practitioners. *Journal of Professional Nursing, 9*(6), 313–326.

Flaskerud, J.H., & Wuerker, A.K. (1999). Mental health nursing in the 21st century. *Issues in Mental Health Nursing, 20*, 5–17.

Friere, P. (1991). *Pedagogy of the oppressed*. New York: Continuum.

Gabel, J. (1997). Ten ways HMOs have changed during the 1990s. *Health Affairs, 16*(3), 134–145.

Gallop, R. (1998). Postdischarge social contact: a potential area for boundary violation. *Journal of the American Psychiatric Nurses Association, 4*(4), 105–110.

Germain, C.P., et al. (1994). Evaluation of a PhD program: paving the way. *Nursing Outlook, 41*, 117–122.

Grace, H.K. (1983). Doctoral education in nursing: dilemmas and directions. In Chaska, N. (Ed.). *The nursing profession: a time to speak up*. New York: McGraw-Hill.

Gutheil, T, & Gabbard, G. (1993). The concept of boundaries in clinical practice: theoretical and risk-management dimensions. *American Journal of Psychiatry, 150*, 188–196.

Haber, J., & Billings, C.V. (1995). Primary mental health care: a model for psychiatric-mental health nursing. *Journal of the American Psychiatric Nurses Association, 1*(5), 154–163.

Hanson, K.S. (1991). An analysis of the historical context of liberal education in nursing education from 1924 to 1939. *Journal of Professional Nursing, 7*(6), 341–350.

Harper, D. (1996). Education for advanced nursing practice. In Hamric, A.B., Spross, J.A., & Hanson, C.M. (Eds.). *Advanced nursing practice: an integrative approach*. Philadelphia: W.B. Saunders.

Huston, C.J., & Fox, S. (1998). The changing health care

market: implications for nursing education in the coming decade. *Nursing Outlook, 46*(3), 109–114.

Johnson, B.S. (1998). The 5 r's of becoming a psychiatric nurse practitioner: rationale, readying, roles, rules, and reality. *Journal of Psychosocial Nursing, 36*(9), 20–24.

Kaufman, A. (Ed.). (1985). *Implementing problem-based medical education.* New York: Springer.

Knowles, M. (1978). *The adult learner: a neglected species* (ed. 2). Houston, TX: Gulf.

Krahenbuhl, G.S. (1998). Faculty work: integrating responsibilities and institutional needs. *Change, 30*(6), 18–25.

Lego, S., & Caverly, S.E. (1995). Coming to terms: psychiatric nurse practitioner versus clinical specialist [point of view]. *Journal of Psychiatric Nurses Association, 1*(2), 61–63.

Lewis, M.L., & Kaas, M.J. (1998). Challenges of teaching graduate psychiatric-mental health nursing with distance education technologies. *Archives of Psychiatric Nursing, 12*(4), 227–233.

Mastrangelo, R. (December, 1993). Merging the NP and CNS roles: will health care reform be the catalyst? *ADVANCE for Nurse Practitioners*, 23–24.

Matteson, P.S. (Ed.). (1995). *Teaching nursing in the neighborhoods: the Northeastern University model.* New York: Springer.

McCloskey, J.C., & Grace, H.K. (1997). Nursing education in transition. In McCloskey, J.C., & Grace, H.K. (Eds.). *Current issues in nursing* (ed. 5). St. Louis: Mosby.

Meleis, A.I. (1992). On the way to scholarship: from master's to doctorate. *Journal of Professional Nursing, 8*(6), 328–334.

Millenson, M.L. (1997). *Demanding medical excellence.* Chicago: University of Chicago Press.

National League for Nursing. (1993). *A vision for nursing education.* New York: Author.

National League for Nursing. (1997). *Nursing data review 1997.* New York: NLN Press.

National Organization of Nurse Practitioner Faculties. (1995). *Advanced practice nursing: curriculum guidelines and program standards for nurse practitioner education.* Washington, DC: Author.

Page, N.E., & Arena, D.M. (1994). Rethinking the merger of the clinical nurse specialist and the nurse practitioner roles. *Image: Journal of Nursing Scholarship, 26*(4), 315–318.

Paterson, B. (1998). Partnership in nursing education: a vision or a fantasy? *Nursing Outlook, 46*(6), 284–289.

Payne, J.L., & Baumgartner, R.G. (1996). CNS role evolution. *Clinical Nurse Specialist, 10*(1), 46–48.

Peplau, H. (1952). *Interpersonal relations in nursing.* New York: G.P. Putnam's Sons.

Pew Health Professions Commission. (1993). *Health professions education for the future: schools in service to the nation.* San Francisco: Author.

Pullen, C., et al. (1994). A comprehensive primary health care delivery model. *Journal of Professional Nursing, 10*(4), 201–208.

Redman, R.W., & Ketefian, S. (1997). The changing face of graduate education. In McCloskey, J.C., & Grace, H.K. (Eds.). *Current issues in nursing* (ed. 5). St. Louis: Mosby.

Shea, C.A. (1994). The three "r's" in nursing education [editorial]. *Journal of Psychosocial Nursing, 32*(5), 7–8.

Shea, C.A. (1995). Laying the groundwork for curriculum change. In Matteson, P.S. (Ed.). *Teaching nursing in the neighborhoods: the Northeastern University model.* New York: Springer.

Shuren, A.W. (1996). The blended role of the clinical nurse specialist and the nurse practitioner. In Hamric, A.B., Spross, J.A., & Hanson, C.M. (Eds.). *Advanced nursing practice: an integrative approach.* Philadelphia: W.B. Saunders.

Skiba, D.J. (1997). Transforming nursing education to celebrate learning. *Nursing and Health Care Perspectives, 18*(3), 124–129, 148.

Smith, L.L., et al. (1997). Nurse-patient boundaries: crossing the line. *American Journal of Nursing, 97*(12), 26–31.

Society for Education and Research in Psychiatric-Mental Health Nursing. (1996). *Educational preparation for psychiatric-mental health nursing.* Pensacola, FL: Author.

Society for Education and Research in Psychiatric-Mental Health Nursing. (1997). *Primary mental health and advanced practice in psychiatric nursing.* Pensacola, FL: Author.

Stuart, G.W. (1997). Recent changes and current issues in psychiatric nursing. In McCloskey, J.C., & Grace, H.K. (Eds.). *Current issues in nursing* (ed. 5). St. Louis: Mosby.

Talley, S., & Caverly, S. (1994). Advanced-practice psychiatric nursing and health care reform. *Hospital and Community Psychiatry, 45,* 545–547.

Trossman, S. (March/April, 1998). Mentoring leads to meaningful relationships, professional growth. *The American Nurse,* 12.

Tusaie-Mumford, K. (1993). Nurse practitioners or clinical nurse specialists? [My side: personal accounts]. *Journal of Psychosocial Nursing, 31*(7), 48.

Vance, C., & Olson, R.K. (1998). *The mentor connection in nursing.* New York: Springer.

Williams, C.A., et al. (1998). Toward an integration of competencies for advanced practice mental health nursing. *Journal of the American Psychiatric Nurses Association, 4,* 48–56.

Wunsch, M.A. (1994). Giving structure to experience: mentoring strategies for women faculty. In Wunsch, M.A. (Ed.). *Mentoring revisited: making an impact on individuals and institutions.* San Francisco: Jossey-Bass Publishers.

Ziemer, M.M., et al. (1992). Doctoral programs in nursing: philosophy, curricula, and program requirements. *Journal of Professional Nursing, 8*(1), 56–62.

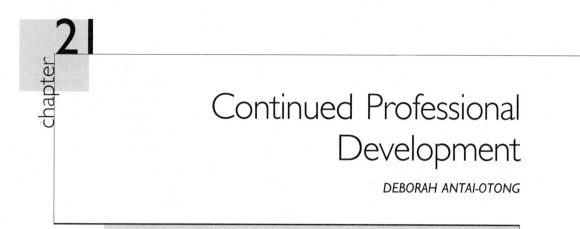

Continued Professional Development

DEBORAH ANTAI-OTONG

chapter 21

■ INTRODUCTION

With movement into the twenty-first century, changing patient populations and their complex needs will challenge advanced practice registered nurses (APRNs) in psychiatric-mental health nursing to respond proactively by staying abreast of contemporary findings in the field through professional development. APRNs recognize the importance of mental and physical health care needs in their quest to provide holistic health care. Thus education for continued professional development must extend beyond biopsychosocial parameters and prescriptive authority and include an appreciation of culture, age, gender, societal issues, marketing, and politics. The educational and professional development of APRNs is a lifelong endeavor. The professional evolution begins with undergraduate education, continues with graduate education, and is governed by professional and personal experiences. This chapter describes the educational needs of APRNs who seek to maintain competency in managing complex patient needs in an ever-changing health care system, and strategies to keep up with events that affect practice issues.

Health care and advanced practice psychiatric-mental health nursing are in the midst of tremendous and far-reaching changes. APRNs are poised to meet these challenges and create roles for the changing health care environment. An integral part of the APRN's role is caring. APRNs are providers and coordinators of care, members of collaborative professional teams, and partners with patients and families (Brackley, 1995). Moreover, they are committed to becoming experts in health

467

promotion and wellness. Historically, APRNs have understood the importance of symptoms and behaviors within the context in which they occur, along with the patient's restorative powers. They now have an even greater holistic appreciation of complex causative favors and interventions needed to promote adaptive responses over time (McBride, 1996). The sheer nature of the attributes of advanced nursing practice contributes to the need to continue to master new strategies and gain new knowledge. These new strategies include interventions that modify complex neurobiologic processes and behaviors, such as medication management, eye-movement desensitization and reprocessing, sleep manipulation, phototherapy, diet modification, and other therapies.

Stakeholders in this rapidly changing health care climate are demanding the highest level of care and positive treatment outcomes. These demands compel APRNs to sharpen and maintain their skills while carving out and articulating their roles to the stakeholders. Maintaining quality standards and achieving positive treatment outcomes require knowledge of the latest developments in neurobiology, technologic advances, life span issues, pharmacology, societal factors, women and children's health, and trends in health care delivery systems. As consumers become more invested in their care, recognizing and addressing their individual needs becomes a greater priority for the APRN. More importantly, as consumers' demands for informed health care become coupled with professional responsibilities and liabilities, there is an urgency for APRNs to master and maintain skills that ensure quality care. Quality care is achievable through educational and clinical experiences, the building blocks of professional development and a productive career.

As the next millennium approaches, the growth of advanced practice psychiatric-mental health nursing will depend upon the APRNs' ability to strategically position themselves and clearly define their roles in the transformed health care system. The role and practice of psychiatric-mental health nursing at the advanced level is often per-

plexing to others, yet it also generates great interest. The attention of stakeholders will continue to expand as the visibility of nurses as primary health care providers becomes more apparent. The stakeholders—consumers, professional nursing organizations, health care insurers and providers—also will have greater expectations of increasing accountability of APRNs for both quality and cost-effective health care. The stakeholders will continue to scrutinize expanding nursing roles and their effects on the quality of care. Therefore it will be important for APRNs to demonstrate their ability to add value. National certification is one process that affords evidence of the APRN's competency in a nursing specialty.

■ CERTIFICATION

Certification refers to a process that validates knowledge and expertise in a practice area or role. Moreover, it is governed by a defined scope of practice and standards that reflect individual qualifications, knowledge, and practice in a specified clinical specialty. It engenders a sense of achievement and reflects a commitment to nursing and continued professional development. Professional distinction and competency, increased job security, and eligibility for third party reimbursement are added benefits of national certification for the individual APRN (see the latest edition of the American Nurses Credentialing Center's [ANCC] *Advanced Practice Board Certification Catalog* [1998a]).

The ANCC was created by the American Nurses Association (ANA) in 1973. It later became a separate entity governing and overseeing its own credentialing programs. Up-to-date information about ANCC activities, accomplishments by volunteers, and certification are available through several media: in the quarterly newsletter, *Credentialing News* (ANCC, 1998b); at the ANCC office in Washington, DC; and on the ANCC Internet website. (See the Resources and Connections section of this chapter.) The ANCC also provides a directory of accredited provider and approver organizations that offer continuing education, as well as providers of independent studies (e.g., Education Design II [EDII]).

In today's health care arena where quality and safe care are a priority, certification connotes a quality improvement process. This quality improvement process also offers evidence to the public and other stakeholders that the APRN has met standards of the profession and competency in a specialty. *Competency* refers to the capacity to perform or respond sufficiently to a given situation. Determining one's competency and need for professional and personal growth is an important hallmark of the APRN. Professional responsibilities to continue to improve extend beyond certification to recertification every 5 years. Recertification is as significant as certification because it enables APRNs to demonstrate continued competency in their specialty. Continuing education (CE) and retesting are the major methods of recertification. CE requirements for recertification are described in the ANCC's *Recertification Catalog*. The requirements for both certification and recertification vary by certification area.

Standards of practice originating from the ANA Congress for Nursing Practice in collaboration with specialty organizations, such as the American Psychiatric Nurses Association (APNA), are the bases of the ANCC credentialing programs. The ANCC is the premier certifying body for advanced practice psychiatric-mental health nursing. There are two certification examinations currently: 1) clinical specialist in adult psychiatric and mental health nursing; and 2) clinical specialist in child and adolescent psychiatric and mental health nursing. In keeping with changes in health care needs and the health care delivery system, educators have developed new master's programs that focus on primary health care. Consequently, the ANCC is designing a new examination for the psychiatric-mental health nurse practitioner. Chapter 20 discusses these programs in greater detail.

The advanced practice of psychiatric-mental health nursing is also contingent on the individual state nurse practice acts and licensure requirements of state boards of nursing. The National Council of State Boards of Nursing (NCOSB) and State Boards of Nursing (SBON) define regulations that enable nurses to practice within their respective states. A survey of the states' CE requirements provides educators with general information about CE requirements for certification and recertification (Yoder-Wise, 1998). Requirements pertaining to APRNs were included in the survey for the first time in 1998. Results from this survey show that most states have CE requirements for certification and APRN licensure. The CE requirements for APRNs, according to most respondents, included courses in specialty areas, such as HIV/AIDS, medical and social effects of substance abuse, and pharmacotherapeutics, particularly in those states with prescriptive authority.

National certification is proving to be a requisite for advanced practice nurse status and licensure in most states. Certification is no longer a luxury or choice but a professional responsibility and commitment to quality and safe health care. Many nursing leaders believe that certification will have a direct effect on practice and quality of care. Certification is an integral aspect of the APRN's preparation for a changing workforce. It parallels insurer, consumer, and legislative demand for positive treatment outcomes and serves as a basis for collaborative relationships.

CONTINUING EDUCATION
Quality Programs

CE is a vital part of the process that enhances development and maintenance of high standards of care in a changing health care environment. Attending quality CE programs is a professional responsibility and integral part of role development. Historically, CE has provided avenues for nurses to enhance practice competencies. This is particularly significant for APRNs whose practice is governed by legal and ethical issues and licensure and certification requirements (Macklin, 1998). The need for specific types of CE depends upon the APRN's specialty area, certification, state licensure requirements, and personal and professional interests.

Ordinarily, the seal of approval by the ANCC, conferred by its Commission on Accreditation (COA), is one of the most recognizable indicators of quality CE programs. The ANCC grants "provider status" to organizations (such as state nurses associations) that offer CE programs after a rigorous application and approval process. Programs offered by ANCC-accredited organizations must meet the test for quality according to criteria established by the COA. The following questions are useful in determining if a CE offering meets the COA criteria (Macklin, 1998):

1. Is this a timely and relevant topic?
2. Do the objectives for this offering meet the needs of the nurse consumer of education?
3. Under which category does this offering fall: Education Design I (planned by others) or Education Design II (self-paced or independent study)?
4. Does the offering meet personal learning needs?
5. What are the credentials of the program's planners?
6. How is the nurse assured that this is a quality educational offering?
7. How will the offering be documented?

Answering these questions will provide basic information about the quality of a CE offering. Paying for CE programs is expensive, especially in a work environment that offers little or no reimbursement as an employee benefit, or does not allow time off to pursue professional activities. This makes it even more important to assess the quality of CE programs, to get good value for the money.

Considering the changes in health care and demands for advanced practice clinical competencies, APRNs can also expect changes in educational requirements for certification and recertification. In the future, 50% of the CE programs taken by the APRN to meet his or her certification or recertification requirement must be offered by ANCC-accredited or other approved providers (ANCC, 1998b). Current ANCC CE requirements parallel changing educational and professional nursing standards. Therefore APRNs seeking certification and recertification should contact the ANCC to obtain the most up-to-date information on the requirements and criteria.

Other avenues for CE include programs offered through numerous journals, such as the *Journal of the American Psychiatric Nurses Association*, and via the Internet. These avenues are particularly convenient for nurses living in remote areas. Other CE opportunities include the use of qualified experts in the field or the study of state-of-the art scientific topics in distance learning programs.

The scope of professional development is broad. The APRN's goals are to acquire and strengthen practice competency, knowledge of the specialty area and clinical practice guidelines, and skills in role development in light of health care delivery trends. The decision to attend or participate in a CE program depends on personal and professional needs. University-based distance learning and correspondence programs, facility-based seminars and workshops, journals and CD-ROM or computer-assisted instructions are resources for professional development. Traditional nursing education programs are also important sources of professional development.

In addition to participating in CE programs for their own professional development, APRNs often design and implement CE programs for others. Designing a CE program involves knowledge of adult learning theories and skills in the areas of learning needs assessment, curriculum design, instructional methodologies, and program evaluation. Box 21-1 provides resources for the planning and implementation of CE programs.

Clinical and Practice Issues

APRNs practice in a wide range of clinical settings, from private group practice, to inpatient institutions, to outpatient agencies. Traditionally, they have provided psychotherapies and patient and

21-1

RESOURCES FOR PLANNING AND IMPLEMENTING CONTINUING EDUCATION PROGRAMS

JOURNALS

Journal of Continuing Education in Nursing
Journal of Nursing Staff Development

BOOKS

Abruzzese, R.S. (1996). *Nursing staff development: strategies for success* (ed. 2). St. Louis: Mosby.

Caffarella, R.S. (1994). *Planning programs for adult learners: a practical guide for educators, trainers, and staff developers.* San Francisco: Jossey-Bass.

Kelly-Thomas, K.J. (Ed.). (1998). *Clinical and nursing staff development: current competence, future focus* (ed. 2). Philadelphia: J.B. Lippincott.

Rodriguez, L., et al. (1996). *Manual of staff development.* St. Louis: Mosby.

Swansburg, R.C. (1995). *Nursing staff development: a component of human resource development.* Boston: Jones & Bartlett.

GUIDELINES AND STANDARDS

American Nurses Association. (1994). *Standards for nursing professional development: continuing education and staff development.* Washington, DC: Author.

American Nurses Credentialing Center. (1998). *Manual for accreditation as a provider of continuing education in nursing.* Washington, DC: Author. (Available in full text at the ANCC website: www.nursingworld.org/ancc)

guidelines enhance treatment efficacy, minimize drug interactions, and promote quality and safe health care. APRNs must acquire competencies in these areas to meet the needs for health promotion, disease prevention, and case management of diverse patient populations. Health assessment, medication management, and alternative therapies are examples of essential clinical competencies that will enhance the role of the APRN. Additionally, APRNs must engage in ongoing professional development to enhance competency in role areas such as political awareness, high technology communication, and marketing of advanced practice services.

Health assessment and medication management. APRNs must obtain the knowledge and skills for primary mental health care, including health assessment and medication management. They must meld these competencies with psychotherapies into a holistic model of care. Health assessment includes taking histories, performing physical examinations, and ordering and interpreting diagnostic studies, such as laboratory tests, electrocardiograms, and serum drug levels. This process also includes making referrals and initiating requests for consultation when appropriate.

Medication management is an integral aspect of primary mental health care requiring monitoring, evaluation, reevaluation, health teaching, and measures to promote adherence to the treatment plan. Collaborative practice models and precepting provide educational opportunities to develop competencies in health assessment and medication management, as do ongoing facility and community educational programs, particularly in pharmacotherapeutics (Hales et al., 1998; Hovey & McEnany, 1996).

The success of a holistic model of care hinges on collaborative relationships with other health care providers, patients, and families. Professional development in the complex role of a primary mental health care provider requires some form of precepting and supervision that involves an experienced collaborator. Clinical supervision is an established interactive process that provides

family education, and they have collaborated with other health care providers to manage the care of diverse patient populations. In comparison, contemporary health care delivery systems focus on community-based primary care, ambulatory and home health settings, and alternative therapies. CE programs that focus on principles of primary care, differential diagnosis, and clinical practice

the necessary guidance and support to the APRN during role transition and further development. In an individualized relationship, the supervisory process becomes an essential quality improvement tool. With medication management, supervision may include weekly meetings for 1 hour focusing on case reviews, practice prescriptive guidelines based on a collaborative relationship, a clearly defined scope of practice, credentialing needs, and the quality improvement process through peer review (Bailey, 1996; Bailey & Synder, 1995). Other resources on medication management in psychiatric nursing include the ANA Task Group on Psychopharmacology's (1994) publication on psychopharmacologic practice (see Chapter 13).

As APRNs move into primary care and community-based settings, they must update these competencies through CE. CE programs that feature neurobiologic technology also enhance the understanding of medications and how they mediate various neurochemical processes that contribute to symptom management. For example, there are the national psychiatric conferences and programs developed through the National Institutes of Health (NIH) and the National Institute of Mental Health (NIMH). NIH and NIMH programs provide the latest research on various psychiatric disorders including schizophrenia, mood and anxiety disorders, and other mental disorders. These programs are excellent examples of federally sponsored conferences for APRNs and nursing educators to enhance their understanding of neurobiologic processes and associated health assessment, medication management, symptoms reduction, disease prevention, and health promotion.

Complementary therapies. Another practice issue affecting health care is the explosion of complementary or alternative therapies. As more consumers turn to alternative forms of treatment, it behooves APRNs to command knowledge of diverse treatment approaches. Consumers are able to purchase various products that improve their health (Eisenberg et al., 1993). These products range from herbs (French, 1996), such as St. John's Wort and primrose, to aromatherapy and dietary supplements. Understanding the significance of these practices enhances the nurse-patient relationship while providing additional therapies. Nursing implications from the advent of these practices include discerning side effects, therapeutic actions, contraindications with traditional treatment, and long-term effects. There are many CE programs about complementary therapies that focus primarily on herbs, aromatherapy, therapeutic touch, biofeedback, eye-movement desensitization reprocessing, and dietary supplements. Faculty for these educational programs includes nurses, dieticians, physicians, and other health care providers. A discussion of the use of complementary therapies by the APRN is found in Chapter 11.

Political savvy. Keeping up with the legislation and political factors that affect nursing lies within the domain of CE. Reams of information about legislative and political issues can be accessed via journals, newspapers, and newsletters, as well as the websites of various nursing organizations including the APNA, ANA, and ANCC. Educational materials about political issues, such as policies related to reimbursement and billing, are found in numerous nursing journals and the political and legislative update sections of websites. For example, the ANA is developing media that educate nurses on Medicare application procedures. There is the Health Care Financing Administration (HCFA) list of local Medicare carriers, which can be accessed on various professional nursing and federal agencies' websites. The ANA's *American Nurse* newspaper, the *American Journal of Nursing,* the *Journal of the American Psychiatric Nurses Association*, the *APNA news*, the *Society for Education in Psychiatric-Mental Health Nursing's News Series*, and the *Legislative Network for Nurses* are examples of nursing media that disseminate political and legislative updates.

Special training in media relations also affords APRNs opportunities to further their political agenda through local, state, and national media. Dealing with the media often requires mentoring and coaching to focus on issues relevant to legisla-

box 21-2

RECOMMENDATIONS FOR MEDIA INITIATIVES

- Obtain training on how to discuss business, management, and policies.
- Develop a local or national nursing directory.
- Work with your public relations department to appoint specific nurse media representatives.
- Establish a network with your local news reporters from television, newspapers, and radio.
- Focus on retitling your role, rather than the physician's, as "primary care provider."
- Educate the media about various health care issues and the roles nurses play in this arena.
- Use various media to advance the nursing role, including business cards and stationary, to increase the visibility of the nursing profession.

From Stewart, 1998.

tive and practice issues (Box 21-2). The ANA has an excellent program, the Nurses Strategic Action Team (NSTAT), which trains nurses to deal with the media and their legislators.

High technology communication. Technologic advances continue to add to the human encounter. Through innovative communication and sharing of knowledge, APRNs can expand their knowledge base. A significant area of professional development is computer and information literacy. The expansion of computer technology affects the dissemination of information across the globe, regardless of boundaries. Computer technology, television, telemedia, and telecomputers are augmenting conventional approaches to patient care. This form of communication provides enormous opportunities to educate patients, families, and communities in new ways. A related technologic advance is the use of the Internet. The Internet links nurses to vast audiences and current information about treatment, psychopharmacology, re-

search findings, distant learning, and educational opportunities (Korniewicz & Palmer, 1997). A discussion of computer technology for information management is found in Chapter 3.

Another technologic forum for professional development and CE is computer-assisted instruction for home study. This individualized approach provides APRNs with a CE program with easy access, interactive format, and immediate feedback. These programs are readily available and provide state-of-the-art CE on various topics including pharmacokinetics, case histories, literature reviews, and interactive test questioning. Overall, this technologic format is a convenient, cost-effective, pragmatic, and exciting CE approach that enables nurses to advance their knowledge and practice skills at home (Calderone, 1994; Neafsey, 1997). This instructional format also enhances nurses' computer skills. Using interactive CD-ROM software, attending advanced computer classes and CE programs, and reading computer journals and newsletters enhances computer literacy. Newsletters and journals (e.g., *Computers in Nursing*) are also important CE resources, and they can be obtained through various organizations including the National League for Nursing's Council on Nursing Informatics.

Many organizations, both nursing and multidisciplinary, provide up-to-date information on legislation, pharmacology, research and treatment of medical and mental disorders, and upcoming advanced practice nursing conferences. This information is found on the Internet and in newsletters, journals, and other media.

Marketing skills. As APRNs expand their clinical expertise, political savvy, and technologic advances, they must also sharpen their marketing skills. Marketing skills provide insight and expertise into political and financial arenas and enable nurses to become key brokers in the health care arena. Nurses must look to their vision, direction, and marketing skills to survive and grow in a competitive health care environment. Achieving success amidst decreasing resources, changing societal needs, and the competitive nature of health care is a challenge for APRNs. Without this knowledge, APRNs will not reap the resources of a changing health care system.

More nurses are entering the business world, establishing their own practices, and managing satellite clinics and networks of services. Therefore CE that enhances business and marketing skills seems prudent. Most nurses have difficulty putting a price on their services. Even more important, most nurses have difficulty discerning what their services are really worth. To thrive in this environment, APRNs need to understand the nature of their business and develop marketing skills that promote their services. Networking with nurses and other health care providers who are consultants and in private practice helps develop marketing and business skills (see Chapter 4).

Similarly, an often forgotten networking tool is the curriculum vitae (CV), or resume, which enables nurses to develop and showcase a chronology of their contributions to the nursing profession and the public. A CV provides a chronologic account of educational preparation; certification information; employment; scholarly activities including publications, grant writing, research, awards, and presentations; and CE or professional development (Hinck, 1997). This invaluable document projects the importance of the APRN's present and future professional career to colleagues and prospective employers. The exercise of updating a CV can also be a source of justifiable pride as the APRN reviews his or her milestones, progress toward goals, and professional accomplishments.

CE topics that enhance professional skills include financial accounting, money management, and retirement planning. Moreover, negotiation, conflict resolution, and time management skills also help APRNs establish and promote collaborative relationships. Likewise, CE programs that focus on reimbursement from private, state, and federal agencies; contractual agreements; and application for provider status build these skills. Marketing and accounting courses can be obtained through community colleges, universities, financial consultants, and medical facilities. Advancing marketing and financial skills promotes a sense of independence, confidence, and knowledge— qualities that are crucial to managing resources, negotiating contracts, and establishing lucrative businesses.

KEEPING CURRENT THROUGH ■ THE LITERATURE

Ever-expanding technologic advances and information systems strengthen the argument to expand the APRN's knowledge base through various means. Keeping current through the literature provides a convenient avenue of professional development and growth. Numerous forms of publications are available to nurses. Publications include journals, textbooks, the Internet, newsletters, CD-ROMs, and videos. Suggested readings for APRNs include major psychiatric nursing journals, various websites, newsletters, newspapers, medical and interdisciplinary journals, and review journals, such as *Journal Watch for Psychiatry*. Educational materials can also be acquired by browsing the Internet for contemporary research findings, consumer information, and upcoming mental health conferences sponsored by nurses and other health and mental health care providers.

The journals and newsletters listed in Box 21-3 provide a wealth of information ranging from managing the care of patients experiencing acute and chronic mental disorders to dealing with pertinent issues related to health care delivery systems. Many of the journals provide evidence-based interventions that enhance practice competencies and holistic treatment planning. Another invaluable resource for APRNs is the monograph, *Report of the APNA Congress on Advanced Practice in Psychiatric Nursing* (APNA, 1997). Major sections of this report include the following:

1. Recognition of the advanced practice nursing role
2. Base for and documenting practice
3. Reimbursement for practice
4. Countering competitive moves
5. Treatment facts

The *Report of the APNA Congress* is a compilation of research-based educational materials and inno-

box 21-3

JOURNALS AND NEWSLETTERS TO KEEP CURRENT

PSYCHIATRIC NURSING

Archives of Psychiatric Nursing
APNA news
Issues in Mental Health Nursing
Journal of Child and Adolescent Psychiatric Nursing
Journal of Psychosocial Nursing and Mental Health Services
Journal of the American Psychiatric Nurses Association
Perspectives in Psychiatric Care
Society for Education in Psychiatric-Mental Health Nursing's News Series

NURSING

American Journal of Nursing
Applied Nursing Research
Clinical Nurse Specialist
Computers in Nursing
Image: Journal of Nursing Scholarship
Journal of Continuing Education in Nursing
Journal of Nursing Administration
Journal of Nursing Education
Journal of Professional Nursing
Nurse Educator

Nurse Practitioner
Nurse Practitioner Forum
Nursing and Health Care
Nursing Economics
Nursing Management
Nursing Outlook
Nursing Research
Research in Nursing and Health

OTHER PSYCHIATRIC

American Journal of Orthopsychiatry
American Journal of Psychiatry
American Journal of Psychotherapy
Biological Psychiatry
Community Mental Health Journal
Harvard Mental Health Letter
Psychiatric Services
Schizophrenia Bulletin

MEDICAL AND OTHER

Journal of the American Medical Association
New England Journal of Medicine
Science

vations provided by advanced practice psychiatric-mental health nursing leaders from around the country. It contains relevant information about practice issues, reimbursement, marketing, and outcome measures (see Appendix E). Accessing research-based data, as in this report and through the literature, improves interventions and promotes quality health care.

SUPERVISION AND ■ PEER CONSULTATION

The concept of clinical or professional supervision is not a new concept. It has been an integral part of the mental health profession for more than 40 years (Stokes, 1969; Poertner, 1986). Professional

supervision is an interactive process that helps APRNs throughout their professional careers. The merit of clinical supervision extends beyond CE, helping to meet criteria for certification and recertification. The supervisee seeks education, consultation, and support from a highly respected and expert colleague or supervisor. Like other CE endeavors, the basis of learning stems from the needs of the supervisee but also involves the needs of the supervisor. The supervisory meetings usually take place weekly for about an hour. Participants review difficult or unusual cases; discuss personal reactions to various relationships; and receive support, guidance, education, and feedback about case reviews. Supervisory relationships are not restricted to APRNs but frequently include other health care providers. APRNs can also attain supervision through groups or with colleagues who share similar needs and interests.

Supervision, like other educational opportunities, occurs in numerous formats. In a study of 61 psychiatric clinical specialists, Pesut and Williams (1990) describe numerous forms of supervision including onsite supervision, review of treatment data, cotherapy with a supervisor, review of progress notes, audiotapes, video tapings, direct supervision, and role-playing. Of these examples, individual supervision, onsite supervision, and review of treatment data were the most common forms of clinical supervision.

Peer consultation is a model for nursing professional development whereby a group of peers meet in regular sessions and share the roles of consultee and consultant among all members on a rotating basis (Shields et al., 1985). Peer consultation in a group context differs from traditional clinical supervision in that the expertise and power are shared among all individuals in the group. Hierarchical relationships are absent, and the accountability for the use of the consultative process for problem solving, support, validation, and professional development is equally distributed among all members. In the peer consultation model, the consultee prepares and delivers a formal presentation of a clinical case, organizational problem, or other professional issue and poses questions for consideration by the consultants. The consultants assist the consultee to clarify the problem or dilemma and to develop additional or alternative questions. The power of the group process is used to synthesize perceptions and insights for the formulation of a collective framework of understanding and professional growth. Finally, the process is summarized and evaluated. A full discussion of the concepts of peer consultation in a group context and detailed guidelines for the development and implementation of a peer consultation group are found in Shields and colleagues (1985).

The success of supervision and peer consultation depends on several factors, including trust, the level of altruism, appreciation and respect of others' clinical competencies, a commitment to patient-focused treatment outcomes, open-mindedness, and assertive communication skills. These supportive and caring environments also promote self-awareness, the crucible of personal growth and professional development (Antai-Otong, 1995). Self-awareness and professional development enable nurses to communicate their expertise effectively in diverse ways, including publication, grant writing, and research studies.

PUBLICATION AND ■ GRANT WRITING
Writing for Publication

Writing for publication enables nurses to disseminate information through various avenues, including writing articles, chapters, monographs, and books; editing books and journals; reviewing books and manuscripts; creating materials for the Internet, CD-ROM, and other forms of technology transfer; making videos and films; and giving scholarly presentations and workshops. The skill of organizing one's thoughts into a coherent presentation of ideas that can be communicated to others is the basic building block of the transfer of knowledge. Writing is its most common form of expression.

Writing is not an easy task, and it requires enormous energy, patience, and the ability to handle negative and constructive feedback. When scholarly, this form of communication enables APRNs to use critical thinking skills and contribute to the success and knowledge of their profession (Axelrod & Cooper, 1994). Through publishing, nurses disseminate research findings, share clinical experiences, analyze basic assumptions, and enhance self-awareness and professional growth.

Moving from a novice to an expert writer is a necessary part of professional growth that often begins by contacting an experienced writer to serve as a coach and mentor. Mirin (1981) outlines the steps for those who wish to pursue writing for publication:

1. Believe in yourself.
2. Find and consult with a mentor or experienced author.
3. Select a topic and journal.
4. Do a literature search and analyze the data.
5. Send a query letter.
6. Develop a topic outline.
7. Write the article.
8. Submit the manuscript.

APRNs should not be surprised if the first submission of their manuscript is not accepted. They should review the editorial comments and use them to revise the manuscript. They might want to consider resubmitting the manuscript to another journal. It can be said that the only manuscripts that are rejected are those that are submitted. The premise of this saying is that APRNs must be willing to take risks and sometimes fail in order to succeed in developing their writing skills.

There is both need and opportunity for the published wisdom of nurses. CE opportunities include national conferences, such as those sponsored by the American Academy of Nursing (AAN), ANA, APNA, SERPN, Sigma Theta Tau International, and annual advanced practice nursing symposia. These programs usually offer courses in writing for publication or opportunities to talk to editors. Reading books on publication is also useful for novices and experienced authors. The fourth edition of *The St. Martin's Guide to Writing* (Axelrod & Cooper, 1994) and the fourth edition of the *Publication Manual* (American Psychological Association, 1994) are resources for prospective writers.

Writing Grant Proposals

Another type of continuing professional development is grant writing. The art and process of grant writing involves knowledge of program, research, and innovation with the goal of procuring funding for a study or project. There are many funding sources that can be accessed on the Internet from various federal agencies, such as the NIMH, private foundations such as the Robert Wood Johnson Foundation, and professional organizations such as research awards from the American Nurses Foundation. Major universities have special resources to help secure extramural funds (e.g., libraries with reference volumes, periodical literature, journals, and the Internet) and departments or offices for research development.

Research and grant writing skills evolve with experience and endure with practice. CE in this area is critical to the advancement of psychiatric-mental health nursing. Nurses can expand these skills by participating on grant writing committees, doing research studies, serving on research review committees, and attending and presenting their work at research conferences. The findings from funded research studies must be integrated into practice guidelines and endorsed by major health care facilities and health maintenance organizations. Results from these studies can be used to validate the cost effectiveness of APRNs while improving the quality of health care. Never before has so much emphasis been placed on research and evidence-based interventions. Efforts to write grants and conduct research are vital to advancing the nursing agenda. Procuring grant money for contemporary research projects, although difficult, yields tremendous dividends for mental health consumers and the nursing profession.

Writing grant proposals is an art and, like writing for publication, requires a preceptor or mentor. The proposal is part of a larger process that evolves over time and includes a collaborative relationship between an organization and a donor. Geever and McNeill (1997) list several tips for successfully writing grant proposals:

1. Organize critical aspects of the project using clear, generic, and simple explanations for the proposal (i.e., major points).
2. Clearly delineate the rationale for the project.
3. Use a visionary approach.
4. Keep it short and to the point, including facts that describe the project, budget, organizational information, and summary.

Grant writing is a scholarly activity. Its value as educational development lies in the unique experience of working with a preceptor or mentor and, over time, becoming the expert and mentor to another generation of nurses.

POST-MASTER'S EDUCATION

Post-master's education, like CE, provides a basis for APRNs to expand their current knowledge and clinical expertise. Unlike CE, post-master's education is a more formal process, involving application and admission to a program at a college or university, matriculation in a curriculum or organized series of courses with grades recorded on a transcript, and a degree or certificate awarded upon graduation. These programs may be degree granting programs, such as a Ph.D. in Nursing, or non-degree as in certificate programs for nurses who already hold a master's degree in nursing and are seeking preparation as NPs.

Doctoral Education

The resolve to advance one's education by obtaining doctorate education is usually based on personal and professional goals. The major benefits of doctoral education are career advancement, social prestige, and personal achievement. For example, most nursing programs in higher education require faculty to have a doctorate in nursing or a related field to hold a tenure-track position. Some individuals pursue a doctorate for self-actualization reasons, such as achieving a life-long goal, sharpening their research skills, or increasing career options. Regardless of the personal reasons for pursuing doctoral education, this scholarly activity enriches the nursing profession. APRNs who have doctoral preparation hold leadership positions in the academic and service arenas, conduct funded research studies as principal investigators, provide expert consultation to groups and organizations, and set the course for the future through their participation in policy-making bodies. These benefits make obtaining a doctorate in nursing a viable and attractive option, extending individual development along the professional continuum.

Doctorally prepared scholars can further enrich the nursing profession by helping others in their quest for doctoral preparation. This process involves creating an academic culture that promotes scholarly development by embracing diversity and establishing collaborative mentorship (Meleis, Hall, & Stevens, 1994). Collaborative mentorship, unlike traditional doctoral education, promotes mutual respect and appreciation and encourages self expression and open communication through scholarly relations. Scholarly relationships imbue confidence and academic freedom to pursue the "truth," as well as reciprocity that advances innovative research. Academic cultures that embrace these concepts make doctoral preparation an attractive and invaluable choice for nurses seeking to expand their professional development. (See Appendix I for a list of nursing doctoral programs).

One area of controversy is the question of whether to pursue doctoral studies in nursing or another discipline. The answer to the question is influenced by the accessibility of program alternatives; the marketability of various degrees in a geographic location; the availability of nursing role models and mentors; requirements for educational qualifications and professional experience; and the abilities, goals, strengths, and socialization of the individual nursing student. Educational opportunities are available to nurses in other disciplines such as clinical psychology, health policy, economics, sociology, education, administration, and information technology.

The decision to pursue a doctoral degree also depends on financial feasibility and time constraints. Currently, most APRNs are extremely busy and find it difficult to fit a full-time program of study into their schedule. Efforts to keep up with the latest technologic advances, newest pharmaceuticals, intricate billing systems for services, and tracking of patient outcomes across settings challenge APRNs to perform at peak levels yet remain safe health care providers. Finding time to seek a doctoral degree may be daunting. High expectations at work, with family and social responsibilities, place tremendous stress on nurses. Therefore part-time, nontraditional, and distance learning programs that meet quality standards of the discipline and the needs of working APRNs may be a solution for those seeking doctoral preparation. Chapter 20 provides further discussion of doctoral education issues.

Non-Degree Programs

Historically, advanced health assessment, pathophysiology, pharmacology, and diagnosis and management of physical illness were not a part of advanced practice psychiatric-mental health nursing's curriculum. Today, these courses are an integral part of the master's curricula of both Clinical Specialist and Nurse Practitioner programs in psychiatric nursing. Many nurses who graduated from programs before the 1990s are now taking these courses through post-master's certification or CE programs.

A major task of APRNs, especially those with preparation as clinical specialists, is to integrate advances in neurobiology and behavioral concepts into practice. Recent legislative changes provide mechanisms for APRNs to obtain prescriptive authority. Post-master's programs are becoming increasingly popular as a way to prepare for certification as an NP and to learn the role of the psychiatric NP. This educational approach has the advantage of meeting various state boards of nursing's regulations in order to hold the NP title and obtain independent practice status and prescriptive authority (Talley & Brooke, 1992). There is also public name recognition for the NP title.

These educational requirements reflect national health care trends and come at a time when concerns about standards of practice are also being addressed. Presently, there is a national movement among boards of nurse examiners, professional organizations, and graduate nursing schools to develop a standard number of practicum hours for advanced practice nursing. Similarly, there is debate over mutual recognition of interstate licensing. The National Council of State Boards of

Nursing is exploring the feasibility of a model of mutual recognition for APRNs moving from one state to another (Yoder-Wise, 1998). The decision to attend a CE program or a post-master's program is affected by the APRN's career goals and current state board of nursing requirements for prescriptive authority, reimbursement guidelines, and other responsibilities.

IMPLICATIONS FOR
■ THE FUTURE

Societal changes, technologic advances, political and legislative issues, and health care stakeholders will continue to have a dramatic effect on psychiatric-mental health nursing. Even more significant are the efforts to build collaborative relationships and become primary health care providers. These reasons and others will compel APRNs to pursue educational opportunities that enhance their competency and increase their knowledge base. Additionally, APRNs moving into the next millennium will be challenged to explore futuristic career and new personal choices. The constant throughout the health care transformation will be professional development and competency, so necessary to managing complex patient populations and building collaborative relationships. APRNs must have a passion for professional development in order to grow both personally and professionally.

RESOURCES AND CONNECTIONS

American Nurses Credentialing Center
1-800-284-CERT
www.nursingworld.org/ancc

National Council of State Boards of Nursing
312-787-6555
www.ncsbn.org

References

American Nurses Association. (1994). *Psychiatric mental health nursing psychopharmacology project.* Washington, DC: Author.

American Nurses Credentialing Center. (1998a). *Advanced practice board certification catalog.* Washington, DC: Author.

American Nurses Credentialing Center. (1998b). *Credentialing news, 2*, 5.

American Psychiatric Nurses Association. (1997). *Report of the APNA Congress on advanced practice in psychiatric nursing*. Washington, DC: Author.

American Psychological Association. (1994). *Publication manual* (ed. 4). Washington, DC: Author.

Antai-Otong, D. (1995). Foundations of psychiatric nursing practice. In Antai-Otong, D. (Ed.). *Psychiatric nursing: biological and behavioral concepts*. Philadelphia: W.B. Saunders.

Axelrod, R.B., & Cooper, C.R. (1994). *The St. Martin's guide to writing, short 4th edition*. New York: St Martin's Press.

Bailey, K.P. (1996). Preparing for prescriptive practice: advanced practice psychiatric nursing and psychopharmacotherapy. *Journal of Psychosocial Nursing, 34*(1), 16–20, 48–49.

Bailey, K.P., & Snyder, M.E. (1995). The implementation of advanced practice psychiatric nurse prescribers: a comprehensive model. *Journal of the American Psychiatric Nurses Association, 1*, 183–189.

Brackley, M. (1995). A framework for developing psychiatric nursing skills. In Antai-Otong, D. (Ed.). *Psychiatric nursing: biological and behavioral concepts*. Philadelphia: W.B. Saunders.

Calderone, A.B. (1994). Computer assisted instruction: learning attitude, and modes of instruction. *Computers in Nursing, 9*, 75–79.

Eisenberg, D.M., et al. (1993). Unconventional medicine in the United States. *New England Journal of Medicine, 328*, 246–252.

French, M. (1996). The power of plants. *ADVANCE for Nurse Practitioners, 4*(7), 16–21.

Geever, J.C., & McNeill, P. (1997). *The Foundation Center's guide to proposal writing, revised edition*. New York: The Foundation Center.

Hales, A., et al. (1998). Preparing for prescriptive privileges: a CNS-Physician collaborative model: expanding the scope of the psychiatric-mental health clinical nurse specialist. *Clinical Nurse Specialist, 12*, 73–82.

Hinck, S.M. (1997). A curriculum vitae that gives you a competitive edge. *Clinical Nurse Specialist, 11*, 174–177.

Hovey, J., & McEnany, G. (1996). Psychobiologic knowledge and prescriptive authority: RX for change in nursing practice. *Journal of the American Psychiatric Nurses Association, 2*, 164–166.

Korniewicz, D.M., & Palmer, M.H. (1997). The preferable future of nursing. *Nursing Outlook, 45*, 108–113.

Macklin, N.R. (1998). Ensuring quality in continuing education. *American Journal of Nursing, 98*(4 Contin. Care Extra Ed.), 60–62.

Meleis, A.I., Hall, J.M., & Stevens, P.E. (1994). Scholarly caring in doctoral nursing education: promoting diversity and collaborative mentorship. *Image: Journal of Nursing Scholarship, 26*, 177–180.

McBride, A.B. (1996). A final word about career development. In McBride, A.B., & Austin, J.K. (Eds.). *Psychiatric-mental health nursing*. Philadelphia: W.B. Saunders.

Mirin, S.K. (1981). *The nurse's guide to writing for publication*. Wakefield, MA: Nursing Resources.

Neafsey, P.J. (1997). Computer-assisted instruction for home study: a new venture for continuing education programs for nursing. *The Journal of Continuing Education in Nursing, 28*, 164–172, 190–191.

Pesut, D.J., & Williams, C.A. (1990). The nature of clinical supervision in psychiatric nursing: a survey of clinical specialists. *Archives of Psychiatric Nursing, 4*, 188–194.

Poertner, J. (1986). The use of client feedback to improve practice: defining the supervisor's role. *Clinical Supervisor, 44*(4), 57–67.

Shields, J.D., et al. (1985). *Peer consultation in a group context: a guide for professional nurses*. New York: Springer.

Stewart, M. (1998). RN=real news: ANA launches comprehensive media initiative to support SNAs, nursing. *The American Nurse, 30*, 20.

Stokes, G.A. (1969). *The roles of psychiatric nurses in community mental health practice*. Brooklyn, NY: Faculty Press.

Talley, S., & Brooke, P. (1992). Prescriptive authority for psychiatric clinical nurse specialists: framing the issues. *Archives of Psychiatric Nursing, 6*, 71–82.

Yoder-Wise, P.S. (1998). State and association/certifying boards CE requirements. *Journal of Continuing Education in Nursing, 29*, 2–9.

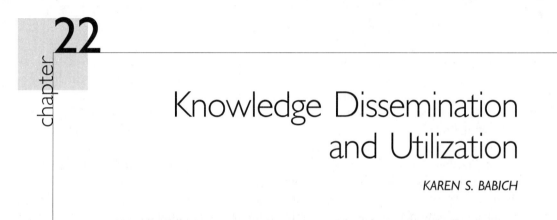

Knowledge Dissemination and Utilization

KAREN S. BABICH

■ INTRODUCTION

Knowledge dissemination and utilization is the study of how information is shared and used. Although the importance of this field of research is acknowledged widely, there is not a clear understanding of what works, for whom it works, and when it works. As a science, knowledge dissemination fits predominately under communication theory and has been used most widely in social marketing and shaping public opinion. Knowledge utilization, on the other hand, requires behavioral change. Change is heavily influenced by motivation, attitudes, and perception, all concepts from the field of social psychology (Green & Johnson, 1996; Patel, 1996).

The purpose of this chapter is to provide the advanced practice registered nurse (APRN) in psychiatric and mental health care with a knowledge base for understanding how health education in-

formation gets transformed from thought to action. Concepts that describe the processes that affect the use of information are drawn from the literature in social psychology and communications theory and discussed in relation to the change process. Although the major focus is on helping the APRN disseminate new information to patients, the process of change described also applies to working with colleagues to advance an evidence-based practice for psychiatric nursing.

INFORMATION AND RESEARCH DISSEMINATION: USING DISSEMINATION ■ STRATEGIES

Sharing health information with consumers and their families to prevent, treat, or cure a disease—historically a key function of the psychiatric nurse—has gained urgency and importance over the past decade because of several far-reaching societal changes. Some of the changes in the nurse's role as communicator stem from the vastly increased demand for information, whereas others reflect a rapidly changing body of knowledge. On the demand side, consumers have become more active participants in their health care. They want to know more about their disease, the treatment options they may have, the cost of treatment, the latest on research advances in understanding and preventing their disease, and with increasing frequency, the genetic risks they and other family members might have for acquiring the disease.

A second momentous societal change is the marked increase in accessibility to information. Coverage of all facets of health and illness, from science to economics to policy, are among the most popular fare of the mass media, and increasing numbers of health consumers are seeking information directly from the professional literature. A burgeoning number of sites on the Internet contain detailed health information and offer opportunities to obtain a wide range of opinions and options through chat rooms and often through direct interactions with experts in a given area. The health care industry is increasingly responsive to the demand for information and has expanded its role from that of "pamphleteer" to being a frequent website sponsor and major distributor of videos concerned with health maintenance and disease management.

A third societal shift that is related to the first reflects changes within the health care delivery system. These changes, which are motivated by efforts to decrease the cost of health care, have transferred some of the burden of health care to consumers and their families. Shortened hospital stays, for example, increasingly require families to care for a member who might still be in an acute phase of the illness and not yet stabilized on medications. System changes are felt as well by health care professionals who, in a limited time frame, are trying to teach consumers or their family members new roles in acute or immediate treatment as well as steps needed to prevent relapse.

On the supply side, advances in technology have accelerated greatly the pace at which scientists are discovering new facts about the neuroscience of the brain. The 1990s, labeled "The Decade of the Brain," provided revolutionary insights into the identification, circuitry, and function of a wide range of neurotransmitters and brain structures that are implicated in mental disorders. Scientific discoveries have led to pharmacologic advances, including the development of new and novel drugs that are more effective in reducing the symptoms associated with chronic and disabling mental disorders, such as schizophrenia and depression. Research also has provided information on both pharmacologic and behavioral interventions with some indication of what works best for whom.

New knowledge is being generated so rapidly that what was considered as best practice during a health professional's formal training is deemed obsolete after 1 or 2 years of practice. Nurses and other health care practitioners cannot plead ignorance of knowledge of new treatments because their contract with society states that they will provide efficient and effective care to help patients achieve maximum levels of health. The *Standards of Clinical Nursing Practice* (ANA, 1991) clearly outline the accountability of every nurse to use new knowledge in practice. The expectation is that the care given will be evidence based (i.e., based on research). However, the existence of research findings that promise to improve the care provided by clinicians and enhance the quality of life for those with mental disorders does not equate necessarily with the communication of that information in a form accessible and immediately applicable to use. As the Agency for Health Care Policy and Research has found with their Guidelines to the Treatment of Depression (Brown, Shye, & McFarland, 1995; Feldman et al., 1998), even when information is communicated in a clear and user-friendly manner, there is no guarantee that it will be used.

Strategies to influence how people think and act have been articulated by philosophers through the ages, but a well-known, *modern* effort to influence the behavior of people based on research findings was the Agriculture Extension Program developed by the U.S. Department of Agriculture (USDA) in the 1920s (Rogers, 1988). Prompted by a need to modernize agricultural practices the Extension Program was intended to encourage farmers to plant corn and other crops more efficiently, to use better seed, to improve irrigation, and otherwise refine the ways of farming they had practiced all their lives. To accomplish this goal, the USDA established field units around the country and assigned to them extension agents who were responsible for bringing new information to farmers and for sharing with the USDA problems from the field that needed to be studied by researchers. The success of the program is evident in its continued existence today, some 70 years later; but from the beginning, more immediate measures of outcome were straightforward. Extension agents were able to readily observe changes in farming practices being used by monitoring the purchase of recommended seed varieties and other tangible markers of change. When the Extension Program itself was evaluated, its success was attributed to the hands-on quality of the dissemination of relevant information. Agriculture extension agents had access to the newest information and could share it readily with others because of their proximity to their audience and the trust gained from living in the community—two factors strongly associated with increased probability that new information will be used.

Lessons gained on the American plains in the 1920s and 1930s proved to be transferable to American cities of the 1980s and 1990s when the acquired immunodeficiency syndrome (AIDS) epidemic underscored the importance of knowledge dissemination and the use of that information (knowledge utilization) in the public health arena. The need to make the public aware of routes of transmission of a potentially deadly disease and the behaviors required for self-protection emerged as a priority on a national agenda that involved government, health care providers, community and advocacy organizations, and individual citizens. The goal of this public health education to change behavior highlighted the complexity of the role of health education in changing behavior and the relative lack of empirical information about the process of change.

Over the past 2 decades, research has yielded frequent—and frequently counter-intuitive—findings about the effectiveness of different approaches to changing sexual practices in high-risk populations. For one, having knowledge about AIDS and how it is transmitted is *not* strongly correlated with engaging in preventive behaviors (Mann, Tarantola, & Netter, 1992). Although knowledge-based behavioral change supports the Western world view that change occurs when logic is provided, it falls short of providing a theory on which to base practice (Helweg-Larsen & Collins, 1997). In reality, these investigators found that change is based more on subjective experience than on objective facts. Contending that measuring the salience of the message to the recipient will have more predictive value of how effective the message is than simply doing a pre-posttest to measure information learned, Helweg-Larsen and Collins urged research colleagues to use persuasion and attitude change theories from social psychology in testing new approaches in AIDS prevention. Less important than whether a person can repeat new information is whether that person believes the information is important to his or her personal well-being.

To understand adequately health promotion and education programs and interventions in AIDS, depression, or any disorder requires an understanding of the components of change as well as a grounding in communications theory. Practitioners must attend to identifying the targets for change, the methods for accomplishing these changes, and the timing and method for evaluating the outcome. The importance of understanding communication and what factors influence behavior change is paramount to APRNs who play a major role in helping people change behavior or learn new behaviors. Perhaps more so than any other specialty area, the provision of psychiatric care has been affected by the changes in the understanding of the risk factors associated with mental illnesses, the growing knowledge base of the neuroscience of the brain, and the demands for documenting outcomes. This means that APRNs are both the recipients of research findings that must be incorporated into practice by either modifying or changing practice, and the transmitters of new information to consumers, family members, colleagues, and other health professionals.

As noted previously, two key components required to understand how the sharing of information gets transferred into changes in behavior are the dissemination process and the utilization process. *Dissemination* characterizes the process by which information is made accessible or available to a target audience. The success of the dissemination effort is measured by the degree to which knowledge becomes available to the target audience *without* regard for what is done with the information (Sechrest, Backer, & Rogers, 1994). *Utilization*, on the other hand, identifies whether the recipient of the information actively decides to use or not to use the information to change a behavior or set of behaviors. The success of knowledge utilization is measured by changes in behavior. Although knowledge dissemination can be discussed as a separate entity from the process of change, it cannot be fully understood without a firm grasp on the components involved in change.

■ THE CHANGE PROCESS

A wide range of self-help programs and professional services exists, all differentially geared for helping people decrease high-risk behaviors and engage in healthier life-styles. Although the various approaches differ in the emphasis placed on particular behaviors, they all engage in three progressive steps: 1) getting the individual or group to perceive the behavior as a problem, 2) motivating the person or group to change the behavior, and 3) helping the person or group to acquire and practice new behaviors. Although other models

exist, the transtheoretical model of change (Prochaska & DiClemente, 1984) is used in this chapter because it provides illuminating detail about variables affecting the movement between stages.

Transtheoretical Model of Change

Prochaska and DiClemente (1984) drew creatively from theories of psychotherapy and behavioral change to develop their aptly labeled *transtheoretical model* to explain the processes used by individuals to change behavior. Their empirical work entailed identifying processes involved in change and then studying the sequence in which they were used. Building on their observations, they have developed a five-stage model of change that involves ten change processes mediated by both self-efficacy and a subjective view of the pros and cons of change.

1. The first stage, the *precontemplative stage*, is marked by the person having no intent to change his or her behavior, either because he or she is unaware of the risk or consequences or is aware and chooses not to change.

2. Stage two, the *contemplation stage*, occurs when a person becomes aware that a problem exists and seriously thinks about modifying the behavior but has not yet made a commitment to do so. Contemplators struggle as they weigh the benefits of change against the amount of effort and loss it will take to overcome the perceived problem.

3. In the *preparation (ready for action) stage*, the individual can specify the plans of action he or she will take within the month; typically, this person already will have taken some significant action in the past year.

4. The person is in the *action stage* when specific overt actions have been taken within the past 6 months and these actions are what professionals would agree are sufficient to reduce the risk of disease (e.g., total abstinence from smoking).

5. In the *maintenance stage* the person works to prevent relapse and is increasingly more con-

fident that the change will continue. Depending on the behavioral change in question this period can last from 6 months to 5 years. Some behavioral changes require a lifetime of maintenance while others, such as the addictions, can be considered to reach a *termination* point (sixth stage) when the person has no temptation to engage in the former behavior and is 100% self-efficacious (Prochaska, Redding, & Evers, 1997).

The time dimension represented by the stages of change constitute a tool, one that provides the APRN with an understanding of when particular shifts in attitudes occur so that the most appropriate information or technique can be used. It is most useful, for example, to present only the pros of changing a behavior during the precontemplation stage and save the negative aspects until the contemplative phase (Prochaska, Redding, & Evers, 1997). How one moves from stage to stage involves processes of change. They are the covert and overt activities that provide the underpinnings and energy for movement from one stage to another. Each process encompasses multiple techniques and interventions to create change. Processes are influenced by a complex, interacting set of beliefs held by an individual that influence whether change in behavior will occur. Beliefs include the following:

- A belief that the behavior to be changed is associated with certain attributes or outcomes
- A belief that significant people approve or disapprove of the behavior and the degree to which one is motivated to please them
- A belief that one does or does not have the capabilities to perform the behavior under a number of different circumstances

The goals of interventions like psychoeducation and psychotherapy are to create a positive valence for the belief in the direction of the desired change by introducing information or providing experiences that fit with processes and stages of change. Prochaska and DiClemente (1984) viewed ten change processes identified from models of psychotherapy as integral to the stages of change. As the event or experience that helps the person move from one stage to another, they are the "hows" of change. Each change process is briefly defined in Table 22-1.

On the basis of 15 years of research on change behaviors in smoking, dieting, exercising, using condoms, relieving psychologic distress, and seeking mammograms, Prochaska, DiClemente, and Norcross (1992) have determined that the processes of change are integrated with the stages of change as seen in Table 22-2. The authors note that "the integration suggests that in early stages, people apply cognitive, affective, and evaluative processes to progress through the stages. In later stages, people rely more on commitments, conditioning, contingencies, environmental controls, and support for progressing toward termination."

Application of Stage and Process to Interventions

Precontemplative stage. People in the precontemplative stage were found to process less information, spend less time and energy in introspection, and not feel concerned about the negative aspects of their problems. They also were less open with significant others about their problems and did little to change their environment. Interventions in this stage are designed to increase awareness (consciousness raising) through providing information about the problem or providing observations, confrontations, and interpretations. The change process, dramatic relief, comes into play when the target of the message experiences emotions related to the problem. For example, a person might feel vulnerable or think he or she is at risk of developing cancer from smoking after seeing a video on autopsies of smokers' lungs. This dramatic response might produce enough of a reaction that the person thinks, "I really should do something about stopping," thus moving him or her from the precontemplative stage to the contemplative stage.

table 22-1

CHANGE PROCESSES

PROCESS	DEFINITION
Consciousness raising	Finding and learning new facts, ideas, and tips that support the healthy behavioral change
Dramatic relief	Experiencing the negative emotions (fear, anxiety, worry) that accompany the risk behavior
Environmental reevaluation	Examining (cognitively and emotionally) the effect of one's behavior on the larger environment, including an awareness of serving as a positive or negative role model to others
Self-reevaluation	Assessing (cognitively and emotionally) one's self-image with and without a particular unhealthy habit
Self-liberation	Believing that one can change and the commitment and recommitment to act on that belief
Counter-conditioning	Learning healthy behaviors that can substitute for problem behaviors
Contingency management	Reinforcing positive change
Stimulus control	Removing cues or avoiding unhealthy habits and adding prompts for healthy behavior
Helping relationships	Seeking and using social support for the healthy behavioral change
Social liberation	Seeing increased opportunity in a social setting to engage in a range of positive behaviors

table 22-2

STAGES OF CHANGE AND CORRESPONDING CHANGE PROCESSES

PRECONTEMPLATION	CONTEMPLATION	PREPARATION	ACTION	MAINTENANCE
Consciousness raising				
Dramatic relief				
Environmental reevaluation				
	Self-reevaluation			
		Self-liberation		
			Contingency management	
			Helping relationships	
			Counter-conditioning	
			Stimulus control	

From Prochaska, Redding, & Evers, 1997.

Contemplative stage. These individuals are most open to consciousness-raising techniques (e.g., observations, confrontations, reading or hearing information on the problem area). With this increased awareness comes a heightened sensitivity to the negative effect related to the negative behavior and a belief that the effect will improve (dramatic relief) with a change in the behavior. They are also more likely to reevaluate their values and problems in relation to their self-identity and to its impact on others (environmental reevaluation) (Prochaska & DiClemente, 1984).

Preparation (ready for action) stage. The cognitive, affective, and analytic components of recognizing a problem and planning corrective action continue through the contemplative and preparation stages. It is the small steps taken toward action that mark this stage. Some of the early actions taken may be counter-conditioning or stimulus control techniques. These techniques are commonly used in weight control and smoking cessation programs as a form of control through avoiding stimuli that are associated with the negative behavior (DiClemente, 1991).

Action stage. As the person begins to believe that he or she has the ability to not engage in the unhealthy behavior and is successful in modifying the conditional stimuli that frequently prompt relapse, there is a sense of self-liberation. It is during this stage that the heaviest reliance on support and understanding from helping relationships occurs.

Maintenance stage. For maintenance to be successful the person needs to assess the conditions under which relapse is likely and develop alternative responses for coping without reverting to "old habits." The strongest reinforcement for maintaining the new behavior and continuing to use counter-conditioning and stimulus control was the sense that one was more the kind of person one wished to be and that the change was also valued by at least one significant other (Prochaska, DiClemente, & Norcross, 1992).

From their research on thousands of self-changers in drug treatment, weight-loss, smoking cessation, and insight programs, Prochaska,

DiClemente, & Norcross (1992) conclude the following:

Efficient self-change depends on doing the right things (processes) at the right time (stages). We have observed two frequent mismatches. First, some self-changers appear to rely primarily on change processes most indicated for the contemplation stage—consciousness raising, self-evaluation—while they are moving into the action stage. They try to modify behaviors by becoming more aware, a common criticism of classical psychoanalysis: Insight alone does not necessarily bring about behavior change. Second, the other self-changers rely primarily on change processes most indicated for the action stage—reinforcement management, stimulus control, counter-conditioning—without requisite awareness, decision making, and readiness provided in the contemplation and preparation stages. They try to modify behaviors without awareness, a common criticism of radical behaviorism: Overt action without insight is likely to lead to temporary change.

The authors further note that therapies that focus on experiential, cognitive, or psychoanalytic methods are most effective during the precontemplative and contemplative stages, whereas more action-oriented therapies, such as existential and behavioral traditions, are more useful during the action and maintenance stages.

■ MOTIVATING CHANGE

The transtheoretical change model is very useful in providing the APRN with a framework for assessing the patient's readiness for change. Although knowing the stage and the processes that help move the person forward are extremely valuable tools, there is still the question of what messages or approaches have the greatest potential of either catching someone's attention to contemplate an issue or taking action necessary to change the situation. Some behaviors are easy to change, whereas others obviously require a great deal of effort. The more central a behavior is to a person's belief and self-image, the more difficult it is to change. Likewise, for addictive substances such as cocaine, alcohol, or cigarettes, the problem is not only the physical craving but also modification of all the environmental cues tied to the addictive behaviors. Regardless of whether the behavioral change will be easy or hard, the first step is always having an awareness of the problem. This is most often referred to as assessing the amount of risk involved in either engaging or not engaging in the behavior.

Perception of Risk

The perception that a given behavior or condition is a risk factor that will lead to a negative outcome (e.g., getting a disease, causing an accident, etc.) is based first on some awareness that there is a stated association or causality between the two events. Examples of this would be the now common knowledge about genetic susceptibility to depression, the link between cholesterol and heart disease, and the involvement of smoking in cancer (Hiatt, 1997). However, knowing that there is a causal link between particular behaviors and a negative outcome does not mean that people necessarily perceive themselves to be at risk. The purpose of health education messages, such as those used in public health campaigns, is not only to increase knowledge about the disease but also to break through denial (the precontemplative stage) by means of motivational messages that appeal to humor or personal values or that engender fear (McCallum, 1995). For example, an antismoking poster pictured a weathered, unkempt, toothless woman smoking a cigarette with a caption that read, "Smoking is glamorous." The message used humor to convey an indirect statement pertaining to values and challenged the notion that a person's appearance is enhanced by smoking.

Fear-appeal messages have an affective component that creates an emotional state that can lead to behavioral change, as noted earlier in discussing dramatic relief as a strategy in the process of change. However, it is not clear whether scare tactics are really effective for long-term change or if they are effective only in motivating the individual to avoid risk. In 1987, the National Heart, Lung, and Blood Institute convened a seminar for media experts to develop guidelines for using fear appeals in their public health campaigns. Basically these guidelines suggest that the user of fear appeals (e.g., exposure to toxic wastes may lead to cancer, eating fats leads to heart attacks, noncompliance with maintenance antidepressant medication leads to relapse) must be aware of the overall effect of the message and that the fear of the problem occurring must not overpower the message about the necessary action to take. The guidelines encourage using appropriate channels such as health care professionals for delivering messages that suggest a threat to someone's well-being but caution that overuse of fear messages will result in desensitization (McCallum, 1995).

Characteristics of the Message

Regardless of whether the message is sent as a public health service announcement or as an instruction to a patient in a therapy session, it must capture the attention of the recipient, be understood, and be readily translatable into a tangible action plan. The motivation to act may not come from the message but from a personal dissatisfaction. The message can reinforce the original belief or provide additional information that allows the person to act, but in some cases, the message itself serves as a stimulus for change. For professional health care providers, the intrinsic motivation to change may come from professional pride that they are providing the best care possible, and thus providers may be more likely to embrace a new procedure or form of delivering care. However, the self-interest factor, such as threats to autonomy or income that may be tied to the change, also need to be taken into account in the way that the change in practice is communicated. Ample evidence exists of the power of well-financed media campaigns to convey negative messages about the personal sacrifice that would result from a change in health care insurance, or more recently, if antismoking legislation were passed. However, negative attitudes about particular types of care or health practices are also conveyed to consumers and their families via health professionals, for example some providers strongly disparage the use of all complementary therapies.

There is no one best way of communicating information. The challenge of deciding what and how much to say, identifying who the audience is, and ascertaining what method should be used reflects the interrelatedness of the message, the sender, and the audience. Based on their classic work, Avorn and Soumerai (1983) suggest that the initial messages should be broad and fairly comprehensive to provide a framework upon which later messages can be understood. Subsequent messages should be simpler but clarify discrete components of the original, broader message. To be effective, Avorn and Soumerai note, dissemination efforts must be characterized by brevity, repetition, and reinforcement. An application of this might be a family session in which the APRN initially provides information about a disorder (e.g., data on its prevalence), what is known about its cause, and the nature and effectiveness of current treatment. A second session might identify those aspects of treatment that seem to most effectively prevent relapse and outline how family involvement fits into this. Subsequent meetings might address questions from the families regarding problems in implementing these activities. It is always wise to remember that most people are likely to respond to efforts directed at changing their behavior if they have some sense of ownership of these efforts.

Availability of new information (e.g., research findings) and the person's accessibility to it clearly are critical elements. Print media have been relied upon most heavily because of their ease in reaching large and dispersed audiences. Providers and administrators have the greatest access to professional journals that address their interests, whereas the general public gets nearly all of its general health-related information through mass media—newspapers, television, and radio. However members of a consumer support group, such as the National Alliance for the Mentally Ill (NAMI), are likely to be familiar with the newest research findings on treatment and hypothesized

etiologies of the diseases of interest. It is a more recent development that the consumer is often as knowledgeable, or more knowledgeable, about treatment options than is the provider (Bourque, 1996; Sechrest, Backer, & Rogers, 1994). On the positive side, this can be a motivating force to encourage providers to keep up-to-date.

It is clear that the Internet already plays a major role in disseminating information, but to what extent it influences behavior and is seen as a credible source of health information is not known. Other important channels for sharing information are professional organizations, networks, and visual media, such as videos, films, and educational television programs.

Characteristics of the Sender

"If a message is to be accepted without undue hesitation and reservations, the credibility of the message source must be beyond question. It must be easily recognized and have a reputation for having been dependably accurate in previous communications" (Sechrest, Backer, & Rogers, 1994). These factors increase the possibility of a user listening to the message, although usually no differentiation is made about the actual source of information. It is more common to say, "I read it in the newspaper or heard it on the radio." However, if a person read that Elvis Presley had been sighted walking on the mall outside the Smithsonian Building by a *Washington Post* reporter, the person might be more likely to believe it and share that information than if he or she read it as a headline in the *National Enquirer* in a grocery store check-out line. Therefore status of the source does matter.

This paradox exists also with the credibility ascribed to research findings. On one hand, research findings are accepted as being the "truth" because scientific methods work to prevent bias. On the other hand, the fact that many studies are conducted in settings from which "typical" patients are excluded because they do not meet protocol criteria and in which conditions differ significantly from those that occur in "front-line" clinical settings makes the research seem less generalizable to a person's own setting and patient population. The more closely the study seems to match the population and setting of the clinician, the more likely he or she is to use the findings (Cronenwett, 1995; Dunn, 1995).

Research findings are much more likely to be used if the researcher is involved in the dissemination effort. Talking directly to potential users is seen as superior to any written forms of communication because it is more flexible, allowing for a more individual response to the intellectual and emotional needs of the users. Dissemination efforts that result in clinicians using a new treatment approach almost always are found to have had an in-house champion. This person must, of course, be seen as credible and be considered an opinion-leader by professional colleagues. Pharmaceutical companies regularly seek opinion-leaders to give talks about new forms of treatment and to advance the use of particular drugs. Opinion-leaders often will be early-adopters of new techniques and will be vocal about the technique's superiority in the treatment of patients. Leaders gather other users and the word continues to spread, but large scale acceptance of changes usually takes years to achieve and continual reinforcement by the advocates (Lomas et al, 1991).

In addressing the question of how to make research findings more accessible for use in nursing practice, Funk, Tornquist, and Champagne (1995) note that it is unlikely that nurses in clinical settings will be able to either obtain the resources necessary to adequately review articles or have the time to do so. They suggest that nursing specialty organizations take on the evaluative function of reviewing articles, determining their merit for implementation into practice, and disseminating this information through regular updates to nurses in practice. The use of specialty organizations to translate research into practice through development of guidelines is also reflected in the 1996 change in the statutory mission of the federal Agency for Health Care Policy and Research (AHCPR). In the past, the AHCPR convened multidisciplinary health professional panels to develop practice guidelines and then published them under the AHCPR's imprimatur. As a result of the change in its mandate, the AHCPR now is responsible for gathering and evaluating all the literature pertaining to treatment of a particular disease, but the task of establishing standards and guidelines for care is the responsibility of professional organizations (AHCPR, 1998). One drawback to this approach is that the cost of developing such guidelines may be prohibitive to smaller specialty organizations in nursing, thus resulting in more well-financed organizations, such as medicine, establishing guidelines for the field.

It seems clear that the amount of information being generated far exceeds the ability of an individual APRN to keep abreast with changes. One solution to this problem has been the work of an international group known as the Cochrane Collaboration Group (1998). This innovative effort is comprised of scientists from all disciplines who have expertise and knowledge of clinical research and practice. They form core interest groups that systematically review all randomized controlled trials published in their interest area throughout the world. Studies that meet scientific standards are plotted on a diagram (Fig. 22-1) indicating whether the treatment was found to be effective. Using a circle with a vertical line through the center to represent the point between effect and no effect, horizontal lines are drawn showing the confidence intervals for the effectiveness of the treatment in each trial. Lines on the left side of the circle indicate treatment effectiveness, and lines on the right side indicate that the treatment did more harm than good. Lines drawn through the middle indicate no difference. The conclusion drawn from the overall analysis of all studies is represented by a diamond either on the right, left, or in the middle. This very effective graphic display allows the APRN to quickly determine if the evidence suggests that the treatment is helpful. The graphic display is accompanied by a written narrative about the review.

Since it was formed in 1993, the Cochrane Collaboration Group has produced over 7000 reports on treatment effectiveness with many more in the pipeline. Of particular interest to APRNs would be the reports published under the fields of schizophrenia, depression, and anxiety. The Collaboration Group also recently added nursing to their list of fields of interest. Regularly updated information related to the work of this group can be found at their website. Because of the rigor of the review, the Cochrane Library is widely used in Europe as a source of determining clinical practice. As more North Americans become involved in this project, it is likely that this model will also be used more widely in the United States. The design of the reviews and the format of disseminating the results have great potential and should certainly be explored as a method for synthesizing the research on effective treatments in mental health care for use by APRNs.

Characteristics of the User

"How-to" manuals for health education campaigns consistently list understanding the target audience

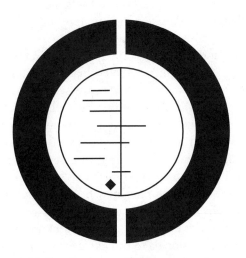

Figure 22-1   Cochrane Collaboration logo representing graphic display of results of research review of clinical research. Courtesy Cochrane Collaboration.

as the first priority (Backer, 1995; Backer & David, 1995; Backer, Rogers, & Sopory, 1992; Sechrest, Backer, & Rogers, 1994). Achieving the bottom-line objective of getting the person to act on new information—that is, to change his or her behavior—requires a good understanding of the barriers that interfere with performing the behavior. Fishbein (1995), in a thorough review of research on behavioral change, identifies eight factors as playing a pivotal role (Box 22-1). Of these, the

---

box 22-1

FACTORS AFFECTING BEHAVIORAL CHANGE

MANDATORY FACTORS

Intention. The person has formed an intent or made a commitment to perform a behavior.
Environmental constraints. There are no environmental constraints that make it impossible for the behavior to occur.
Ability. The person has the skills necessary to perform the behavior.

INFLUENCING FACTORS

Anticipated outcomes. The person believes that the advantages of performing the behavior outweigh the disadvantages (i.e., the person has a positive attitude about changing the behavior).
Norms. The person perceives more social pressure to perform the behavior than to not perform the behavior.
Self-standards. The person perceives that performance of the behavior is more consistent than inconsistent with his or her self-image or that its performance does not violate personal standards that activate negative self-sanctions.
Emotion. The person's emotional reaction to performing the behavior is more positive than negative.
Self-efficacy. The person perceives that he or she has the capabilities to perform the behavior under a number of different circumstances.

Adapted from Fishbein, 1995.

first three—1) having a strong positive intention to perform the behavior in question, 2) having the skills necessary to carry out the behavior, and 3) being in an environment free of constraints on the targeted behavior—are most important. Fishbein notes that these three behaviors are both necessary and sufficient for behavioral change to occur. The other five factors—4) anticipation of positive outcomes, 5) social pressure based on group norms, 6) agreement with one's personal values, 7) positive emotions, and 8) perceived capability to perform the task are seen as influencing the strength of the direction of intention. That is, the valence of each can either strengthen or weaken the person's decision about changing.

These points are addressed in Funk, Tornquist, and Champagne's (1995) study of the barriers and facilitators of using research. Approximately 1000 clinical nurses were asked what they perceived as problems in using research in their practice. Although significant numbers identified a lack of awareness of research findings and a lack of skill in evaluating research as a barrier, the overwhelming majority believed that the environmental constraints would not allow them to implement a "new approach." Thus a first step in working with groups resistant to changing practice or learning new skills is to gain a clearer idea of what they perceive to be environmental constraints. This usually can be done through the use of focus groups to get clarification of the issues.

In an interesting article on disseminating research findings to nurses in practice, Cronenwett (1995) points out that one method of decreasing resistance is by providing more exposure to research articles. She hypothesizes that familiarity with research topics gained through searching databases, reading journals, or attending conferences is correlated with increased readiness to try new approaches when the research eventually warrants such a change. That is, just being familiar with current problems being addressed through research alerts the APRN to alternative solutions to handling clinical problems. She suggests several methods for keeping up with the new findings published in the plethora of journals. Some examples are membership in and attendance at conferences held by professional associations and group efforts, such as journal clubs and work-based research interest groups.

Nutbeam (1996), in examining the structural barriers that keep research findings from being implemented, notes that peer-reviewed journals that require published articles to include a "so what?" section are a boon to the APRN because they force researchers to think more carefully about the use of their findings. Nutbeam also advocates the use of brief reports and case studies in journals for two purposes: 1) to speed up reporting of preliminary results, and 2) as a method to encourage practitioners to submit short reports on how well the research-based approach worked in their setting.

Another method frequently used to increase public and professional awareness of new information and to help consumers ascertain if they are at risk for (or may have) a particular disease is the use of national screening programs, such as the National Depression Screening Day (NDSD). The NDSD is an annual event designed to increase recognition of depression in the general population and to facilitate access to appropriate health care for those with symptoms of depression. Magruder and colleagues (1995) used the Zung Self-Rating Depression Scale to evaluate the success of this program in identifying depressed individuals. They found that of the 4109 screened, 76.6% had at least minimal depressive symptoms. Over half (53.3%) had moderate symptoms of depression, and 22.6% had scores indicating severe depression. The authors hypothesize that one of the reasons for such high rates may be that people who attend NDSD events already have some awareness that they are depressed and are seeking mental health professionals to discuss their symptoms in an anonymous and free setting. Unfortunately, what is *not* known from this study is whether those counselled to seek treatment actually followed through with the referrals made at the time of the screening test.

In one of the few studies that has looked at the effects of health teaching on behavioral change concerned with risk behaviors for AIDS in severely mentally ill (SMI) adults living in the inner city, Kelly and colleagues (1997) conclude that the combination of teaching risk-reduction skills and then encouraging participants to advocate behavior change to their friends strengthens SMI adults' capacity to change their behavior. The total study group comprised 104 severely mentally ill men and women with a primary diagnosis of schizophrenia (19%), mood disorder (58%), anxiety disorder (11%), and either personality disorder or substance abuse (11%). These persons were randomly assigned to one of three conditions. 1) a single AIDS education session, 2) a seven-session cognitive-behavioral HIV risk-reduction group intervention, or 3) a seven-session group intervention that combined the risk-reduction intervention with training to act as a risk-reduction advocate to friends. Although all subjects exhibited change at follow-up on risk reduction, self-efficacy, and positive intent regarding condom use, the greatest change occurred in group three. Group three reported greater reductions in rates of unprotected sex and had fewer sexual partners at follow-up. The authors attribute the success of this approach to the principle of cognitive dissonance that states that "persons who publicly endorse a cause tend to shift their personal beliefs in the direction of their public statement to reduce cognitive dissonance or to bring their private beliefs into congruence with their public statements" (Kelly et al., 1997). They also suggest that acquiring the skill of being able to make convincing statements about endorsing change to others may have affected their own intent and belief about their ability to do the behavior they were endorsing to others.

Other characteristics of the interaction between the user and the change message that seem to have positive bearing on successful implementation are as follows:

- Ideas used in the form originally presented tend to be relatively easy to implement (Larsen, 1985).
- The ease with which the adopter can see how it is done with practice and understands the need for change, the greater the chance of implementation (Bell et al., 1994).
- The relevance of the new information to addressing a specific problem increases the likelihood that it will be used (Funk et al., 1995).
- If the degree of change required is small or can be done incrementally, it is more likely to be implemented (Fishbein, 1995).
- It is easier to adopt behaviors that require little response cost (less of the self) or only require individual change rather than a larger group of individuals or system change (Backer, Rogers, & Sopory, 1992).
- There is a clear relative advantage over the old way (Backer, Liberman, & Kuehnel, 1986).
- The person has the ability to do the new behavior. Individuals will avoid activities they think exceed their capabilities (Fishbein, 1995; Medder et al., 1997).

Fig. 22-2 displays the relationship between the stages of change (the behavioral processes that influence the direction of change) and summarizes some of the interventions APRNs can use in working with people to expedite the integration of new behaviors. In the diagram, the change process is represented by a circle with arrows in both directions to indicate a cycle that has movement in both directions. It serves as a reminder of the cyclic nature of change, where the steps may be repeated numerous times before the behavior can be permanently maintained. The process of forming an intent to engage in a behavior, plus overcoming any environmental constraints and developing the skills necessary to do the new behaviors, is the process that underlies the transfer of new findings from research into practice.

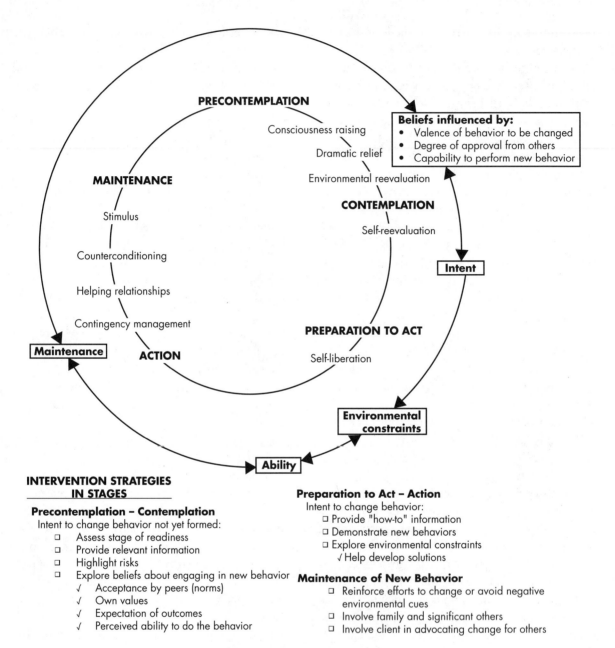

Figure 22-2 Stages of change and factors that influence its direction.

IMPLICATIONS FOR
■ THE FUTURE

The overall goal of clinical research is to improve health care. To accomplish this, research findings must be disseminated through journal articles, presentations at conferences, media coverage, and word-of-mouth. In the case of new treatments, this information has traditionally been disseminated to health care professionals who integrate the new findings into their practice and make the new treatments available to consumers. However, increased accessibilty to information through technology; active, vocal advocacy groups; and a societal expectation of having evidence of positive results have increased the demand for research-based, state-of-the-art health care. It also has increased the need to understand how to disseminate health information most effectively in order to produce changes in the care APRNs provide and in consumers' health practices.

APRNs must take a more active stance in using and disseminating research in their clinical practice and teaching roles. In particular, it will be important to critically evaluate research results that are derived from standard models or theories that may have become outdated, refuted, or simply not relevant for a patient population or specific case. This will require a proactive search for data and timely information from various sources. Given the lengthy time frame from research proposal and scientific study to publication of the results in refereed journals, APRNs cannot rely solely on these scientific publications for knowledge about evidence-based interventions and state-of-the-art practice. At the same time, APRNs must scrutinize new scientific developments that are touted on the Internet and other public media. Adopting practices wholesale that lack rigorous corroboration or are reported from the early stages of experimentation will not advance best practice and may in fact cause harm.

Appropriate dissemination and utilization of research will continue to be a delicate balance between practicing innovatively to improve the quality of mental health care and resisting the temptation to jump too soon on the bandwagon of the latest scientific study. In deciding about research and what will work in advanced practice, ultimately there is no substitute for the APRN's thorough knowledge of the specific needs of her or his patients and their beliefs, preferences, and unique capabilities to learn new behaviors for a healthier lifestyle.

RESOURCES AND CONNECTIONS

JOURNALS

Knowledge: Creation, Diffusion, Utilization (now called *Science Communication Patient Education and Counseling*)

INTERNET CONNECTIONS

Agency for Health Care Policy and Research (AHCPR) www.ahcpr.gov/clinic/evidence.htm

Center for Mental Health Services (CMHS) www.mentalhealth.org
Established the Knowledge Exchange Network as a one-stop national clearinghouse for free information about mental health, including publications, references, and referrals to local and national resources and organizations.

Healthfinder www.healthfinder.gov or www.web.health.gov/healthypeople
A gateway consumer health and human services information website from the U. S. government. Healthfinder can lead you to selected online publications, clearinghouses, databases, websites, and support and self-help groups, as well as the government agencies and not-for-profit organizations that produce reliable information for consumers and health professionals.

National Women's Health Information Center (NWHIC) www.4women.gov
A one-stop gateway for women's health resources and materials for consumers and professionals.

Cochrane Collaboration Group www.cochrane.co.uk
The Cochrane Library is an electronic publication designed to supply high-quality evidence to inform people providing and receiving care and those responsible for research, teaching, funding, and administration at all levels.

National Institute of Mental Health www.nimh.nih.gov
Information on specific mental disorders, diagnosis, and treatment; "Mental Illness in America" Consensus Conference proceedings; NIMH long range plans and research reports; publications order forms; quicktime videos; anxiety disorders and depression information; and other resources.

MENTAL HEALTH FAX4U

Can be accessed by calling 301-443-5158 at the NIMH headquarters in Rockville, Maryland. Users must call from either a fax machine that is equipped with a telephone handset or a computer with both a modem and telephone handset. Documents currently available through MENTAL HEALTH FAX4U include NIMH grant announcements for the scientific community, description of NIMH studies needing patients, and the text of NIMH publications for the general public about mental disorders and the brain.

References

Agency for Health Care Policy and Research (AHCPR). (1998). www.ahcpr.gov/clinic/evidence.htm.

American Nurses Association. (1991). *Standards of clinical nursing practice.* Washington, DC: American Nurses Publishing.

Avorn, J., & Soumerai, S.B. (1983). Improving drug-therapy decisions through education outreach: a randomized controlled trial of academically based "detailing." *New England Journal of Medicine, 308,* 1457–1463.

Backer, T.E. (1995). Assessing and enhancing readiness for change: implications for technology transfer. In Backer, T.E., David, S.L., & Soucy, G. (Eds.). *NIDA research monograph: reviewing the behavioral science knowledge base on technology transfer.* Rockville, MD: DHHS, NIH, NIDA, NIDA Research Monograph.

Backer, T.E., & David, S.L. (1995). Synthesis of behavioral science learnings about technology transfer. In Backer, T.E., David, S.L., & Soucy, G. (Eds.). *NIDA research monograph: reviewing the behavioral science knowledge base on technology transfer.* Rockville, MD: DHHS, NIH, NIDA, NIDA Research Monograph.

Backer, T.E., Liberman, R.P., & Kuehnel, T.G. (1986). Dissemination and adoption of innovative psychosocial interventions. *Journal of Consulting and Clinical Psychology, 54*(1), 111–118.

Backer, T.E., Rogers, E.M., & Sopory, P. (1992). *Designing health communication campaigns: what works?* Newbury Park: Sage Publication.

Bell, S., et al. (1994). Implementing a research-based protocol: an interactive approach. *AACN: Clinical Issues, 5*(2), 147–151.

Bourque, N.M. (1996). Searching for the knowledge to heal: improving the links between medical research and the consumer. *Canadian Journal of Public Health, 87*(2), S68–S70.

Brown, J.B., Shye, D., & McFarland, B. (1995). The paradox of guideline implementation: how AHCPR's depression guideline was adapted at Kaiser Permanente Northwest Region. *Journal of Qualitative Improvement, 21*(1), 5–21.

Cochrane Collaboration Group. (1998). www.cochrane.co.uk.

Cronenwett, L.R. (1995). Effective methods for disseminating research findings to nurses in practice. *Nursing Clinics of North America, 30*(3), 429–438.

DiClemente, C.C. (1991). Motivational interviewing and the stages of change. In Miller, W.R., & Rollnick, S. (Eds.). *Motivational interviewing: preparing people for change.* New York: Guilford Press.

Dunn, S.M. (1995). Barriers and challenges in training health care providers for patient education. *Patient Education and Counseling, 26,* 131–138.

Feldman, E.L., et al. (1998). Clinical practice guidelines on depression: awareness, attitudes, and content knowledge among family physicians in New York. *Archives of Family Medicine, 7*(1), 58–62.

Fishbein, M. (1995). Developing effective behavior change interventions: some lessons learned from behavioral research. In Backer, T.E., David, S.L., & Soucy, G. (Eds.). *NIDA research monograph: reviewing the behavioral science knowledge base on technology transfer.* Rockville, MD: DHHS, NIH, NIDA, NIDA Research Monograph.

Funk, S.G., Tornquist, E.M., & Champagne, M.T. (1995). Barriers and facilitators of research utilization: an integrative review. *Nursing Clinics of North America, 30*(3), 395–407.

Green, L.W., & Johnson, J.I. (1996). Dissemination and utilization of health promotion and disease prevention knowledge: theory, research and experience. *Canadian Journal of Public Health, 87*(2), S11–S17.

Helweg-Larsen, M., & Collins, B.E. (1997). A social psychological perspective on the role of knowledge about AIDS in AIDS prevention. *Current Directions in Psychological Science, 6*(2), 23–26.

Hiatt, R.A. (1997). Behavioral research contributions and needs in cancer prevention and control: adherence to cancer screening advice. *Preventive Medicine, 26,* S11–S18.

Kelly, J.A., et al. (1997). Reduction in risk behavior among adults with severe mental illness who learned to advocate for HIV prevention. *Psychiatric Services, 48*(10), 1283–1288.

Larsen, J.K. (1985). Effect of time on information utilization. *Knowledge: Creation, Diffusion, Utilization, 7*(2), 143–159.

Lomas, J., et al. (1991). Opinion leaders vs. audit and feedback to implement practice guidelines: delivery after previous cesarean section. *Journal of the American Medical Association, 265,* 2202–2207.

Magruder, K.M., et al. (1995). Who comes to a voluntary

depression screening program? *The American Journal of Psychiatry, 152*(11), 1615–1622.

Mann, J.M., Tarantola, D.J.M., & Netter, T.W. (Eds.). (1992). *AIDS in the world.* Cambridge, MA: Harvard University Press.

Medder, J., et al. (1997). Dissemination and implementation of putting prevention into family practice. *American Journal of Preventive Medicine, 13*(5), 345–351.

McCallum, D.B. (1995). Risk communication: a tool for behavioral change. In Backer, T.E., David, S.L., & Soucy, G. (Eds.). *NIDA research monograph: reviewing the behavioral science knowledge base on technology transfer.* Rockville, MD: DHHS, NIH, NIDA, NIDA Research Monograph.

Nutbeam, D. (1996). Improving the fit between research and practice in health promotion: overcoming structural barriers. *Canadian Journal of Public Health, 87*(6), S18–S23.

Patel, V. (1996). Cognition and technology in health education research. *Canadian Journal of Public Health, 87*(2), S63–S67.

Prochaska, J.O., & DiClemente, C.C. (1984). *The transtheoretical approach: crossing traditional boundaries of change.* Homewood, IL: Dorsey Press.

Prochaska, J.O., DiClemente, C.C. & Norcross, J.C. (1992). In search of how people change: applications to addictive behaviors. *American Psychologist, 47*(9), 1102–1114.

Prochaska, J.O., Redding, C.A., & Evers, K.E. (1997). The transtheoretical model and stages of change. In Glanz, K., Lewis, F.M., & Rimer, B. (Eds.). *Health behavior and health education: theory, research and practice.* San Francisco: Jossey-Bass Publishers.

Rogers, E.M. (1988). The intellectual foundation and history of the agricultural extension agent model. *Knowledge: Creation, Diffusion, Utilization 9*(4), 492–510.

Sechrest, L., Backer, T.E., & Rogers, E.M. (1994). Synthesis of ideas for effective dissemination. In Sechrest, L., et al. (Eds.). *Effective dissemination of clinical and health information, AHCPR.* Pub. No. 95-0015, Rockville, MD: Agency for Health Care Policy and Research

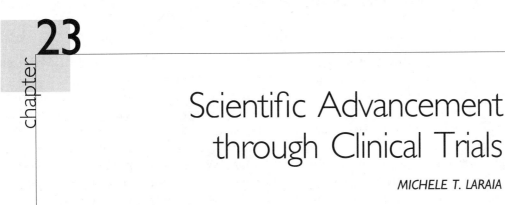

■ INTRODUCTION

The *clinical trial* is considered to be the strongest research approach for a scientific investigation, designed to determine the efficacy and safety of a prospective intervention or treatment. These interventions can encompass biomedical, psychologic, or social frameworks. The intervention can include a drug therapy, a nondrug therapy, a therapeutic program, a type of treatment setting, or combinations of these. In the health field, the randomized controlled trial (RCT) is the gold standard underlying the testing of treatments that have widespread acceptance in medical and nursing practice. It is the research method used to determine whether a proposed treatment has the following characteristics:

1. Effective against a particular illness
2. Effective in a particular population
3. More effective than no treatment
4. More beneficial than available standard treatments
5. A risk/benefit ratio assessible for each individual consumer of the treatment.

In mental health care, the psychopharmacologic clinical trial is the underlying method of scientific inquiry for every new drug for the treatment of psychiatrically ill patients.

The "Decade of the Brain" turned a significant corner in the understanding of the biologic bases for mental health and illness and in the clinical applicability of psychobiologically-based interventions, the most prolific of which have been psychotropic drugs. Although there are important nondrug treatments available for psychiatrically ill patients, psychopharmacologic treatments have come to dominate the compendium of interventions available to mental health practitioners and consumers of mental health services.

In today's mental health care arena, particularly in managed care settings where short-term treatments are facilitated, the advanced practice registered nurse (APRN) will spend a significant amount of time in the treatment, training, evaluation, and policy development regarding the myriad issues involved in the prescription, administration, evaluation, integration, outcome assessment, and economics associated with the use of psychopharmacologic agents in the treatment of persons with mental illness. The succinct evaluation and appropriate application of cutting-edge information in the scientific literature is an essential skill for competent, ethical, and reimbursable health care. Thus these skills are critical for the continued advancement, credibility, and leadership of the APRN in the current sophisticated and competitive health care environment.

Clinical trial methodology underscores the vast majority of interventions that reach widespread acceptability in the health field, and the issues in this chapter can apply to clinical trials of any type of treatment. However, it is the current standard for mental health practitioners to include psychopharmacologic interventions when considering the possible treatments available for a patient suffering from mental illness, and psychopharmacologic interventions consume the vast majority of clinical trial report space in the scientific literature. Thus the APRN is in a multifaceted role

requiring complex and sophisticated judgments and must do the following:

- Determine if, and then which, psychopharmacologic agents are appropriate for an individual patient.
- Identify target symptoms and design the application and evaluation specific for each drug.
- Teach patients, families, and colleagues the goals, risks, benefits, and alternatives for each drug, as well as the underlying neurobiology.
- Integrate and balance psychopharmacology into the multifaceted treatment and educational plan for each patient.
- Monitor the scientific literature in order to evaluate the post-marketing phase of each drug, as well as the potential of experimental agents as they progress through the clinical trials phases and come to market.
- Interact with ongoing psychopharmacologic clinical trials as a source of patient referral to clinical trials programs or as a member of an RCT team.

The primary goal of this chapter is to assist the APRN in the successful fulfillment of these functions by providing a frame of reference for the process involved in understanding the development of drugs—from custom design in the laboratory, to clinical testing programs with human subjects, to evaluation and approval by the Food and Drug Administration (FDA). It will also allow the APRN to better judge RCT reports of all types, but particularly psychopharmacologic interventions, in order to remain current in the field and to determine applicability of findings for use in clinical practice.

THE CLINICAL TRIAL: A ■ BRIDGE TO TREATMENT

A clinical trial is a prospective experiment designed to determine the efficacy of the interventions by using the scientific method (Box 23-1) to compare one or more interventions with a central group. These principles apply to any situation in which the issue of who is exposed to which condi-

box 23-1

THE SCIENTIFIC METHOD

- *Construct a hypothesis* based on what is known or believed about the phenomenon to be investigated.
- *Design an experiment* to test (disprove) the hypothesis.
- *Perform the experiment.*
- *Observe and record the results obtained.*
- *Do the data support the hypothesis?* If so, the hypothesis is strengthened. If not, revise the hypothesis and begin again.

tion is under the control of the experimenter and the method of assignment is through randomization (Wassertheil-Smoller, 1995). This methodology and the regulations governing drug RCTs arose from the need to provide the public with drugs distributed for general consumption that would have known efficacy and safety profiles and to provide the pharmaceutical companies with a forum for producing the most reliable products possible.

The nature of clinical drug testing has evolved from the often dangerous auto-experimentation and direct human screening methods to the theoretically sophisticated and highly specialized RCT. This rigorous method has all but replaced the occasionally exciting but always inefficient serendipitous treatment discovery. Using well established scientific rules, early RCTs targeted therapeutic efficacy and product safety as primary goals. By the 1960s, the RCT had become the norm in pharmaceutical research. More recently, the evolution of the clinical trial has been affected by several additional methods that have emerged as essential considerations in bringing new pharmacologic agents to market. These include the following:

1. *Computer modeling* has become a highly-functional drug-design tool. If the structure and function of an endogenous enzyme, transmitter, or receptor are known, then a theoretical compound can be efficiently custom-designed to effect the desired biologic response with state-of-the-art computer programming techniques. The future of drug development also promises further advances from biotechnology, such as peptide mimics, which survive the stomach's acidity, allowing more products to be taken by mouth and making drugs available to more people in more diverse settings. The futuristic science of nanotechnology allows scientists to grasp, maneuver, and alter single designer molecules, eliminating the presence of impurities from drug compounds and allowing them to go directly to the desired biologic target site. Long before new drug testing expends the resources required for preclinical phases of development, these technologies will bring the experimental compound to the cutting edge of the molecular foundations of neuroscience. Bleidt and Montagne (1996) foresee the future role of pharmaceutical research and development as one that will evolve from creating new products that duplicate and compete with older ones to developing products that are unique and thus have no competition.

2. *Pharmacoeconomics* and *health outcomes research* have come to be recognized as scientific disciplines. The inclusion of these methods in the analyses of clinical trials data as well as postmarketing surveillance studies are now common critical components contributing to the understanding of the overall effect of drug therapies on society. The clinical trial must be able to document a cost-effectiveness/cost-benefit analysis (formal methods of determining whether a medical intervention is worth doing based on costs compared with benefits) as well as rapid, measurable, replicable treatment outcomes. It must be demonstrated that a new product can optimize significant aspects of patient care in naturalistic clinical settings. Only then will it be considered an essential drug treatment and thus included in an institu-

tion's formulary and reimbursed in today's managed health care environment.

3. *Bioethics* and *quality of life measures* are now required considerations in the plans to test new products and bring them to the point of generalized human consumption. Concerns for ethical treatment, effects of treatment on lifestyle, and patient satisfaction have reached respectable proportions in today's competitive, consumer-oriented marketplace and are championed by patient advocacy groups as well as professionals in health care and related fields.

4. *Data collection technologies* are evolving. Measurement and rating scale formats are expanding from the traditional "paper and pencil" tests and the newer computer-administered scales, to the increasing use of interactive voice response (IVR) technology. This latest data-collection technique, which uses recorded instructions over the telephone to facilitate longitudinal monitoring of patients without requiring office visits or study personnel, has well-documented reliability and validity (Kobak et al, 1996).

5. The *multicenter clinical trial* (MCT), a relatively recent development, is an experiment involving more than one clinical facility (sometimes up to several dozen across the country), each of which must train a research team, recruit patients, and conduct the study under one commonly agreed-upon research protocol. The patients are actually participants in one large study; data from each site are combined into one large database for statistical analysis, and the results can be generalized to a more diverse population. The MCT is more difficult and costly to manage and must incorporate automated data entry and management programs as well as rapid communications technologies for its success. The MCT is quickly becoming the mainstay of the pharmaceutical industry's drug development and approval efforts for its advantage of greatly increasing the number of patients enrolled in a study in a relatively short period of time, thus accelerating the testing process for a particular drug.

6. Perhaps not surprisingly, the *area* or *project team* concept has been established within the pharmaceutical industry to meet the growing demands of the drug development process. The project team consists of representatives from a variety of disciplines, including chemistry, biology, pharmacology, law, toxicology, medicine, epidemiology, statistics, and marketing. These multidisciplinary industry teams are now considered necessary to drive the development process from beginning to end, to maintain continuity throughout the clinical trials process, to recommend termination of a drug in development if there is sufficient negative evidence, and thus to ensure efficient, successful outcomes of pharmaceutical drug development.

7. A *progression of RCTs* is required to fully evaluate a potential new drug. In the past, costly retrials were often necessary to answer important unanticipated questions that emerged during the final analysis of a completed series of trials for a drug. Today's economic imperative has stimulated the use of efficient, cost-effective statistical solutions to this dilemma (Cohen & Posner, 1995; Kupfer et al., 1994; Prien & Robinson, 1994). Examples are the *response-adaptive* and *interim-analysis* designs (modify, abbreviate, or even terminate a particular trial as data are collected based on incremental gains in knowledge as the trial progresses); the *chain of evidence* method (progressively larger and more complex trials are built upon information gained from simpler, preliminary trials); *meta-analysis* (unrelated trials with similar goals and methods can be analyzed as one large study, providing additional conclusions about the accumulated but separate evidence about a treatment); and the *Bayesian approach* (as the sequencing of experiments progresses for a drug, efficacy from each trial is quantified, becoming the next "current state of knowledge," and thus the forerunner of the next trial design). Sophisticated statistical applications are increasingly used and included in RCT reports.

THE DRUG DEVELOPMENT
■ AND APPROVAL PROCESS

The U.S. drug approval system is one of the most rigorous in the world. On average, it takes $500 million and 15 years for an experimental drug to progress from initial laboratory testing to clinical approval for human use. For every 5000 compounds that enter preclinical testing, only one ever reaches market. In 1996, there were over 80 drugs in clinical trials for psychiatric illnesses (Siegfried, 1996). The length of time and financial expenditure required for such a process have intermittently been targeted by persistent elements of social control. Some examples are the plea to accelerate the testing process for drugs that treat HIV and other life-threatening illnesses and rare diseases in the 1980s, and the outcry to tighten drug testing regulations that occurred during the fen-phen recall in the 1990s. The process of clinical drug research is evolving, and changes are

constantly being proposed from many sectors. Finding the sophisticated balance between providing needed treatments with expediency and ensuring their risk/benefit ratios with confidence is an accomplishment that requires a blend of interactions from the special interest perspectives of many different groups, including health professionals and the lay public, as well the scientific, pharmaceutical, and governmental communities. Thus understanding the drug development and approval process (Fig. 23-1) is the responsibility of everyone who administers and consumes pharmaceutical products.

After completing preclinical testing, the pharmaceutical company, called the *study sponsor*, files an Investigational New Drug (IND) application with the FDA, whose primary mission is consumer protection, to begin to test the drug in humans. Additionally, the IND and the proposed research protocol must be approved by the Institutional Review Board (IRB) where the clinical trial will

	Early research/ preclinical testing	IND TO FDA	PHASE I	PHASE II	PHASE III	NDA TO FDA	FDA		PHASE IV
Years	6.5		1.5	2	3.5		1.5	15 Total	
Test population	Laboratory and animal studies		20 to 80 healthy volunteers	100 to 300 patient volunteers	1000 to 3000 patient volunteers		Review process and approval		Additional postmarketing testing required by FDA
Purpose	Assess safety and biologic activity		Determine safety and dosage	Evaluate effectiveness and look for side effects	Confirm effectiveness, monitor adverse reactions from long-term use				
Success rate	5000 compounds evaluated		5 enter trials				1 approved		

Figure 23-1   Drug development and approval process. (From Siegfried J: *PhRMA*, 1996.)

be conducted. The sponsor submits progress reports to the FDA at intervals throughout the conduction of the study. After completion of phases I through III of the development and approval process, a New Drug Application (NDA), which contains all the scientific information that was gathered, is filed with the FDA if the data successfully demonstrate efficacy and safety. These applications can run 100,000 or more pages, and although by law the FDA has 6 months to review the NDA, the average review time for compounds approved in 1996 was approximately 18 months (Siegfried, 1996). The drug is then marketed, the sponsor continues to submit periodic reports to the FDA, and some drugs require additional studies to evaluate long-term effects. The roles of clinical trial participants are outlined in Table 23-1.

Regulations Governing Clinical Trial Research

There is a large volume of federal regulations for clinical research and drug development that is updated annually. Other jurisdictions may also affect the conduct of a trial, such as state laws, local public health codes, and institutional policies. The *Code of Federal Regulations* and the *Federal Register* are available in most medical and legal libraries. Topics such as protection of human subjects, informed consent procedures (Box 23-2), good clinical practice (standards for the conduct of clinical trials with investigational new drugs), and guidelines for monitoring clinical investigations are just several that may be of interest to the APRN. Rosenbaum (1995)

---

box 23-2

ELEMENTS OF INFORMED CONSENT FOR HUMAN RESEARCH

The following information shall be provided to each subject considered for a research study:

- An explanation of the part of the study that is research, and the purposes, duration, and procedures to be followed
- A description of any foreseeable risks or discomforts, benefits that may be expected, and alternative procedures or courses of treatment
- A statement describing the extent to which confidentiality of records will be maintained, including a disclosure of who may inspect the records, such as the FDA
- Discussion of whether compensation or treatment is available if there should be an injury to the subject, as well as where further information can be obtained
- A list of contact persons for answers to pertinent questions about the research or research subjects' rights and whom to contact in the event of research-related injury to the subject

- A statement that participation is voluntary, that refusal to participate or withdrawal from the study will not jeopardize any benefits or care to which the subject is otherwise entitled
- When appropriate, the informed consent should also contain the following:
  - A statement that there may be unforeseeable risks associated with the research.
  - Circumstances under which the investigator may terminate the subject's participation without regard to the subject's consent
  - Costs to the subject as a result of participation
  - Any consequences from a subject's decision to withdraw and procedures for orderly termination by the subject
  - A statement that the subject will be notified of significant new findings that may occur during the study that may relate to the subject's willingness to continue
  - The approximate number of subjects involved in the study

Modified from *Federal regulations pertaining to informed patient consent*, Subpart B, 46 FR 8951, Jan 27, 1981, 50.25: Elements of Informed Consent.

table   23-1

ROLE OF CLINICAL TRIAL PARTICIPANTS

PARTICIPANTS	ROLE
FDA	The Food and Drug Administration is the agency of the federal government with oversight responsibility for premarketing clearance of all new drug products, regulation of all drug labeling and prescription drug advertising, regulation of manufacturing, regulation of bioequivalence standards, postmarketing surveillance, and determination of orphan drug designation (treats illnesses affecting fewer than 200,000 people), entitling the manufacturer to tax cuts and exclusive marketing rights.
CDER	The FDA's Center for Drug Evaluation and Research reviews and approves all new drug products, including prescription and nonprescription drugs.
IRB	The Institutional Review Board is composed of a diverse group (health care providers appointed by the institution and local community volunteers) who must determine that the study is scientifically valid, the benefits outweigh the risks, enrollment criteria are ethical, the subjects are adequately informed, the study is monitored for continued safety, and subject confidentiality is maintained.
Sponsor	The sponsor is the corporation or institution initiating the IND application for a new drug. The sponsor is responsible for the integrity of the trial and for the results, is financially and legally liable for the trial, and receives financial incentives and rewards if the new product is successful.
Monitor	Employed or contracted by the sponsor, the monitor visits multicenter study sites regularly and reviews protocol compliance, adherence to regulations, patient enrollment, safety, progress through the study, and quality of data (sources, collection procedures, case report forms and record keeping, database, etc.).
Investigative team	The principal investigator, co-investigators, and research team (one of whom serves as the study coordinator) is usually a reputable group of the institution's interdisciplinary experts, including researchers and clinicians with experience in the illness under study and the classification of the proposed new drug therapy, statisticians, data collectors and data base managers, grant and financial managers, and ancillary personnel. The team is responsible for recruiting and enrolling subjects, conducting the trial, maintaining the integrity of the protocol, ensuring the care and safety of the subjects, ensuring the quality of the data, and complying with federal and local regulations and institutional policies.
Subjects	Subjects are human volunteers who are either healthy (phase I) or patients with specific conditions (phases II to IV). They must be capable of giving informed consent (understanding the purpose of the study, the risk/benefit ratio, the study requirements of them, any financial costs or benefits to them for participating, and, for patients, currently available alternatives to the experimental treatment, and any risks associated with delaying current treatment).

provides a succinct reference guide to FDA regulations.

Several trends for the future of drug development have begun in the 1990s and promise to continue into the next century. These include the following:

1. Conceptualization and implementation of postmarketing surveillance systems (the clinical experience component of drug testing) to detect problems with short- and long-term use of newly marketed drugs in clinical and community settings.

2. Harmonizing the drug research, development, and approval processes around the world in an effort to decrease costs and increase marketability of new drug products. Several difficult issues to be addressed include conflicting regulatory demands; differences in informed consent ethics and diagnostic and treatment criteria; cultural influences of lifestyle, diet, and belief systems; and general differences in health from country to country.

METHODOLOGIC ISSUES IN ■ CLINICAL TRIAL RESEARCH

The psychiatric literature presents numerous reports of clinical trials, many of which can only be considered preliminary after careful evaluation. Before a clinical trial can be considered successful, with credible and applicable results that are ready for clinical integration, the knowledgeable clinician must assess several important elements when reading clinical trial reports and comparing them with each other and with standard treatments. Several of the most essential issues to consider when critically reading this literature are discussed in this section.

Importance of the Trial

For the trial to be approved, the *research question* must be important, and the results must have a high likelihood of a positive effect on clinical care. Is the clinical disorder to be treated of sufficient

prevalence (anxiety), or if the prevalence is low, is it of sufficient societal effect (Alzheimer's disease) to warrant such extensive use of research resources? Are existing interventions in some way insufficient in terms of efficacy, safety, or cost? Does the intervention to be tested flow from the existing state of knowledge, have a sound theoretical framework, and have a sufficiently high probability of doing more good than harm?

Clozapine, the first atypical antipsychotic drug, is the product of such a line of thinking. Schizophrenia, an illness that affects a relatively small group of people (1% of the general population, or an incidence of 300,000 in the United States) yet has a devastating effect on individuals and society (33 billion dollars total economic cost per year in the United States), has been insufficiently treated in most people with conventional antipsychotic drugs for the past 40 years. The basic science phase of the development of clozapine used existing information about the neurocellular functions of the typical antipsychotics (the "dopamine hypothesis"), added new information from the neurosciences about the interactions of neurotransmitters with each other (the balance of dopamine and serotonin), receptor physiology (such as D_1 and D_2), and functional interrelationships between the temporal lobes (limbic system) and the frontal lobes (neocortex) in the pathophysiology of this severe brain disease (the "dysregulation hypothesis of schizophrenia"). What resulted is a novel drug that has revolutionized both the psychopharmacologic treatment of schizophrenia as well as the next era of antipsychotic drug research. Because clozapine has better efficacy than the traditional antipsychotic drugs in treatment-resistant schizophrenia, the risk/benefit ratio, even in light of this drug's significant adverse effects and cost of treatment, has been acceptable for a subpopulation of severely ill patients with schizophrenia who had been insufficiently treated with traditional antipsychotics.

Antipsychotic drug clinical trials to date have resulted in several new atypical drugs with a better safety profile than clozapine, yet with significant efficacy and safety advantages over the traditional drugs for many patients with schizophrenia. Some antipsychotic agents currently in clinical trials do not attribute their proposed efficacy to the dopamine system, pursuing a more novel biologic path than marketed drugs thus far. The increased understanding of the interactions of biology and the psychosocial environment have followed neuroscientific developments, and an exciting line of research addressing early detection and intervention, and even prevention strategies in children at high risk for schizophrenia, is emerging in the literature. It is a challenge for the APRN to expediently evaluate and appropriately integrate this information into the clinical arena.

Clarity of the Research Question

The research question of the trial needs to be both appropriate and unambiguous. Does the trial attempt to *explain* how a treatment produces its effects or whether it can work (only subjects most likely to comply with and respond to the trial should be recruited)? The *explanatory* trial requires frequent, close monitoring and measurements, unlike usual clinical practice, and thus can obtain relatively quick results with relatively small numbers of study patients, although its applicability may be limited. Thus when the clinician integrates these study results, there should be an expectation of logistical challenges.

Does the trial attempt to *manage* all the consequences of treating an illness as close to routine clinical practice as possible in order to determine whether the treatment works ("all comers," including patients with poor compliance and previous treatment failures, are accepted into the trial to best assess the usefulness of a particular approach in the real clinical world)? The *management* trial can be fraught with intrusions of extraneous outside variables; therefore it takes a larger patient population over a longer time frame to control for these variables in order to determine treatment efficacy and safety. It also takes special-

ized statistical considerations to handle missing data, but its results are more readily applicable to clinical settings in general.

Validity of The Trial

To be valid, the trial must have defined and limited bias (conscious and unconscious). Does the design of the trial measure what it was intended to measure and are the inferences from the trial true (internal validity)? Can the trial results be generalized to settings or samples beyond those represented in the trial (external validity)? Has the trial been designed to diminish confounding variables? Confounding leads to bias—a conclusion that differs systematically from the truth because of distortions in patient selection, data collection, and final analysis.

The following are the three most important elements used to control bias and thus enable the statistical testing of hypotheses of a clinical trial.

Blindedness. The patient (single-blind study) or both the patient and the members of the research team or independent outcome raters (double-blind study) do not know to which study group the patient has been randomly assigned (experimental or comparison). If the blind is broken, either by accident or deliberately (as in the case of a patient emergency), while the patient and researchers are active in the study (or in multicenter psychopharmacologic research, before the final submission of data to the FDA for drug approval), the patient, the patient's data, and sometimes the investigator are eliminated from the study.

Concurrent controls. For the most powerful trial results, a new drug is tested against one or more known quantities, or *controls*, usually a placebo and/or another drug that is similar to the study drug and that has known efficacy in treating the illness under investigation (usually called a *comparison group*). *Concurrent* means that the controls were included in the experiment and tested at the same time and in the same way as the experimental drug.

The double-blind placebo-controlled clinical

trial has long been considered an imperative element in controlling bias that can occur from the expectation that the experimental drug will have particular assumed effects or from changes in behavior that can occur simply from the knowledge that one is in an experiment (the Hawthorn effect). The placebo is an inert substance that looks like the drug being tested. It is used as a placebo-control for one study group throughout the course of the study, in an initial "drug washout period" as a transition for subjects who have been treated with medication up until their enrollment in a clinical trial, or when the trial calls for a blinded "placebo lead-in" for the baseline assessment of symptomatology before administration of the experimental drug. Recently, there has been increasing concern that the use of placebos in clinical trials may actually cause more harm than good in some cases, and thus the risk/benefit ratio for each study population and each individual patient must be carefully considered (Addington et al., 1997; Orr, 1996). A placebo may actually cause an increase of severity in some illnesses for some patients by inordinately delaying or withholding active treatment, such as in patients with a "first-break" schizophrenia or in patients with depression and increased risk factors for suicide. A placebo control may also cause additional expense if an exacerbation of symptoms causes a loss of work productivity in some outpatients or necessitates inpatient hospitalization for a portion of the study.

Randomization. There are two reasons to randomize a clinical trial: 1) to control for differences in patient entry characteristics that may influence the trial outcome (it is important to ensure that the study groups are initially comparable so that differences between groups over time can be assumed to be due to the effect of the intervention), and 2) to allow for the use of powerful statistical tests of comparison to analyze the trial data.

It must become a matter of chance, a "lottery" or "coin toss," that determines which patient receives a given treatment, so every patient must have an equal chance of being assigned to either the experimental or control groups. It is assumed that the average effect of a given drug will be the same regardless of which randomly selected group of patients receives it. Because it is not known which variables may affect the outcome of the trial, this process ensures an approximately equal distribution of variables among the groups to be studied so that differences in outcome can be attributed to the treatment and not to different characteristics of the groups. This prevents distortion by known as well as unknown variables by ensuring the equal distribution of subjects among treatment groups. These may include subject demographics, concurrent illnesses or treatments, individual belief systems, or early developmental experiences.

In cases where it is feared that the groups may become unequal in that one or more variables are known to potentially affect the study results, these can be taken into account by several techniques in addition to simple randomization:

1. *Stratifying* a variable (gender, for example, becomes 2 strata, men and women) and then randomizing to a trial group from within each strata maintains a balance of this potentially confounding variable within each trial group (all the men are given an equal chance of being assigned to one of the trial groups, and all the women are given an equal chance of being assigned to one of the trial groups; thus each gender will be proportionately represented in each trial group).

2. Another form of stratification is *matching*. Patients in each group may be matched on certain characteristics to patients in each other group. These characteristics are regarded by the investigator as likely to affect the trial results if by chance the groups become uneven for this variable. Examples are severity of illness, previous exposure to psychopharmacologic agents, abnormal MRI scans, patient age or race, etc.

The scientific reason for randomization in clinical trials is that it is one of the underlying assumptions to be met by many statistical techniques before they can be used to make valid hypothesis tests of the trial data. The FDA recognizes this and generally refuses to approve nonrandomized or incorrectly randomized trials as primary evidence of efficacy and safety (Wooding, 1996). The study report should include a succinct yet complete description of randomization procedures along with all other procedures used to ensure the validity of the trial. Additional control techniques to ensure validity for clinical trials include the following:

- Any additional therapeutic procedures are avoided during the trial or occur equally in the experimental and comparison groups.
- When possible, the subject has not been previously exposed to the study procedure.
- Only the experimental, not the control (comparison), subjects receive the test procedure.
- Standardized tests and procedures should be used throughout the trial, and interrater reliability should be achieved between all study raters within each study site as well as across sites in multicenter trials.
- Specific statistical tests can also be used during the data analysis phase of the trial to adjust for baseline characteristics that are known to affect outcome and that were not initially stratified.
- Potential investigator conflicts of interest (such as background, training, and sources of research support), which may influence the research design or conduct of the study, are clearly stated in the research report.
- Clear pathogenic hierarchies are used so that the occurrence of a major event (such as a successful suicide), which may preclude the subsequent occurence of a lesser event (such as a decrease in depression), is not considered in isolation. Otherwise, if suicide is simply dismissed by the researchers as an occasional unfortunate outcome of depression, an experimental drug that may actually stimulate suicidal events in some depressed patients could be mistaken for a drug that only causes an antidepressant effect in most.
- Investigators are increasingly pressured to clarify whether the data in a published report is the full analysis of a progression of RCTs for a drug or a smaller part of a larger research effort, thus preliminary rather than complete.

The applicability of clinical trial results to the clinical setting depends on the trial's success in detecting, assessing, and diminishing potential biases that might result in misleading conclusions. Most successful RCTs demonstrate *efficacy* (the treatment can attain its stated goal in optimal circumstances) rather than *effectiveness* (the treatment does more good than harm when used in clinical circumstances for a particular patient). This is because RCTs apply the treatment to a narrow spectrum of patients and deliver care in a very controlled fashion, optimizing the chances of demonstrating treatment benefit. The clinician must use judgement to determine generalizability of the trial results when applying the treatment in actual practice.

Appropriateness of Patient Selection Criteria

The patient inclusion/exclusion criteria must strike a balance between efficient recruitment and generalizability, or external validity. A clinical trial will not succeed if it does not recruit appropriate subjects in sufficient numbers or if the results cannot be applied to populations beyond the study sample. A clinical trial must be efficient in every aspect of its design and conduct in order to succeed. It is important from an economic as well as a compassionate perspective to answer the study question with as small a number of study subjects as is required to demonstrate a statistically significant between-group difference. Thus the important question becomes which patients and how many of them will be needed to successfully complete the trial.

Patient definition and screening for relevant information during the recruitment process are frequently among the most complex components of the trial, requiring clinical experience with the population from which the patients are to be selected, clinical judgment to keep patients safe during their participation in the trial, and research expertise in order to remain true to the focus of the study from which the inclusion/exclusion criteria have emerged. Several questions to consider when evaluating the selection of clinical trial subjects in order to decide to whom the conclusions may apply include the following:

1. *Was a clear, standard diagnostic nomenclature system used as a defining factor for the study sample?* It is imperative in any study of human subjects to define the diagnostic classification that must be met by every study subject in a trial. This is the first step in defining the parameters of a trial's subject homogeneity. The more similar the subjects are to each other on as many appropriate characteristics as possible, such as severity of illness and anticipated prognosis, without inordinately restricting the population pool from which the sample can be selected, the more clear-cut and unambiguous the demonstration of efficacy. For example, a study treating people with depression must be clear in defining whether it is major depression, dysthymia, or depression as a subclinical mood state. Psychopharmacologic clinical trials invariably use the current edition of the *Diagnostic and Statistical Manual of Mental Disorders* (APA, 1994) to ensure that study patients meet criteria for the disease for which the drug is being tested.

2. *Have the sample characteristics been justified?* One of the limitations of a homogeneous study sample is that it limits generalizability. For example, until recently, psychopharmacologic studies were conducted with medically healthy middle-class adult white men. Only now is it being realized the extent to which the extrapolation of data generated in this fashion has been confusing and potentially dangerous when applied to other clinical trial samples, such as women, ethnic and racially diverse people, elders, children, and people with multiple concomitant illnesses and treatments (Herz, 1997).

Drug considerations such as dose levels and schedules, side effect profiles, drug interactions, and belief systems have complicated the application of psychopharmacologic clinical trial results in clinical arenas with diverse clinician and patient populations. For federally funded research, the government now requires a justification for systematically eliminating study subjects based on gender, age, ethnic and racial background, and religious preference (Hohmann & Parron, 1996). At the least, the study report should document exclusions of patients who would otherwise be eligible and other nonentrants (such as refusals) in the discussion on sample characteristics in order to diminish investigator bias in subject selection.

Adequacy of Sample Size

The study sample size is one of the most important underlying features of the reliability (the study results can be reproduced) of the trial. Also, if the sample size is so low that differences in variables cannot be detected or cannot reach statistical significance, or that only huge effects (uncommon in health care in general) can be detected, the findings of the trial are meaningless (Gould, 1995; Shih & Quan, 1997). Adequate statistical power can only be reached when the sample size is adequate to answer the study questions. *Statistical power* is the probability that a real effect will be detected if there is one, and sufficient power is dependant upon determining the number of study subjects required for an adequate power analysis. Box 23-3 provides a brief list of components necessary to determine the minimum number of study subjects and thus will assist the reader of clinical trials literature to make a judgment regarding the clinical applicability of significant study findings based on statistical power.

Clarity of Patient Trajectories

The trial report should help the reader understand the intended time line and procedural progression through the study for each subject. The report should also be very clear about how variations in this progression were handled from a statistical as well as an interpretive perspective. The best way to handle missing data from patients who have been randomized but were terminated early or from protocol violations by the research team is controversial and complicated. Even though every effort is made to establish the eligibility of patients before randomization, to prevent subject withdrawal, and to include all enrolled participants in the analysis, this is never the case in any clinical trial with human subjects. The study sample at the initiation of study participation is never the same as the study sample of completers because of several issues all resulting in incomplete data sets. However, it is the initial study sample that

most closely reflects the population for purposes of generalizability. The reader of this literature should be able to understand from the report how missing data occurred and what systematic decisions were made about how to adjust for it (was the subject dropped, was the last rating carried forward, was an intention-to-treat analysis or covariate adjustment used, etc) and then make a best judgment about the study findings based on the implications of each of these decisions (Gibaldi, 1996).

A working vocabulary will be helpful when critiquing this issue in RCT reports:

1. *Inclusions.* Depending on the context in which this term is used in the report, it can include

---

box 23-3

COMPONENTS NECESSARY TO ESTIMATE CLINICAL TRIAL SAMPLE SIZE

The clinical trial must have the following components to determine the minimum required numbers of subjects:

1. A defined, measurable outcome variable is selected.
2. Relevant statistical properties (distribution, average, standard deviation, etc.) of the outcome variable have been assessed in previous research (pilot data or a previous clinical trial).
3. The properties entered into the power equation depend on an index at stake (e.g., for differences between averages of this outcome variable, an estimate of the standard deviation is imperative).
4. The statistical technique selected is appropriate to test differences between the experimental and control group on this outcome variable in terms of averages, proportions, etc.
5. The level of significance is stated (usually 5%: p = .05; or 1%: p = .01). This is the risk one is willing to take that an observed difference in the outcome variable is not caused by dif-

ferences in the experimental and control groups, but rather by some other chance influence.

6. The direction of the test of significance is stated as one-tailed or two-tailed.
7. The minimum effect thought to be a realistic success (effect size) is stated.
8. The desirable power is stated. This is the probability one wants to have that this minimum effect also shows up statistically (i.e., leads to rejection of the null hypothesis of no relation).
9. The following relationships must exist:
   a. The lower the level of significance, the more patients are needed.
   b. The smaller the effect size, the more patients are needed.
   c. The higher the power, the more patients are needed.
   d. The more outcome variables of interest, the more patients are needed.
   e. The more interventions, or groups, to be compared, the more patients are needed.

Modified from Kluiter & Wiersma, 1996.

people who are recruited from the target population, screened, or agree to participate; or baseline data collected, randomized, and entered into the study. It implies that they began double-blind treatment. However, it could also refer to the group of people included in the analysis who may not match the randomization group entered into the study.

2. *Exclusions.* Exclusions are people who do not meet entry criteria at the screening period, thus do not sign an informed consent, and are not randomized. This last point is important statistically since the lack of randomization does not bias group comparisons; however, from an interpretive standpoint, a follow-up of excluded people (as well as people who met criteria but refused to consent) and a comparison of them to the study groups may help the investigator better understand how the natural course of events may have affected the study sample, and thus the study outcome, and perhaps the generalizability of the results.

3. *Ineligibility.* Enrolled participants who then were either withdrawn before study completion or excluded from the analysis of the response variable data are considered ineligible. This usually implies that a protocol violation was found to have occurred (exclusionary information was obtained after randomization, clerical, lab, or entry assessment error, etc.). The decision to keep these patients in the study is an economical and a clinical one—if the study site can afford it, perhaps they might benefit from continued study participation. The decision to exclude them from the analysis to determine treatment effect is a statistical one—they no longer match the study sample on some important factor.

4. *Nonadherence.* Nonadherence refers to enrolled participants who are withdrawn from the study (referred to as *drop-outs*) as a result of the patient's failure to follow study requirements (refusal to take double-blind medications as prescribed or to abstain from excluded concomitant treatments, failure to attend study rat-

ing sessions or complete required rating scales, etc.). Subjects in the control arm of the study who begin to follow the treatment strategy are called *drop-ins*. Nonadherence may result from loss of interest on the part of the participant, decisions made by the participant's primary care or referring health care provider, exacerbation or remission of the patient's symptoms or adverse effects from the study, etc. Whether these subjects are included in or withdrawn from analysis of the study group to which they were randomized can lead to bias, and a careful judgment must be made to determine how these decisions might effect the interpretation of results.

Additional issues that should be included in the report accompanied by discussions of possible implications include the following:

1. *Use of rescue medications.* Standard prn treatments are allowed in some studies for subjects who experience severe symptom exacerbation while on blinded treatments.

2. *Inclusion of ancillary studies.* Add-on procedures to the study protocol that answer additional research questions on the same study sample may affect the study results.

3. *Code-breaking events.* The blind intervention is unveiled prematurely to intervene in the treatment of the patient for safety reasons, or the blind is inadvertently broken by the patient or a research team member.

Consideration of Pharmacologic Issues

Despite the wide acceptance of the RCT in psychopharmacology research, results are reported in the aggregate, and there is always an unexplained variation of a drug's effects in individual patients. It is likely that these individual variations can be at least partly explained by pharmacologic factors. RCTs cannot address intrinsic (pharmacodynamic) factors such as differential patient responses to the same dose of the same drug that occur at the level of the receptor. Pharmacokinetic (absorption, distribution, metabolism, and excretion) differences in drug response, on the other hand, can be measured and documented in the well-designed RCT. Clinical trial reports should include a discussion of these factors and their clinical applicability. These study data translate directly to clinical practice as the likely effects of individual patient age, gender, diet and meal patterns, general health, and concomitant treatments are included in new product information.

■ CLINICAL TRIAL DESIGNS

There are several designs that are used in psychopharmacologic trials. Each one has advantages and disadvantages, and each one presents a different slant on the study results. A working knowledge of the more frequently used designs is useful in the evaluation of trial reports. In each of the following models, *population* refers to both the 1) target population (the population one wishes to generalize to, such as all people with the illness under study), and 2) study population (all the people with the illness under study who are within reach of the study, such as all people who present for treatment of the illness at a hospital or center where a trial is being conducted). *Study sample* refers to the members of the study population who are recruited for the trial, meet criteria, and agree to participate.

Parallel Designs

Two or more treatments are compared with one another in the same trial. Ideally, a four (or more) treatment parallel design is used. Although in psy-

chiatry it is more common to find one experimental and one control (or comparison) group used for the purposes of practicality, the more complex designs are more desirable for their stronger results.

This design has the following elements:
1. An experimental treatment is compared with one or more standard treatments of known efficacy, as well as to a placebo answering the following questions:
    a. Does the experimental drug work?
    b. How does it compare with the currently available standard drugs used to treat the same illness?
    c. Does the experiment give reasonable results that can be trusted?

This last question affirms the reliability of the trial procedures if the standard drugs prove to be significantly more effective than the placebo, as they should.
2. Each subject is randomized to only one of the treatments, or one at a time.
3. The trial groups are run concurrently and the experiment is completed in a reasonable amount of time to control for bias inherent in the passage of time. Examples of historical bias are inordinate subject attrition from relocation, illness, death, or lack of efficacy; significant changes in patients' lives that may confound the illness under investigation; changeover in investigators that may confound interrater reliability; changes in economics that may adversely affect funding streams; and highly competitive drugs that may reach the market first. An example of the parallel design model can be seen in Fig. 23-2.

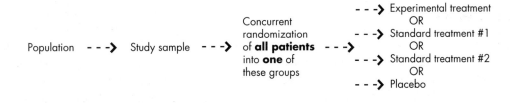

Figure 23-2 Parallel design model.

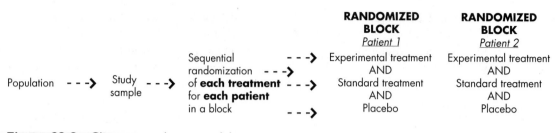

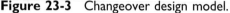

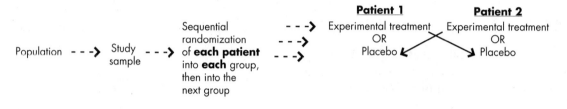

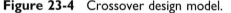

Figure 23-3 Changeover design model.

Figure 23-4 Crossover design model.

Changeover Designs

Two or more treatments are given sequentially to each patient in the trial, and the order of the treatments is randomized for each patient. A randomized block design is commonly used in changeover studies in which the patients form the blocks. Each patient is his or her own control as well as a comparison for other patients in the trial.

The issue of a potential confounding factor from being in the previous group if the treatment were an active compound must be addressed in changeover designs, particularly in psychopharmacologic trials. Thus it is common to see fewer groups and the use of a double-blind placebo lead-in between groups as a treatment washout. An example of the changeover design model can be seen in Fig. 23-3.

Crossover Designs

More commonly, a crossover design is used in psychopharmacologic clinical trials that use two groups, the experimental group and usually a placebo, although one standard treatment can be used instead. Each patient is randomly assigned to one of the groups for a designated period of time, and then is crossed-over to each of the other groups, one at a time. The same issue of potential confounds from previous treatments also applies to the crossover design in psychopharmacologic trials. Again, fewer groups and a double-blind placebo washout between groups are possible methods to adjust for this problem. An example of the crossover design model can be seen in Fig. 23-4.

Crossed Parallel Design with Two Factors

A parallel design can possess more than one *factor* (a controlled experimental entity, or treatment), such as drugs, as well as other treatments, such as different drug doses. In this design, it is possible to determine the efficacy of the experimental drug compared with the standard drugs and with placebo. It is also possible to make a determination about the effects of various dose ranges (called a *dose response* or *dose-finding trial*). An example of the crossed parallel design with two factors model can be seen in Fig. 23-5.

This design is frequently used in psychopharmacologic research in an effort to ask as many

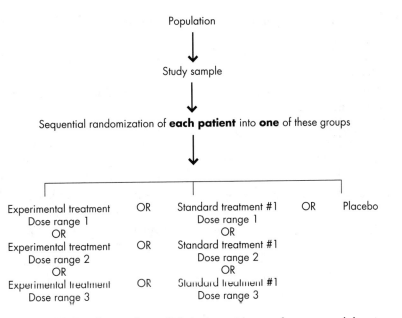

Figure 23-5 Crossed parallel design with two factors model.

important questions as possible in the context of one large clinical trial. The need for a particularly large patient sample is often a disadvantage of this design.

■ CLINICAL TRIAL OUTCOMES

In RCT research, the research questions and the study objectives determine what to measure, which tools to use, and when to measure in order to test the independent variable, or treatment. Trial designs use some system to measure outcome variables (called *end points* or *effect variables*). The study outcome is no more useful than the quality of the measurements.

RCT Measurement Issues

Assessment and change measures usually focus on combinations of several domains of dependent variables:

1. Signs and symptoms of illness within the context of a diagnosis
2. Concomitant issues such as quality of life, functional status, and overall health
3. Treatment effects (both efficacy and side effects)
4. Biologic correlates of illness and clinical change

The number of constructs that can be measured is dictated by the projected size of the study sample in order to ensure statistical significance (the more constructs measured, the larger the sample must be). The rating tools selected should reflect the construct of interest and a blend of state-of-the-art scales, a tie-in to current and past trials for comparisons, both clinician-rated and patient self-report scales with standardized reliability (including demonstrated interrater reliability) and validity, and utility in the clinical setting. Frequency of measurement is affected by the intended use of the scales, predicted biologic and clinical change trajectory of the experimental drug as well as any comparison treatments, and the feasibility of the measurement schedule for the research participants.

The first data-collection point (pretest) ideally should occur after the patient has completed screening, informed consent, and randomization procedures and is ready to begin the test (initiate treatment). The data collection should be repeated at least once more at a predetermined point after the results of the treatment should have occurred (posttest). Most trials of any length include additional measures at intervals throughout the patient's progression within a group (repeated measures). A clinical trials measurement time line is shown in Fig. 23-6. The pretest for each patient occurs at the time of enrollment into the study (and again before every initiation into another trial group, such as occurs in crossover designs). The posttest occurs at the end of each study group, at the termination of the study, or at the time a patient may drop out. Additional posttest measures are usually taken after patients complete the double-blind portion of the study and are in a follow-up phase of the trial. It is not usual, but is ideal, to repeat measures at some point after the end of the trial on a random sample of subjects to ensure health status, to check for long-term outcome, and to ensure that subjects have received active treatment for their illness after the trial.

Clinical Trial Hypothesis Testing

Empirical research requires expertise in conceptual, theoretical, and statistical skills and the proper communication of results. The reader of

the scientific report must assess these results critically and place them in a context in which to interpret and make best use of the findings. The more clinically experienced the reader, the more critically the report will be interpreted and applied if the results are believable.

A key to the statistical interpretation of clinical trials research is to remember that experimental design studies use directional null-hypotheses significance tests as the core to understanding the significance of the findings. It is therefore important to interpret the statistical findings and make a judgment about their clinical applicability to practice. In the context of a well-designed and well-managed study and after accepting the fact that one can never be absolutely certain that accepting or rejecting a hypothesis is correct (evidence from a sample never completely represents the whole population), the reasoning behind directional null-hypothesis significance tests is as follows:

1. Assume that the hypothesis of no difference (null) is true (it is easier to test for one value [0% difference] than to anticipate and test for each and every possible difference).
2. Collect the data and observe the differences, if any, between groups.

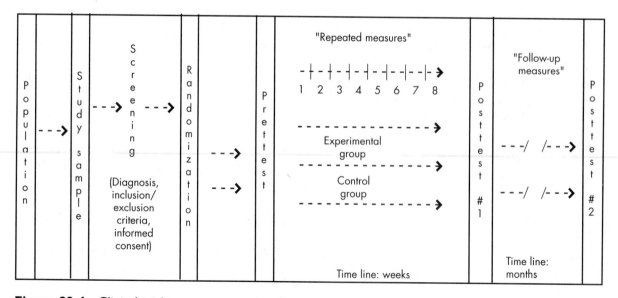

Figure 23-6 Clinical trials measurement time line.

3. Ask how likely it is that by chance alone these results would occur (*p* value) if the null hypothesis is true (there is no difference between groups).

4. Reject the null hypothesis and accept the alternative hypothesis if it is not likely that these results would arise by chance; therefore there is a true difference between groups.

5. Determine the clinical implications of an incorrect assumption (an error).

   a. *Type I error.* This occurs when the null hypothesis is rejected in favor of the alternate hypothesis (it is concluded that the drug is effective when there is no true difference between groups). The probability of making a type I error is known as *alpha*, the significance level of a statistical test. If a result is reported significant at the .05 level (*p* = .05), it means that the probability of making a type I error (thinking a drug works when it does not) is 5% or less.

      Clinical implications of a type I error. The drug will be accepted as an efficacious treatment when in fact it does not work. In mental health care, receiving no treatment or ineffective treatment can significantly affect the safety, life satisfaction, and disease progression for many patients. The rules of the FDA are set up to lower the probability of making a type I error to minimize having ineffective drugs on the market (Wassertheil-Smoller, 1995).

   b. *Type II error.* This occurs when the null hypothesis is not rejected (the drug is declared ineffective when there actually is a true difference between groups that was not detected). The risk of making a type II error is the *power* of the trial, known as *beta*.

      Clinical implications of a Type II error. A drug that is beneficial will be judged to be ineffective and will not be used. In mental health care, since many patients currently suffer dose-limiting side effects, incomplete response, symptom breakthrough, and progression of illness, in the context of today's best interventions, the loss of any improved

treatment would be a serious one. Additionally, pharmaceutical companies guard against making a type II error in order to not overlook efficacious drugs that they can market.

6. If the alternative hypothesis is accepted, is it one-tailed or two-tailed (is there a direction to the difference)? A clinical trial is designed to test a particular hypothesis, and direction of the findings can be clinically relevant. Direction is expressed as one- versus two-tailed tests:

   Example. Research report: The experimental drug was significantly superior to placebo in decreasing depression ($p < 0.05$, one-tailed test).

   Hypothesis #1:

   H_O (null)   Mean depression rating score in the treatment group = mean depression rating score in the control group

   H_A (alternate)   Mean depression rating score in the treatment group is less than the mean depression rating score in the control group

   In this example, to reject the null hypothesis and consider the drug to be effective, the difference between the experimental group and the control group must not just be significant, but the direction of the difference matters as well. The experimental antidepressant drug must not only be different from the placebo, but it must also be "better than" the placebo—the mean depression score must have fallen, not risen. Only one direction will prove successful for the treatment. This is a one-tailed test.

   In the example above, it is also of interest to know if the successful drug has different effects based on sample characteristics, such as gender:

   Hypothesis #2:

   H_O (null)   Mean depression rating score for women in the treatment group = mean depression rating score for men in the treatment group

H_A (alternate)   Mean depression rating score for women in the treatment group is different from the mean depression rating score for men in the treatment group

In this example, the null hypothesis is rejected in favor of the alternative either if the mean for women was sufficiently greater or lower than the mean for men. The direction of the difference is not specified. This is a two-tailed test. A two-tailed test postulates that the response rate in the treatment group can be either larger or smaller than the response rate in the control group. This test of significance is used most often in biomedical research because it is difficult to know in which direction a difference may turn out to be, although it requires a larger sample size than a one-tailed test to determine significance.

7. Determine the clinical relevance of statistically significant study results. Statistical significance is only the beginning of the judgment needed to make inferences about the study effects and their clinical importance when applied to the population beyond the study sample. Clinical trial findings cannot be evaluated in the absence of a clinical treatment context. The determined level of clinical significance is affected more by the sample size, measurement, and study design than by the clinical importance of the effect. The descriptive statistics accompanying the research report should support the statistical test results in determining relevance and applicability to a particular clinical population.

Additionally, some journals have increased their standards for trial reports to include the name of the statistical test, the numeric value of the test statistic, degrees of freedom, or n, as appropriate, the p value, point estimates, and confidence intervals, as well as graphic displays of the data as aids in determining clinical importance of study findings. When the point estimate (the observed result) is placed within a confidence interval (CI, another measure of uncertainty), the reader is provided with the best estimate of the size of a difference. The p value (conveys information about the level of doubt, not the magnitude of clinical importance) and the CI are related arithmatically. Thus in the context of a well-designed and well-managed study, if the 95% CI excludes 0 (the null hypothesis), the value of the point estimate falls close to the middle of the CI, and $p = .05$, then the results are very powerful. This information permits readers to use their own judgment regarding the value of the smallest clinically important difference in making treatment decisions (Friedman, Furberg, & DeMets, 1996; Borenstein, 1997).

Evaluating Clinical Trials

Investigators have an obligation to review their study and its findings critically and to present sufficient information so that readers can properly evaluate the trial (Friedman, Furberg, & DeMets, 1996). When evaluating a clinical trial report, the APRN can use a variety of methods (Bigby & Gradenne, 1996; Chalmers et al., 1992; Murphy & Albers, 1992; Greenhalgh, 1997; Guyatt, Sackett, & Cook, 1993; Sindhu, Carpenter, & Seers, 1997) but must rely most heavily on two things: an understanding of the most salient clinical trial issues and a sophisticated vision of how particular trial results would apply in the clinical arena based on one's education and experience in treating patients in the same target population as those in the study (Yastrubetskaya, Chiu, & O'Connell, 1996; Preskorn, 1997).

Many of the issues covered in this chapter are outlined in Table 23-2. This may serve as an informal "report card" for the APRN to use as a standard from which to best judge the thoroughness, quality, and believability of the progression of trials for a new treatment. These issues form the springboard from which the APRN can begin to consider the clinical applicability of a new drug.

table 23-2

REPORT CARD FOR CLINICAL TRIAL EVALUATION: DOES IT MAKE THE GRADE?

LEVEL	EVIDENCE	VALUE	GRADE
I	Large randomized controlled clinical trial with clear results and low risk of error: • Standard diagnostic nomenclature was used • Theoretical framework underlying experimental treatment was identified • At least one standard treatment comparison group was used • A placebo control group was used • Variables were controlled • Patient recruitment, selection criteria, and group characteristics were discussed • Randomization methods were described • Sample size estimate was discussed • Special populations were discussed • Risk/benefit ratio of treatment was discussed • Patient compliance in the treatment groups was discussed • All patients who entered the study were accounted for, and trajectories were clear • All clinically relevant outcomes were reported (mortality and morbidity) • Clinical applicability of experimental treatment was discussed (bioethics, quality of life, outcomes, costs, treatment settings, etc) • More than one study site in more than one geographic region was used • Study sites were diverse (e.g., types of facilities, reimbursement sources, catchment areas, access to services, etc.) • Report of the statistical analysis was adequate to understand clinical significance • Limitations of the study were discussed • Investigator conflict of interest issues were disclosed *Value*: Subtract ½ pt for each missing item; *Grade*: Subtract total from highest value (100).	100	A
II	Small randomized controlled clinical trial with uncertain results and moderate- to high-risk of error • Use checklist above	90	B
III	Nonrandomized, contemporaneous controls	85	B-
IV	Nonrandomized, historical controls	80	C
V	Case series study • No controls	75	C-
VI	Anecdotal report	70	D

ROLE OF THE APRN IN ■ CLINICAL TRIAL RESEARCH

There are many important roles to be filled in clinical trials research, and the well-qualified APRN can accomplish most of them. Essential elements for successful participation in a clinical trial are to be very well prepared for and mentored into a particular role, to make a nursing contribution to the discovery of the scientific knowledge, and to both give and receive appropriate credit for that participation. Each member of the research team may be required to negotiate such things as investigator status, participation in protocol design, inclusion of discipline-specific theoretical frameworks, planning and analysis meetings, and authorship in trial publications. There may be several funding, policy, and credentialling constraints at the level of Principal Investigator for a psychopharmacologic clinical trial in many settings. Nonetheless, it is a worthy aspiration for the seasoned APRN who has been a co-investigator, particularly with doctoral preparation, seminal publications, a funding background, and institutional support. The paucity of nurse scientists at the investigative level of RCT research is a failure on the part of the federal government, the pharmaceutical industry, research institutions, and scientific investigative teams to appreciate the considerable and evolving potential of the APRN as an independent mental health clinician, educator, and researcher. It is also a failure of the nursing profession to adequately appreciate the importance of this research method, as well as a failure to address these difficult issues assertively, politically, and repeatedly.

A reasonable place to attain expertise in this arena is membership in the IRB, which, by law, must be composed of experienced clinicians and not just research scientists. Many university and medical center IRBs have rotating memberships and a knowledgeable and helpful staff, and they provide excellent experience in evaluating research protocols. See Chapter 19 for a discussion of IRBs.

Another introductory role for nurses is that of data collector. The data collector is frequently the clinician who interfaces between research requirements and clinical care for the patient participating in a research trial. The role of clinical trials coordinator can also be a richly rewarding career choice for nurses as well as a significant contribution to scientific inquiry (Di Giulio et al., 1996; Kenkre, 1997; Molloy & Laraia, 1996; Pelke & Easa, 1997; Raybuck, 1997).

IMPLICATIONS FOR ■ THE FUTURE

According to Polit and Hungler (1997), the general purpose of nursing research is to answer questions or solve problems of relevance to the nursing profession. The nursing research literature exemplifies the struggle to integrate the various important methodologies into the best scientific approach for the acquisition of knowledge (Champagne, Tornquist, & Funk, 1997; Poole, 1996; Sandelowski, 1996). Unfortunately, RCTs are a relatively rare event in the psychiatric nursing research literature, yet they are considered by most of the scientific community to be a "gold standard" method of inquiry. The nursing community in general, but particularly APRNs, continue to struggle with the integration of information attained by non-nursing disciplines into the art and science of nursing practice. The recent national debate about whether nurse practitioners (NPs) and prescribing clinical nurse specialists are stepping beyond their discipline by asking for reimbursement for "doctor's work" is at the heart of the issue of who "owns" and can thus use the results of scientific discovery for the betterment of humankind. This is an interesting contemporary debate in light of scientific results from a now classic clinical trial documenting the comparable effectiveness and patient satisfaction of physicians and NPs in a primary care practice (Spitzer et al, 1974).

Equally important is the need for nursing interventions to be evaluated in RCT study designs to meet established scientific criteria for efficacy. Psychiatric-mental health nurses cannot claim to provide quality, cost-effective care if they cannot demonstrate efficacy outcomes using accepted scientific methods. The use of RCTs directly informs evidence-based practice, and psychiatric-mental health nurses should subject their own interventions and treatment strategies to investigations of necessary scientific rigor. This may, in fact, be the next frontier of APRN research.

There are several reasons for nursing to increase its visibility in the clinical trial arena, in any role:

1. *Credibility*. The profession must stand toe to toe with scientists from all disciplines to lay claim to the scientific process that underlies the expansion of knowledge in health care.

2. *Quality of the discovery*. If the nursing profession does not lend the special aura of nursing theory, context, consciousness, and interpretation to the process of scientific inquiry, than the information used to prevent and treat illness will not be as holistic as possible. Specifically, nursing interventions will not be integrated in the larger scientific knowledge base used in the diagnosis and treatment of mental illness.

3. *Quality of nursing practice*. Without a grounding in quantitative experimental design methods, nursing practice will continue to struggle with challenges to nursing care efficacy and effectiveness and questions about the reality of evidence-based psychiatric nursing practice.

In 1994, the ANA Psychopharmacology Task Force reviewed the national psychiatric nursing environment for neuroscientific and psychopharmacologic content (ANA, 1994). This report compelled educational institutions with nursing programs, nursing authors and publishers, and nursing conference sponsors to not only increase the content of these areas for nurses, but to facilitate, encourage, and demand that *nurses* teach, write, present, and research these critical content areas. It is likely true that for nursing to be able to embrace this complex, dramatically prolific body of knowledge, it must be represented in sufficient volume in the works produced by and representing the nursing discipline. It can no longer be necessary or acceptable for APRNs to have to consistently review the works of other disciplines to keep current with advanced nursing practice. There have been great strides made in these areas since the ANA report, and continued vigilance on the part of APRNs will continue to move the specialty forward in these areas.

Educational programs, texts, books and journals, conferences and presentations, and distance learning offerings that target the APRN in psychiatric-mental health nursing have the mandate to put forward this agenda. The APRN should assess educational and media events as well as professional association agendas for research-based neuroscientific and psychopharmacology content for the following components:

- Neuroscientific underpinnings of the targeted illness as well as the indicated drug treatments
- Overview of the Phase III (efficacy and safety) and Phase IV (postmarketing surveillance) clinical trials producing information about the drug
- Clinical assessments, drug applications, treatment integration strategies, and alternative treatments
- Rational prescribing practices
- Review of current pertinent Phase III clinical trials in the field
- Information that incorporates a nursing perspective and includes nurses in the display of the work

In addition to federal regulations for clinical trials, additional resources found in newsletters and on the Internet that should be helpful as sources of information for the APRN are shown in the Resources and Connections section that follows. It must then be the APRN who uses, integrates, and disseminates this information for nurses, for patients, and for clinical practices.

RESOURCES AND CONNECTIONS

RESOURCE	**SOURCE**
Code of Federal Regulations; The Federal Register (also, see local medical and legal libraries)	**The Superintendent of Documents** Attn: New Orders Box 371954 Pittsburgh, PA 15240-7954 GPO: 202-512-1800
Guidelines for the monitoring of clinical investigations; information sheets	**Bioresearch Program Coordinator** HFC-230 5600 Fisher's Lane Rockville, MD 20857
Audit/inspection resource guides available for sponsors, investigators, and IRBs	**National Technical Information Service** 5285 Port Royal Road Springfield, VA 22161 703-487-4650
Good Clinical Practices packet; IRB information sheet; General Considerations for the Clinical Evaluation Of Drugs; Guidelines for Investigators brochure; Guidelines for the Conduct of a Study	**Center for Drug Evaluation and Research** Executive Secretariat Staff (HFD-8) 5600 Fisher's Lane Rockville, MD 20857 301-594-1012
Many guidelines and summaries of information sheets are available in book form and on CD-ROM (call 301-443-6770 for CD-ROM) from the FDA	**Food and Drug Administration** FOI Staff, HFI-35, Room 12A-16 5600 Fisher's Lane Rockville, MD 20857 301-443-6310
Psychiatric Research Report: Quarterly newsletter that provides information on meetings, funding, legislation, and research training	**Psychiatric Research Report, APA Office of Research** 1400 K Street, NW Washington, DC 20005 Fax: 202-789-1874 Email: sferris@psych.org
CenterWatch Newsletter (monthly) and CW Weekly (fax letter): Sources of timely business news for the clinical trials industry as well as grant leads for investigators from all specialities	**CenterWatch** 581 Boylston Street, Suite 407 Boston, MA 02116 617-247-2327 Fax: 617-247-2535
The Blue Sheet: A weekly newsletter devoted to specialized health care policy and research information. Topics alternate and include clinical trials, research and grants administration, funding, bioethics, the IRB, public health, genetics, alternative medicine, Capitol Hill legislative updates, etc.	**Health Policy & Biomedical Research News FDC Reports, Inc.** 5550 Friendship Blvd, Suite One Chevy Chase, MD 20815-7278 301-657-9830 Fax: 301-656-3094

INTERNET AND ONLINE SERVICES

Legi-Slate online service: Complete and updated Federal Register and Code of Federal Regulations. Call 1-800-877-6999 to subscribe to this listserv

CenterWatch Clinical Trials Listing Service: Resource for patients interested in participating in RCTs and for professionals.
www.centerwatch.com
Email: cntrwatch@aol.com

Community of Science (COS): Descriptive list of federally funded research in the United States; indexing and online search and retrieval capabilities; science policy updates
Available through member universities:
cos.gdb.org

Electronic Nursing Ladder: Information, Cyber-Courses, and links
www3.uchc.edu/~uchclib/eduoff/nnre.html

PharmInfoNet: Pharmaceutical Information Network: Nervous System Disease and Mental Health Center
www.pharminfo.com
www.pharminfo.com/disease/mental.html

Society for Clinical Trials: Dedicated to the development and dissemination of knowledge about clinical trials
members.aol.com/sctbalt/index.htm

UCSF Library and Center for Knowledge Management: Research Investigators Handbook
www.library.ucsf.edu/ih

Center for Clinical Trials, The Johns Hopkins Medical Institutions: Promotes clinical trial methodology
www.jhsph.edu/Research/Centers/CCT/backgrou.htm

Food and Drug Administration: Human drugs, medical devices, medical products reporting, new drug development in the United States
www.fda.gov

Office of Research Integrity (ORI): Promotes integrity in research; oversees PHS research activities: NIH, CDC, SAMHSA, AHCPR, FDA (except regulatory activities)

DHHS Office of the Secretary, *ORI Newsletter*
5515 Security Lane, Suite 700
Rockville, MD 20852
ori.dhhs.gov

National Institute of Mental Health (NIMH): Research activities, clinical studies, search the studies
nimh.nih.gov

Agency for Health Care Policy and Research (AHCPR): Makes practical, science-based health care information easily available
www.ahcpr.gov
Email: Info@ahcpr.gov

References

Addington D, et al. (1997): Placebos in clinical trials of psychotropic medication, *Canadian J Psychiatry, 42*, 3.

American Nurses Association. (1994). *Psychiatric mental health nursing psychopharmacology project.* Washington, DC: American Nurses Publishing.

American Psychiatric Association. (1994). *Diagnostic and statistical manual of mental disorders* (ed. 4). Washington, DC: American Psychiatric Press.

Bigby, M., & Gradenne, A.S. (1996). Understanding and evaluating clinical trials. *Journal of the American Academy of Dermatology, 34*, 555–594.

Bleidt, B., & Montagne, M. (1996). *Clinical research in pharmaceutical development.* New York: Marcel Dekker.

Borenstein, M. (1997). Hypothesis testing and effect size estimation in clinical trials. *Annals of Allergy, Asthma, and Immunology, 78*, 5–11.

Chalmers, T.C., et al. (1992). Clinical trials: a readers' guide. *Patient Care, 11*, 85–102.

Champagne, M.T., Tornquist, E.M., & Funk, S.G. (1997). Achieving research-based practice. *American Journal of Nursing, 97*, 16AAA–16DDD.

Cohen, A., & Posner, J. (1995). *A guide to clinical drug research.* Boston: Kluwer Academic Publishers.

Di Giulio, P., et al. (1996). Expanding the role of the nurse in clinical trials: the nursing summaries. *Cancer Nursing, 19*, 343–347.

Friedman, L.M., Furberg, C.D., & DeMets, D.L. (1996). *Fundamentals of clinical trials* (ed. 3). St. Louis: Mosby.

Gibaldi, M. (1996). Failure to comply: a therapeutic dilemma and the bane of clinical trials, *Journal of Clinical Pharmacology, 36*, 674–682.

Gould, A.L. (1995). Planning and revising the sample size for a trial. *Statistics in Medicine, 14*, 1039–1051.

Greenhalgh, T. (1997). How to read a paper: papers that report drug trials. *British Medical Journal, 315*, 480–483.

Guyatt, G.H., Sackett, D.L., & Cook, D.J. (1993). For the evidence-based medicine working group: users' guide to the medical literature. II. How to use an article about therapy or prevention. A. Are the results of the study valid? *Journal of the American Medical Association, 270*, 2598–2601.

Herz, S.E. (1997). Don't test, do sell: legal implications of inclusion and exclusion of women in clinical drug trials. *Epilepsia, 38*, S42–S49.

Hohmann, A.A., & Parron, D.L. (1996). How the new NIH Guidelines on Inclusion of Women and Minorities apply: efficacy trials, effectiveness trials, and validity. *Journal of Consulting and Clinical Psychology, 64*, 851–855.

Kenkre, J. (1997). Running a clinical trial. *Practice Nurse, 4*, 380–384.

Kluiter, H., & Wiersma, D. (1996). Randomized control trials of programmes. In Knudsen, H.C., & Thornicroft, G. (Eds.). *Mental health services evaluation*. London: Cambridge University Press.

Kobak, K.A., et al. (1996). Computer-administered clinical rating scales: a review. *Psychopharmacology, 127*, 291–301.

Kupfer, D.J., Kraemer, H.C., & Bartko, J.J. (1994). Documenting and reporting the study results of a randomized clinical trial (spicy meatballs, not pablum). In Prien, R.F., & Robinson, D.S. (Eds). *Clinical evaluation of psychotropic drugs: principles and guidelines*. New York: Raven Press.

Molloy, M.A., & Laraia, M.T. (1996). Nursing and psychopharmacologic clinical research. *APNA News, 8*, 3.

Murphy, P.A., & Albers, L.L. (1992). Evaluation of research studies. Part I. Randomized trials. *Journal of Nurse-Midwifery, 37*, 287–290.

Orr, R.D. (1996). Guidelines for the use of placebo controls in clinical trials of pharmacologic agents. *Psychiatric Services, 47*, 1262–1264.

Pelke, S., & Easa, D. (1997). The role of the clinical research coordinator in multicenter clinical trials. *Journal of Obstetric, Gynecologic, and Neonatal Nursing, 26*, 279–285.

Polit, D.F., & Hungler, B.P. (1997). *Essentials of nursing research: methods, appraisals, and utilization*. Philadelphia: J.B. Lippincott.

Poole, K. (1996). A re-examination of the experimental design for nursing research. *Journal of Advanced Nursing, 24*, 108–114.

Preskorn, S.E. (1997). The appearance of knowledge. *Journal of Practical and Behavioral Health, 7*, 233–238.

Prien, R.F., & Robinson, D.S. (1994). *Clinical evaluation of psychotropic drugs: principles and guidelines*. New York: Raven Press.

Raybuck, J.A. (1997). The clinical nurse specialist as a research coordinator in clinical drug trials. *Clinical Nurse Specialist, 11*, 15–19.

Rosenbaum, D. (December, 1995). Reference guide to FDA regulations. *The Monitor*, 1–4.

Sandelowski, M. (1996). Using qualitative methods in intervention studies. *Research in Nursing and Health, 19*, 359–364.

Shih, W.J., & Quan, H. (1997). Testing for treatment differences with dropouts present in clinical trials: a composite approach. *Statistics in Medicine, 16*, 1225–1239.

Siegfried, J.D. (1996). *New medicines in development for mental illness: the drug development and approval process*. Washington, DC: Pharmaceutical Research and Manufacturers of America.

Sindhu, F., Carpenter, L., & Seers, K. (1997). Development of a tool to rate the quality assessment of RCTs using Delphi technique. *Journal of Advanced Nursing, 25*, 1262–1268.

Spitzer, W.O., et al. (1974). The Burlington randomized trial of the nurse practitioner. *The New England Journal of Medicine, 290*, 251–256.

Wassertheil-Smoller, S. (1995). *Biostatistics and epidemiology: a primer for health professionals* (ed. 2). New York: Springer-Verlag.

Wooding, W.M. (1996). *Planning pharmaceutical clinical trials: basic statistical principles*. New York: John Wiley & Sons.

Yastrubetskaya, O., Chiu, E., & O'Connell, S. (1996). Is good clinical research practice for clinical trials good clinical practice? *International Journal of Geriatric Psychiatry, 12*, 227–231.

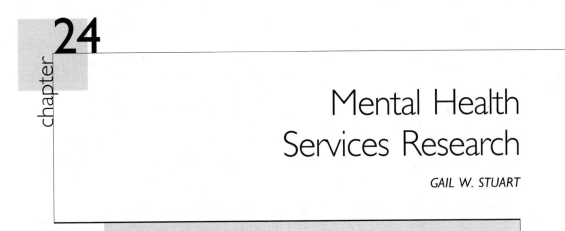

Mental Health
Services Research

GAIL W. STUART

■ INTRODUCTION

Health services research is a relatively new field of inquiry, although its origins may be traced back to the early 1900s in the United States (Anderson, 1991). The lead federal agency for support of formal health services research activities, the National Center for Health Services Research and Development (NCHSRD), was established in 1968. During the following years, many other federal agencies (including the Veterans Administration, Health Care Financing Administration [HCFA], National Institute of Mental Health [NIMH], and National Institute of Aging, among others) as well as private foundations (e.g., the Robert Wood Johnson Foundation, Commonwealth Fund, Milbank Memorial Fund, and Pew Foundation) assumed a greater role in supporting the design and conduct of health services research

activities. The first national meeting of the Association for Health Services Research (AHSR) and the Foundation for Health Services Research (FHSR) was held in Chicago in June 1984. In 1989, the NCHSRD received a substantial boost in funding for patient outcomes and medical effectiveness research as a result of major outcomes research bills introduced by Congress, and the agency itself was subsequently renamed the Agency for Health Care Policy and Research (AHCPR) to reflect its more policy-oriented focus. Health services research is increasingly making contributions to the design and evaluation of health policies and programs at the federal, state, and local levels, such as Medicaid and Medicare payment systems, provider reimbursement, and clinical practice guidelines (Brown, 1991; Roper, 1997).

Mental health services research, as a subset of

health services research, is also an emerging field of study that has come into its own only within recent years. It is supported in large part by the NIMH and the Center for Mental Health Services (CMHS), which is part of the Substance Abuse and Mental Health Services Administration (SAMHSA) of the U.S. Department of Health and Human Services (USDHHS). The Center for Mental Health Services (CMHS), in partnership with states, leads national efforts to demonstrate, evaluate, and disseminate service delivery models to treat mental illness, promote mental health, and prevent the development or worsening of mental illness when possible. The CMHS oversees a variety of service-

box 24-1

PROGRAMS SUPPORTED BY THE CENTER FOR MENTAL HEALTH SERVICES

NATIONAL MENTAL HEALTH SERVICES KNOWLEDGE EXCHANGE NETWORK (KEN)
PO Box 42490
Washington, DC 20015
www.mentalhealth.org.

KEN provides a "one-stop" gateway to a wide range of resources on mental health services, including technical assistance centers; federal, state, and local mental health agencies; other national clearinghouses and information centers; mental health organizations and professional associations; and consumer and family advocacy organizations. An electronic bulletin-board service (18007902647), with the access password "public," is available through personal computers, public libraries, universities, educational organizations, and state and local health or mental health departments.

COMMUNITY MENTAL HEALTH SERVICES BLOCK GRANTS
Federal partnership with states that include the following:
- Infrastructure building financial support for program startups, improving rural service access, and management information systems (MIS).
- Services integration, support, and coordination of children's mental health; medical, dental, and education services; and assessment of special population needs.

CHILDREN'S MENTAL HEALTH SERVICES DEMONSTRATION PROGRAM
Provides grants and technical assistance to support community-based services for children, adolescents, and young adults and their families with severe behavioral or mental disorders.

PLANNING AND SYSTEM DEVELOPMENT PROGRAM FOR CHILDREN (CASSP)
Provides grants to improve systems of care for children and adolescents and their families with or at risk for developing severe mental, behavioral, and emotional disturbances.

ACCESS TO COMMUNITY CARE AND EFFECTIVE SERVICES AND SUPPORTS (ACCESS)
Tests promising approaches to integrating treatment, housing, and support services for homeless persons with mental illnesses.

DUAL DIAGNOSIS TREATMENT DEMONSTRATION PROGRAM
Creates and evaluates effective treatment interventions for co-occurring substance abuse and serious mental illness in homeless adults through a collaboration with the Center for Substance Abuse Treatment (CSAT).

related programs and conducts several programs mandated by Congress. Some of these are listed in Box 24-1.

Just as mental health care has changed radically in the past 15 years, research into mental health services effectiveness has also come of age and contributed significantly to improvements in qual-

ity of care. The mental health community has documented the broad scope and effects of mental illness, the extent of treatment (and the gaps in treatment), and the fact that the efficacy of mental health treatment is generally equal to or superior to treatment efficacy in other sectors of health care as seen in Table 24-1 (NAMHC, 1993). For

NATIONAL RESOURCE CENTER ON HOMELESSNESS AND MENTAL ILLNESS

Develops and disseminates effective approaches to providing services and housing to homeless persons with mental illnesses.

PROJECTS FOR ASSISTANCE IN TRANSITION FROM HOMELESSNESS (PATH)

Provides a variety of treatment formula grant awards to the states for homeless people with mental illnesses and co-occurring substance abuse problems, including treatment, support services in residential settings, and coordination of services and housing.

COMMUNITY SUPPORT PROGRAM (CSP)

Works with states to improve treatment, housing, and support services for adults with severe mental illnesses to enable them to carry out daily living activities in their communities.

HIV/AIDS DEMONSTRATION PROGRAM

Provides mental health services for individuals, their families, and others who experience severe psychologic distress as a result of positive HIV antibody testing and those with HIV/AIDS.

MENTAL HEALTH STATISTICS IMPROVEMENT PROGRAM

Helps states to collect and analyze data on mental illnesses and to increase the comparability and utility of mental health statistics. Guidance and technical assistance are provided on the

design, structure, content, and use of information systems.

NATIONAL REPORTING PROGRAM

Provides the foundation and impetus for data-collection activities with a focus on services and organizations. Extensive statistical publications are produced including the recent *Mental Health, United States, 1994.*

PROTECTION AND ADVOCACY PROGRAM

Funds formula grants to states to develop programs that protect and advocate for the legal rights of people with mental illnesses and investigate incidents of abuse or neglect in facilities that care for or treat such individuals.

PREVENTION AND PROGRAM DEVELOPMENT

Provides information and technical assistance to public and private agencies wishing to improve mental health services delivery to special populations, including women, minority groups, and those residing in the criminal justice system and rural areas.

CHILDREN'S MENTAL HEALTH PUBLIC EDUCATION CAMPAIGN—CARING FOR EVERY CHILD'S MENTAL HEALTH: COMMUNITIES TOGETHER

Sponsors a 4-year national public education campaign to increase awareness about the emotional problems of children and adolescents and gain support for needed services.

example, studies of the efficacy of mental health treatment have established the effectiveness of care for various illnesses such as depression, anxiety, and schizophrenia, as well as the effectiveness of particular interventions, including pharmacotherapy, psychotherapy, family group treatments, and assertive community treatment.

24-1

PSYCHIATRIC TREATMENT EFFICACY

DISORDER	TREATMENT SUCCESS RATE (%)
Panic disorder	80
Bipolar disorder	80
Major depression	65
Schizophrenia	60
Obsessive-compulsive disorder	60
Cardiovascular treatments	
Atherectomy	52
Angioplasty	41

Mental health services research is designed to produce useful, actionable conclusions. It is intended to go beyond abstract discussions and to assertively participate in practice and policy by providing information that will eventually lead to improvements in the mental health of individuals, families, and communities. It is research that should be useful to individual mental health care consumers, purchasers of mental health care services, providers of mental health care, designers of mental health plans, and health care policy makers.

DEFINING MENTAL HEALTH
■ SERVICES RESEARCH

Research in mental health services is performed in response to stated or perceived needs for information to guide social action. It is more complex than laboratory research where methods are easily stated and variables such as temperature and chemical compounds can be accurately measured and specified. In contrast, in mental health services research, quality care is difficult to define and a challenge to measure, and the intervening variables are numerous and multifaceted.

As evident in Fig. 24-1, disciplinary research

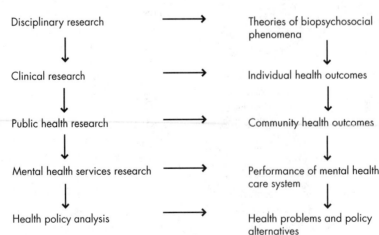

Figure 24-1 Comparison of mental health services research with other types of study.

is primarily concerned with the development and testing of theories to explain biopsychosocial phenomena. Clinical research is typically limited to health-related outcomes and predictors for individual patients, whereas public health research focuses on many of these same outcomes but does so at the level of populations in the community. In contrast, mental health services research applies the theories and methods that have evolved within these other areas of study to investigate problems related to the performance of the mental health care system. Mental health services research incorporates these knowledge bases but also more broadly acknowledges the array of nonmedical (social, economic, and organizational) factors that can affect the operation and outcomes of the mental health care system. Mental health services research also incorporates health program evaluation, which is concerned with assessing the effect of specific policies and programs (such as reimbursement mechanisms or consumer cost-sharing provisions) on a defined policy outcome of interest (such as cost containment). In fact, the evaluation of the implementation and effect of mental health care programs (such as assertive community treatment teams, multisystem therapy, or outreach efforts for rural populations) has been a major component of mental health services research (Brown et al., 1997; McDonel et al., 1997; Mowbray et al., 1997). To the extent that such evaluations are directed toward assessing specific policies or programs, they may provide direct input to related health policy analysis efforts (Bird et al., 1998). Finally, policy analysis draws upon the fund of knowledge generated by disciplinary, clinical, and mental health services research to clarify concerns about current policies (such as insurance coverage), compare new policy alternatives (such as mental health parity health insurance proposals), and make recommendations to national, state, and local decision makers.

Research Focus

Mental health services research produces knowledge about the performance of the mental health care system with respect to the objectives of effectiveness, efficiency, and equity (Aday et al., 1993) where:

1. *Effectiveness* concerns the benefits of mental health care measured by improvements in health;
2. *Efficiency* relates these health improvements to the resources required to produce them;
3. *Equity* assesses whether the benefits and burdens of mental health care are fairly distributed.

The effectiveness of mental health care concerns the benefits of care as measured by improvements in people's health. Improvements in health not only include the sum of the individual benefits (i.e., reduced mortality rates, increased life expectancies, and the decreased prevalence of disease) but also refer to more general indicators of quality of care, including increased economic productivity, enhanced well-being, and improved quality of life.

A second major objective of the mental health care delivery system is the drive for efficiency. When mental health care is viewed as an output, it is referred to as *production efficiency*, defined as producing services at least cost. An example of production efficiency is when a mental health program attempts to deliver the same level of services at lower cost by decreasing the overall number of staff or by substituting less qualified and less expensive staff for more qualified and more expensive staff (such as replacing psychiatric nurses with counselors or social workers). When mental health care is viewed as an input in the production of health improvements, it is referred to as *allocative efficiency,* defined as maximizing health given constrained resources. An example of allocative efficiency is the inclusion of routine screening for depression in a primary care practice. Allocative efficiency depends on the relative cost and effectiveness of mental health care in improving health. Ultimately, maximizing health requires both production and allocative efficiency.

Equity is concerned with adequate access and the fair distribution of the benefits and burdens (including the costs) of mental health care among groups or individuals. However, what is fair will differ depending on who is making the judgment and the values that person or group of people hold. For example, for some people the personal freedom to choose from several different options and to decide the kind of care they want without being dictated by anyone else is of utmost importance. Others would define fairness more in terms of the costs and outcomes for society as a whole: Is everyone being treated equally? Are those who need it most being helped? Is the well-being of society as a whole enhanced? Are the benefits on average for each person maximized? Clearly, one of the most difficult problems for contemporary American society lies in the enactment of mental health care equity in a political arena that is characterized by self-serving values, irrational prejudices, and conflicting ideologies.

There are two ways of relating the effectiveness, efficiency, and equity objectives. One is to attempt to determine which is a better criterion in evaluating the performance of the mental health care system. This is a value question that is subject to differing views of the nature of health care and the role of the mental health care system. As such, it has been suggested that this answer is perhaps best left to the political process. The second way is to observe how these objectives complement or conflict with each other in mental health research. For example, the three objectives are often complementary, as when improving mental health care effectiveness while holding resources constant increases efficiency, and increases in efficiency create opportunities for improved effectiveness and equity. However, the objectives may also be in conflict, as when maximizing effectiveness by allocating additional resources to improve mental health conflicts with efficiency if the cost of the resources is very high relative to their effectiveness. Also, maximizing effectiveness and efficiency by distributing resources to persons who would gain the most may be inequitable if the policy leads to a very uneven distribution. This can occur, for example, if a mental health care system decides to allocate most of its resources to persons with first episodes of acute psychiatric illness, knowing that rates of response and recovery will be high among this group, and in turn allocates few resources to services for the chronic and severely mentally ill where rates of response and recovery will be lower.

Thus identifying appropriate trade-offs among the three objectives is an important product of mental health services research. Assuming that all three are important objectives, a key question for decision makers in comparing policy alternatives is the degree to which one objective must be sacrificed to achieve the others.

Research Process

Mental health services research is inherently *inter-disciplinary* in focus. Its purpose is to develop more comprehensive knowledge that offers a better understanding of the research problem than any single discipline could develop alone (Kahn & Prager, 1994). It draws upon and applies theories and methods from an array of disciplines, including sociology, political science, epidemiology, demography, economics, law, medicine, nursing, and psychology among others. Each discipline, such as psychiatric-mental health nursing, views problems through the unique lens of the theories and conceptual models embedded in its particular field of study. Also, each discipline has associated methods commonly used in pursuit of disciplinary knowledge. Mental health services research benefits from bringing these diverse perspectives together to more fully analyze and understand the dimensions of complex research problems. Thus it offers a rich research opportunity for advanced practice registered nurses (APRNs) in psychiatric and mental health care. The process of this interdisciplinary teamwork has been summarized as one of development, maturation, and success (Kahn, 1993) and is highlighted in the example presented in Box 24-2.

Comparison with Policy Analysis

Research in mental health services resembles policy research in that it is performed in response to stated or perceived needs for information to guide social action. *Policy analysis* has been defined in terms of two principal objectives: (1) the production of information relevant to policy making, and (2) the development of reasonable arguments translating the information into recommendations for governmental action (Dunn, 1981). The distinction that has been drawn between mental health services research and policy analysis is that the first objective (the *production* of knowledge) defines the primary contributions of mental health services research and the second (the *application* of knowledge) represents the primary contributions of health policy analysis to governmental decision making (Aday et al., 1993).

The first objective most directly mirrors the goal of mental health services research that is concerned with generating knowledge about the implementation and effect of specific mental health programs and policies. The principal questions and issues addressed are factual or objective: to document the scope or origins of a problem and the probable effectiveness of alternatives for addressing it. The second objective extends beyond the role traditionally assumed by mental health services research. It attempts to justify the relevance of particular types of research, weigh the evidence, and construct a logical case to policy makers regarding the significance of a problem or the utility of specific programs or policies for addressing it. The primary emphasis is on providing a logical, well-documented rationale for evaluating the adequacy of existing policies and choosing one alternative over another in the light of the competing health policy goals of effectiveness, efficiency, and equity.

■ THEORETICAL MODELS

A core element of mental health research is the use of a theoretical or conceptual model. One model that is generally regarded as exemplary in the field has been developed by Barbara Starfield (1992). She proposes that every health care system has two main goals. The first is to optimize the health of the population by employing the most

---

box 24-2

BUILDING INTERDISCIPLINARY MENTAL HEALTH SERVICES RESEARCH TEAMS

In this article, Dr. Merwin, a psychiatric nurse researcher, describes the experience of developing an interdisciplinary research team to study the effects of using different combinations of registered nurses and unlicensed mental health workers on the outcomes of 1) length of inpatient stay, 2) percentage of patients readmitted to inpatient care shortly after discharge, 3) percentage of patients using emergency room care for psychiatric problems after discharge, 4) cost of care, and 5) percentage of patients discharged against medical advice. The creation of roles for research team members, the development of working relationships, and the evolution of additional research projects are discussed. Her recommendations for creating interdisciplinary research teams include the following:

- Recognize the different "cultures" of different disciplines, particularly as they relate to authorship rules, sharing of findings before publication, and style of writing.
- Clarify professional expectations and goals of team members before initiating the project.
- Use interpersonal relationship skills to promote open, clear communication, acknowledging different styles and approaches based on both personality and disciplinary training.
- Expect to make compromises as a preferred resolution strategy when dealing with such issues as ownership of data, supervision of research assistants, and choice of computer programming languages or software packages.
- Build on individual competencies and interests based upon each individual's background and area of expertise.
- Ensure that each team member maintains the ability to choose whether to participate in each new project, building on the concept of academic freedom which acknowledges the autonomy of the individual researcher.

From Merwin, 1995.

current knowledge about promoting health, treating illness, and minimizing disability. The second goal is to minimize the disparities across population subgroups to ensure equal access to health services and the ability to achieve optimal health outcomes. As such, each health services system has three main components: structural, process, and outcome (Donabedian, 1966). The components have been conceptualized in a variety of ways (Mitchell, Ferketich, & Jennings, 1998). Fig. 24-2 shows the components and elements that comprise each one as identified by Starfield.

Structure of a Health Services System

The component of structure allows the system to provide services. Structure describes the "setting in which medical care takes place and the instrumentalities of which it is the product" (Donabedian, 1966). Structural elements involve both capital and operating expenses, as well as expenditures by patients of time and money to use the mental health system. Structural factors have been the focus of most evaluations of mental health services and usually have been the basis for estab-

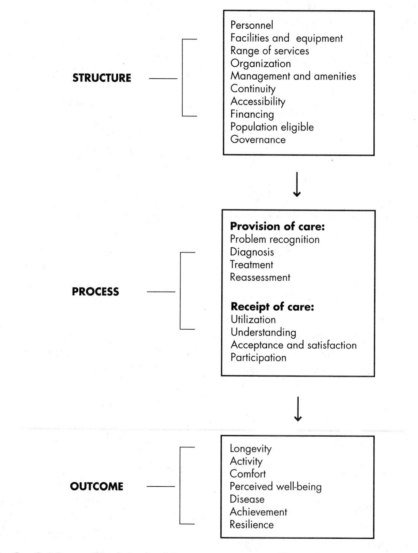

Figure 24-2 Starfield's model of the health services system. (From Starfield, B. [1992]. *Primary care: concept, evaluation and policy.* Oxford, England: Oxford University Press.)

lishing standards of care, even though there is often little support for their validity. For example, assertions are made about specific nurse-patient ratios required for "good" nursing care, and the fact that "sound" record-keeping reflects quality care.

There are ten main structural elements:

1. *Personnel.* Those involved in providing the services, their education, and their training.

2. *Facilities and equipment.* The buildings (e.g., hospitals, clinics, or health centers) and offices, as well as the physical components of the facilities (e.g., laboratory instruments and technology for diagnosis or therapy).

3. *Range of services provided by facilities.* This range of services may vary from community to community, but every facility has made decisions about what kinds of services will be available and what will not be available. The range of services provided is an important consideration in recent demonstrations of integrated mental health delivery systems for children and the severely mentally ill.

4. *Organization of services.* Do the personnel work in groups or alone? What are the mechanisms for ensuring accountability, and who is responsible for providing the different aspects of care?

5. *Management and amenities, including characteristics of services other than those directly related to clinical care.* Are laboratory results reported in a timely fashion? Are patients treated with courtesy and respect?

6. *Mechanisms for providing continuity of care.* Continuity is usually provided in the form of practitioners or teams of practitioners who serve as the primary contact for the patient (such as case managers), but sometimes the only mechanism for continuity is some form of written record.

7. *Mechanisms for providing access to care.* There is no point to having personnel, facilities, and equipment if they cannot be reached by persons who need them. There are several types of accessibility: accessibility in time (the hours of availability such as evenings and weekends), geographic accessibility (adequacy of transportation and distance to be covered), and psychosocial accessibility (language and cultural facilitators or barriers to communication between personnel in the facilities and patients).

8. *Arrangements for financing.* What is the method of payment for services, and how are the personnel remunerated for their work? Of all of the structural features, this is the most likely to differ across countries and is therefore of great interest for cross-national comparative studies.

9. *Delineation of the population eligible to receive services.* Each unit of the mental health services system should be able to define the community it serves and should know its important sociodemographic and health characteristics. Members of the population should be able to identify their source of care and be aware of its responsibility for providing required services. This structural feature is a critical element for mental health care, especially for vulnerable populations such as children, the elderly, and the severely mentally ill.

10. *Governance of the health system.* Health systems differ in their accountability to those they serve. Often they do not involve the consumers of mental health services in decisions about the way services are organized or delivered. Sometimes community councils serve in an advisory capacity, but seldom is responsibility for organizational governance and decision-making shared or assumed by the community boards of mental health delivery systems.

Processes of a Health Services System

The component of *process* includes the activities of both the health care provider as well as the patient, consumer, or recipient of care. Providers must first recognize the needs existing in both the community and individual patients. This feature is knows as *problem (or needs) recognition.* The problem may be a symptom, sign, abnormal laboratory test, previous but relevant item in the history of the patient or the community, or need for an indicated preventive procedure. After recognizing the problem, the health professional generally formulates a *diagnosis*. This is necessary to move to the next step in the process of care, which is implementing an appropriate strategy for *treatment and management*. After that, the provider must allow for *reassessment* of the problem to determine if the original recognition of the problem, diagnosis, and treatment regimen were adequate. At this point, the process of care is started on a new cycle of monitoring and surveillance, with recognition of the problems as they currently exist.

The processes of care that reflect how people interact with the health system are also important. First, people decide whether and when to *utilize* the mental health care system. If they do use it, they come to an *understanding* of what providers offer them. They then decide whether they will accept the providers' recommendations and the extent to which they will *participate* in the treatment process. Specifically, they can decide to comply and carry through with the provider's recommendations, to modify them in ways they see fit, or to disregard them partly or completely. Finally they decide how *satisfied* they are with their care. Theoretically, effective care should result when appropriate care is given by the provider (correct problem recognition, diagnosis, treatment, and reassessment) in partnership with the patient, who uses, accepts, understands, and complies and is satisfied with treatment recommendations.

Outcome of Care in the Health Services System

The component of outcome is the ultimate test of a health care system, and it includes the various indicators of health status. There are many ways to consider outcome of care. Starfield's conceptualization is focused on the individual level of analysis and identifies seven components of health status:

- *Longevity*. The most common measure of health status, especially at the population level, is longevity, or life expectancy, and its converse, mortality. An important characteristic of the health of individuals is their life expectancy; the average life expectancy in a population is an important descriptor of the health status of a nation. Mental health care systems influence life expectancy, which is also affected by such other determinants as genetic structure, the social and physical environment, and personal behaviors.
- *Activity*. The second component of health status is the nature of activity of the individual or population. Relevant qualities include those pertaining to the kinds of disability that affect the individual and, on the population level, the proportion of the population that can carry on with normal activities.
- *Comfort*. This includes pain, distress, or other physical and emotional sensations that interfere with work and pleasure.
- *Perceived well-being and satisfaction*. This characteristic connotes how people view their own health and the extent to which they are satisfied with it.
- *Disease*. This involves the presence of conditions recognized as potentially or actually interfering with the well-being of individuals or the population; it includes mental as well as physical pathology.
- *Achievement*. This reflects the positive aspects of health that must be considered in achieving what the World Health Organization (WHO) has defined as "a state of well-being." Achievement signifies the level of development or accomplishment and the potential for future development of better health.
- *Resilience*. This characteristic of health also pertains to a state of well-being. It refers to the ability to cope with adversity and measures the potential for resisting a range of possible threats to health. Ability to respond constructively to stress may be measured by physiologic techniques, psychologic techniques, or evidence that certain defenses known to increase resistance are present or have been provided. The

prototype of biologic resilience is the state of being appropriately immunized against preventable diseases. A second measure of resilience is the attainment of certain nutritional standards. A third measure is the performance of certain health behaviors known to reduce the likelihood of disease, an example of which is stress management.

Unit of Study

The structure, process, and outcomes of medical care can be studied at either the micro level (individual patient, provider or institutional) or the macro level (system or community). An exclusive focus on one level of analysis may fail to acknowledge the existence or consequences of the other. For example, commitments to developing medical technologies or procedures to optimize individual patient outcomes may fail to consider whether these are the best investments to enhance the health and well-being of the population as a whole. On the other hand, a macro-level look at aggregate indicators of health status (suicide rates in the elderly) and measures of system performance (undetected rates of depression in the elderly) may fail to appreciate fully the underlying role that personal lifestyle practices (drinking), social behavior (elder abuse), and attitudes (negative perceptions about growing old in American society) play in affecting individuals' health status.

Specifically, different images of effectiveness emerge when viewed through macro-level lenses focusing on changes in the *population's* health compared with a micro-level look at outcomes for individual *patients*. Also, the production efficiency of individual health care providers does not necessarily lead to allocative efficiency in the health care marketplace. Finally, yardsticks of fairness may be applied in assessing the extent to which either individual institutions (hospitals or clinics) or the delivery system as a whole measure up in terms of the equity objective. Thus a truly inclusive theoretical model for engaging in mental health services research would expand upon Starfield's conceptualization and include the macro-

level aspects of health policy, effectiveness, efficiency, and equity as components of structure, process, and outcome, since these elements reflect the social context in which mental health services research is imbedded. The expanded model, as seen in Fig. 24-3, now allows for research on the many factors and relationships affecting health care.

In summary, a theoretical framework for engaging in mental health services research, whether it focuses on the individual, the community, or the entire population, should take into account at least some aspects of the structure, process, and outcome of the mental health delivery system. Although it is true that studies that consider a combination of these elements are not easily accomplished, they should be of high priority because they are likely to illuminate the mechanisms by which mental health care influences health status.

■ RESEARCH METHODS

There are many different methods associated with mental health services research. However, given the complex issues facing the field, most research questions cannot be addressed by relying on a single method. Mental health services research designs have to be flexible and innovative in order to examine the full scale of contemporary problems. The multimethod approach appears to be an effective response because it is capable of combining different methods in ways that offset strengths and weaknesses against each other, producing a multilayered analysis. Some of the types of research methods commonly used in the field are described in this section.

Types of Research

Descriptive research. Health policy and planning require a sound understanding of the current health status of populations and their relevant social groupings. This entails mental health research focused on analyzing the general population and specific individuals or groups within it, which is most commonly provided through de-

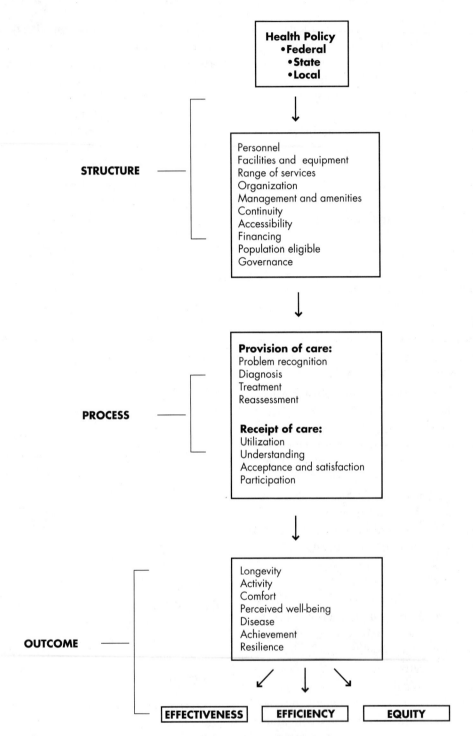

Figure 24-3 Expanded model for health services research.

scriptive research. In the health arena, epidemiologic research tends to fulfill this function, and descriptive epidemiologic research is often used to make choices in setting policy objectives and strategic targets.

Explanatory research. The distinction between explanatory research as providing explanations for patterns of health and disease and the descriptive type as discussed previously is one of gradation. In explanatory research, however, examination of the factors underlying patterning is the primary objective. For example, research concerned with the inequalities of mental health care focuses on explaining the reasons for inequalities and how inequality manifests itself in health and disease, whereas research influenced by anthropology attempts to illuminate the cultural factors in the epidemiology of mental illness. Explanations of patterns of health and illness within and between social groups are complex, depending on an interplay of variables that are environmental, economic, social, cultural, and psychologic. The relevance of this type of detailed and multifaceted research lies in posing the question as to whether mental health services are responsive to the needs of populations and individuals and whether mental health services are taking into account potential inequalities in services received.

Strategic research. *Strategy* can be defined as a pattern in a stream of decisions or as a pattern in a stream of actions. As a result, strategic research has either concerned itself with the concept of decision and the outcomes of decision or with the links and discontinuities between decision and implementation. Decision modeling and meta-analysis are some examples of strategic research (Adams, Freeman, & Lewis, 1996). Decision modeling attempts to structure problems of decision making under terms of uncertainty. It often results in the formulation of decision trees, which when clinically focused are also called *treatment algorithms*. A decision tree describes the major factors involved in decision making and are widely used to model screening and testing decisions.

---

box 24-3

EVALUATING META-ANALYSIS REVIEW ARTICLES

1. Were the questions and methods clearly stated?
2. Were comprehensive search methods used to locate the relevant studies?
3. Were explicit methods used to determine which articles were included in the review?
4. Was the methodologic quality of the primary studies assessed?
5. Were the selection and assessment of the primary studies reproducible and free from bias?
6. Were the differences in individual study results adequately explained?
7. Were the results of the primary studies combined appropriately?
8. Were the reviewers' conclusions supported by the data cited?

From Adams, Freeman, & Lewis, 1996.

Meta-analysis is the quantitative synthesis of the results of a systematic overview of previous studies. Systematic overviews are a way of collating and synthesizing all the available evidence on a particular scientific question, often resulting in an overall estimation of the effectiveness of a particular treatment. This is done by performing a stratified analysis of the results of available studies and weighing the studies so that the larger, more statistically powerful studies are given more weight. The validity of such a quantitative approach, however, rests upon the method with which the studies have been selected and the completeness of the evidence in the systematic review. Questions that nurses who read meta-analysis review articles should ask are listed in Box 24-3. Although meta-analyses are difficult to undertake, there is clear acceptance of this research method as a way of investigating the effectiveness of interventions in the field of mental health. This endeavor has been facilitated by the establishment of the Cochrane Center in 1992 in Oxford England, which produces systematic reviews of research on all aspects of health care. This initiative has now developed into the Cochrane Collaboration (Box 24-4), which is an international network with centers in Australia, Canada, Denmark, Italy, the Netherlands, the United Kingdom, and the United States. The Cochrane Collaboration is also discussed in Chapter 22.

An extension of strategic research is the so-called *future scenarios research*, which is a way of identifying key mechanisms that will affect the development of a particular field in the mid to longer-term future. Markov models, for example,

---

Box 24-4

THE COCHRANE COLLABORATION

MISSION STATEMENT

The Cochrane Collaboration is an international organization that aims to help people make well-informed decisions about health care by preparing, maintaining, and promoting the accessibility of systematic reviews of the effects of health care interventions. It is a not-for-profit organization.

PRINCIPLES

The Cochrane Collaboration's work is based on eight key principles:

- *Collaboration* by internally and externally fostering good communications, open decision making, and teamwork.
- *Building on the enthusiasm of individuals* by involving and supporting people of different skills and backgrounds.
- *Avoiding duplication* by good management and coordination to maximize economy of effort.
- *Minimizing bias* through a variety of approaches such as scientific rigor, ensuring broad participation, and avoiding conflicts of interest.
- *Keeping up to date* by a commitment to ensure that Cochrane Reviews are maintained through identification and incorporation of new evidence.
- *Striving for relevance* by promoting the assessment of health care interventions using outcomes that matter to people making choices in health care.

- *Promoting access* by wide dissemination of the outputs of the Collaboration, taking advantage of strategic alliances, and promoting appropriate prices, content, and media to meet the needs of users worldwide.
- *Ensuring quality* by being open and responsive to criticism, applying advances in methodology, and developing systems for quality improvement.

THE COCHRANE LIBRARY

This is the main output of the Collaboration, updated quarterly and distributed on an annual subscription basis on disk, CD-ROM, and via the Internet. Several databases are included in *The Cochrane Library*. One of them, *The Cochrane Database of Systematic Reviews*, contains Cochrane reviews, and another, *The Cochrane Controlled Trials Register*, is a bibliographic database of controlled trials. The *Database of Abstracts of Reviews of Effectiveness* (DARE) includes structured abstracts of systematic reviews, and *The Cochrane Review Methodology Database* is a bibliography of articles on the science of research synthesis. Three review groups that may be of particular interest to APRNs:

- Dementia and Cognitive Impairment Group
- Depression, Anxiety, and Neurosis Group
- Schizophrenia Group.

From Chalmers, 1993.

are used to predict the long-term outcomes of treatment (Keeler, 1995). These models are a technique for analyzing events that repeat, such as mental health treatment, or events that play out over a long period of time, such as the progression of severe mental illness. They are simple and powerful tools since they allow one to assess the outcome implications of data-based or hypothetical transition probabilities. The future scenario approach can also explicitly link itself with policy making because one of its aims is to lay the foundation for long-term policy. The consequences of the scenarios are worked out in terms of organizational impact, policy control, financing, information systems, expertise, and effectiveness. These are then extrapolated to the full public health territory before drawing final conclusions that are to inform policy decisions. This type of strategic research directly attempts to influence its use at a high level of decision making and policy analysis.

Evaluation research. Evaluation is a complex exercise, which not only includes assessing outcome and effects, but can also be concerned with understanding the nature and variability of implementation, barriers to implementation, or unanticipated effects. An example of a psychiatric nursing outcome study conducted in England (Gournay & Brooking, 1994, 1995) is presented in Box 24-5. However, not all evaluation research succeeds in capturing this complexity, and as a result it often fails to make an effect on policy makers and managers. Evaluation research has a better chance to be used if it is considered as an integral part of the development process and serves as a feedback loop for decision making. Evaluative study designs can be broadly grouped into three kinds (Wing, 1996):

- Clinical audits that compare clinical procedures for individual patients against normative standards such as clinical guidelines or peer review
- Monitoring that involves routine or special collection of data that can subsequently be used as part of comparative hypothesis-testing, although with less control over key variables
- Focused research that uses quasi-experimental

---

box 24-5

RANDOMIZED CONTROLLED TRIAL OF COMMUNITY PSYCHIATRIC NURSING IN PRIMARY CARE

This study was carried out in six health centers in North London with a total of 36 general practitioners (GPs) and 11 community psychiatric nurses (CPNs). Using a randomized controlled trial, 177 patients were randomly allocated to continuing GP care or to two conditions of community psychiatric nursing intervention (one immediate, a second occurring after a 12-week waitlist period). A range of measures for symptoms and social function were used, and ratings were carried out at assessment in 24 weeks. Although patients improved on all measures, over time there was no difference between the group of patients receiving GP care and patients seen by the CPN. Improvements seemed to be independent of the amount of contact. Dropout rates from CPN intervention were high (50%). CPN dropouts were more disabled to start with but did as well as CPN treatment completers. There was no evidence that referral to a CPN saved GP time. An economic analysis showed that patients receiving CPN intervention experienced less absence from work, and this resulted in a benefit. However, the cost per quality adjusted life year by intervening with this group of patients was several times more than for intervening with the seriously mentally ill. The researchers concluded that if one considers both the clinical and economic results of the study taken with other evidence from the literature, there seemed to be little justification for CPNs continuing to work in this area.

---

or experimental comparisons to test specific hypotheses.

A significant part of this last type of focused evaluation research is the emergence of outcomes research. Outcomes can be either positive or negative, ranging from complete health to death. With the increasing emphasis on effectiveness and efficiency, there is strong pressure to further develop and apply outcomes research that can inform both clinical and health policy decision making. Three of the main types of outcome studies that occur in psychiatric research, all of which are designed to improve patients' health through better clinical care, are as follows (Kashner, Rush, & Altshuler, 1997):

- *Efficacy studies* to determine if a treatment developed in the basic sciences will work in a controlled clinical setting when used by an expert for subjects who meet scientific disease criteria.

- *Effectiveness studies* to determine what works in actual clinical care settings, on whom, and under what circumstances. There are many reasons why treatments shown to be efficacious in the laboratory (i.e., in efficacy studies) may not work in actual clinical practice. For instance, clinicians may not properly understand the treatment, or patients may fail to comply with it. Effectiveness studies explore the feasibility that new procedures will be accepted by practicing clinicians and patients.

- *Cost studies* measure the value society assigns to the health resources that, in turn, are used to produce medical products. Resources include the professional's time, other staff time, supplies, administrative activities and support, equipment, office and building space, and building maintenance. Medical products include procedures, activities, home and outpatient visits, inpatient days, and other health care products that are intended to help patients.

Efficacy studies imply that clinical strategies can achieve their stated goal of improving clinical outcomes when used in optimal circumstances. *Effectiveness studies* require evidence that the clinical strategy does more good than harm when used in the specific clinical circumstance applicable to a particular patient. The major difference, therefore, between efficacy and effectiveness is the difference in both the type of patient to which the clinical

strategy would be applied and the nature of the system delivering care. Most clinical studies, particularly randomized controlled trials (RCTs), demonstrate efficacy rather than effectiveness because they apply the therapy to a narrow spectrum of homogeneous patients and deliver care in a very controlled fashion, both of which optimize the chances of demonstrating benefit. Nonetheless, RCTs are the "gold standard" method in terms of internal validity (Detsky, 1995). Whether the results of a study supporting the efficacy of a particular intervention are applicable to other patients in other more naturalistic health care settings is a matter that often requires judgment concerning generalizability or external validity. Sometimes in mental health services research, evidence from RCTs is supplemented by evidence from other studies using nonexperimental designs that occasionally involve large administrative databases (such as Medicare or Medicaid). At the present time, however, there is no standard approach to integrating information aimed at maximizing the internal validity or efficacy of RCTs with that aimed at establishing external validity.

In fact, outcome evaluations and audits are relatively rare in psychiatry. A substantial expansion in epidemiologically based, naturalistic, observational, structure-process-outcome data collection in routine psychiatric practice is essential to identify treatment allocation biases and reasons for expected and unexpected outcomes. Identified causes of undertreatment can then lead to detailed clinical guidelines. Similarly, experimental evaluation should take place in routine clinical practice settings, with change in structure, process, and outcome as the objective. Ultimately, the results of both experimental and observational outcome studies on service users should converge, permitting outcomes to be the ultimate indicator of quality (Brugha & Lindsay, 1996).

Finally, *cost studies* are of four types and these are described in Box 24-6. Although cost studies are an important aspect of mental health services research, one must carefully consider whether, in fact, a cost analysis is needed. Before selecting a

box 24-6

TYPES OF COST STUDIES

1. *Cost-effectiveness studies.* The evaluation of alternatives according to both their costs and their effects with regard to producing some outcome or set of outcomes.
2. *Cost-benefit studies.* The evaluation of alternatives according to a comparison of both their costs and benefits when each is measured in monetary terms.
3. *Cost-utility studies.* The evaluation of alternatives according to a comparison of their costs and the estimated utility or value of their outcomes. Both cost-benefit and cost-effectiveness approaches require specific types of quantitative data to implement their evaluations. In contrast, cost-utility analysis permits a wide range of qualitative and quantitative data to inform the decisions. However, the subjective nature of such analyses often limits their value.
4. *Cost-feasibility studies.* The estimation of only the costs of an alternative to determine whether it can be considered. That is, if the cost of an alternative exceeds the budget and other resources that are available, then there is no point in doing further analysis.

From Levin, 1983.

particular cost analysis technique, it is important to go through the following procedure (Levin, 1983):

1. A formal identification of the problem
2. Consideration and selection of alternatives to be analyzed
3. Recognition of one's audience and their needs
4. Selection of appropriate modes of analysis
5. Discussion of feasibility of conducting the analysis
6. Assessing whether results are likely to be worthwhile

Given the limits on resources, it is not surprising that research on the cost-effectiveness of health care is in great demand. The cost-effectiveness analysis framework has been suggested as appropriate to help with resource allocation decisions involving the delivery of nursing care and improving the overall quality of clinical care (Stone, 1998). While in the past nursing research has not emphasized cost-effectiveness research, the time has come for nurses to take a more active role in this area (Allred et al., 1998; Siegel, 1998). Nurses are particularly well positioned to evaluate health care practices and contribute to the dialog about their value. Perhaps, most importantly, cost-effective research studies of nursing interventions can demonstrate the value of nursing as compared with other uses of society's health care resources.

Developmental research. Research using a developmental approach is geared toward advancing the discussion and implementation of service provision models. It focuses on assessing the application of theory to practice and assists in remodeling particular approaches by a critical analysis of the interpretation and achievement of objectives. This type of research builds on a dialog between researchers and policy makers. By its very nature, developmental research is used almost immediately. Precisely because of these characteristics the potential value of the research is great. It can serve to advance discussions between the different parties involved in the implementation of mental health care in the community. On one hand, it pushes back the boundaries of knowledge; on the other hand, it remains in close contact with current practice, which means that the research can form the bridge between the present and the future.

Methodologic research. The complexity of health services management, coupled with the wide range of problems faced in health and disease, often leads to the realization that current research methods are inadequate in solving contemporary issues. Methodologic research attempts to fill this void by testing new methods. Its distinction from fundamental scientific research is that the need to search for new methods is prompted by the policy or management agenda, and close collaboration between decision makers and researchers is crucial if this type of methodologic work is to be used.

A key area for methodologic research is in the area of needs assessment (Thornicroft, Phelan, & Strathdee, 1996). No established methods exist, in large part because "need" has been variously defined. One's definition in part depends on who is defining need—the consumer, the provider, or the payer. Also, need can be broadly seen as holistic health and autonomy or as the more narrow ability to benefit from health care. Depending on the theoretical underpinnings of the concept of need, methods have ranged from relying on a formal, standardized, and objective measurement of need using tools that are validated and tested, to more contextual and subjective descriptions by those "in need." The pattern that seems to be emerging is one that combines the formal and informal assessment of need, and there is some acknowledgment that there is no methodologic consensus. Clearly, the science of measuring need is underdeveloped, and there is a search for methods in the field of mental health services research that are scientifically grounded and provide results that can be translated into policy and strategic decision making.

IMPLICATIONS FOR ■ THE FUTURE

For APRNs interested in mental health services research, this could be the best of times. Major experimentation in health and social programs, such as in Medicaid and Medicare, coupled with unprecedented levels of change in health care markets create the opportunity for a wide range of research questions and initiatives related to what works, what does not work, and how current mental health delivery systems can be improved. However, if psychiatric nurse researchers and others do not rise to this challenge, it could be the worst of times. The need is to conduct studies that lead to useful, actionable conclusions, to go beyond

abstract discussions and obscure investigations and aggressively participate in practice and policy by providing information that will lead to improvements in the mental health of populations.

The dangers are many. One is that there is a tendency in the research community to re-prove what is already known, as in studies showing that people who are without health insurance have poorer health outcomes or that the seriously mentally ill dominate the lower socioeconomic groups. Another danger is that the research community sometimes studies things that seem to have little practical value, such as studies with interventions that are so complex, impractical, or expensive that they cannot possibly be implemented in real service delivery settings. A final danger is that researchers may focus on obscure issues that have nothing to contribute to those problems that matter most to public and private decision makers, consumers, and payers. The bottom line, therefore, is that mental health services research has to produce useful research, and the results of the research need to be translated into forms that can be easily understood and used in policy and practice arenas.

Future challenges for mental health services research loom large and embrace issues that are intellectual, informational, financial, clinical, and political in nature (Ginzberg, 1991). Perhaps the most basic challenge to the field is that mental health services research is only recently emerging as an academic discipline and it suffers from problems shared by other fields that are interdisciplinary in nature. The fact remains that academia is likely to remain discipline-centered, and few researchers in the field, including psychiatric nurse researchers, have received a doctorate in health services research. Thus the field must attract and retain investigators from other disciplines. Furthermore, mental health services research does not fit easily into the existing academic establishment. Health services research programs may be located in medical schools, schools of public health, or policy centers, as well as in other academic subdivisions, although at this time, none are known to exist in schools of nursing. Finding a safe and appropriate niche within the discipline-bound academic environment clearly presents a major challenge for supporting this type of research activity.

There is broad agreement within the health services research community that another problem for the field is the lack of adequate databases. Although model building is possible in the absence of data, model testing is not. Significant advances can be made if there can be agreement in the field as to the types of data that need to be collected and a universal system for collecting them. While the design and implementation of mechanisms for collecting data, organizing them for use, and making them readily accessible in the mental health services community still lie in the future, it is an essential task if mental health services research is to realize its potential.

Another issue for the field lies in the financial arena. Funding for mental health services research has been stimulated by the NIMH and facilitated by congressional enactment of a 15% set-aside for such research within the NIMH budget. The developing momentum for services research has led to such projects as the Patient Outcomes Research Teams (PORTs) on illnesses such as schizophrenia and new research centers at a number of academic institutions and in the public sector. More recent research is being performed in the research departments of managed care organizations and pharmaceutical companies. However, as the momentum for mental health services research has grown, so has the competition for NIMH grants. It is now estimated that only 10% to 20% of services research grant applications are successful. This number is comparable with other areas of NIMH-funded research, although it is lower than the 30% to 31% success rates of the NIH. In addition, although the FY99 budget proposal gives the NIH an increase of more than $1 billion ($702 million of which will go toward investigating the causes of and treatment for mental illness), no increase was proposed for the Center for Mental Health Services. Thus there has been federal resistance to appropriating substantial sums of money for better data systems, training grants for young health services investigators, and research focused on service delivery rather than basic science.

Another concern is clinical in nature, as evident by the wide gaps that exist between the demonstrated efficacy of mental health treatments and their effectiveness seen in that which is provided as "usual care." Despite advances, the field lacks definitive evidence linking specific interventions with specific stages in the course of different psychiatric illnesses. Additionally, relatively less is known about mental health promotion and mental illness prevention. Potentially, however, these last areas may result in the greatest gains related to mental health care. A related challenge arises from the rapidly changing mental health care landscape, which is driven in large part by the increased use of managed care strategies and by federal efforts to reduce the deficit by decreasing spending for Medicare and Medicaid. Because Medicaid finances 30% to 50% of community mental health services, the increased use of HMOs to provide all Medicaid health care and the increased use of carve-out Medicaid managed care approaches in mental health are significant trends. Specifically, there are many concerns about the effects of managed care on the clinical care of persons with psychiatric and mental health problems (see discussion in Chapter 2).

A final challenge for the field is that the findings from mental health services research may not have the effect they could have on policy formulations because of the vast array and competing agendas of special interest groups, political lobbies, and the media, as well as other participants. The American health care sector is characterized by great scope and diversity in the number of parties involved in the financing, provision, and control of mental health care services, and one of the realities of mental health services research is that it often illuminates unpleasant realities that are often seen as the enemy rather than the ally of progress. Clearly, mental health services research cannot resolve issues of values, public need, resource allocation, economic revenues, or the like. It can, however, point the way to initial steps that may improve the mental health of people in a constrained fiscal and social environment.

In spite of these challenges, mental health services research has demonstrated its capacity to make important and continuing contributions to the improved understanding of how the mental health delivery system operates and how it can be made to perform more effectively, efficiently, and equitably for the benefit of individuals, families, and groups. Thus advances in the field have set the stage for future work as new knowledge and changes in the organization of mental health service delivery are leading to considerable interest in using mental health services research as an important and powerful tool in improving treatment outcomes and the quality of mental health care.

RESOURCES AND CONNECTIONS

JOURNALS

Journal of Behavioral Health Services and Research

WEBSITES

Agency for Health Care Policy & Research (AHCPR) www.ahcpr.gov
American College of Mental Health Administration www.acmha.org
Association for Health Services Research www.ahsr.org
Centers for Disease Control & Prevention (CDC) www.cdc.gov
Center for Mental Health Services (CMHS) www.samhsa.gov/cmhs/cmhs.htm
Cochrane Collaboration www.cochrane.org
General Accounting Office (GAO) www.gao.gov
Health Care Financing Administration (HCFA)—The Medicare/Medicaid Agency www.hcfa.gov
Internet Grateful Med igm.nlm.nih.gov

National Institutes of Health (NIH)—Guide to Grants and Contracts Database www.med.nyu.edu/nih-guide.html
National Institute of Mental Health (NIMH) gopher.nimh.nih.gov
Knowledge Exchange Network (KEN) www.mentalhealth.org
Substance Abuse & Mental Health Services Administration (SAMHSA) www.samhsa.gov

References

Aday, L.A., et al. (1993). *Evaluating the medical care system: effectiveness, efficiency and equity.* Ann Arbor, MI: Health Administration Press.

Adams, C., Freeman, N., & Lewis, G. (1996). Meta-analysis. In Knudsen, H.C., & Thornicroft, G. (Eds.). *Mental health service evaluation.* Cambridge, UK: Cambridge University Press.

Allred, C., et al. (1998). Cost-effectiveness analysis in the nursing literature, 1992-1996. *Image: Journal of Nursing Scholarship, 30*(3), 235–242.

Anderson, O.W. (1991). *The evolution of health services research: personal reflections on applied social science.* San Francisco: Jossey-Bass.

Bird, D.C., et al. (1998). Rural models for integrating primary care and mental health services. *Administration and Policy in Mental Health, 25*(3), 287–308.

Brown, L.D. (1991). Knowledge and power: health services research as a political resource. In Ginzberg, E. (Ed.). *Health services research: key to health policy.* Cambridge, MA: Harvard University Press.

Brown, T.L., et al. (1997). Multisystemic treatment of violent and chronic juvenile offenders: bridging the gap between research and practice. *Administration and Policy in Mental Health, 25*(2), 221–238.

Brugha, T. S., & Lindsay, F. (1996). Quality of mental health service care: the forgotten pathway from process to outcome. *Social Psychiatry and Psychiatric Epidemiology, 31*, 89–98.

Chalmers, I. (1993). The Cochrane Collaboration: preparing, maintaining and disseminating systematic reviews of the effects of health care. In Warren, K.S., & Mosteller, F. (Eds.). Doing more good than harm: the evaluation of health care interventions. *Annals of the New York Academy of Science, 703*, 156–163.

Detsky, A.S. (1995). Evidence of effectiveness: evaluating its quality. In Sloan, F.A. (Ed.). *Valuing health care: cost, benefits, and effectiveness of pharmaceuticals and other medical technologies.* New York: Cambridge University Press.

Donabedian, A. (1966). Evaluating the quality of medical care. *Milbank Memorial Fund Quarterly, 44*(3), 166–206.

Dunn, W.N. (1981). *Public policy analysis.* Englewood Cliffs, NJ: Prentice-Hall.

Ginzberg, E. (1991). *Health services research: key to health policy.* Cambridge, MA: Harvard University Press.

Gournay, K., & Brooking, J. (1994). Community psychiatric nurses in primary health care. *British Journal of Psychiatry, 165,* 231–238.

Gournay, K., & Brooking, J. (1995). The community psychiatric nurse in primary health care: an economic analysis. *Journal of Advanced Nursing, 22,* 769–778.

Kahn, R.L. (1993). *An experiment in scientific organizations (MacArthur Foundation occasional paper).* Chicago, IL: MacArthur Foundation.

Kahn, R.L., & Prager, D.L. (1994). Interdisciplinary collaborations are a scientific and social imperative. *The Scientist, 8*(14), 12.

Kashner, T.M., Rush, A.J., & Altshuler, K.Z. (1997). Managed care and the focus on outcomes research. *Journal of Practical Psychiatry and Behavioral Health, 3*(3), 135

Keeler, E. (1995). Decision trees and Markov models in cost-effectiveness research. In Sloan, F.A. (Ed.). *Valuing health care: cost, benefits, and effectiveness of pharmaceuticals and other medical technologies.* New York: Cambridge University Press.

Levin, H.M. (1983). *Cost-effectiveness: a primer.* Newbury Park: Sage Publications.

McDonel, E.C., et al. (1997). Implementing assertive community treatment programs in rural settings. *Administration and Policy in Mental Health, 25*(2), 153–173.

Merwin, E. (1995). Building interdisciplinary mental health service research teams. *Issues in Mental Health Nursing, 16,* 547–554.

Mitchell, P.H., Ferketich, S., & Jennings, B.M. (1998). Quality health outcomes model. *Image: Journal of Nursing Scholarship, 30*(1), 43–46.

Mowbray, C.T., et al. (1997). Harbinger. I: the development and evaluation of the first pact replication. *Administration and Policy in Mental Health, 25*(2), 105–123.

National Advisory Mental Health Council. (1993). Healthcare reform for Americans with severe mental illness: report of the Advisory Mental Health Council. *American Journal of Psychiatry, 150,* 1447.

Roper, W.L. (1997). The new environment for health services research: private and public sector opportunities. *Health Services Research, 32*(5), 549–556.

Siegel, J. (1998). Cost-effectiveness analysis and nursing research—is there a fit? *Image: Journal of Nursing Scholarship, 30*(3), 221–222.

Starfield, B. (1992). *Primary care: concept, evaluation and policy.* Oxford, England: Oxford University Press.

Stone, P. (1998). Methods for conducting and reporting cost-effectiveness analysis in nursing. *Image: Journal of Nursing Scholarship, 30*(3), 229–234.

Thornicroft, G., Phelan, M., & Strathdee, G. (1996). Needs assessment. In Knudsen, H.C., & Thornicroft, G. (Eds.). *Mental health service evaluation.* Cambridge, UK: Cambridge University Press.

Wing, J. (1996). Research designs for the evaluation of services. In Knudsen, H.C., & Thornicroft, G. (Eds.). *Mental health service evaluation.* Cambridge, UK: Cambridge University Press.

Envisioning the Future in Mental Health Care

LUC R. PELLETIER, ELIZABETH C. POSTER, CAROLE A. SHEA,
GAIL W. STUART, and MARILYN P. VERHEY

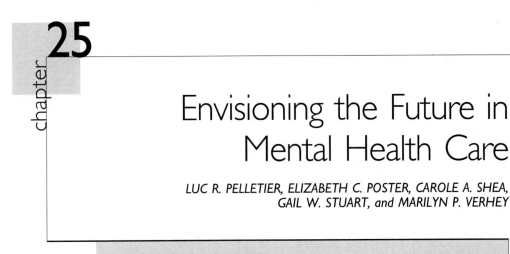

■ INTRODUCTION

The future of advanced practice nursing is bright and expansive if advanced practice registered nurses (APRNs) seize the opportunities and do so together as part of a strategic, organized initiative. For future success, strength in numbers cannot be overemphasized since the necessary strategies will rely on consensus about direction and a pooling of advanced practice nursing resources. In conceptualizing and developing this book, the edi-

tors examined pages of manuscripts and reviewed source documents. They became intimately familiar with current state-of-the-art products and procedures regarding the health care environment, clinical practice, and professional scholarship as it relates to advanced practice nursing in psychiatric and mental health care. In writing this chapter, the editors propose to forecast a future direction for the specialty, given its enormous evolution to date. In consideration of all that has been presented thus far in this book, the editors believe that in the future, it is likely that the following will occur:

- Strategic partnerships will grow.
- Privatization of health care will decline.
- Focused factories will take the place of vertically integrated systems of care.
- The focus on quality and outcomes will continue.
- The information superhighway will expand capabilities and create new challenges.
- Genetics and vulnerability markers will lead to new formulations of mental illness.
- Advances in psychopharmacology and psychosocial treatments will expand rapidly.
- Holistic, coordinated care activities will leverage the preoccupation with cure.
- The number of APRNs will continue to increase.
- The viability of the psychiatric specialty will be threatened.
- Options for learning will expand beyond national boundaries.
- More opportunities for entrepreneurship will evolve.
- Research opportunities will abound.
- The paradigm of scholarship in psychiatric-mental health nursing will continue to evolve.

APRNs have a wonderful opportunity to take advantage of all of these events. By participating in the shaping of the health care environment, researching and applying the science of nursing care to the mentally ill, and developing their professional competencies through life-long learning, APRNs will continue to influence and improve the lives of patients, families, and communities.

THE HEALTH
■ CARE ENVIRONMENT

Strategic Partnerships Will Grow

Future mental health delivery systems will include the development and maintenance of strategic partnerships between managed care and community-based provider groups. Such partnerships are built on the premise that clinical decisions should be made as close to the patient's care as possible (Bigelow, Pelletier, & Beaudin, 1996). With the advent and growth of managed care legislation to protect patients' rights, the pendulum will swing back in favor of consumers and providers and thus be a benefit to APRNs. Successful partnerships will be the result of these key factors (Lipson, 1997):

1. The collaborating partners must learn as much as they can about each other—their organization, terminology, goals, missions, and values.
2. Both entities must be willing to cast aside business-as-usual attitudes and truly think outside the box.
3. Organization partners must be willing to invest time in meeting regularly to discuss progress, pitfalls, and barriers to success.
4. Various payment and reimbursement structures must be investigated.
5. Information systems must be developed to support all aspects of the operation.
6. Continuous quality improvement must be a foundational component of the program.

APRNs in solo and group practice have an opportunity to form strategic alliances with both individual employers and managed care entities. Current options such as joining provider panels and contracting for individual programs and services will become more common. APRNs will "sell" their worth and value by providing payers with evidence that their services result in efficient and effective clinical outcomes and patient satisfaction.

Privatization of Health Care Will Decline

The mid-1980s and the 1990s saw the increase in privatization of public programs, including Medicare and Medicaid. However, the systems of the future may be less likely to include such arrangements, sending the locus of control back to provider organizations instead of private, for-profit companies that currently operate managed care enterprises. Some of these for-profit companies have not realized their anticipated profits since the care required and the costs associated with the care far exceeded projections (Ray, 1998). Restrictions on profit margins also made the public sector contracts less attractive. "The inescapable fact about HMOs is that they are businesses—often accountable to shareholders—and they must closely examine the bottom line" (Ellerman, 1998). Health maintenance organizations (HMOs) in some states have withdrawn from the market because reimbursement rates set by the states were not enough to cover the care for high-risk populations who require protracted care management and a myriad of services and programs. In the mental health arena, TennCare Partners, the Medicaid program in Tennessee, was plagued with access and financial problems. The procurement of Medicaid business was uncertain in the 1990s and even influenced some states to continue managing their own programs rather than establish partnerships with managed behavioral healthcare organizations (MBHOs). There are several examples, such as Tennessee, Ohio, and Montana, in which the states abandoned their plan for Medicaid carve-outs because of local political pressure or pricing issues during the procurement process. States have often made changes to their programs after implementation, which shifted the control of the program from an MBHO back to the community-based programs and services (Mental Health Weekly, 1998a, 1998b; Shinkman, 1998).

APRNs have traditionally cared for vulnerable populations and the disenfranchised covered by public programs, such as Medicaid and Medicare. In winning reimbursement for services in the 1990s, APRNs will continue to provide services to the chronically mentally ill in the twenty-first century. Mohr (1998) proposes that APRNs become activists, especially in the fight for parity of coverage, and suggests specific actions that nurses might take as the pendulum shifts back to providers. She recommends that APRNs do the following:
- Develop diagnosis-specific treatment protocols.
- Write opinion/editorials and letters-to-the-editor expounding upon various issues related to the provision of mental health services.
- Conduct information programs at hospitals,

schools, homeowners associations, churches, senior centers, etc.
- Contact the media and act as media spokespersons on issues related to mental health.
- Empower clients and families to also become activists.

Focused Factories Will Replace Vertical Integration

Vertical integration of health care services (the centralization of different businesses and services within a single organizational entity) was a strategic method adopted by many health care systems in the 1980s and 1990s. However, this strategy has not proved to be the answer to an ailing service industry. As described by Chandler and Daems (1980), vertical integration started as a means for companies to internalize their activities and transactions with other companies so they could operate more profitably by controlling costs through a centralized hierarchy rather than with decentralized market mechanisms. In a 1996 survey of 37 HMOs owned by vertically integrated systems, financial results decreased significantly for 18 of these organizations as a result of integration (Kertesz, 1996). The reason for less-than-desired results may in part have been due to the leadership acumen (or lack thereof) of the chief executive officers (CEO) and other senior management in these organizations (Ray, 1998). In a 1993 survey, a majority of CEOs affirmed that they did not have the requisite knowledge and skills required for the new health care environment (Heidrick & Struggles, Inc., 1993). In addition to leadership problems, organizational barriers to effective vertical integration included 1) the merger of different cultures (physicians, hospitals, and insurers), 2) the reconciliation of different types of personalities, 3) the development of new payment methods for the required units, and 4) the need for the creation of a mutually agreeable business plan (Burns & Thorpe, 1993).

A new concept similar to "centers of excellence" is gaining attention as a health system of the future. Herzlinger's concept of "niche" or "focused factories" bears mention as a growth potential for APRNs. Based on the operational definition of "simplicity and repetition breed competence" (Skinner, 1974), focused factories are organizations that thrive because of "consistency, reliability, clear standards, and low costs" (Herzlinger, 1997). Instead of being broad in scope, focused factories develop core competencies and excel in a few areas. This concept is easily adaptable to APRN practice.

With the swing of the pendulum back to community-based quality care, there is a potential benefit for both consumers and providers. For example, using the focused factory concept, an APRN-managed clinic that focuses primarily on depressive disorders, hiring only expert clinicians proven to be effective at treating such disorders, could be successful in meeting the needs of a community. With a focus on one diagnosis, the organization could build an operating system that treats patients with similar conditions using standard protocols to achieve consistent results. Results or clinical outcomes would be measured routinely using reliable and valid tools, and program effectiveness would be communicated throughout the organization to its patients, families, and payers. Standard protocols or practice guidelines would be tested and refined in real time. Furthermore, the publishing of these positive clinical outcomes would add to the body of scientific knowledge related to care provided by APRNs. Over time, the organization would be able to "improve the relationship between cost and output, and not [only] to reduce costs" (Herzlinger, 1997).

APRNs could also gain status by acquiring chief operating officer (COO) positions in health systems or hospitals. Given their experience in clinical services, management, and systems theory and practice, APRNs possess the perfect skill set to "make sure all parts of the system are working together. That means knowing from a clinical perspective the processes and systems the organization needs to move forward" (Sloane, 1998). Similarly, with organizational experience as highly competent COOs, APRNs could be positioned perfectly to compete for CEO and other senior management offices in health care organizations.

Focus on Quality and Outcomes Will Continue

Health systems will continue to fund internal quality management departments and activities. Having reached the height of a "national commitment to the measurement, improvement, and maintenance of high quality care for all Americans" (Advisory Commission on Consumer Protection and Quality in the Health Care Industry, 1998), the focus on quality will be scrutinized by federal, state, and local constituents. These internal programs will be maintained, in part, as a result of continuing pressures to meet external regulatory standards, but also to serve as internal organizational compliance checks. The late 1990s saw the advent of compliance and ethics officers in large health care organizations as a result of large-scale, highly publicized fraud investigations by the U.S. Department of Health and Human Services. Health systems of the future will have ethics, business conduct, and quality and outcomes measurement as a critical part of their overall operations strategy. Chief Quality Officers will sit at the senior management table and guide the organization in its efforts to prove quality and value to its customers, consumers, other stakeholders, and the public-at-large.

Nurses have traditionally been a strong force as quality professionals. Many have sought certification in health care quality. The APRN who is also a quality professional has the potential to influence the development of comprehensive quality management and improvement programs, clinical outcomes initiatives, and practice guideline development efforts. The APRN is particularly suited to this role since he or she has the knowledge, skills, and abilities to assess an organization or system, identify process flows, and determine required changes in workflow to enhance system performance.

Information Superhighway Will Expand Capabilities and Create New Challenges

The information technology explosion will continue to heavily influence the development of advanced practice nursing in psychiatric and mental health care. Health care environments will increasingly depend on national databases of information for decision making and policy development. Jones (1997) forecasts that the information infrastructure required for managed care will need data in three key areas: 1) purchasing decisions, 2) policy making and public-private partnerships, and 3) health care administration. Contributing to and using regional and national aggregated patient information databases will position APRNs to increase their professional power in these arenas of managed care. The APRNs of the future must increase their participation in the major initiatives in national data sets and develop a unified approach in the use of standardized nursing languages. Their input will be critical in defining what information is collected and how it is used and disseminated. Access to large databases will further nursing research in population-based care and health services research.

The information superhighway will also become increasingly traveled by patients and their families. Alessi, Huang, and Quinlan (1997) offer a view of how information technology will influence psychiatry in the year 2005. In their projections, they describe "The End of the Reign of the Omniscient Psychiatrist," a scenario that highlights several important assumptions for APRNs as well. These assumptions include the following:

- Individuals will become much more informed as consumers of mental health services.
- Individuals will be able to access a provider profile from a national database.
- Videoconferencing will be used for consultation regarding complicated psychiatric conditions and treatments.
- Patients will become experts in their conditions, in part through the use of Internet-based mental health information.

Alessi and colleagues assert that the relationship between the patient and psychiatric care provider will be strengthened by reviewing and discussing information. The APRN is in a favorable position to assist in the empowerment of patients and families. APRNS are experts in using and evaluating information for the development of treatment plans for mental illness and the promotion of mental health care.

■ CLINICAL PRACTICE

Genetics and Vulnerability Markers Will Lead to New Formulations of Mental Illness

Mental illness places an enormous burden of suffering on patients and families throughout the world. It also creates a large economic burden, costing billions of dollars for treatment, disability, and lost productivity. Thus identifying ways to prevent it, detect it early, and improve treatment will continue to be at the top of national health priorities in the years to come. However, cutting edge research in the field promises to change the now familiar landscape. For example, findings about genetics, plasticity, and vulnerability markers may reframe how mental illness is diagnosed and treated as reflected in current research. Consider the answers to the following questions (Kupfer, 1996):

- How do genes, biology, and the environment work together in dynamic ways over time to influence each other in normal and pathologic development?
- What are the implications of the concept of brain "plasticity" for psychotherapeutic and other interventions?
- How do emerging insights into vulnerability and susceptibility change our understanding of psychiatric illness and the nature of patient education?

Some researchers predict that genetics will revolutionize psychiatric care (Barondes, 1998). At the very least, modern genetic technology is increasingly capable of finding relevant susceptibility genes. Even though many genes may play a role in a particular disease, finding just one can lead to practical benefits. For this reason, the genetics of mental illness will continue to be a major priority for the National Institute of Mental Health (NIMH) and for many biotechnology and pharmaceutical companies. Most psychiatric illnesses are probably not only polygenic but also heterogeneous, meaning that the gene combinations that increase susceptibility are different in different families and populations. Thus gene discovery will probably lead to the identification of new subtypes and classifications of many mental illnesses. In fact, the entire approach to psychiatric diagnosis may change. Although interviews with patients will remain the most important diagnostic tool, DNA testing will also be important. DNA tests for a mental illness may be made available to relatives of people with the disorder to find out whether they too have inherited the vulnerability. Such information could lead some people to take preventive measures as effective ones become identified.

Yet another future development will be the tendency for the field to think in developmental terms, both in behavioral environmental spheres as well as neurobiologic ones. This reflects the emerging concept of "plasticity," which suggests that early events, whether biologic or environmental, do not establish fixed patterns. Rather, a "window of opportunity" continues to exist and remains malleable throughout the later years of development (Kupfer, 1996; Lieberman, Sheitman, & Kinon, 1997). Future research will uncover which neurobiologic processes are time dependent versus those that demonstrate plasticity over time, as well as how control over psychosocial and environmental domains, such as body or social rhythms, can induce or delay the onset of a disorder. These findings will allow for the identification of potential biologic or vulnerability markers that may suggest a predisposition for a future illness, as well as the development of new treatments that cut across traditional biologic and psychosocial boundaries.

Some researchers believe that it is not too farfetched to examine hypotheses that link infectious diseases to mental illness (Hooper, 1999). The seminal work of Paul Ewald (1993) about the evolution of infectious diseases and a new "germ theory" may hold promise in the not too distant future. Although still in the theoretical stage, Ewald is combining his study of biologic infectious agents and epidemiologic research to detect evolutionary patterns in chronic conditions such as Alzheimer's disease, AIDS, schizophrenia, cancer, and arthritis. If clinical evidence were to substantiate Ewald's hypothesis that infectious processes cause some chronic illnesses, a new generation of antibiotics could be developed with the possibility of effective treatment and cure of some of the world's greatest scourges. This kind of radical thinking takes courage and persistence. For example, it has taken many years for the medical community to accept the research finding that duodenal ulcers are not stress-induced but are caused by a common bacteria that is effectively treated with a course of antibiotics. Even today, only slightly more than half of practicing physicians treat these ulcers effectively based on research evidence (Hooper, 1999).

This "brave new world" of clinical science has major implications for APRNs in the future. First is the task of staying abreast of this emerging science. Second is the task of translating this information to improve patient and family education so that they can adjust their lifestyles and seek treatment when their symptoms first begin to occur. Screening children for biologic or vulnerability markers can lead to preventive strategies as well as early detection and intervention activities. Genetic counseling by APRNs can inform, correct misperceptions, and relieve fears. Support, counseling, and follow-up services based on new findings in the field can assist patients and families in coping with a psychiatric diagnosis, the risk family members face, and life decisions that may follow.

Advances in Psychopharmacology and Psychosocial Treatments Will Expand Rapidly

The proliferation of new psychopharmacologic agents for the treatment of mental illness will continue in the years ahead and will permit a more tailored treatment of mental illness (Schultz, 1997). These medications will have wider therapeutic indices, lower side effect profiles, more positive effects on neurotransmitter regulation, more extensive routes of administration, and advantages in cost-effective clinical care. The implications of such developments for APRNs are clear. Psychiatric nurses must continue to stay abreast of all aspects of these new medications as they receive Food and Drug Administration (FDA) approval and become available to patients. Increasingly, APRNs will be asked to provide information and education on these treatments and prescribe them if appropriate. Knowledge of new drug efficacy and effectiveness and new drug-old drug interactions must be an essential part of the APRN's clinical practice. This can be accomplished by attending a graduate program that has a strong psychopharmacology component in the curriculum, practicing according to guidelines published in the field, and participating in yearly educational programs to update one's psychopharmacology knowledge base.

The increase in precision in psychopharmacology will also bring about a concomitant precision in psychosocial interventions. As these medications shed light on the human mind, they allow psychosocial interventions to be used in more prescriptive and focused ways. For example, new investigations are reporting that medications and psychosocial interventions can have a synergistic effect that enhances treatment efficacy and may forestall potential relapse. Specifically, cognitive-behavioral treatments will grow in popularity since they reflect brief and relatively low-cost interventions that have proven repeatedly to be effective in a variety of psychiatric disorders as described in Chapter 9.

The future of psychosocial treatments will also be based on the importance of perceived self-efficacy or the belief in one's personal capabilities. As such, self-efficacy regulates human functioning in four major ways: cognitive, motivational, mood or affect, and behavior (Bandura, 1997). It is known, for example, that belief in a person's own ability to cope with sources of stress reduces biologic reactions that can impair immune function. Also, efficacy beliefs largely determine whether people consider changing their health habits and whether they succeed in making and maintaining change. Finally, perceived self-efficacy also helps to prevent existing illness from becoming worse.

In a future in which people will live longer with multiple chronic illnesses, the importance of having people exercise control over events and reactions that affect their health will be critical (Zauszniewski, 1995). The mastery of this aspect of enhancing behavior change in patients presents one of the brightest opportunities for APRNs in psychiatric and mental health care. Taking advantage of this opportunity, however, requires that APRNs master advanced cognitive and behavioral psychotherapy techniques—techniques that may not be taught currently with rigor or precision in clinical nurse specialist (CNS) graduate programs and are almost never included in sufficient depth in psychiatric nurse practitioner (NP) graduate programs. However, each of these psychosocial treatment modalities have descriptive manuals and treatment protocols and need to be an essential part of the APRN's clinical skills. APRNs today and in the future need *more* rather than *less* intense education and clinical experience in the very specific, complex, and rigorous therapeutic treatments available to patients who have a mental illness. Thus, as discussed in Chapter 20, the specialty will need to seriously evaluate what is being taught in CNS and NP graduate programs and how well this prepares graduates to truly meet the needs of populations at risk.

Holistic, Coordinated Care Will Leverage the Preoccupation with Cure

The past 50 years in American medicine have been dominated by curative activities, often through the use of high technology in tertiary care facilities. At the cusp of the millennium it is now evident that more people are living longer lives, often with chronic illnesses that can be managed but not necessarily cured. Thus increased emphasis will be placed on providing "care" rather than "cure" through coordinated, community-based clinical management (Lindemann, 1996).

A related challenge is that of helping patients assume greater responsibility for their own health. These changes can play to the very strengths of psychiatric APRNs who have a long tradition of caregiving, health care coordination, clinical management, and community outreach. However, it is also evident that these same activities are being assumed by other types of providers in a health care environment with contained and limited resources. A typical example of this is the role of case manager, which from one setting to another may vary greatly in assigned activities, educational preparation, level of expertise, and salary remuneration. To move confidently into the future, APRNs need to document both their skills and the cost effectiveness of the care they provide. They might also consider expanding their entrepreneurial skills to create psychiatric care centers where such needs of patients and families can be met with APRNs planning, implementing, and evaluating the care provided.

A final aspect of evolving expectations of patients is the phenomenon of growing interest in complementary and alternative health care. This reflects a holistic world view of health and illness that is outside the biomedical mainstream of Western medicine. This trend is easily measured in dollars and cents. One third of adult Americans, most of whom pursue traditional health care treatment as well, spend an estimated $13.7 billion a year out of pocket on complementary or alternative therapies. In addition, more than 1000 homeopathic medicines are sold over the counter, along with a wide variety of vitamins, minerals, herbal remedies, fat burners, passion promoters, and bee pollen (Langone, 1996).

Federal funding to study the efficacy of alternative treatment is likely to increase in the future. In the fall of 1998, the Office of Alternative and Complementary Medicine of the National Institutes of Health (NIH) was raised to the status of a National Center for Complementary and Alternative Medicine (NCCAM). The NCCAM's mission is "the conduct and support of basic and applied research and training, and will disseminate information on complementary and alternative medicine (CAM) to practitioners and the public" (NCCAM, 1998). Effectiveness research is a primary objective of the NCCAM. The funding for the NCCAM has increased from $2 million in 1993 to $50 million for fiscal year 1999. This funding has been due largely to the popularity of complementary and alternative medicine with U.S. citizens.

The reasons for selecting nontraditional care are many and include a fear of harm and intrusion by traditional medicine, easier access, lower cost, greater personal control, fewer adverse effects, medical disenchantment, and loss of faith in medical science's promises of health and freedom from disease and disability. Perhaps even more importantly, it may be that the traditional health care establishment has placed too much emphasis on high technology at the expense of attending to basic human needs related to understanding, compassion, and care (Donley, 1998). Clearly this trend can help lead nurses back to their roots in the nurse-patient relationship. It also suggests, however, that APRNs must go beyond the descriptive and often anecdotal discussions of the nurse-patient relationship from the past. They must document and validate both the attributes and the important outcomes associated with the nurse-patient therapeutic alliance, since this is the essence of evidence-based psychiatric nursing practice.

■ PROFESSIONAL SCHOLARSHIP

Number of APRNs Will Continue to Increase

In the future, the number of APRNs is projected to continue to increase, despite small fluctuations in enrollments from year to year (NLN, 1997). There will also be an increase in psychiatric-mental health APRNs from the 7958 who were certified specialists (CSs) in adult or child and adolescent psychiatric-mental health nursing in 1998, according to the American Nurses Credentialing Center's Associate Registrar (Brown, 1998). This number represents 7020 adult CSs and 938 child and adolescent CSs. Yet with the closure of many psychiatric-mental health CNS programs and the opening of psychiatric-mental health NP and blended role CNS/NP programs, there will be a shift in the APRN's educational background. This new APRN may well fill the gaps in providing comprehensive primary health care for the mentally ill. As this vulnerable population ages, those with mental illness are more likely to have comorbid physical illnesses, especially of a serious and chronic nature. Prevailing beliefs about the value of shared decision making, self-care, and self-efficacy will make the care for these individuals even more complex and call for even better communication and relationship skills on the part of the APRN. In essence, while more has been added to the role and functions of the psychiatric NP-prepared nurse, all the knowledge and competencies of the CNS-prepared nurse are still very necessary. With substantive changes in role preparation and practice expectations, the new APRN will need to partner with academic faculty and service providers to conduct much needed clinical outcome studies. Educators will have to concentrate on demonstrating effective educational outcomes that meet the needs of advanced practice students, health care services, and society.

Over the next 10 years, professional scholarship can increase dramatically as APRNs work together in their professional organizations to provide leadership and resources to increase research and outcome evaluation. As noted in Chapter 22, there are those already advocating for specialty organizations to take on the evaluative function of reviewing the scientific evidence-based literature and disseminating those findings with merit for application in the field. Also, the federal Agency for Health Care Policy and Research (AHCPR) is moving toward gathering, evaluating, and disseminating the literature related to specific conditions. While psychiatric nursing organizations have already taken the responsibility to establish standards and guidelines for care, they will assume a far more active role in determining research priorities and national multisite studies for the future.

Viability of the Specialty Will Be Threatened

Increasing the desirability of graduate education for APRNs will be critical for survival of the specialty. As discussed in Chapter 20, this is both an immediate and a long-term problem that will require attention to recruitment into bachelor as well as master's nursing degree programs. In its national survey (Barrell, Merwin, & Poster, 1997), the Society for Education and Research in Psychiatric Nursing (SERPN) found that 77% of APRNs are currently between 40 and 59 years of age, and only 15.6% of the APRNs are under 39 years of age. Without major changes in this demographic trend of the aging APRN, professional scholarship activities in the specialty are at severe risk.

It is common knowledge that the longer a faculty member waits to publish his or her dissertation after receiving a doctoral degree, the less likely it is that the research will be published. It takes many years to develop an active research program, and generally, it is the faculty rather than the clinical role that allows for the support and flexibility of time, as well as the expectation of scholarship, to be successful in this area. Today, the average age of faculty members is 55 years (AACN, 1998a). Without an infusion of doctorally prepared faculty, graduate programs will not be able to provide the education and mentoring for future generations of APRNs. Unless nurse scientists prepare for their careers at an earlier age, their research programs will not develop their full scientific potential. Without solid research and innovative teaching, the discipline will not flourish.

Despite federal funding efforts to encourage more nurses with ethnically diverse backgrounds to choose nursing as a career, the rate of minorities entering nursing has stagnated (NLN, 1997). This inverse trend of a fast-growing, more diverse patient population and a less diverse provider population lessens the viability of the specialty too. Without appropriate role models who share a similar cultural and ethnic background, the nursing workforce has difficulty attracting and retaining minorities. Furthermore, the discrepancy comes at a time when consumers are demanding culturally competent care from providers who can translate their needs accurately and sensitively when they seek care (Andrews, 1992). APRNs in psychiatric and mental health care have a special obligation to provide care that respects the sociocultural aspects of mental health and illness. They also have special expertise as Madeleine Leininger, an internationally known anthropologist and psychiatric nurse, has shown in her work in developing transcultural nursing.

What would generate an increased number of nurses entering the specialty, becoming both master's and doctorally prepared, and integrating scholarship into their multiple roles? With closure of graduate programs, there may be a backlash in meeting the mental health needs, particularly of children, adolescents, and families, if master's-prepared APRNs are not available. The government may be pressured to step in once again (as in the late 1960s) to dramatically increase federal funding for substantial traineeships for advanced specialty nursing education. This national strategy

has been used successfully to alleviate a potential shortage of APRNs in the past. With the increasing emphasis on the mental health needs of children and those with chronic and severe mental illness, new master's-degree programs will need to open. Paralleling the federal funding, the demand for APRNs will also increase salaries and make the specialty a more desirable career option for young women and men.

Options for Learning Will Expand Beyond National Boundaries

Learning will become a way of life. It is projected that the average person will have three or more different careers over the course of his or her life. Because of massive changes in the world of work brought about by new information and technology, whole industries will be created and others will change radically or disappear in a single generation. Therefore people will have to be ready to move in new directions and to learn new roles and skills.

Nurses are fortunate because there are so many roles, specialties, and settings in which they can practice nursing. They can change the focus of their practice and still remain in nursing. However, as nursing comes of age as a true scientific discipline, assuming a new role or moving to a different practice environment will require re-training, re-tooling, and perhaps formally re-educating to become a competent, accountable professional. In the future, "a nurse is a nurse is a nurse" will most definitely *not* be the refrain of most employers. The practice of nursing will still be varied—with specialists and generalists, those who are cross-trained, and those who are expert in a specific area—but all will be well prepared. Competition from other providers will help to instill a drive for excellence in those who are seeking new positions. A better-educated patient population will demand competence from providers of care.

In addition to the formal programs in universities, continuing education through professional associations, and certificate programs as discussed in Chapters 20 and 21, there will be an exponential increase in the number of programs and learning opportunities through the Internet and through university-sponsored distance learning courses (Rothert, Talarczyk, & Awbrey, 1997). In the past, these offerings were directed to the needs of those in rural areas or at some distance from the campus. Now learning through courses posted on websites and by searching for specific topics on the Internet has become a method of choice for many individuals who are self-directed learners. Given the busy lives that most working professionals lead, the ability to access information and study at a convenient time is very enticing. Quality is only one of the issues that attend this alternative to the faculty-led lecture on campus. However, most experts believe that these issues will be solved in time as alternative learning methods move into the mainstream of education (Clark, 1997; Skiba, 1997).

In graduate clinical education, two of the burning issues are 1) Who will precept students in the future? and 2) How will students learn requisite psychomotor skills in the intensely competitve managed care environment? Students from different health professions programs, in seeking clinical practice experience, must vie with those in their same discipline as well as other disciplines, including medicine, for the same choice practicum sites and experienced preceptors. The mid-level providers (NPs, CNSs, and physician assistants [PAs]), who have traditionally volunteered to be preceptors for graduate health professions students, are under tremendous pressure to "be productive and bill for services." They claim that they do not have time to deliver services *and* teach and mentor students on a volunteer basis and that they must be paid for this professional activity. Nursing deans believe this is not only a "dereliction of professional duty" but very short-sighted. They ask service administrators, if there is no investment in clinical training now, where the agency's future qualified providers will come from. Most nursing programs do not have a budget to support direct payment to preceptors or their agency and

feel that to do so would set an untenable precedent. One solution may be the "pass-through" of Medicare funds to support clinical education in graduate nursing. Currently, graduate medical education (GME) is supported by Medicare payments to hospitals for training of resident physicians. Organized nursing will continue to work with legislative advocates to introduce bills into Congress to redirect Medicare funding to nursing and allied health (AACN, 1998b). Given its successful track record in securing reimbursement for APRNs who provide Medicare services, as described in Chapter 7, nursing may score another victory in the fight for a portion of GME Medicare funds.

Another difficulty to overcome is the teaching of psychomotor skills, particularly physical examination and diagnosis in primary health care. As these skills have become incorporated into the practice of all APRNs and must be taught in sufficent depth to graduate a proficient APRN, again the competition for clinical sites and appropriate patient populations is great. Some graduate programs are beginning to employ "standardized patients" (i.e., professional actors or trained individuals who serve as patients for the students to interview and examine). The cost is borne by the program or in some cases by the student. The advantage to this approach is that the "patient" can give feedback to the student from the patient's perspective and participate in a debriefing after the session to increase the student's understanding of how he or she provides care. The disadvantage is that this type of learning is a simulation, not reality. Other methods of learning about psychomotor skills include computer-assisted instruction programs, video conferencing, and virtual reality experiences. As the financial cost of these alternatives to "real-life" situations comes down and the sophistication and complexity of the technology increases, there will be a much greater reliance on these teaching methods in the future (Clark, 1997). Faculty members as well as students will have to adjust their teaching and learning methods to fit with these clinical practice tools so that encounters with patients can be productive for the students and beneficial to the patients.

Another method of learning involves travel to other countries and cultures. Just as the United States has experienced a big wave of foreign visitors and immigrants, more Americans are traveling abroad to vacation and study. Many nurses are bringing their expertise in American nursing to exchange with health professionals in other lands, who have much to teach them about health care in their countries, indigenous healers, time-tested theories and therapies, and translated versions of the American system of health care (Fenton, 1997). Nurses may be sponsored by the Carnegie, Rockefeller, and W.W. Kellogg Foundations; Fullbright Fellowships; federal programs of exchange; and university sabbatical leave funds. Although international exchange programs for undergraduate students have existed for many years, more opportunities that combine learning with service in another country will be developed for graduate students. Exposure to different people and cultures is professionally broadening and personally enriching. As globalization accelerates, there will be a need to develop universal certifications and readily reciprocal licensing mechanisms to allow the free flow of providers across state and national boundaries. In the developed world, the European Economic Union could be a testing ground for these mechanisms and transcultural nursing.

Currently, there is no substitute for "being there," but in the future there may be virtual reality environments that will allow students, faculty members, and health care providers to immerse themselves in a different culture and community. In the meantime, email, video conferencing, and other electronic technology help APRNs initiate and maintain relationships with their counterparts all over the world.

More Opportunities for Entrepreneurship Will Evolve

In the future, APRNs will enhance clinical trials by taking an entrepreneurial approach. APRN-owned and -operated research consulting firms and care delivery systems will supplement the academic centers' clinical trials. Because they are not funded from grants, but rather paid a fee by contracting agencies or individuals, their clinical trial management approach will provide an opportunity for many nurses who want to blend research, administration, and consultation. One of their functions will be to assess services by conducting field and in-house monitoring to ensure protocol and regulatory compliance, collection of data, and auditing. Additional aspects of their work will be consulting to assist clients in strategic planning and systems analysis, as well as coordination of services, from Investigational Review Board (IRB) submission and budget development to staff education.

Similarly, in the education arena, there are many opportunities for consultation about program development based on clinical and systems expertise. As academic programs respond to the challenge to modernize (i.e., become outcome-oriented and cost-effective), APRNs with experience in making system-wide changes and setting human resources policies will be in great demand. Other teaching initiatives for APRNs will include contracting with health care organizations as outsource providers to deliver staff development and continuing education programs. This too will require knowledge of the clinical state-of-the-art and modern teaching technologies and methods. Making immediate connections and forming egalitarian relationships will be an important part of the transformed learning process (Gaines & Baldwin, 1996). Psychiatric APRNs will draw on their special talents to quickly assess learning needs and form alliances between the teacher/consultant and the student/client.

Research Opportunities Will Abound

As predicted for managed care/provider partnerships, research partnerships will also evolve to continue the investigation of evidence-based practice. As recently as June 1998, the AHCPR and the American Association of Health Plans (AAHP) announced a collaboration that would allocate an award of $8.5 million to six research teams. The overall purpose of the grants will be to study the effect of certain policies, procedures, and techniques used by managed care organizations to effect positive clinical outcomes. The focus will be on the chronically ill, to show evidence on how specific strategies for managing and financing care affect quality (AHCPR, 1998). The increased funding of the NIH and the NIMH paves the way for continued research opportunities for APRN scientists. Academic medical centers will move in the direction of applying health services research to the populations they serve. The growth of health services research programs that began in the late 1990s will continue to provide practical research findings to the care of specific populations, including patients suffering from mental illness.

In whichever venue APRNs choose to practice, they will need to continue to confirm their value. Continued research will need to highlight cost, quality, and value of APRN services compared with other mental health providers. These evidence-based studies will need to be done nationally. They must also generate region-specific information to assist local APRNs to prove their worth and value in the competitive health care market. Evidence-based research specific to the services provided by APRNs will need to be disseminated widely and will inform the future development of interdisciplinary practice guidelines.

Paradigm of Scholarship Will Continue to Evolve

Traditionally, the concept of scholarship has been interpreted as the pursuit of new knowledge through the conduct of research. The work of Boyer (1990) has produced an expanded view of scholarship that presents an evolving paradigm comprised of four elements: the scholarship of discovery, the scholarship of integration, the scholarship of application, and the scholarship of teaching.

The *scholarship of discovery* is the most similar to the concept of scholarship as the advancement of knowledge through research. Chapter 23 addresses the important role of APRNs in the conduct of clinical trials. It is vitally important that APRNs continue to engage in research for the discovery of new knowledge that will benefit patients, their families, and the health care system.

The *scholarship of integration* involves making connections across disciplines, making interpretations of knowledge, and finding meaning in what has been discovered through research. The role of the APRN in the health care environment (in Unit One) and as a clinical practitioner (in Unit Two) is informed by the outcomes of the scholarship of integration. Chapter 24 provides examples of mental health services research.

The *scholarship of application* focuses on how knowledge is applied responsibly in problem solving at the individual and institutional levels. For APRNs, the scholarship of application connects theory with clinical practice and the health care environment. Chapter 22 provides specific strategies for scholarly endeavors through the application of research in practice. Additionally, the chapters in Units One and Two apply nursing and interdisciplinary knowledge to the role of the APRN.

The Pew Health Professions Commission (PHPC, 1998), in its fourth and final major report, recommends that health service delivery be reconsidered in fundamental ways. The four challenges initially identified by the PHPC, which are still relevant for today and the future, include the following:

1. Reconsider the nature of health care work.
2. Restructure how health professionals are regulated to promote independence in practice and ensure that credentials fit the new work.
3. Ensure an adequate supply of manpower to meet the needs of consumers, but not an oversupply, which would result in waste.
4. Realign training and education to more closely match the ever-changing care delivery system.

Moreover, the PHPC proposes 21 competencies for health professionals in the twenty-first century. These are listed in Box 25-1. Specific recommendations were also made for advanced practice

box 25-1

PEW HEALTH PROFESSIONS COMMISSION: 21 COMPETENCIES FOR THE TWENTY-FIRST CENTURY

1. Embrace a personal ethic of social responsibility and service.
2. Exhibit ethical behavior in all professional activities.
3. Provide evidence-based clinically competent care.
4. Incorporate the multiple determinants of health in clinical care.
5. Apply knowledge of new sciences.
6. Demonstrate critical thinking, reflection, and problem-solving skills.
7. Understand the role of primary care.
8. Rigorously practice preventive health care.
9. Integrate population-based care and services into practice.
10. Improve access to health care for those with unmet health needs.
11. Practice relationship-centered care with individuals and families.
12. Provide culturally sensitive care to a diverse society.
13. Partner with communities in health care decisions.
14. Use communication and information technology effectively and appropriately.
15. Work in interdisciplinary teams.
16. Ensure care that balances individual, professional, system, and societal needs.
17. Practice leadership.
18. Take responsibility for quality of care and health outcomes at all levels.
19. Contribute to continuous improvement of the health care system.
20. Advocate for public policy that promotes and protects the health of the public.
21. Continue to learn and help others learn.

From PHPC, 1998. Reprinted with permission.

nursing (PHPC, 1998). These include the following:

- Reorient advanced practice nursing education programs to prepare APRNs for the changing situations and settings in which they are likely to practice.
- Regardless of payer source, federal funding for graduate medical education should be made available to support the training of APRNs and other non-physician providers.
- Develop standard guidelines for advanced practice and reinforce them with curriculum guidelines, examination requirements, and accreditation regulations.
- Emphasize the practice styles that are a critical part of advanced practice nursing, including the emphasis on preventive and health-promoting interventions and attention to psychosocial, environmental and resource factors.

The *scholarship of teaching* is defined as a dynamic process that connects the teacher's understandings with the learner's (Gaines & Baldwin, 1996). Good teaching requires that teachers are constant learners as well. It involves not only transmitting knowledge but also transforming and extending it. Chapters 20 and 21 focus on the scholarship of teaching and learning, but pearls of wisdom are sprinkled throughout the book. In the ever-changing health care environment and with the rapid expansion of knowledge in psychiatric and mental health care, the commitment of APRNs to a lifetime of learning and teaching is a fundamental requirement for the provision of quality patient care.

■ CONCLUSION

The future of advanced practice psychiatric-mental health nursing is bright and broad. The blueprint for its art and science has been formed and fostered by psychiatric nurses in the past 100 years and still serves the specialty well. APRNs who have a profound understanding and appreciation for the transformations in the health care environment, clinical practice issues, and professional scholarship will have the strength and creativity to ignite the spark that will produce a better system of quality mental health care for individuals, families, and populations.

References

Advisory Commission on Consumer Protection and Quality in the Health Care Industry. *The challenge and potential for assuring quality health care for the 21st century.* [On-line, p. 1] Available: www.ahcpr.gov/qual/21stcena.htm, accessed 8/19/98.

Agency for Health Care Policy and Research. (June 22, 1998). *AHCPR teams with AAHP Foundation to improve care for the chronically ill.* [Press Release]. Rockville, MD: Author. [Online] Available: www.ahcpr.gov/news/press/aahppr.htm.

Alessi, N., Huang, M., & Quinlan, P. (1997). 2005: information technology impacts psychiatry. In *Computers, the patient and the psychiatrist: American Psychiatric Press Review of Psychiatry.* Washington, DC: American Psychiatric Press.

American Association of Colleges of Nursing. (1998a). With demand for RNs climbing and shortening supply, forecasters say what's ahead isn't typical "nursing shortage." *Issue Bulletin.* Washington, DC: Author.

American Association of Colleges of Nursing. (1998b). Managed care constraints stir debate on preceptor reimbursement. *Issue Bulletin.* Washington, DC: Author.

Andrews, M.M. (1992). Cultural perspectives on nursing in the 21st century. *Journal of Professional Nursing, 8*(1), 7–15.

Bandura, A. (1997). *Self-efficacy: the exercise of control.* New York: W.H. Freeman.

Barondes, S. (1998). *Mood genes: hunting for origins of mania and depression.* New York: W.H. Freeman.

Barrell, L.M., Merwin E.L., & Poster E.C. (1997). Patient outcomes used by advanced practice psychiatric nurses to evaluate effectiveness of practice. *Archives of Psychiatric Nursing, 11*(4), 184–197.

Bigelow, J., Pelletier, L.R., & Beaudin, C.L. (1996). Trends in behavioral health benefit management: ensuring accountability through quality improvement. *Managing Employee Health Benefits, 4*(3), 20–26.

Boyer, E.L. (1990). *Scholarship reconsidered: priorities of the professoriate.* San Francisco: Jossey-Bass.

Brown, J. (1998). Personal communication.

Burns, L.R., & Thorpe, D..P. (1993). Trends and models and physician-hospital organization. *Health Care Management Review, 18*(4), 7–20.

Chandler, A., & Daems, H. (Eds.). (1980). *Managerial hierarchies.* Cambridge, MA: Harvard University Press.

Clark, C.E. (1997). New teaching strategies and technologies. In McCloskey, J.C., & Grace, H.K. (Eds.). *Current issues in nursing* (ed. 5). St. Louis: Mosby.

Donley, R. (1998). The alternative health care revolution. *Nursing Economic$, 16*(6), 298–302.

Ellerman, S. (1998). Cutting off care: HMOs re-evaluate their programs for the poor. *NurseWeek, 11*(16), 9.

Ewald, P. (1993). *Evolution of infectious disease.* New York: Oxford University Press.

Fenton, M.V. (1997). Development of models of international exchange to upgrade nursing education. In McCloskey, J.C., & Grace, H.K. (Eds.). *Current issues in nursing* (ed. 5). St. Louis: Mosby.

Gaines, S., & Baldwin, D. (1996). Guiding dialogue in the transformation of teacher-student relationships. *Nursing Outlook, 44*(3), 124–128.

Heidrick & Struggles, Inc. (1993). *Leading change.* Chicago: Author.

Herzlinger, R.E. (1997). *Market driven health care: who wins, who loses in the transformation of America's largest service industry.* Reading, MA: Addison-Wesley.

Hooper, J. (1999). A new germ theory. *Atlantic Monthly, 283*(2), 41–53.

Jones, L.D. (1997). Building the information infrastructure required for managed care. *Image: Journal of Nursing Scholarship, 29,* 377–382.

Kertesz, L. (June 17, 1996). Systems begin pruning HMOs from holdings. *Modern Healthcare,* 77.

Kupfer, D.J. (1996). Developmental plasticity: is it the plastics of the 90's? In *Advancing research in developmental plasticity: integrating the behavioral science and the neuroscience of mental health.* Proceedings from the NIMH Conference held May 12, 1996. Washington DC: US Government Printing Office.

Kupfer D.J. (1997). *Our scientific revolution in psychiatry: pitfalls and caveats.* Presented at the Annual Meeting of the American Psychiatric Association, San Diego, CA.

Langone, J. (1996). Challenging the mainstream. *Time Magazine, 148*(14), 40.

Lieberman, J., Sheitman, B., & Kinon, B. (1997). Neurochemical sensitization in the pathophysiology of schizophrenia: deficits and dysfunction in neuronal regulation and plasticity. *Neuropsychopharmacology, 17*(4), 205–229.

Lindeman, C.A. (September, 1996). Curriculum changes needed in nursing education. *The American Nurse,* 6.

Lipson, D.J. (1997). Medicaid managed care and community providers: new partnerships. *Health Affairs, 16*(4), 100–101.

Mental Health Weekly. (1998a). Changes to TennCare Partners program bring relief to BHOs. June 1, 1998, p. 1.

Mental Health Weekly. (1998b). Corrective actions put fate of Montana contract in question. August 10, 1998, p. 1.

Mohr, W.K. (1998). Managed care and mental health services: how we got to where we are. *Journal of the American Psychiatric Nurses Association, 4*(5), 159–160.

National Center for Complementary and Alternative Medicine (NCCAM). (1998). [On-line] Available: www.altmed.od.nih.gov/nccam/about/general.shtml

National League for Nursing. (1997). *Nursing data review 1997*. New York: Author.

Pew Health Professions Commission. (1998). *Executive summary: recreating health professional practice for a new century*. [On-line] Available: futurehealth.ucsf.edu/pdf_files/rept4.pdf

Ray, C.G. (1998). How CMHCs are taking on a new role (and a new name). *Behavioral Health Management, 18*(6), 14–15.

Rothert, M.L., Talarczyk, G.J., & Awbrey, S.M. (1997). Distance learning: an integral part of transforming the university and nursing education. In McCloskey, J.C., &

Grace, H.K. (Eds.). *Current issues in nursing* (ed. 5). St. Louis: Mosby.

Schulz, S.C. (1997). The brave new world of psychopharmacology. *The Leifer Report, Special Edition*, 29–31.

Shinkman, R. (1998). Montana sours on managed care. *Modern Healthcare, 28*(37), 26, 28.

Skiba, D. (1997). Transforming nursing education to celebrate learning. *Nursing and Health Care Perspectives, 18*(3), 124–129, 148.

Skinner, W. (May-June, 1974). The focused factory. *Harvard Business Review*, 113–122.

Sloane, T. (1998). Reinventing the COO: after being down and out, the position is back—but with some changes. *Modern Healthcare, 28*(27), 30–32.

Zauszniewski, J.A. (1995). Theoretical and empirical considerations of resourcefulness. *Image: Journal of Nursing Scholarship, 27*(3), 177–180.

APPENDIXES

APNA Position Statements

Report

Education

Other

Psychiatric-Mental Health Nursing Practice

Psychiatric-mental health nursing focuses on the "promotion of optimal mental health, the prevention of mental illness, health maintenance, management of, and/or referral of mental and physical health problems, the diagnosis and treatment of mental disorders and their sequelae, and rehabilitation" (Haber & Billings, 1993).

The clinical practice of psychiatric nursing occurs at two levels—basic and advanced. At the basic level, registered nurses work with "individuals, families, groups, and communities to assess mental health needs, develop diagnoses, and plan, implement, and evaluate nursing care. Basic level nursing practice is characterized by interventions that promote and foster health, assess dysfunction, assist clients to regain or improve their coping abilities, and prevent further disability" (ANA et al., 1994). These interventions focus on psychiatric-mental health clients and include health promotion, preventive interventions, and health maintenance; assessment, screening, and evaluation; management of a therapeutic environment; assisting clients with self-care activities; administering and monitoring psychobiological treatment regimens; health teaching, including psychoeducation; crisis intervention and counseling; and case management. Psychiatric nurses work in a variety of inpatient and outpatient settings such as full or partial hospitals; community-based or home care programs; and local, state, and federal mental health agencies.

Registered nurses who seek additional education and obtain a master's or doctoral degree can become advanced practice nurses in the specialty (psychiatric-mental health clinical nurse specialists or psychiatric nurse practitioners). After postmaster's supervised clinical practice, they can become certified as specialists in adult or child and adolescent psychiatric-mental health nursing. In addition to the functions performed at the basic level, these advanced practice nurses assess, diagnose, and treat psychiatric disorders and potential mental health problems. They provide the full range of primary mental health care services to individuals, families, groups, and communities; function as psychotherapists; and in some states have the authority to prescribe medications. Psychiatric-mental health nurses in advanced practice are qualified to practice independently to offer direct care services in settings such as agencies, communities, homes, hospitals, and offices. Some psychiatric-mental health clinical nurse specialists practice consultation/liaison nursing, delivering direct mental health services to physically ill patients or consultation to staff in general medical settings.

There are two principal arrangements for the clinical practice of advanced practice psychiatric nurses:

1. *Organized care systems.* In these arrangements in which a full continuum of care services is provided in a variety of settings, nurses are paid or reimbursed for their services on a salaried, contractual, or fee-for-service basis.
2. *Self-employment.* Self-employed nurses generally offer a full range of care, from acute inpatient to community-based services, directly to the consumer. Payment arrangements include direct fee-for-service or reimbursement through a third party payer such as an insurance or a managed care company.

Psychiatric-mental health nurses at either level of practice may focus their clinical activities on different populations (child and adolescent, older adults, families); on specific mental health problems (violence, substance abuse, severe and persistent mental illness); on targeted patient outcomes (clinical, functional, perceptual) in a cost-effective manner; or on different aspects of mental health such as health promotion, illness prevention, and rehabilitation. Psychiatric-mental health nurses provide individualized care, focusing on the whole person, the family, or the community. In addition to their direct care activities, they can function as case managers, serve as consultants, or engage in research. Because of their broad background in biologic, pharmacologic, sociologic, and psychologic sciences, psychiatric-mental health nurses are a rich resource as providers of psychiatric-mental health services and patient care partners for the consumers of those services.

References

American Nurses Association (1994). *A statement on psychiatric-mental health clinical nursing practice and standards of psychiatric-mental health clinical nursing practice.* Washington, DC: American Nurses Publishing.

Haber, J., & Billings, C. (1993). Primary mental health care: a vision for the future of psychiatric-mental health nursing. *ANA Council Perspectives* 2(2), 1.

Prescriptive Authority for Advanced Practice Psychiatric Nurses

■ INTRODUCTION

In increasing numbers, states are legislating prescriptive practice authority for advanced practice nurses, including those who are psychiatric-mental health clinical nurse specialists and psychiatric nurse practitioners. The intent of this legislation is to increase access to health care and to utilize nurses to their full capacity as accessible, cost-effective, full-service providers. Each state, when determining rules and regulations to govern prescriptive authority for advanced practice nurses, specifies the requirements that a nurse must meet to qualify for this aspect of practice. In general, state statutes or rules and regulations grant prescriptive authority to nurses who provide evidence of "advanced educational preparation, proof of certification from a national certifying body, a specified number of recently acquired hours of pharmacology preparation, and evidence of continuing education in the pharmacotherapeutics related to the nurse's specialty area of practice" (Talley & Brooke, 1992).

■ PURPOSE

The purpose of this document is to do the following:
- Provide a statement of support for prescriptive practice by psychiatric nurses in advanced practice.
- Offer guidance to regulatory and legislative bodies with regard to the appropriate requirements that states should set for granting of prescriptive authority to advanced practice psychiatric nurses (psychiatric-mental health clinical nurse specialists and psychiatric nurse practitioners).

■ BACKGROUND

Prescription of psychoactive medications and the adjunctive pharmacologic agents that ameliorate side effects of these medications is recognized as a highly specialized nursing function. Prerequisite competencies for prescriptive activities include knowledge of neuroscience related to drug action and disorder pathology; understanding the dynamics and kinetics of psychopharmacologic agents and their actions; and competency in clinical case management, including assessment, diagnosis, treatment, and evaluation. The prescription of psychoactive medication also relies on knowledge of health status, coexisting physical conditions and/or medications, and other information necessary to provide a holistic plan of care for psychiatric-mental health patients in today's society (ANA, 1994).

■ POSITION

The American Psychiatric Nurses Association supports the granting of prescriptive authority to psychiatric nurses who meet the following qualifications:
- Licensure as a registered nurse (or advanced practice registered nurse) by a state board of nursing
- Master's degree in the field
- Certification as a specialist by the American Nurses Credentialing Center

- Demonstrated competence in physical assessment, neuroscience, and clinical psychopharmacology

ADVANCED EDUCATIONAL ■ PREPARATION

"The Psychiatric-Mental Health Advanced Practice Registered Nurse is a licensed registered nurse (RN) who is educationally prepared at a master's level, at a minimum, and is distinguished by a "depth of knowledge of theory and practice, supervised clinical practice, and competence in advanced clinical nursing skills. The psychiatric-mental health advanced practice registered nurse has the ability to apply knowledge, skills, and experience autonomously to complex mental health problems" (ANA et al., 1994).

PROFESSIONAL ■ CERTIFICATION

Among the over 40,000 clinical nurse specialists currently in practice across the United States, close to 7000 are credentialed at the national level by the American Nurses Credentialing Center as certified specialists (RN,CS) in adult and/or child and adolescent psychiatric-mental health nursing. However, not all of these advanced practice psychiatric nurses have prescriptive authority. In some states, legislation does not yet recognize psychiatric clinical nurse specialists as eligible to prescribe; in other states prescriptive authority is legalized, but not all eligible nurses have selected this intervention for their practice.

To be certified for advanced practice, the psychiatric nurse must meet the educational and clinical practice requirements of the American Nurses Credentialing Center. Nurses who meet all qualifications and pass the national certifying examination are awarded certification for 5 years as a certified specialist in either adult or child and adolescent psychiatric nursing. To maintain certification, the nurse must complete the certification renewal process (ANCC, 1995).

■ CONTINUED EDUCATION

To qualify to prescribe psychoactive medications in either a complementary or substitutive authority arrangement, advanced practice psychiatric nurses should successfully complete speciality-focused graduate level nursing courses (or their equivalent) in physical assessment, neuroscience, and clinical psychopharmacology. Demonstrated competence in these designated areas is necessary preparation for expansion of the advanced practice psychiatric nurse's role to include prescriptive authority. It is appropriate to expect that ongoing demonstration and documentation of competence through recertification or continuing education constitute a requirement for renewal of approval for prescriptive authority.

References

American Nurses Association. (1994). *Psychiatric Mental Health Nursing Psychopharmacology Project*. Washington, DC: American Nurses Publishing.

American Nurses Association (1994). *A statement on psychiatric-mental health clinical nursing practice and standards of psychiatric-mental health clinical nursing practice*. Washington, DC: American Nurses Publishing.

American Nurses Credentialing Center. (1995). *ANCC 1995 certification catalog*. Washington, DC: Author.

Talley, S., & Brooke, P. (1992). Prescriptive authority for psychiatric clinical specialists: framing the issues. *Archives of Psychiatric Nursing, 6*(2), 71–82.

Psychiatric-Mental Health Nurse Roles in Outcomes Evaluation and Management

■ INTRODUCTION

Outcome evaluation and management (OEM) is an accountability method that can be used to drive the process of balancing quality and cost of clinical health care service delivery. The collection and interpretation of outcome data are critical to survival within the health care system. As the evolving managed health care system continues to build momentum, it is imperative that the American Psychiatric Nurses Association (APNA) promote OEM as a strategy that will demonstrate efficacy of and enhance accountability and legitimacy for psychiatric-mental health nursing practice.

BACKGROUND AND ■ FRAMEWORK

OEM is a multidimensional process that can be studied using a framework for health care evaluation research that employs the concepts of structure, process, and outcomes (Bloch, 1975; Donabedian, 1976). The effect of setting- and provider-specific variables (structure) upon provider actions (processes) can be related to changes in the recipient of care (outcomes) through this evaluation method. Outcomes are studied at individual and population levels. These concepts will improve practice by enhancing understanding of the context within which treatment and services are provided. OEM will aid in developing and contributing to nursing knowledge through theory development and testing.

Psychiatric-mental health nurses have critical roles in OEM at both the basic and advanced levels. At the basic level, psychiatric-mental health nurses are at the forefront of clinical care delivery, often providing a wide range of direct and indirect services to individuals, families, and communities. At the advanced level, psychiatric-mental health nurses may be involved in both direct and indirect clinical service provision as well as in the analysis of aggregate data to evaluate programs of clinical care for targeted, "at risk" populations.

The ANA *Standards of Care* (1994) provides guidance and direction for psychiatric-mental health nursing practice. We must rely on our unique contributions in varied levels and specialty areas to provide the wide range and mix of services that are crucial in today's complex health care environment. Psychiatric-mental health nurses as a specialty group are uniquely poised to provide the type of collaborative, integrative, and multi-level clinical care service delivery that will be critical to successful psychiatric programs in the next decade.

■ POSITION

The APNA believes that outcome evaluation offers a critically important approach in determining the "value" of psychiatric-mental health nursing practice. It is essential that psychiatric-mental health nurses play key roles in addressing this effort. The APNA supports the following efforts:

- Involve APNA members in OEM at the local, state, and national levels.
- Appoint APNA members to national task forces, committees, and policy-setting groups that are

creating the agenda for outcome evaluation and management.

- Provide psychiatric-mental health nurses with education on utilizing outcome evaluation measures in the context of an interdisciplinary team within a variety of patient care settings.
- Establish guidelines for the selection of outcome evaluation tools, services, and techniques for psychiatric-mental health care.
- Promote the use of valid and reliable data for the measurement and evaluation of nursing-sensitive indicators within the provision of psychiatric-mental health services.
- Collaborate with the American Nurses Association, the Society for Education and Research in Psychiatric Nursing (SERPN), and other psychiatric-mental health nursing organizations in collecting, measuring, and interpreting psychiatric-mental health nursing-sensitive indicators.

References

American Nurses Association. (1994). *A statement on psychiatric-mental health clinical nursing practice and standards of psychiatric-mental health clinical nursing practice.* Washington, DC: American Nurses Publishing.

American Nurses Association. (1995). *Nursing care report for acute care.* Washington, DC: American Nurses Publishing.

American Nurses Association. (1996a). *Nursing quality indicators: definitions and implications.* Washington, DC: American Nurses Publishing.

American Nurses Association. (1996b). Nursing quality indicators: guide for implementation. Washington, DC: American Nurses Publishing.

Bloch, D. (1975). Evaluation of nursing care in terms of process and outcomes: issues in research and quality assurance. *Nursing Research, 24*(4), 256–263.

Center for Mental Health Services. (1996). *Consumer-oriented mental health report card.* Washington, DC: U.S. Department of Health and Human Services, Substance Abuse and Mental Health Services Administration.

Donabedian, A. (1966). Evaluating the quality of medical care. *Milbank Memorial Fund Quarterly, 44,* 166–196.

Mark, B. (1995). The black box of patient outcomes research. *IMAGE: Journal of Nursing Scholarship, 27*(1), 42.

Merwin, E., & Mauck, A. (1995). Psychiatric nursing outcome research: the state of the science. *Archives of Psychiatric Nursing, 9*(6), 311–331

Sederer, L., & Dickey, B. (Eds.). (1996). *Outcome assessment in clinical practice.* Baltimore, MD: Williams & Wilkins.

Sperry, L. (1997). Treatment outcomes: an overview. *Psychiatric Annals, 27*(2), 95–99.

Roles of Psychiatric-Mental Health Nurses in Managed Care

■ INTRODUCTION

Managed care has become a financing reality in health care as payers have developed strategies to curtail costs and improve the provision of care. *Managed care* is defined as "a system of managing and financing health care delivery to ensure that services provided to managed care plan members are necessary, efficiently provided and appropriately priced. Through a variety of techniques, such as pre-admission certification, concurrent review, financial incentives or penalties, managed care attempts to control access to provider sites where services are received, contain costs, manage utilization of services and resources, and ensure favorable patient outcomes. The term covers a broad spectrum of arrangements for health care delivery and financing, including managed indemnity plans (MIP), health maintenance organizations (HMO), preferred provider organizations (PPO), point of service plans (POS), as well as direct contracting arrangements between employers and providers" (Hart, 1995).

Assumptions about managed care include the following:

1. Based on a health (rather than illness) paradigm
2. Increases client access to appropriate (mental health) services
3. Ensures cost effectiveness through the development of clear boundaries with regard to targeting, planning, and delivering needed (mental health) services
4. Ensures quality control through a utilization review process
5. Offers availability of a choice of providers based on the type of care required (ANA, 1993)
6. Support for a meaningful participation of consumers and families in the redesign, implementation, evaluation, and monitoring of the managed care system is encouraged (NAMI, 1995).

■ BACKGROUND

At the beginning of 1996, it was estimated that more than 124 million Americans, or 44% of the population, were covered by some type of managed care plan. It is predicted that within the next 10 years, 90% of the health care in the United States will be provided in a managed care environment. Managed care is also making headlines because it is driving massive changes in professional practice, the definition of mental disorders, the nature of professional accountability, the allocation of professional resources, and the relationship of mental health professionals to one another (Shore & Beigel, 1996). The goal of managed care is not only to lower costs but also to ensure that maximum value is received from the resources used in the production and delivery of health care services to the population (Hicks, Stallmeyer, & Coleman, 1993).

■ POSITION

The American Psychiatric Nurses Association (APNA) believes that registered nurses in both basic and advanced practice roles utilize culturally competent standards in their practice and bring great value to the managed care arena through their rich blend of knowledge, skills, and expertise (WICHE, 1997). It is essential that managed care companies recognize the considerable expertise that psychiatric-mental health nurses contribute to the health care setting and maximize the full potential of nursing roles to best improve the process and outcomes of behavioral health care provided to consumers and their families across the life span.

■ DESCRIPTION

Psychiatric-mental health nurses at both the basic and advanced practice levels are uniquely qualified to serve in both indirect and direct care roles within managed care systems. Nurses alone among the various mental health disciplines combine the biopsychosocial knowledge, psychopharmacologic competency, and physical and psychiatric assessment skills with an intrinsic perspective of patient advocacy and 24-hour accountability. Psychiatric nurses are expert at evaluating complex psychiatric, substance abuse, and physical health needs and problems of patients over the life span. Nurses assess and treat psychosocial consequences of physical illness (APNA, 1997). Further, the American Nurses Association "endorses the utilization of psychiatric-mental health nurses as highly qualified professional participants in both indirect and direct care roles within psychiatric-mental health managed care systems. As the managed care industry evolves, we believe that it will be important for the professional to monitor the operationalization of the managed care concept to assure that its original objectives are fulfilled" (ANA, 1998). Because there is great variability of nursing activity based on service setting and geographic location, the advanced practice nurse and basic nurse may assume a number of roles in managed care systems. These include the following (Stuart, 1997):

- *Psychiatric-mental health nurse.* Nurses with various levels of preparation serve as direct care providers in contracted facilities and practices. These roles include staff nurses; managers and administrators; practitioners in psychiatric home health and community mental health settings; primary care providers; and independent providers of psychotherapy to individuals, groups, and families across the life span. The advanced practice registered nurse in psychiatric-mental health (APRN-PMH) has prescriptive authority in most states, but all registered nurses administer and monitor pharmacologic agents and monitor their effects.

- *Care manager.* Nurses in this role assess patients, develop treatment plans, and coordinate resources and care provided by others. The care manager also manages patient needs and resources episodically and is skilled in managing psychiatric rehabilitation and relapse prevention.

- *Assessment, evaluation, triage, and referral nurse.* In this role, the nurse evaluates patients in direct encounters or by telephone to triage the patient to the most appropriate level of care, including referrals to credentialed providers, contracted facilities, and community resources.

- *Utilization review nurse.* Many managed care companies employ psychiatric nurses to function as utilization reviewers in which they review aspects of the patient's care and influence decisions about treatment assignment. In this role they serve as "gatekeepers" to mental health services.

- *Patient educator.* Some settings hire nurses with responsibility assigned to them for patient and family education. This role has grown with an emphasis placed on patient-compliance and disease-management programs. In public sector programs, this role could include prevention, education, and outreach.

- *Risk manager.* Nurses who work as risk managers are charged with the task of decreasing the probability of adverse outcomes related to patient care. They engage in identifying risk factors, individual and system-wide problems, corrective actions, and the implementation of strategies to reduce risk and prevent loss.

- *Chief quality officer.* Nurses have assumed primary responsibility for formulating and implementing comprehensive quality management and improvement programs for managed care companies. They train other staff onsite and synthesize data related to performance improvement, outcomes management, and other health services research activities.

- *Marketing and development specialist.* Some psychiatric nurses work in the managed care growth areas of sales (proposal writing), marketing, and program development. In these roles, they interface with consumers, employers, providers, and regulators, and they make recommendations for furthering the mission and goals of the managed care organization.

- *Corporate manager and executive.* Psychiatric nurses are also present in middle management positions and in senior management positions where they participate in the development of corporate policy and strategic planning. Nurses hold positions in various departments, including provider relations, quality management, care management/clinical operations, service operations, and clinical/medical affairs.

References

American Nurses Association. (1993). *Position statement: psychiatric mental health nursing and managed care.* www.nursingworld.org/readroom/position/practice/prpsymen.htm

American Nurses Association. (1998). ANA board adopts nursing's principles for managed care environment. *The American Nurse,* January/February, 19.

American Psychiatric Nurses Association. (1997). *Advanced practice registered nurses in psychiatric and mental health care.* [Brochure]. Washington, DC: Author.

Hart, S. (1995). *ANA managed care curriculum for baccalaureate nursing programs.* Washington, DC: American Nurses Publishing.

Hicks, L.L., Stallmeyer, J.M., & Coleman, J.R. (1993). *Role of the nurse in managed care.* Washington, DC: American Nurses Publishing.

National Alliance for the Mentally Ill. (1995). *NAMI's principles for managed care.* [Brochure]. Arlington, VA: Author

Shore, M., & Beigel, A. (1996). Sounding board: the challenges posed by managed behavioral healthcare. *New England Journal of Medicine, 334*:116.

Stuart, G.W. (1997). Professional associations and managed care: how four provider groups are helping their members. *Behavioral Healthcare Tomorrow,* August, 41–44, 85.

WICHE. (1997). *Cultural competence standards in managed mental health care for underserved/underrepresented racial/ethnic groups.* (WICHE no. 97MO4762401D). Boulder, CO: Author.

Internet Resources

Agency for Health Care Policy and Research (AHCPR) (www.ahcpr.gov/)

American Association of Health Plans (www.aahp.org)

American Nurses Association (www.nursingworld.org)

American Psychiatric Nurses Association (www.apna.org)

Institute for Behavioral Healthcare (www.ibh.com)

National Committee for Quality Assurance (NCQA) (www.ncqa.org)

Psychotherapy Finances and Managed Care Strategies (www.psyfin.com)

American Managed Behavioral Healthcare Association (AMBHA) (www.ambha.org)

Selected Bibliography

Chisholm, M., et al. (1997). Quality indicators for primary mental health within managed care: a public health focus. *Archives of Psychiatric Nursing, 11*(40), 167–181.

Goodman, M., Brown, J.A., & Deitz, P.M. (1996). *Managing managed care II: a handbook for mental health professionals* (ed 2.). Washington, DC: American Psychiatric Press.

Haber, J., & Billings, C. (1995). Primary mental health care: a model for psychiatric-mental health nursing. *Journal of the American Psychiatric Nurses Association, 1,* 154–163.

Mason, D.J., et al. (1997). Managed care organizations' arrangements with nurse practitioners. *Nursing Economic$, 15*(6), 306–314.

Novartis. (1997). *A thru Z: managed care terms.* Bronxville, NY: Medicom International.

American Association for Marriage and Family Therapy, et al. (1997). *Your mental health rights: a joint initiative of mental health professional organizations.* [Brochure]. Washington, DC: Authors.

Measuring Outcomes in APRN-PMH Practice

III-A MEASURING OUTCOMES IN APRN-PMH PRACTICE
■ WORK GROUP

Chair: Deborah Antai-Otong, MS, RN, CS
Recorder: Susan Simmons-Alling, MSN, RN, CS
Carolyn L. Anich, APRN, CS
Andrea C. Bostrom, PhD, RN,
Document Preparation
Colleen S. Brems, MN, RN, CS
Ann M. Derrick, APRN, MS, CS
Carolyn Niziolek, RN, MS, CS
Margaret M. Pfeiffer
R. M. Scott Purol, MN, RN, CS
George Byron Smith, RN, MS, CS
Gail A. Staudt, MSN, RNC, CS
Mary Walker, MA, RN

QUESTIONS TO BE
■ ADDRESSED:

- Is there a need to develop a national database on impact of care provided by APRNs?
- If so, what information needs to be collected?
- Should we use standardized outcome measures?

■ BELIEF STATEMENT:
Introduction

The profession and consumers are requesting that psychiatric mental health services be empirically based to recognize the value of their delivery of services. Nurses are directly concerned with the well-being of their clients regardless of where in the continuum of care the services are delivered.

Advanced Practice Registered Nurses (APRNs) are major providers of ambulatory health care and therefore must assume a leadership role in measuring the quality of their services as well as documenting their worth. One weakness of existing databases is the lack of complete coverage in service provider related to identity, location, and sample served. Existing data systems are weak on measures of symptomatology, levels of functioning, and perceptual outcomes. The purpose of this document is to provide support for a national database to include clinical, functional, and financial outcomes and patient satisfaction.

Measuring Outcomes for Advanced Practice Registered Nurses in Psychiatric-Mental Health Nursing

Changes in the health care system since 1990 are necessitating increased efforts to systematically evaluate treatment outcomes. These changes affected many areas of society. Policy makers became acutely aware of health care's costs and its inexorable increases as a percentage of gross domestic product. The federal government attempted to rein in the cost of Medicaid and Medicare. Insurance companies followed prepayment procedures begun by the federal government in the 1980s. Health maintenance organizations (HMOs) pointed the way to managed care. For-profit corporations purchased hospitals and HMOs and demonstrated that costs could be cut. Health care professionals protected their practice domains with varying degrees of success. Health care purchasers (businesses, insurance companies, and consumers) wondered if they were receiving their money's worth. As a result of these changes, containing costs and protecting the market share must be coordinated with maintaining quality.

Nurses, like other health care professionals, are finding it necessary to validate their importance in the health care system. Credentialing, competency, and reimbursement for professional services require quality review and justification of outcome. Where advanced practice registered nurses (APRNs) provide clinical services that compete with other professionals, client outcomes that are at least equivalent to and in some dimensions better than other providers' outcomes must be demonstrated. This is particularly true for advanced practice registered nurses in psychiatric and mental health nursing (APRN-PMH).

Mental health treatment is complex. Several health care disciplines besides nursing deliver mental health treatment and are reimbursed. These include psychiatrists, psychologists, and social workers. Over 200 models of therapy are practiced across these disciplines (Burlingame et al., 1995). Similarly, over 200 diagnoses are treated (American Psychiatric Association [APA] et al., 1994). Many measures are available to assess psychiatric illnesses, their progression, and the functioning of those afflicted. These, however, range from complex, costly, and expensive rating scales to simplistic, idiosyncratic, and untested tools. In general, what needs to be assessed as outcomes and how to do this assessment remain unclear.

What is becoming clear, however, is that outcome assessment needs to be done (Burlingame et al., 1995). Mental health treatment is a growing proportion of health care expenditures. This is the case because there are more practitioners, so less stigma of mental health problems and the universal nature of problems like depression have been recognized. Another factor necessitating outcome assessment is the change in expectations of accrediting bodies, like the Joint Commission on the Accreditation of Healthcare Organizations, which now require monitoring of patient care. Finally,

a shift to managed care is occurring in federal, state, and many insurance programs. This shift creates competition to demonstrate cost containment and quality of outcome in order to receive approval or funding from these programs.

The purpose of this document is to clarify for APRNs-PMH how to demonstrate the achievement of outcomes comparable with those of other practitioners. In addition, APRNs-PMH need to demonstrate the unique and valuable services that nurses provide. Nurse psychotherapists are "especially suited to provide culturally relevant nursing therapy, integrating physical and mental concepts and involving and managing the family, milieu, and other social systems" (Hogarth, 1991, p. 312).

Nurses address issues of health behavior and illness prevention, assist with identifying social roles and supports for maintaining or changing these over the developmental stages, and sustain client efforts to overcome the complexities of day-to-day living and the inertia that challenges these efforts. All of these outcomes need to be evaluated. Therefore, along with other practitioners in the mental health field, nurses need to examine the impact of their interventions on symptoms, symptom clusters, and satisfaction.

Assessment of Outcomes

Outcomes Traditionally outcome investigations have focused on research protocols and patient satisfaction. The former primarily examined discrete symptom changes (e.g., responses to a particular medication or treatment activity). The latter examined the structure and process of treatment encounters (e.g., the promptness of treatment or the courtesy of staff). These remain important; however, outcomes also should focus on 1) symptoms, symptom clusters, and their progression over time; 2) functional status related to the ability to participate in day-to-day living; 3) patient satisfaction; and 4) family satisfaction.

Many assessment instruments are available to evaluate symptoms. Selected instruments should be consistent with symptom clusters as outlined in the *Diagnostic and Statistical Manual of Mental Disorders* (DSM-IV) (APA, 1994). APRNs-PMH should become most familiar with instruments that assess the diagnoses they most commonly treat. These include depression, anxiety, personality disorders, eating disorders, bipolar disorders, and schizophrenia. Outcome assessments of symptoms should examine initial symptomatology and be sensitive to an observable change in symptoms (clinician or significant other assessment) and a subjective change in symptoms (client assessment).

Fewer instruments are available for functional assessment. This is a complex area and of particular importance for nurses. Nurses typically have focused on such activities of daily living as bathing, eating, and sleeping, but "functioning" is a much broader concept. Sederer, Dickey, and Hermann (1996) suggest that functioning includes "the capacity to function within a family, community, or work environment or to exist independently, without undue burden on the family and the social welfare system" (p. 2). This includes the ability to know oneself and to assess for signs of relapse, to care for one's home, to obtain and manage income, to engage community agencies, and to become engaged in activities that enhance quality of life (such as family, leisure, and work).

Both patient and family satisfaction should be assessed. Patients need not only be happy with the structure and process of treatment, but they should also feel that they obtained the service for which they engaged the APRN-PMH. While this may include relief of symptoms, the patient's definition of satisfaction may include much more. At the very least it may mean a "subjective sense of health and well-being" (Sederer et al., 1996, p. 2). For the family, satisfaction may also be defined by the particular desires of the family unit. Satisfaction for families, however, is complicated by the confidentiality requirements for identified patients. For some families, satisfaction may be limited to the structure and process of the therapeutic encounter because the client is unwilling to engage the family beyond that. For others, feedback on symptoms, progress, and the match between these and expectations may be easily obtained.

Outcome measures Several considerations need to be incorporated into the selection of actual assessment instruments. These can be classified by the practicality of their use and the psychometric properties of the actual scale (Vermillion & Pfeiffer, 1995; Burlingame et al., 1995). Practicality includes the ease of use, the acceptance by practitioners and patients, and cost. Psychometric properties include standardization, reliability, validity, and sensitivity.

On a practical basis, it is important that the instrument is easy to use. This means that it is brief though inclusive, that it can be easily administered, and that it can be easily scored. Paper and pencil tests are best if they can be completed during a brief pre-therapy wait and scored by a scanner and/or computer. Interpretation should be relatively simple or clear, and the tests should be easy to obtain and in the public domain whenever possible. If they must be purchased, then they should be as inexpensive as possible. Outcome measures should not add to the paperwork of the clinicians (Burlingame et al., 1995).

Selected instruments should be standardized with normative data from samples similar to the patients seen by the clinician. It is important that instruments not be idiosyncratic or individually developed because these are not likely to be comparable to measures used by other clinicians or agencies. There needs to be evidence that reliability has been evaluated and that coefficients are acceptable for both internal consistency (coefficient alpha = .80 or better) and test-retest reliability (correlation = .70 or better) (Burlingame et al., 1995). It also is important that there is evidence of sensitivity (i.e., that the instrument is able to detect actual changes in patient symptoms, functioning, and satisfaction) (Vermillion & Pfeiffer, 1995).

References

Abraham, I.L. (1991). The Geriatric Depression Scale and Hopelessness Index: longitudinal psychometric data on frail nursing home residents. *Perceptual & Motor Skills,* 875–88.

Acorn, S. (1993). Use of the brief psychiatric rating scale. *Journal of Psychosocial Nursing 31*(5), 9–12.

American Psychiatric Association. (1994). *Diagnostic and statistical manual of mental disorders* (ed. 4). Washington, D.C.: Author.

Andreasen, N.C. (1982). Negative symptoms of schizophrenia: definition and reliability. *Archives of General Psychiatry, 39,* 784–788.

Andreasen, N.C. (1984a). *Scale for the assessment of negative symptoms (SANS).* Iowa City: CID.

Andreasen, N.C. (1984b). *Scale for the assessment of positive symptoms (SAPS).* Iowa City: CID.

Attkisson, C.C., & Greenfield, T.K. (1996). The client satisfaction questionnaire (CSQ) scales and the service satisfaction scale-30 (SSS-30). In Sederer, L.I., & Dickey, B. (Eds.). *Outcomes assessment in clinical practice.* Baltimore: Williams & Wilkins.

Beck, A.T., & Steer, R.A. (1993). *Manual for the Beck Depression Inventory.* San Antonio: Psychological Corporation.

Beck, A.T., Steer, R.A., & Garbin, M.G. (1988). Psychometric properties of the Beck Depression Inventory: twenty-five years of evaluation. *Clinical Psychology Review, 8,* 77–100.

Brink, T.L., et al. (1982). Screening tests for geriatric depression. *Clinical Gerontologist, 1,* 37–43.

Burlingame, G.M. (1995). Pragmatics of tracking mental health outcomes in a managed care setting. *Journal of Mental Health Administration, 22,* 226–236.

Eisen, S.V. (1995). Assessment of subjective distress by patients' self-report versus structured interview. *Psychological Reports, 76,* 35–39.

Eisen, S.V. (1996). Behavior and Symptom Identification Scale (BASIS-32). In Sederer, L.I., & Dickey, B. (Eds.). *Outcomes assessment in clinical practice.* Baltimore: Williams & Wilkins.

Eisen, S.V., Dill, D.L., & Grob, M.C. (1994). Reliability and validity of a brief patient-report instrument for psychiatric outcome evaluation. *Hospital and Community Psychiatry, 45,* 242–247.

Garner, D.M. (1996). Eating disorder inventory-2 (EDI-2). In Sederer, L.I., & Dickey, B. (Eds.). *Outcomes assessment in clinical practice.* Baltimore: Williams & Wilkins.

Garner, D.M. (1993). *Eating disorder inventory-2 professional manual.* Odessa, FL: Psychological Assessment Resources.

Garner, D.M., Olmstead M.P., & Polivy, J. (1983a). Development and validation of a multidimensional eating disorder inventory for anorexia nervosa and bulimia. *International Journal of Eating Disorders, 2*(2), 15–34.

Garner, D.M., Olmstead, M.P., & Polivy, J. (1983b). The

eating disorder inventory: a measure of cognitive-behavioral dimensions of anorexia nervosa and bulimia. In Darby, P.L., et al. (Eds.). *Anorexia nervosa: recent developments in research.* New York: Alan R. Liss.

Goodman, W.K., et al. (1989). The Yale-Brown Obsessive Compulsive Scale: development, use, and reliability. *Archives of General Psychiatry, 46,* 1006–1011.

Goodman, W.K., et al. (1989). The Yale-Brown Obsessive Compulsive Scale: validity. *Archives of General Psychiatry, 46,* 1012–1016.

Hamilton, M. (1959). The assessment of anxiety states by rating. *British Journal of Medical Psychology, 32,* 50–55.

Hamilton, M. (1960). A rating scale for depression. *Journal of Neurology, Neurosurgery, and Psychiatry, 23,* 56–62.

Hamilton, M. (1967). Development of a rating scale for primary depressive illness. *British Journal of Social and Clinical Psychology, 6,* 278–296.

Hogarth, C.R. (1991). *Adolescent psychiatric nursing.* St. Louis: Mosby.

Jones, S.H., Thornicroft, G., Coffey, M., & Dunn, G. (1995). A brief mental health outcome scale: reliability, and validity of the global assessment of functioning (GAF). *British Journal of Psychiatry, 166,* 654–659.

Kovacs, M. (1992). *Children's Depression Inventory manual.* North Tonawanda, N.Y.: Multi-Health Systems, Inc.

Murphy. M.F., & Moller, M.D. (1993). Relapse management in neurobiological disorders: the Moller-Murphy Symptom Management Assessment Tool. *Archives of Psychiatric Nursing, 7,* 226–235.

Overall, J.E., & Gorham, D.R. (1962). The Brief Psychiatric Rating Scale. *Psychological Reports, 10,* 799–812.

Overall, J.E., & Gorham, D.R. (1988). The Brief Psychiatric Rating Scale (BPRS): recent developments in ascertainment and scaling. *Psychopharmacology Bulletin, 24,* 97–99.

Sederer, L.I., Dickey, B., & Hermann, R.C. (1996). The imperative of outcome assessment in psychiatry. In Sederer, L.I., & Dickey, B. (Eds.). *Outcomes assessment in clinical practice.* Baltimore: Williams & Wilkins.

Sederer, L.I., & Dickey, B. (1996). *Outcomes assessment in clinical practice.* Baltimore: Williams & Wilkins.

Steer, R.A., & Beck, A.T. (1996). Beck Depression Inventory (BDI). In Sederer, L.I., & Dickey, B. (Eds.). *Outcomes assessment in clinical practice.* Baltimore: Williams & Wilkins.

Tarell, J.D., & Schulz, S.C. (1988). Nursing assessment using the BPRS: a structured interview. *Psychopharmacology Bulletin, 24,* 105–111.

Vermillion, J.M., & Pfeiffer, S.I. (1995). Treatment outcome and continuous quality improvement: two aspects of program evaluation. *Psychiatric Hospital, 24,* 9–14.

Ware, J.E. (1996). The MOS 36-item short-form health survey (SF-36). In Sederer, L.I., & Dickey, B. (Eds.).

Outcomes assessment in clinical practice. Baltimore: Williams & Wilkins.

Ware, J.E., Kosinski, M., & Keller, S.D. (1994). *SF-36 physical and mental component summary measures—user's manual.* Boston: New England Medical Center. The Health Institute.

Ware, J.E., Snow, K.K., Kosinski, M., & Gandek, B. (1993). *SF-36 health survey manual and interpretation, guide.* Boston: New England Medical Center. The Health Institute.

Wilier, B., Ottenbacher, K.J., & Coad, M.L. (1994). The community integration questionnaire: a comparative examination. *American Journal of Physical Medicine and Rehabilitation, 73,* 103–111.

Wilier, B., et al. (1993). Assessment of community integration following rehabilitation for traumatic brain injury. *Journal of Head Trauma Rehabilitation, 8*(2), 75–87.

Yesavage, J.A., et al. (1983). Development and validation of a geriatric depression screening scale: a preliminary report. *Journal of Psychiatric Research, 17,* 37–49.

SERPN Position Statement: Graduate Educational Preparation for Psychiatric-Mental Health Nursing Practice

WHEREAS, advanced practice psychiatric nurses possess knowledge and skills to effectively address mental health needs of individuals, families, and communities, and

WHEREAS, access to mental health care is limited by state and federal regulations and other special interest groups, and

WHEREAS, external forces determine who provides and is reimbursed for services as well as the scope and extent of such services, and

WHEREAS, there is considerable lack of clarity regarding titles and definitions of advanced practice nurses, and

WHEREAS, the need for mental health services has increased and the supply of graduates prepared in the specialty of psychiatric nursing has not kept pace with the demand, and

WHEREAS, there is a need for research addressing the efficacy, quality, and cost effectiveness of psychiatric nursing care as an essential element of healthcare reform,

Therefore Be It Resolved That:

Psychiatric nursing programs support the American Nurses Association's position that education

From Society for Education and Research in Psychiatric-Mental Health Nursing. (1996). *Educational preparation for psychiatric-mental health nursing practice.* Pensacola, FL: Author.

for advanced nursing practice take place in Master's degree programs.

Practice sites in home care, managed care settings, schools, industry, and primary care clinics be developed to expand access to advanced psychiatric nursing care.

Psychiatric nursing services provided by advanced practice nurses be reimbursed by private, state, and federal health insurance plans.

Psychiatric nursing organizations and state boards of nursing continue to collaborate to define the scope of advanced psychiatric nursing practice and to attain advanced practice privileges.

Faculty in schools of nursing and providers of nursing service collaborate in the development of aggressive strategies for recruitment into the specialty.

Research be conducted to investigate the efficacy, quality, and cost effectiveness of advanced practice psychiatric nursing, and

Be It Further Resolved That:

Programs preparing advanced practice psychiatric nurses address the following:

The development, utilization, and evaluation of conceptual frameworks that guide assessment and intervention strategies for underserved populations and populations at risk for mental illness.

The development of practicum experiences and sites that reflect multicultural concerns and emerging trends in the delivery of psychiatric care.

The expansion of the scope of practice to include a focus on primary prevention in the area of mental health.

The inclusion of educational and collaborative modes of working with clients and their families.

The inclusion of both direct (assessment, intervention) and indirect (consultation, case management, supervision) advanced practice roles.

The inclusion of biological and pharmacological content as fundamental to advanced practice.

The inclusion of health assessment skills, with emphasis on those skills most pertinent to the care of those with or at risk for a mental illness.

The inclusion of mental health aspects and psychiatric complications of physical illnesses.

The analysis of the legal and ethical problems associated with the expansion of the role and scope of practice of the advanced practice nurse.

The analysis of existing mental health policy and participation in the development of new policy initiatives.

The integration of content on cost benefit analysis, fiscal resources, and the impact of economic realities on mental health services.

The expansion of the focus and methodologies of psychiatric nursing research to include outcome and intervention studies.

The collaboration with consumer groups in the development of curricula for advanced nursing practice.

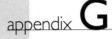

appendix **G**

SERPN Guidelines for Graduate Education in Psychiatric-Mental Health Nursing (PMHN)

Position Statement (1)

The utilization, evaluation, and conceptualization of intervention strategies used with persons with mental illness and persons/populations at risk for mental illness

CORE CONTENT	ESSENTIAL PMHN CONTENT	CLINICAL SKILLS
Introduction to concepts, theories, and models	Theories related to the neurobiological aspects of mental illness	Reflect and document theory, practice, and research integration in clinical practice
Epidemiology		
Diagnostic reasoning	Developmental theories and models	
Systems theory	Psychotherapy theories and models	

Position Statement (2)

The development of practicum experiences and sites that reflect multicultural concerns and emerging trends in the delivery of psychiatric care

CORE CONTENT	ESSENTIAL PMHN CONTENT	CLINICAL SKILLS
Community assessment	Assessment of community mental health needs	Demonstrate ability to access and collaborate with community groups
Sociocultural theories	Ethnic and cultural aspects of accessing and collaborating with specific populations for mental health care	Document an identifiable number of clinical practice hours in nontraditional community sites
Community as client	Traditional and nontraditional community practice sites	
	Emerging service delivery models	

581

Position Statement (3)

The expansion of the scope of practice to include a focus on primary prevention in the area of mental health

CORE CONTENT	ESSENTIAL PMHN CONTENT	CLINICAL SKILLS
Health promotion	Diagnostic characteristics of specific psychiatric illnesses	Identify clients at risk and plan and implement intervention strategies
Levels of prevention	Risk factors associated with psychiatric illnesses	
	Prevention and mental health promotion	

Position Statement (4)

The inclusion of educational and collaborative modes of working with clients and their families

CORE CONTENT	ESSENTIAL PMHN CONTENT	CLINICAL SKILLS
Teaching/ learning process	Collaboration	Document continuing client and family involvement in the planning and implementation of care

CORE CONTENT	ESSENTIAL PMHN CONTENT	CLINICAL SKILLS
	Psychoeducation	Plan and implement psychoeducation approaches with psychiatric clients and families

Position Statement (5)

The inclusion of both direct (assessment, intervention) and indirect (consultation, case management, supervision) advanced practice roles

CORE CONTENT	ESSENTIAL PMHN CONTENT	CLINICAL SKILLS
	Comprehensive psychiatric mental health history	Demonstrate ability to perform rapid assessment
	Psychiatric interviewing	Demonstrate ability to diagnose intervene, and manage common and recurrent psychiatric symptoms/ conditions
	Diagnostic classification systems related to psychiatric illness	Provide care for psychiatric patients that addresses initial contact,

CORE CONTENT	ESSENTIAL PMHN CONTENT	CLINICAL SKILLS
		comprehensive, coordinated, and continuous care
	Psychiatric formulations underlying treatment plans	
	Psychotherapeutic treatment modalities	
	PMH Consultation/ Liaison theory	
	Clinical supervision	
	Clinical case management	
	Boundary issues related to direct and indirect advanced practice	
	Primary psychiatric care as a first line provider	

CORE CONTENT	ESSENTIAL PMHN CONTENT	CLINICAL SKILLS
Pharmacology	Psychopharmacology as outlined on page 23 of the psychopharmacology document*	Demonstrate knowledge of the clinical principles of psychopharmacology guidelines outlined in the psychopharmacology document* pp. 41–45

*American Nurses Association (1994). *Psychiatric mental health nursing psychopharmacology project.* Washington, DC: American Nurses Publishing.

Position Statement (7)

The inclusion of health assessment skills, with emphasis on those skills most pertinent to the care of those with or at risk for a mental illness

CORE CONTENT	ESSENTIAL PMHN CONTENT	CLINICAL SKILLS
Physical assessment	Differential diagnosis	Demonstrate the ability to screen for physical abnormalities
Comprehensive history taking		
Diagnostic reasoning		

Position Statement (6)

The inclusion of biological and pharmacological content as fundamental to advanced practice

Position Statement (8)

The inclusion of mental health aspects and psychiatric complications of physical illnesses

CORE CONTENT	ESSENTIAL PMHN CONTENT	CLINICAL SKILLS
Comprehensive health assessment	Comprehensive psychiatric assessment	Demonstrate performance of differential diagnosis of physical/mental illness
Physical assessment	Diagnosis of common physical illnesses that mimic psychiatric illnesses and common psychiatric symptoms that occur in physical illness	Use appropriate referral sources for physical symptoms/illnesses and provide follow-up care

Position Statement (9)

The analysis of the legal and ethical problems associated with the expansion of the role and scope of practice of the advanced practice nurse

CORE CONTENT	ESSENTIAL PMHN CONTENT	CLINICAL SKILLS
Legal basis and legal boundaries of advanced practice nursing	Advanced PMHN certification and licensure (e.g., Nurse Practice Act; Standards for Advanced PMHN)	Identify legal and ethical issues in direct and indirect practice
Ethical aspects of advanced practice nursing	Forensic issues, (e.g., prediction of violence, duty to warn)	Seek expert guidance in regard to identified legal and ethical problems
Prescriptive authority	Boundary issues related to direct and indirect PMHN practice	
	Confidentiality and its limits	
	Informed consent	
	Contracting for service provision	

Position Statement (10)

The analysis of existing mental health policy and participation in the development of new policy initiatives

CORE CONTENT	ESSENTIAL PMHN CONTENT	CLINICAL SKILLS
Health policy dictates practice	History of mental health legislation	Analyze a public policy for its impact on mental health
Practice influences health policy	Mental health policy practice implications	
Legislative process	Mental health policy and social climate	Analyze a mental health policy for its impact on practice

Position Statement (11)

The integration of content on cost benefit analysis, fiscal resources, and the impact of economic realities on mental health services

CORE CONTENT	ESSENTIAL PMHN CONTENT	CLINICAL SKILLS
Economics of health care		
Fiscal consequences of public policy	Fiscal consequences of public policy on mental health service delivery	Write a contract with a third party provider for the delivery of mental health services
Principles of managed health care	Principles of behavioral health care	
Cost benefit analysis	Cost benefit analysis related to psychiatric services	Perform a cost benefit analysis for a psychiatric intervention
	Contracting with health-care providers	

Position Statement (12)

The expansion of the focus and methodologies of psychiatric nursing research to include outcome and intervention studies

CORE CONTENT	ESSENTIAL PMHN CONTENT	CLINICAL SKILLS
Graduate level research course	Intervention research related to psychiatric treatment	Use intervention research findings in planning care
	Outcomes research related to psychiatric treatment	Identify common basic outcome measurement tools for PMHN core

Position Statement (13)

The collaboration with consumer groups in the development of curricula for advanced nursing practice

CORE CONTENT	ESSENTIAL PMHN CONTENT	CLINICAL SKILLS
	Knowledge of mental health consumer/advocacy groups	Demonstrate knowledge of collaborative strategies in working with consumer/advocacy groups
	Functions of advisory boards	

Recommendations for Clinical Hours: (ORIGINAL)

(1) A minimum of 500 hours of clinical experience which may include a maximum of 100 hours of clinical supervision (i.e., individual and/or group supervision provided by a qualified faculty member or certified specialist in PMHN).

(2) Core content must be taught by a qualified faculty member with specialization in PMHN.

(3) Curricula are designed to prepare students to meet the qualifications for certification in PMHN as proposed by the American Nurses Credentialing Center.

(4) The advanced practice psychiatric nurse is prepared to practice consistent with the Advanced Practice Standards in the *Statement on PMH Clinical Nursing Practice and Standards of PMH Clinical Nursing Practice*,* which is different from primary care nurse practitioners who work with psychiatric populations.

*American Nurses Association. (1994). *A statement on psychiatric-mental health clinical nursing practice and standards of psychiatric-mental health clinical nursing practice*. Washington, DC: American Nurses Publishing.

Colleges with Psychiatric-Mental Health Nursing Master's Programs

COLLEGE	TYPE OF PROGRAM
ALABAMA	
University of Alabama at Birmingham	CNS and NP
University of South Alabama College of Nursing	CNS and Teaching/Education
ALASKA	
University of Alaska, Anchorage	CNS
ARIZONA	
Arizona State University	CNS, NP, and Post-Master's/NP
University of Arizona	NP, Post-Master's/NP
ARKANSAS	
University of Arkansas for Medical Sciences, College of Nursing	CNS and NP
CALIFORNIA	
Azusa Pacific University	CNS
California State University at Long Beach	NP
California State University at Los Angeles	CNS
University of California	CNS and NP
University of California Center for Health Sciences	CNS
COLORADO	
University of Colorado School of Nursing	CNS
CONNECTICUT	
Fairfield University	CNS
St. Joseph College Nursing Division	CNS
University of Connecticut	CNS
Yale University	CNS
DISTRICT OF COLUMBIA	
Catholic University of America	CNS and NP
FLORIDA	
Florida International University	CNS, NP, Post-Master's/NP, and Teaching/Education
Florida State University	CNS

University of Florida College of Nursing	NP
University of Miami	NP
University of South Florida	CNS and NP

GEORGIA

Georgia College	CNS and Teaching/Education
Georgia State University	CNS
Medical College of Georgia	CNS and Teaching/Education
Valdosta State University College of Nursing	CNS

HAWAII

University of Hawaii	CNS

ILLINOIS

Governors State University	CNS and Teaching/Education
Northern Illinois University	CNS
Rush University	CNS
Southern Illinois University School of Nursing	CNS, Teaching/Education, and Nurse Administration
St. Xavier College	CNS, Teaching/Education
University of Illinois College of Nursing	CNS

INDIANA

Ball State University	Teaching/Education
Indiana University School of Nursing	CNS and Post-Master's/NP
Valparaiso University	CNS

KANSAS

University of Kansas School of Nursing	CNS
Wichita State University	CNS

KENTUCKY

University of Kentucky College of Nursing	CNS and Post-Master's/NP

LOUISIANA

Louisiana State University Medical Center	CNS
Northwestern State University	CNS

MAINE

University of Southern Maine	CNS

MARYLAND

University of Maryland at Baltimore	CNS

MASSACHUSETTS

Boston College	CNS and Post-Master's/NP
Massachusetts General Hospital Institute	
Northeastern University	CNS and NP
University of Massachusetts—Amherst	CNS, NP, and Teaching/Education
University of Massachusetts—Lowell	NP

MICHIGAN

Grand Valley State University - Kirkhof School	CNS and Teaching/Education
University of Michigan	CNS
Wayne State University	CNS

MINNESOTA

University of Minnesota School of Nursing	CNS

MISSISSIPPI

University of Southern Mississippi	CNS

MISSOURI

St. Louis University School of Nursing	CNS
University of Missouri—Columbia	CNS, Teaching/Education, Nurse Administration

MONTANA

Montana State University	CNS

NEBRASKA

University of Nebraska	CNS

NEW HAMPSHIRE

Rivier College	NP

NEW JERSEY

Rutgers—The State University of New Jersey	CNS and NP

NEW MEXICO

New Mexico State University	CNS and Teaching/Education
University of New Mexico	CNS and Teaching/Education

NEW YORK

Adelphi University	Teaching/Education
College of Mt. St. Vincent	CNS
Columbia University School of Nursing	NP and Post-Master's/NP
Hunter College—City University of New York	CNS
Pace University	CNS
Russell Sage College	CNS, NP, and Post-Master's/NP
State University of New York at Buffalo	CNS
State University of New York—Stony Brook	NP and Post-Master's/NP
Syracuse University	CNS
University of Rochester	CNS

NORTH CAROLINA

East Carolina University	CNS
University of North Carolina at Chapel Hill	CNS
University of North Carolina at Charlotte	CNS
University of North Carolina at Greensboro	CNS

OHIO
Case Western Reserve University	CNS, NP, and Post-Master's/NP
Kent State University	CNS, NP, Post-Master's/NP, and Teach/Education
Medical College of Ohio School of Nursing	CNS and Teaching/Education
Ohio State University College of Nursing	CNS
University of Akron College of Nursing	CNS and Teaching/Education
University of Cincinnati College of Nursing and Health	CNS

OKLAHOMA
University of Oklahoma Health Sciences Center	CNS and Teaching/Education

OREGON
The Oregon Health Sciences University	CNS, NP, and Post-Master's/NP

PENNSYLVANIA
Temple University College of Allied Health Professionals	CNS
University of Pennsylvania	CNS
University of Pittsburgh School of Nursing	CNS and NP
Villanova University	CNS

PUERTO RICO
Catholic University of Puerto Rico	CNS and Teaching/Education
University of Puerto Rico	CNS and Teaching/Education

RHODE ISLAND
University of Rhode Island	CNS

SOUTH CAROLINA
Medical University of South Carolina College of Nursing	CNS
University of South Carolina College of Nursing	CNS, NP, and Teaching/Education

TENNESSEE
University of Tennessee College of Nursing	NP
University of Tennessee at Knoxville	CNS
Vanderbilt University	CNS and Post-Master's/NP

TEXAS
Texas Woman's University College of Nursing	CNS
University of Texas Health Science Center	CNS, NP, and Teaching/Education
University of Texas Health Science Center (San Antonio)	CNS
University of Texas at Arlington School of Nursing	NP, Post-Master's/NP, and Teaching/Education
University of Texas at Austin School of Nursing	CNS
University of Texas at El Paso School of Nursing	CNS and NP
University of Texas at Tyler School of Nursing	CNS

UTAH
University of Utah	NP and Post-Master's/NP

VIRGINIA

Hampton University	Teaching/Education
University of Virginia	CNS and NP
Virginia Commonwealth University Medical College	CNS

WASHINGTON

Gonzaga University	CNS and Teaching/Education
Intercollegiate Center for Nursing Education	CNS
Seattle Pacific University	CNS and Teaching/Education
University of Washington	CNS and NP

WISCONSIN

University of Wisconsin at Madison	CNS and Teaching/Education
University of Wisconsin—Milwaukee	CNS

From *Annual guide to graduate nursing education.* (1996). New York: National League for Nursing.

Nursing Doctoral Programs in the United States

Alabama

University of Alabama at
 Birmingham
School of Nursing UAB
1701 University Blvd
Birmingham, AL 35294-1210

Arizona

University of Arizona
College of Nursing
1305 North Martin Ave.
PO Box 210203
Tucson, AZ 85721-0203

Arkansas

University of Arkansas for Medical
 Sciences
College of Nursing
4301 W. Markham St., Slot 529
Little Rock, AR 72205-7199

California

University of California—
 Los Angeles
School of Nursing
700 Tiverton Ave.
Box 951702
Los Angeles, CA 90095-1702

University of California—
 San Francisco
School of Nursing
3rd and Parnassus
San Francisco, CA 94143-0604

University of San Diego
Philip Y. Hahn School of Nursing
5998 Alcala Park
San Diego, CA 92110-2492

Colorado

University of Colorado Health
 Science Center
School of Nursing
4200 East Ninth Ave., Box C288
Denver, CO 80262-0288

Connecticut

University of Connecticut
School of Nursing
U-26, Rm. 113
231 Glenbrook Rd.
Storrs, CT 06269-2026

Yale University
School of Nursing
100 Church St. South
PO Box 9740
New Haven, CT 06536-0740

District of Columbia

The Catholic University of
 America
School of Nursing
620 Michigan Ave., N.E.
Washington, DC 20064

Florida

Barry University
School of Nursing
11300 N.E., 2nd Ave.
Wiegand 133
Miami Shores, FL 33161-6695

University of Florida
College of Nursing
P.O. Box 100197, JHMCH
Gainesville, FL 32610-0197

University of Miami
School of Nursing
P.O. Box 248153
Coral Gables, FL 33124-3850

University of South Florida
College of Nursing
12901 Bruce B. Downs Blvd,
MDC Box 22
Tampa, FL 33612-4766

Georgia

Georgia State University
College of Health Sciences
School of Nursing
P.O. Box 4019
Atlanta, GA 30302-4019

Medical College of Georgia
School of Nursing
997 St. Sebastian Way
Augusta, GA 30912-4206

Illinois

Loyola University of Chicago
Marcella Niehoff School of
 Nursing
6525 N. Sheridan Rd.
Chicago, IL 60626-5385

Rush University
School of Nursing
1743 Harrison St.
Chicago, IL 60612-7350

University of Illinois at Chicago
College of Nursing M/C 802
845 South Damen Avenue
Chicago, IL 60612-7350

Indiana

Indiana University
School of Nursing
1111 Middle Dr.
Indianapolis, IN 46202-5107

Iowa

University of Iowa
College of Nursing
Room 101F NB
Iowa City, IA 52242-1121

Kansas

University of Kansas Medical
  Center
School of Nursing
3901 Rainbow Blvd.
Kansas City, KS 66160-7500

Kentucky

University of Kentucky
College of Nursing
315 CON/HSLC Building
760 Rose St.
Lexington, KY 40536-0232

Louisiana

Louisiana State University Medical
  Center
School of Nursing
1900 Gravier St.
New Orleans, LA 70112-2262

Maryland

The Johns Hopkins University
School of Nursing
525 North Wolfe St.
Baltimore, MD 21205-2110

University of Maryland
School of Nursing
655 West Lombard St.
Baltimore, MD 21201-1579

Massachusetts

Boston College
School of Nursing
140 Commonwealth Ave.
Cushing Hall
Chestnut Hill, MA 02167-3812

University of
  Massachusetts—Lowell
Department of Nursing
One University Ave.
Lowell, MA 01854

Michigan

University of Michigan
School of Nursing
400 North Ingalls St., Room 1320
Ann Arbor, MI 48109-0482

Wayne State University
College of Nursing
5557 Cass Ave.
Detroit, MI 48202

Minnesota

University of Minnesota
School of Nursing
6-101 Weaver-Densford Hall
308 Harvard St. S.E.
Minneapolis, MN 55545-0342

Mississippi

University of Southern Mississippi
College of Nursing
SS Box 5095
Hattiesburg, MS 39406-5095

Missouri

Saint Louis University
School of Nursing
3525 Caroline St.
St. Louis, MO 63104-1099

University of Missouri—Columbia
Sinclair School of Nursing
8215 School of Nursing Building
Columbia, MO 65211

University of Missouri—
  Kansas City
School of Nursing
2220 Holmes
Kansas City, MO 64108-2676

University of Missouri—St. Louis
Barnes College of Nursing
8001 Natural Bridge
St. Louis, MO 63121-4496

Nebraska

University of Nebraska Medical
  Center
College of Nursing
600 South 42nd St.
Omaha, NE 68198

New Jersey

Rutgers—The State University of
  New Jersey
College of Nursing
Ackerson 102
180 University Ave.
Newark, NJ 07102

New York

Adelphi University
School of Nursing
P.O. Box 516
Garden City, NY 11530

Binghamton University
Decker School of Nursing
P.O. Box 6000
Binghamton, NY 13902-6000

Columbia University
Department of Nursing
630 West 168th St.
New York, NY 10032

New York University
Division of Nursing
429 Shimkin Hall
50 West 4th St.
New York, NY 10012

State University of New York at
  Buffalo
School of Nursing
1030 Kimball Tower
3425 Main St.
Buffalo, NY 14214-3079

Teacher's College—Columbia
  University
Program in Nursing Education
525 West 120th St.
Box 150
New York, New York 10027

University of Rochester
School of Nursing
601 Elmwood Ave., Box 703
Rochester, NY 14642

North Carolina
University of North
  Carolina—Chapel Hill
School of Nursing
107 Carrington Hall CB#7460
Chapel Hill, NC 27599-7460

Ohio
Case Western Reserve University
Frances Payne Bolton School of
  Nursing
10900 Euclid Ave.
Cleveland, OH 44106-4904

Kent State University
School of Nursing
Henderson Hall
Kent, OH 44242

Ohio State University
College of Nursing
1585 Neil Ave.
Columbus, OH 43210-1289

University of Akron
College of Nursing
209 Carroll St.
Akron, OH 44325-3701

University of Cincinnati
College of Nursing and Health
3110 Vine St.
Cincinnati, OH 45219

Oregon
Oregon Health Sciences University
School of Nursing
3181 S.W. Sam Jackson Park Road
Portland, OR 97201-3098

Pennsylvania
Duquesne University
School of Nursing
600 Forbes Ave.
Pittsburgh, PA 15282

Unniversity of Pennsylvania
School of Nursing
420 Guardian Dr.
Philadelphia, PA 19104-6096

University of Pittsburgh
School of Nursing
3500 Victoria St.
Pittsburgh, PA 15261

Widener University
School of Nursing
One University Place
Chester, PA 19013-5792

Rhode Island
University of Rhode Island
College of Nursing
White Hall
2 Heathman Rd.
Kingston, RI 02881-0814

South Carolina
University of South Carolina
College of Nursing
Pickens & Green St.
Columbia, SC 29208-9998

Tennessee
University of Tennessee at
  Knoxville
College of Nursing
1200 Volunteer Blvd.
Knoxville, TN 37916-4180

University of
  Tennessee—Memphis
College of Nursing
877 Madison Ave., Suite 620
Memphis, TN 38163

Vanderbilt University
School of Nursing
21st Ave. S., 111 Godchaux Hall
Nashville, TN 37240-0008

Texas
Texas Woman's University
College of Nursing
P.O. Box 425498
Denton, TX 76204-5498

University of Texas at Austin
School of Nursing
1700 Red River
Austin, TX 78701-1499

University of Texas Health Science
  Center—Houston
School of Nursing
1100 Holcombe Blvd., Suite 5500
Houston, TX 77030

University of Texas Health Science
  Center—San Antonio
School of Nursing
7703 Floyd Curl Drive
San Antonio, TX 78284-7942

Univeristy of Texas Medical
  Branch at Galveston
School of Nursing
301 University Blvd., Route J-29
Galveston, TX 77555-1029

Utah
University of Utah
College of Nursing
105 2000 E. Front
Salt Lake City, UT 84112-5880

Virginia
George Mason University
College of Nursing and Health
  Science
4400 University Dr.
Fairfax, VA 22030-4444

University of Virginia
School of Nursing
McLeod Hall, Box 1
Charlottesville, VA 22903-3395

Virginia Commonwealth University
School of Nursing
1220 East Broad St.
P.O. Box 980567
Richmond, VA 23298-0567

Washington

University of Washington
School of Nursing
Box 357260
Seattle, WA 98195-7260

Wisconsin

University of Wisconsin at Madison
School of Nursing
600 Highland Ave.
Madison, WI 53792-2445

University of
  Wisconsin—Milwaukee
School of Nursing
P.O. Box 413
Milwaukee, WI 53201-0413

Publications of the American Nurses Association (ANA)

Psychiatric Mental Health Nursing Psychopharmacology Project

This book (winner of the 1994 AJN Book of the Year Award) is the report of the ANA Psychopharmacology Task Force (1992-1994). Part I analyzes how psychiatric nursing as a specialty prepares and updates nurses in the neurosciences, and particularly in psychopharmacology. Schools of nursing, psychiatric nursing journals, psychiatric nursing conferences, computer resources, consumers of psychiatric nursing care, practicing psychiatric nurses from around the country, and psychiatric nursing leaders contributed to this section. Part II contains the Psychopharmacology Guidelines for Psychiatric Mental Health Nurses developed by the Task Force. The Guidelines are also reproduced, along with a brief summary, in a handy detachable booklet at the back of the Report. This information is designed to be used as a tool for psychiatric nurses to determine their knowledge and skill in this important area and to design a plan for their continued growth in this field.

Health Care Reform: Essential Mental Health Services

This paper was written by Judith Krauss, RN, MSN (1993) for the ANA Council on Psychiatric and Mental Health Nursing and the Coalition of Psychiatric Nursing Organizations. It provides nursing's plan for mental health care reform in the following areas: primary care and mental health services; universal access to a basic mental health benefits package; structure and financing of the public mental health system for long-term care; and managed care. In addition, it defines risk groups for mental illness and selectively reviews the literature on psychiatric nursing practice research.

A Statement on Psychiatric-Mental Health Clinical Nursing Practice and Standards of Psychiatric-Mental Health Clinical Nursing Practice (1994)

This book is the latest revision of the ANA *Statement and Standards of Psychiatric-Mental Health Nursing Practice*. It provides definitions and descriptions of basic and advanced psychiatric-mental health nursing practice. It delineates the scope, functions, roles, and practice settings of the clinical practice of psychiatric-mental health nurses. It establishes the standards of clinical practice and professional performance for the specialty. Thus it provides clinicians, consumers of services, policy makers, insurers, and the public with information about the roles and responsibilities of psychiatric-mental health nurses across the continuum of care.

To purchase any of the publications listed, please contact the American Nurses Association at
ANA Publications
600 Maryland Avenue, S.W.
Suite 100 West
Washington, D.C. 20024-2571
Phone: 202-651-7000
Fax: 202-651-7001

APNA Items for Purchase

SLIDE KITS

Each contains over 40 full-color slides, detailed text to accompany each slide, an extensive reference list, appendixes with helpful tables and checklists, and a quiz for 2.4 continuing nursing education contact hours.

Biology, Brain, and Behavior: A Psychiatric Nursing Perspective

Provides an in-depth review of the relationship of biology, brain, and behavior and relates it to the psychiatric illnesses of schizophrenia, depression, panic disorder, and Alzheimer's dementia.

Managing the Symptoms of Schizophrenia: A Nursing Perspective

Provides a detailed framework for applying the biopsychosocial model to one particularly debilitating disease: schizophrenia.

BROCHURES
Mental Health Care: A Consumers Guide (Consumer Brochure)

Supported by a grant from the W.K. Kellogg Foundation, this brochure is a practical tool for consumers in today's confusing health care arena, covering the ins and outs of finding a mental health care provider, what to expect from treatment, and what types of payment options are available. The Guide provides essential information to consumers and their families for understanding the elements of quality mental health care.

Advanced Practice Registered Nurses (APRN) in Psychiatric and Mental Health Care (APRN Brochure)

This brochure is perfect for individuals interested in psychiatric nursing or individuals who are unfamiliar with the profession. The brochure includes information on what APRNs are, what clinical services they can provide, and why to choose an APRN for mental health services.

VIDEO TAPES
The Nurse/Patient Relationship

In this classic teaching video, Hildegard Peplau RN, EdD, FAAN, explains and demonstrates her timeless theory of the nurse-patient relationship, which has served as a major foundation of psychiatric nursing theory.

Dialogue with Hildegard Peplau

This interview with the "mother of psychiatric nursing" was conducted at the APNA's 1992 Annual Conference.

Choice and Challenge: Caring for Agressive Older Adults Across Levels of Care

This training program illustrates common problems and provides practical solutions to a variety of real-life problems experienced by older adults and their care providers. This curriculum uses a combined approach:
- 23-minute documentary-style training tape
- 20 pages of handouts
- Continuing education credits

  The video and printed material are designed for nurses, nursing assistants, and other professionals and paraprofessional health care providers who provide direct services to behaviorally impaired and agressive older adults in diverse settings.

REPORTS AND GUIDES
Report of APNA Congress on Advanced Practice in Psychiatric Nursing

This report details the work of the 50 state representatives who attended the Congress in July of

1996. The goal of the Congress was to develop a strategic plan that addressed issues of survival for the psychiatric nurse profession. The report is a compilation of activities and provides an arena for involvement for interested individuals.

Legislative Guide/Advocacy Guide

This handbook was designed to provide basic information about the APNA's government relations grassroots network. Included is information on getting organized, answers to some frequently asked questions, tips on effective communication with Congress, tips on educating members about Congress, and information about becoming an APNA state legislative affiliate.

For information about how to order these products, see the American Psychiatric Nurses Association website (www.apna.org) or contact the APNA directly at:

American Psychiatric Nurses Association
1200 19th St, NW, Suite 300
Washington, DC 20036
Phone: 202-857-1100
Fax: 202-429-5112

Index